Treatment of Stuttering

Established and Emerging Interventions

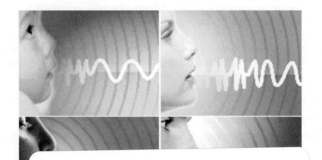

Barry Guitar, PhD

Department of Communication Sciences
University of Vermont
Burlington, Vermont

Rebecca McCauley, PhD

The Ohio State University
Department of Speech & Hearing Science
Columbus, Ohio

 Wolters Kluwer | Lippincott Williams & Wilkins
Health
Philadelphia · Baltimore · New York · London

MW

Acquisitions Editor: Peter Sabatini
Senior Product Manager: Heather Rybacki
Associate Product Manager: Kristin Royer
Marketing Manager: Allison Noplock
Designer: Doug Smock
Manufacturing Coordinator: Margie Orzech-Zeranko
Typesetter: Cadmus Communications
Printer & Binder: C&C Offset Printing

First Edition

Library of Congress Cataloging-in-Publication Data

Treatment of stuttering : established and emerging approaches / editors, Barry Guitar, Rebecca McCauley. — 1st ed.

  p. ; cm.

Includes bibliographical references and index.

ISBN 978-0-7817-7104-7

1. Stuttering—Treatment. 2. Speech therapy. I. Guitar, Barry. II. McCauley, Rebecca Joan, 1952-
[DNLM: 1. Stuttering—therapy. WM 475 T7837 2010]

RC424.T6984   2010

616.85'5406—dc22   2009016518

DISCLAIMER

Care has been taken to confirm the accuracy of the information present and to describe generally accepted practices. However, the authors, editors, and publisher are not responsible for errors or omissions or for any consequences from application of the information in this book and make no warranty, expressed or implied, with respect to the currency, completeness, or accuracy of the contents of the publication. Application of this information in a particular situation remains the professional responsibility of the practitioner; the clinical treatments described and recommended may not be considered absolute and universal recommendations.

The authors, editors, and publisher have exerted every effort to ensure that drug selection and dosage set forth in this text are in accordance with the current recommendations and practice at the time of publication. However, in view of ongoing research, changes in government regulations, and the constant flow of information relating to drug therapy and drug reactions, the reader is urged to check the package insert for each drug for any change in indications and dosage and for added warnings and precautions. This is particularly important when the recommended agent is a new or infrequently employed drug.

Some drugs and medical devices presented in this publication have Food and Drug Administration (FDA) clearance for limited use in restricted research settings. It is the responsibility of the health care provider to ascertain the FDA status of each drug or device planned for use in their clinical practice.

To purchase additional copies of this book, call our customer service department at **(800) 638-3030 or fax orders to (301) 223-2320. International customers should call (301) 223-2300.**

Visit Lippincott Williams & Wilkins on the Internet: http://www.lww.com. Lippincott Williams & Wilkins customer service representatives are available from 8:30 am to 6:00 pm, EST.

CCS0809

6/16/10

We want to dedicate this book to four men who have taught us that there are no more important research questions in speech-language pathology than those designed to improve treatments:

In memory of Dick Curlee and Charles Van Riper and in gratitude to Ralph Shelton and Larry Shriberg

PREFACE

This book is a beginning. It was written for students, teachers, clinicians, and those who stutter, to provide an update about a selected group of stuttering treatments for preschoolers, school age children, adolescents, and adults. Thirty-three authors, including ourselves, combined their talents in chapters that lay out the details of treatment, analyze the evidence for treatment effectiveness, and describe the process of an evidence-based approach to practice—including information about assessment.

The overview chapters at the beginning of each major section in the book provide a summary of basic concepts critical to understanding the nature of interventions for stuttering, methods to evaluate them, and evidence based practice in this area. Each of the eleven treat-ment chapters include key principles, primary goals for clients, as well as the theoretical and empirical bases for each approach and a case study of a client for whom the treatment was considered appropriate and effective. Each treatment chapter is also accompanied by video segments that demonstrate the authors' intervention. The video segments are available on thePoint site.

In this status report on stuttering treatment as of 2009, we have undoubtedly left out many effective approaches and approaches that are being developed to achieve that status. We hope the future and therefore future editions will bring more clinicians and clinical researchers who document their interventions and gather data on their outcomes.

ACKNOWLEDGEMENTS

Many people have helped us bring this book to life.

We would like to thank the thirty-one authors who responded with grace and energy to our initial invitations and our subsequent suggestions for revisions, additions, and deletions. We are also indebted to three people who did crucial work beyond the text: Our colleague (and chapter co-author) Melissa Bruce has created clear and cogent PowerPoint slides for many chapters of the book; our student Heather Fjeld has constructed fair and balanced quizzes to motivate students; Carroll Guitar has managed references, permissions, and helped with editing; Katherine Askinazi has been a wizard with video editing.

Our publisher Lippincott, Williams & Wilkins has provided a host of talented people who have encouraged and advised us. Peter Sabatini has been a major support ever since he read our proposal and set forth a plan to make the book a reality. Kristin Royer, as our most recent managing editor, has given us a keen sense of deadlines and has helped us solve many problems. Andrea Klingler got us off to a good start as our first managing editor. We are grateful to Jen Clements who turned our primitive drawings into artful illustrations and to Ed Shultes and Freddie Patane who have educated us in the art of videography. We would like to thank Allison Noplock, Marketing Manager, for her early involvement and continuing support to make this book available to a wide audience. Finally, we would like to express our appreciation to Ruth Einstein of Cadmus Communications, who patiently guided us through the process of correcting the page proofs.

CONTRIBUTORS

Anne K. Bothe, PhD
Professor
Department of Communication Sciences
and Special Education
University of Georgia
Athens, Georgia

WillieBotterill, MSc
Consultant Speech and Language Therapist
The Michael Palin Centre
Finsbury Health Centre
London, United Kingdom

Melissa C. Bruce, MS
Clinic Director
Department of Communication
Sciences and Disorders
University of Houston
Houston, Texas

Edward G. Conture, PhD
Professor and Director, Graduate Studies
Department Hearing and Speech Sciences
Vanderbilt University
Nashville, Tennessee

AshleyCraig, PhD
Professor of Behavioural Sciences
Department of Health Sciences
Faculty of Science, University of Technology
Sydney, Australia

JohnEllis, MS, PhD candidate
Speech-Language Pathologist
Department of Speech, Language &
Hearing Sciences
University of Colorado
Boulder, Colorado

Harald A. Euler, PhD
Professor
Department of Economics, Institute
of Psychology
University of Kassel
Kassel, Germany

David L. Franklin, PsyD
Clinical Psychologist
University of California, Irvine Medical Center
Orange, California

Sheryl R. Gottwald, PhD
Assistant Professor
Department of Communication Sciences and
Disorders
University of New Hampshire
Durham, New Hampshire

Barry Guitar, PhD
Professor
Department of Communication Sciences
University of Vermont
Burlington, Vermont

Ergi Gumusaneli, MD
University of California, Irvine
Orange, California

Elisabeth Harrison, PhD
Senior Lecturer
Department of Linguistics
Macquarie University
Sydney, Australia

Janis Costello Ingham, PhD
Professor
Department of Speech and Hearing Sciences
University of California, Santa Barbara
Santa Barbara, California

Roger Ingham, PhD
Professor
Department of Speech and Hearing Sciences
University of California, Santa Barbara
Santa Barbara, California

Elaine Kelman, MSc
Consultant Speech and
Language Therapist
The Michael Palin Centre
Finsbury Health Centre
London, United Kingdom

Sarita Koushik, MSLP (C)
Speech Pathologist, PhD Candidate
Montreal Fluency Center
Montreal, Quebec

Robert Kroll, PhD
Executive Director, The Speech and
Stuttering Institute
Adjunct Faculty, University of Toronto
Toronto, Ontario

Gerald A. Maguire, MD
Associate Professor of Clinical Psychiatry
Associate Dean, CME College of Medicine
University of California, Irvine Medical Center
Orange, California

Rebecca McCauley, PhD
Professor, Department of Speech & Hearing Science
The Ohio State University
Department of Speech & Hearing Science
Columbus, Ohio

Katrin Neumann, MD
Professor, Director of the Department for
Phoniatry and Pediatric Audiology
Goethe-University of Frankfurt
Main, Germany

Sue O'Brian, PhD
Speech Pathologist and Research Officer
Australian Stuttering Research Centre
Faculty of Health Sciences
The University of Sydney
Lidcombe, Australia

Mark Onslow, PhD
Professor and Director
Australian Stuttering Research Centre
The University of Sydney
Lidcombe, Australia

Ann Packman, PhD
Australian Stuttering Research Centre
The University of Sydney
Lidcombe, Australia

Kristin M. Pelczarski, MA
Speech-Language Pathologist
Department of Communication Disorders
Children's Hospital of UPMC
Pittsburgh, Pennsylvania

Ryan Pollard, PhD
Speech-Language Pathologist
Department of Speech,
Language & Hearing Sciences
University of Colorado
Boulder, Colorado

Robert W. Quesal, PhD
Professor

Department of Communication Sciences and
Disorders
Western Illinois University
Macomb, Illinois

Peter R. Ramig, PhD
Professor and Associate Chair
Department of Speech, Language &
Hearing Sciences
University of Colorado
Boulder, Colorado

Corrin Richels, PhD
Adjust Assistant Professor
Department of Early Childhood, Special Education,
and Speech-Language Pathology
Old Dominion University
Norfolk, Virginia

Glyn Riley, PhD
Professor Emeritus, California State University
Fullerton, California
Consultant, University of California Medical
Treatment of Stuttering Program
University of California, Irvine
Irvine, California

Charles M. Runyan, PhD
Professor and Graduate Coordinator
Department of Communication Sciences
and Disorders
James Madison University
Harrisonburg, Virginia

Sara Elizabeth Runyan, MA
Professor Emeritus
Department of Communication Sciences
and Disorders
James Madison University
Harrisonburg, Virginia

Lori Scott-Sulsky, MSc
Speech-Language Pathologist
Speech and Stuttering Institute
Toronto, Ontario

Rosalee C. Shenker, PhD
Founder and Executive Director
Montreal Fluency Center
Montreal, Quebec

J. Scott Yaruss, PhD
Associate Professor
Department of Communication Science
and Disorders
University of Pittsburgh
Pittsburgh, Pennsylvania

CONTENTS

CHAPTER **1**

How to Use This Book

Rebecca J. McCauley and Barry E. Guitar

CHAPTER OUTLINE

STUDENTS
    Chapters You May Be Most Interested In
    Chapter Components to Be Sure to Read
    Additional Resources
PEOPLE WHO STUTTER
    Chapters You May Be Most Interested In
    Chapter Components to Be Sure to Read

    Additional Resources
PARENTS OF CHILDREN WHO STUTTER
    Chapters You May Be Most Interested In
    Chapter Components to Be Sure to Read
FACULTY
    Chapters You May Be Most Interested In
    Chapter Components to Be Sure to Read

W e want this book to be valuable to all readers interested in stuttering treatment—either because they want to learn more about how best to help people who stutter, because they stutter themselves, or because they have someone close to them who stutters. Nonetheless, we recognize that not all readers will have the same level of interest in all aspects of the book. Therefore, in this chapter, we want to suggest how four different audiences might best use this book. You probably fit into one of these categories:

- Students of speech-language pathology
- Adolescents and adults who stutter
- Parents of children who stutter
- Professors who teach students about stuttering

We first offer sets of questions that readers may want to ask themselves or others—either before or during their reading, or as they act on what they have read. Next, we point out the chapters, as well as subsections within chapters, that may be of greatest interest. Finally, we identify additional resources, such as websites, videos, books, and articles, that may have special value for that specific group of readers.

You may want to read our suggestions for different groups of readers to obtain a broader perspective. However, our intuitions cannot be expected to work for every reader, so you may want to skip our suggestions altogether and dive into the rest of the book. Regardless of your choice, we hope you will find this chapter and the book as a whole organized so that you

can easily find the information that you most need.

STUDENTS

You may be looking at this book for the simple reason that it is required reading. Obviously, that's not the most compelling motivation. On the other hand, you may be reading this book because you have been assigned a client who stutters this very semester who will need your help. If that is the case, let's get you right into the thick of the action—solving the clinical puzzle of which treatment to choose.

Choosing a treatment will require you to consider your client's needs, the evidence supporting competing treatments, and your clinical abilities. Some of your client's needs will be identified as part of your evaluation. Others can be anticipated based on readings you will do about the nature of stuttering and how it changes over the course of a stutterer's life. Evidence about competing treatments boils down to *what* works for *which* clients *when*. To help you get that information from this book, authors have provided a summary of the strongest evidence for their treatments, and we, as editors, have compared the evidence across treatments vying for your attention. Clinical abilities may be something that you believe lie more in your future than in your present. However, as a product of growing up and learning to relate to people, you have already begun to develop the core abilities on which you will build. This book will help you learn about methods you will use with people who stutter by reading about treatments and seeing them in action on the video clips which are on publisher's website (which is called thePoint).

CHAPTERS YOU MAY BE MOST INTERESTED IN

Although we think that you should be interested in every chapter in the book, we would like to provide you with a little more guidance than just saying "read everything." Although your professor may have strong ideas about the order in which you should read chapters and even which ones you should read, you might benefit more from pre-reading parts of the book in an order that you think best suits you. For example, you may be helped by getting a sense of the *organization* of each treatment chapter and *principles of treatment* by reading Chapter 2 and then reading our overviews of the three major sections (Chapters 4, 8, and 13).

Next, you may want to read Chapter 3, "Indirect Treatment of Childhood Stuttering: Diagnostic Predictors of Treatment Outcome," to understand how evidence-based practice guides the clinician in choosing the treatment that holds the most promise for an individual client. In case you didn't know, evidence-based practice (EBP) alludes to procedures used to guide clinical practice that combine research evidence with clinical expertise and client values. Reading the treatment chapters in the order they appear may make the most sense because you will see that there is a shifting of goals from curing early stuttering to coping with chronic stuttering. Once you know about the details of treatments, the final two chapters (Chapters 19 and 20) will make sense. Chapter 19 explores neurophysiologic explanations of how treatments work and is the most ambitious chapter in the book. Chapter 20 pulls together the common themes from preceding chapters and then suggests what needs to be done to improve existing treatments and develop new ones to address unmet client needs.

CHAPTER COMPONENTS TO BE SURE TO READ

As a student reading this book, you are beginning your training as a scholar, but you are also becoming a clinician. With this book, we hope to help you see that these roles can be one and the same.

To begin, read the introduction to each treatment chapter to orient yourself. Some treatments are strictly behavioral; others involve cognitive procedures as well. One treatment included in this book uses medication, whereas another employs an electroacoustic device. You need to start with a sense of what each treatment involves before you can evaluate its potential effectiveness or imagine yourself implementing it.

As a scholar, you will need to develop your critical thinking skills. An important place to start would be the section of each treatment chapter that describes the theoretical basis, or theory, from which the treatment was developed. What is a theory, you ask? One writer has described it this way: "Theory gives the researcher a structured perspective without which collected facts are only the ditty bag of an idiot, filled with bits of pebbles, straws, feathers, and other random hoardings" (Lynd, 1939, p. 183).

As a crude example of a theory of stuttering, one of us (Barry, in case you were wondering) developed an idea when he was an adolescent who stuttered that not showering after gym class reduced his stuttering for the rest of the day. Now, this represents something like a theory—it provided him with an explanation for something he thought he had experienced, it gave him a plan for how to address his stuttering, and it made him feel a little more in control of the situation. However, this is not the kind of theoretical basis that we think you should be looking for. In fact, Barry eventually came to the conclusion (as you may have already) that this theory stinks.

A better theory than this one would be one that describes a mechanism by which the intervention should result in a change in stuttering (e.g., because of how it affects the physiology, beliefs, or learning of the person who stutters). For example, the diagnosogenic theory of stuttering (Johnson et al., 1942) postulated that stuttering was precipitated by parents' overreaction to their child's normal disfluencies. The mechanism by which this was believed to work was that the parents' constant correction of their child's disfluencies resulted in the child's negative anticipation and tension that, over time, led the child to manifest struggle, escape, and avoidance behaviors as part of a habitual pattern—that is, full-blown stuttering. The treatment based on this theory followed closely from the hypothesized mechanism: Parents were taught to re-evaluate what they thought to be stutters as normal speech disruptions. In other words, they learned to view these disfluencies nonjudgmentally, thereby allowing the child to respond to his own disfluencies in an accepting manner that promoted relaxed, fluent speech.

As you can see, in the second example, the theory involves a tight linkage between how a phenomenon was believed to occur and how it was treated. Sadly, the beautiful diagnosogenic theory was destroyed by a series of homely facts. Among these was the assumption that the speech disfluencies of children diagnosed by their parents as stuttering were the same as those of children never receiving that diagnosis (Johnson & Associates, 1959). The homely fact that the disfluencies of these two groups of children were indeed quite different was uncovered by McDearmon (1968), who re-examined the very data reported by Johnson et al. Now, although we are clearly taking the diagnosogenic theory to task, we are doing so to reveal one of the chief virtues of a scientific theory—that is, because it generates testable hypotheses, it can be disproven. Figure 1.1 illustrates the relationships among theories, hypotheses, tests of hypotheses (experiments), findings resulting from the experiments, and feedback to disprove, support, or modify the theory.

With a critical eye, you will want to examine the theoretical basis section of each chapter. Consider which hypotheses arising from the theory have actually been studied by the developer and which additional hypotheses could be—or even should be—studied to improve the treatment, the theory, or both.

ADDITIONAL RESOURCES

Packman, A., & Attanasio, J. (2004). *Theoretical Issues in Stuttering*. London: Routledge Press. (This book provides a good description of what theories are and what they do to further scientific research. Major theories of stuttering are discussed and analyzed.)

The Stuttering Homepage. Available at http://www.mnsu.edu/comdis/kuster/stutter.html (This website provides links for parents to talk to other parents as well as links for stutterers of all ages to chat with one another. There is also a wealth of informational material on stuttering written from both scientific and humanistic perspectives.)

Schneider, P. (n.d.). *Transcending Stuttering: The Inside Story*. New York: National Stuttering Association. (This DVD was made for and by people who stutter. It provides a personalized view of what it's like to deal with stuttering over a lifetime.)

PEOPLE WHO STUTTER

As a person who stutters, you may have many different reasons for reading this book. You may just be curious about current approaches to treatment. Or you may be considering treatment, possibly for the first time or after having previous therapy. If you have had therapy before and it was effective, you may be interested in the latest information on it or in seeing whether there are new strategies to help you better retain its benefits. If you have participated in treatment before but felt that it did not work or that its effects were not long lasting, you may be looking for a better alternative. On the other hand, you may want to improve your speech, but for various reasons, you want to do it on your own. Most people find it helpful to have a coach or therapist to guide and support them, but some are so highly motivated and self-directed that they can accomplish a great deal by themselves. If this is your situation, you may be able to extract key ideas that seem appropriate to you and be able to put together a program of self-therapy.

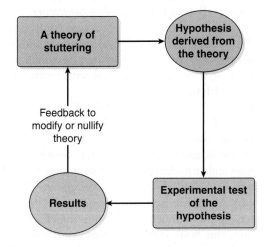

Figure 1.1. Relationship among theory, hypothesis, tests of hypothesis, results, and feedback.

Regardless of what your reasons are for reading this book, you should know that speech-language pathologists are currently thinking about their work with clients in terms of EBP. In EBP, clinicians are instructed to link three sources of information as they join with clients to plan treatments. As the name implies, one of these sources is the evidence offered in various places (including this book) about how well a treatment works. The second source is the clinician's own clinical expertise, and the third is the preferences, values, and needs of you, the client. Although good clinicians have always attempted to meld these sources of information to best meet a client's needs, the explicit nature of this kind of thinking within EBP emphasizes the clinician's obligation to understand what matters most to you as you work together to improve your communication. In the form shown in Figure 1.2, we suggest some questions that you may want to ask yourself to learn more about your own preferences and values. If you are actively considering therapy, you may want to share this form with potential therapists you might interview to help you reach a decision about undertaking treatment with them. Alternatively, if you are considering working on your speech independently, you may still find this form useful. It may help you decide what bothers you the most about your stuttering so that you can attack it strategically.

CHAPTERS YOU MAY BE MOST INTERESTED IN

As an adolescent or adult, you will probably find chapters in Section III (Chapters 13 to 17) to be of greatest interest. These chapters deal with four interventions developed for people who stutter. In Chapter 13, we offer an overview of these interventions. In that chapter, we identify common philosophies and procedures as well as unique features. We also comment on the overall strength of existing evidence to support claims that each intervention is effective for a wide range of stutterers. Reviewing this short chapter first should give you a sense of which interventions might be of greatest interest to you and, therefore, the order in which you might read them.

Besides the introductory chapter and the treatment chapters in Section III, there are two other chapters in the book—Chapters 2 and 18—that we think you may want to consider reading. However, they are likely to be a bit cumbersome, with more references and more abstract discussions than you may be interested in. In Chapter 2, we describe a model of treatment and discuss the different kinds of problems that tend to go along with stuttering. In Chapter 18, Anne Bothe and her colleagues discuss how developers of treatments can provide the best possible evidence that their treatment works. Because all of the authors in other parts of the book may refer to some of these same concepts, you may want to look at these chapters before you go on to the treatment chapters in Section III. However, you may just want to be aware that these chapters are there and go back to them if you would like to understand an aspect of stuttering treatments in greater detail.

CHAPTER COMPONENTS TO BE SURE TO READ

Table 1.1 lists the contents of those sections we think may prove of special interest to you. In addition, the table presents questions you may want to ask yourself as you read those sections. Each of these sections, as well as others, is described in greater detail in Chapter 2.

ADDITIONAL RESOURCES

National Stuttering Association. Available at http://www.nsastutter.org/ (This is a website run by people who stutter for people who stutter. It contains links to chat rooms for people who stutter as well as links for information about stuttering and stuttering therapy.)

Schneider, P. (n.d.). *Transcending Stuttering: The Inside Story*. New York: National Stuttering Association. (This DVD was made for and by people who stutter. It provides a personalized view of what it's like to deal with stuttering over a lifetime.)

Guitar, B., & Guitar, C. (2005). *If You Stutter: Advice for Adults* (revised). Memphis: Stuttering Foundation. (This book offers advice from professionals and people who stutter about techniques and attitudes to deal with stuttering.)

Fraser, M. (n.d.) *Self-Therapy for the Stutterer* (10th ed.). Memphis: Stuttering Foundation. (Written by the founder of the Stuttering Foundation, this book contains recommendations for working on one's own stuttering from someone who learned to manage his own stuttering.)

Client Preferences for Stuttering Treatment

Treatment format/duration

Treatment is typically conducted in either a short-term or long-term format. Which of the following better meets your needs:

(a) Weekly one-hour sessions conducted over a longer period of time (e.g., a year)

(b) Daily sessions of several hours each conducted over a shorter period of time (e.g., several weeks)

(c) Some combination of the above

Goals of treatment

How important are the following goals: *rank from 1 (not important) to 5 (very important)*

Very fluent speech	1	2	3	4	5
Feeling of control of stuttering	1	2	3	4	5
Ease of participation in most or all speaking situations	1	2	3	4	5

Ease of speaking in specific situations:

Talking on the telephone	1	2	3	4	5
Introducing myself or others	1	2	3	4	5
Conversations with friends	1	2	3	4	5
Conversations with strangers	1	2	3	4	5
Talking to supervisor	1	2	3	4	5
Talking to co-workers	1	2	3	4	5

Nature of Treatment

Circle your preferences for the nature of therapy:

Type: individual OR group OR combination

Focus: stuttering severity OR feelings about stuttering OR combination

Other Aspects of Therapy to ask about

Cost of Treatment

Cost per session

Cost of total treatment

Insurance coverage

Treatment Cost

Time or number of sessions to achieve treatment goals

Time or number of sessions for maintenance or follow-up treatment

Figure 1.2. Client preferences for stuttering treatment.

Table 1.1. *Book Sections and Related Questions to Consider for People Who Stutter*

Section	Content	Questions to consider
Practical requirements	Resources, such as time, equipment, and clinical expertise, required for the treatment	• Does this treatment require more time than I have available or that I want to spend on my stuttering—either in treatment sessions themselves or in independent work outside of these sessions? • How will I be able to tell if a clinician has the appropriate expertise to work with me using this approach?
Key components	Treatment procedures, including who will be involved	• Do I think I can participate in this treatment as it is described? • Do I need more information about certain aspects of the treatment before I can feel comfortable about embarking on it?
Tailoring the treatment to the individual client	How the treatment is modified to address the specific needs of individuals whose culture or circumstances are different from those for whom the treatment was first developed	• Do I have specific needs that may be different from other clients because of my cultural or language background, education, or views? • Is my background similar to those for whom the treatment was developed or for whom the authors suggest modifications?
Application to a specific client	A case study describing one person's successful experience with the intervention	• Does the description make this sound like it would be appropriate for me?

PARENTS OF CHILDREN WHO STUTTER

As parents of a child who stutters, you may be reading this book in hopes of identifying the most effective treatment for your son or daughter. This book is divided into separate sections for preschool children and school-age children, so the age of your child will determine where to look. You may also be seeking advice about what you should be doing to help your child. Although none of the chapters directly address this last issue, you can extract ideas about what you should do from most chapters. These ideas will work best when you are working with a clinician who is guiding the treatment. However, in some cases—particularly for environmentally based treatments like those described in Chapters 6 and 7—you will be able to get ideas about changes that you can make in your child's environment that may help him or her become more fluent.

There is one more point to address before we talk about specific chapters. You, the parents, are the most important agents in the treatment of your child. You have a tremendous wealth of knowledge about him or her, and you are with your child many, many more hours per week than the clinician. Wise clinicians will be eager to form a good working relationship with you because their alliance with you is critical for the effectiveness of the treatment. In order for that alliance to be as powerful as possible, one of your roles will be to help the clinician understand your goals for your child. For example, if you know about a particular situation in which your child is most penalized for his stuttering, you should bring it to the attention of your clinician. If it is more important for you to have your child speak out than to have your child speak perfectly, you should make that known as well. If you believe that something you have done either caused the stuttering or made it worse, let your clinician know—not only will it be safe, but it will also feel good to have done. Reading these chapters will help you appreciate what your clinician may be trying to achieve.

Table 1.2. *Book Sections and Related Questions to Consider for Parents of Children Who Stutter*

Section	Content	Questions to consider
Practical requirements	Resources, such as time, equipment, and clinical expertise, required for the treatment	• Are we as a family able to commit the time, energy, and probable expense required by this approach? • Are we able to find a clinician close by who is sufficiently trained in this approach? If so, are we comfortable with that clinician?
Key components	Treatment procedures, including who will be involved	• Do we feel that this approach will involve us to the degree and in the way we want to be involved? • Do the procedures as described make sense to us as ways to help our child over the problems we think matter? • Do the goals of this approach match our goals in seeking treatment for our child? • Do we think our child will respond well to this approach?
Tailoring the treatment to the individual client	How the treatment is modified to address the specific needs of individuals whose culture or circumstances are different from those for whom the treatment was first developed	• Are there elements of this approach that make us uneasy and that are not addressed in this section? • Is this treatment flexible enough to fit our child's and our family's needs?
Application to an individual client	A case study describing one person's successful experience with the intervention	• Does this example help us come up with additional questions for the clinician about the procedures and how they will be used with our child?

CHAPTERS YOU MAY BE MOST INTERESTED IN

Start with the overview chapter for the age group appropriate for your child—Chapter 4 for preschool children and Chapter 8 for school-age children. Based on what you learn in the chapter, you will probably have a good idea about which treatments seem most suited to your child.

Among those features that may affect your decisions would be how and to what extent parents are involved in treatment. In general, the younger the child is, the more the parents are involved in therapy. Nonetheless, some treatments ask more of parents than others, and different approaches involve parents differently.

In the preschool section, Chapter 3—which focuses as much on assessment as it does on treatment—involves the parents primarily in interactions with other parents and does not ask the parent to be the primary therapist. At the other extreme, Chapter 7 describes an approach that entails the parent doing daily therapy with the child, with guidance from the clinician provided during weekly visits by the parent and child to the clinician's office. The two other approaches—in Chapters 5 and 6—fall somewhere in between.

In the school-age section, Chapters 10, 11, and 12 involve the clinician as the primary therapist for the child, with parents participating in activities that transfer the child's skills to the home environment. Chapter 9 presents a parent-administered approach for school-age children and, like the preschool version in Chapter 7, parents conduct the treatment but with greater input from the child and continuing guidance from the clinician.

CHAPTER COMPONENTS TO BE SURE TO READ

Start with the following sections: Practical Requirements; Key Components; Tailoring the Treatment to the Individual Client; and Application to an Individual Client. These sections are described in Table 1.2, along with questions you may want to consider as you read them. If you read these sections and are interested, you may want to look at the scientific support for the intervention in the theoretical and empirical basis sections.

FACULTY

As a faculty member reading this book for the first time, you are probably interested in seeing how it meets your students' needs and fits your perspectives on stuttering treatment. Although we have tried to shape this book so that it addresses the academic and clinical needs of a wide array of students and the perspectives of a wide range of faculty, we understand that you will be the final judge. Therefore, in this section, we will simply point out aspects of the book that we think you will find most helpful in your work with students.

CHAPTERS YOU MAY BE MOST INTERESTED IN

Chapter 2 is designed to provide an overview of the book's content within the context of a model of treatment. That model is based on one proposed by Marc Fey and his colleagues for treatment of language disorders (McCauley & Fey, 2006). This framework serves to highlight commonalities across interventions in a way we hope you will find helpful. It also introduces the International Classification of Functioning, Disability, and Health (World Health Organization, 2002) so that student readers will be sensitized to differences in outcome focus, such as goals related to quality of life versus goals related to speech production.

Reading the three section overviews (Chapters 4, 8, and 13) will give you a sense of the range of interventions we have included for preschoolers, school-age children, and adolescents and adults. This should help you decide what chapters to have students focus on and the extent to which you will want to supplement this text with readings about treatments that we did not include. As a further aid to your course planning, you may want to peruse the short list of suggested readings associated with each of the treatment chapters to decide whether you wish to add those to your students' reading lists.

Chapter 19 contains a review of existing evidence about the neural processes associated with stuttering and how these might be affected by successful treatment. Depending on your students' background and the extent to which you have decided to focus on the neurophysiologic nature of stuttering, you may want to ask your students to read this chapter first. It will probably be one of the most challenging and maybe even most exciting chapters in the book.

Chapter 20 will help students process the book as a whole and develop their own thinking about next steps in this area.

CHAPTER COMPONENTS TO BE SURE TO READ

You can easily direct students' attention to specific content areas because of the use of uniform subsections. For example, if you are particularly interested in the evidence base for each intervention, each chapter includes a subsection with that title. In addition, the chapter Overviews, Summaries, and Key Words can be highlighted as study aids. We are hoping that this book will help you teach your students critical thinking skills. Most fundamentally, each chapter can be used to teach students about the quality of empirical support provided for a treatment.

Here are three examples of activities to teach critical thinking:

- Some treatments only have evidence supplied by the developers of the treatment themselves, whereas others will have that evidence as well as evidence provided by independent clinician-researchers. See how many treatments in the book have both kinds of evidence.
- Within each larger section (e.g., Interventions for Preschool Children), students could compare treatments, which is a task of greater complexity because different kinds of limitations may exist for individual treatments that make their comparison more challenging.
- Another example of a critical thinking exercise would involve students working in groups developing research designs to improve the empirical basis supporting an individual treatment. Although authors will have been asked to discuss such plans in the chapter subsection titled "Future Directions," they will often not have done so in a very thorough way or for the full range of possible clients.
- In a related exercise, for each chapter, students could identify the assumptions of the theory on which a treatment is based; sometimes these are stated directly, and sometimes they are implicit to the discussion.

CHAPTER 2

Introduction to *Treatment of Stuttering: Established and Emerging Interventions*

BARRY E. GUITAR AND REBECCA J. McCAULEY

CHAPTER OUTLINE

THE PURPOSE OF THIS BOOK

Our purpose in writing this book is to introduce clinicians and students to evidence-based practice in stuttering and to stimulate future research on the interventions described here. In addition, we hope to give people who stutter and their families information about some of the interventions that they may be offered.

To make this book as current as possible, we have invited 12 groups of authors to write chapters about treatments they have recently developed or tested. In addition to these chapters, we include a chapter by Bothe and her colleagues that describes the current state of evidence-based practice in stuttering and a chapter by Neumann and Euler that discusses neurophysiologic correlates of stuttering treatment. We also provide overview chapters for each of the major sections of the book and a final summary chapter. The major sections are organized by the age level of the client: (a) preschoolers, (b) school-age children, and (c) adolescents and adults.

HOW TREATMENTS ARE DESCRIBED IN THIS BOOK

Authors' descriptions were guided by a template to make the information readily accessible to readers and to encourage similar coverage of topics across treatments. Thus, this template was designed to make sure that readers will learn enough about each treatment to determine its practical requirements, theoretical orientation, empirical evidence base, and the clients for

whom it was developed. With this information in hand, readers can evaluate its likely value for their own clients. The template components are similar to those used in a recent text on the treatment of language disorders in children (McCauley & Fey, 2006) but have been modified to ensure their relevance to stuttering in both children and adults. The components of the template are listed in Table 2.1.

Each treatment chapter includes a brief **Introduction** to the treatment, including a summary of its major theoretical and empirical underpinnings and the population for which it was intended. The introduction is followed by a longer discussion of **Theoretical Bases**, in which the authors describe the view of stuttering that guided the development of their treatment, as well as the most relevant principles of treatment. In addition, the specific treatment focus (e.g., increase in fluency versus reduction of stuttering) is described in this section.

The next section, **Empirical Basis for Use**, highlights the best research and clinical evidence available to support the value of the intervention for at least one group of clients. The kinds of evidence typically regarded as valuable in the support of treatment validity are reviewed in Chapter 18, so it may be worthwhile to read that chapter prior to reading treatment chapters. That background prepares readers to evaluate the evidence offered by chapter authors in relation to the population with which they work.

Even before that chapter, however, we want to introduce you to three terms that will help

Table 2.1. *Template Components*

Section	Content
Introduction	A brief summary of the treatment approach, including the population for which it was designed, principles guiding its development, and its methods
Theoretical Basis	A description of the conceptualization of stuttering on which the treatment is based, other aspects of its rationale, and long-term goals (e.g., reduction of disfluency, modification of secondary characteristics, and/or reduction of negative attitudes and feelings)
Empirical Basis	Detailed discussion of research supporting the effectiveness of the treatment that includes a discussion of the quality of evidence and the size of treatment effects (where available)
Practical Requirements	Summary of resources needed to implement the treatment, including time demands, training or expertise required of the clinician, and any materials or equipment needed
Key Components	A description of the approach that includes treatment procedures, stages, goals, and participants
Assessment Methods to Support Ongoing Decision Making	A description of methods to be followed by the clinician to assess the treatment's immediate and long-term effectiveness and to guide adaptations of procedures when these are needed to improve effectiveness
Tailoring the Treatment to the Individual Client	A description of ways in which a treatment can be modified to meet the needs of a client and his/her family; for example, a treatment might be modified by taking into consideration cultural or personal factors affecting social roles and interaction patterns
An Example of the Treatment's Application to an Individual Who Stutters	A description of the choice and implementation of the treatment for an individual, problem-solving that occurred during the implementation, and resulting outcomes
Future Directions	Discussion of the kinds of studies required to strengthen the evidence base for this treatment
Suggested Readings	Key references that provide in-depth discussion of aspects of the treatment, such as its procedures or empirical base

you get a head start on understanding evidence supporting a treatment's efficacy. We will take a few paragraphs to do so, which makes the introduction to the section on empirical basis for use the longest by far. We are aware that introducing some meaty concepts at this point could take your attention away from getting an overall sense of how chapters are organized. However, because we believe the Empirical Basis section is really one of the most important to be found in each of the treatment-oriented chapters, we want to be sure you are in the best position possible to appreciate its content, and we are willing to take a little detour to make sure that happens.

To begin, we want to introduce three important concepts: statistical significance, effect size, and clinical significance. Put simply, here is what each concept means. *Statistical significance*

relates to whether a finding seems to be real (i.e., probably not related to chance). *Effect size* is a calculation that can be made from study results to help determine whether the difference between two conditions, or the relationship between two variables, appears to be big enough to have some importance. Finally, *clinical significance* demands not only that a finding is unlikely to be a result of chance and of a certain magnitude, but also that the finding relates to an outcome measure or measures that have the kind of impact the client and clinician are looking for (e.g., reduced stuttering, improved attitudes toward public speaking, maintenance of a low percentage of stuttering lasting over a year, etc.).

A little more background about the kind of studies that may be done to show that a treatment is valuable may help you see how these three terms are related to one another but also different in important ways. First, studies used to support stuttering treatments will often take the form of a comparison between two groups. Sometimes one group is given treatment and the other is not given treatment (or is not given treatment until after the study is over). At other times—and this is better—the two groups are given two different treatments; we say that this is a more interesting study because it provides you with information not only about whether it is better to do something than nothing, but also about which of the two "things to do" (which treatment) seems better for the kinds of individuals who participated in the study. (Although it will not be discussed here, note that for the comparisons to be meaningful, it would be important to have the individuals in each of the two groups be as similar to one another as possible. Otherwise, the comparison may have a certain outcome simply because, for example, one group had individuals with more severe stuttering or other problems, which might make their treatment more difficult. Understanding this helps one understand many of the steps that are taken in designing treatment studies and why they are hard to design.)

Imagine that you are conducting a study to support a new treatment for adults who stutter. You recruit two groups of very similar individuals (e.g., in terms of stuttering severity and age). You provide them with two treatments—one that you have just devised (the Super Method) and another that has been used before (the Standard Method). For purposes of this discussion, let's imagine that you only looked at one outcome measure—that is, some aspect of stuttering that one would consider wanting to change with treatment, for example, percentage of syllables stuttered (%SS). Now imagine that at the beginning of the study, both groups had approximately the same level of stuttering—let's say an average of 10.2% SS for the Super group and 10.5% SS for the Standard group.

At the end of treatment, you found that participants in the Super group now had an average of 8% SS and participants in the Standard group now had an average of 11% SS. Hmm, what do you make of that? Indeed, in terms of raw numbers, it appears that the Super group did better than the Standard group. Yet, as you think about it, you realize that the difference is pretty small and may have been due to chance, especially because you remember the fact that there was variability in %SS in each group to begin with. Statistical significance information provided for the statistical difference test you performed (probably a t-test or an analysis of variance) would tell you how unlikely it is that the difference was due to chance. For our purposes here, let's say that it was significant at the .01 level. That would mean that for a difference in scores of that magnitude for groups of that size showing that level of variability within groups, there was only one chance in a hundred that it would occur by chance. Neat! It seems like your treatment is better!

However, is the size of the difference between the Standard group and Super group very important? It was only 3% after all. Clearly, it seems more important for groups starting out with a mean %SS of approximately 10% than for groups starting with a much higher %SS, such as 50%, in which case 3% might seem like a very small change. **Effect size** is a statistical strategy for estimating how important—or substantively significant (Dollaghan, 2007)—a finding might be.

There are several types of effect size measures. Which one is used in a given study depends on aspects of the study's design. Nonetheless, an effect size measure is always intended to give you information about how important the finding is likely to be. In treatment studies, like the one we just described, in which two groups are compared, one of the most—if not *the* most—commonly used effect size measures is Cohen's *d*. Nonetheless, regardless of what measure is used, if an effect size is available, it can help the consumer of the research begin to get a handle on how much this research should influence his or her decision about choosing or recommending a particular treatment.

Recommendations are available for how to gauge effect size measures (e.g., see Table 2.2). However, effect sizes also have to be considered in terms of related treatment studies; for example, if a moderate effect size is better than any that has been achieved in treatments for similar study participants, the finding associated with it should receive lots of attention. Another matter affecting how to interpret an effect size concerns how reliable the measure is as an estimate—a matter that we will not go into here, but that readers may wish to look into further (e.g., Dollaghan, 2007; Robey, 2004).

Table 2.2. *Rule of Thumb Characterization of Cohen's* d *as an Indication of Effect Size (Cohen, 1992)*

Characterization	Value of *d*
Small	.2
Medium	.5
Large	.8

The third term we introduced earlier is **clinical significance**. Returning to our example, imagine that the better outcome in %SS found for the Super treatment group compared with the Standard treatment group was both statistically significant and associated with a moderate effect size. The question still remains of whether or not that finding truly matters clinically—to the clinician and, more importantly, to the individual who might be considering participating in the treatment.

At this point, *which* outcome measures were used in the treatment study and *when* they were used can figure prominently in the decision about whether your findings favoring the Super treatment over the Standard treatment will really be clinically significant. To an adult who stutters and is focused on stuttering less and who cares a great deal about the short-term outcomes, your findings would probably be considered clinically significant. However, to another adult who stutterers but is interested in more enduring changes in communicative effectiveness as well as stuttering less frequently over the longer term, your study's results are not as clinically significant. Additional outcome measures looking at whether that degree of change in stuttering also resulted in changes in self-perceptions of communicative effectiveness and at how durable the changes in any outcomes measures were would be incredibly valuable in helping answer questions about clinical significance and your new Super Method of treatment.

Readers should favor those treatments for which stronger evidence bases are provided—that is, those supported by studies with findings that are both clinically significant (to the reader) and statistically significant. However, even treatments with a strong evidence base will have limitations in their applicability to some individual clients. Thus, readers may be reasonably drawn to promising interventions in early stages of development that appear more relevant. Such interventions, however, warrant special cautions in their application. For example, not only should clinicians warn a client about a treatment's limitations, but also they should be particularly scrupulous in assessing the treatment's effectiveness with that client.

One way in which clinicians might achieve more rigorous assessment of outcomes for their own clients is by enlisting a colleague to administer and score one or more systematic outcome measures to limit the action of unconscious bias on ongoing assessment (Dollaghan, 2007). Although this would be an ideal strategy to use for every client, a clinician may need to be cautious in requesting use of other clinicians' time for fearing of exhausting their goodwill. Thus, situations in which a controversial intervention is used may represent the kind of extraordinary circumstance that will call forth the generosity and interest of colleagues with stuttering expertise and reward them for their efforts by having them learn from your experience.

The **Practical Requirements for the Treatment** section describes real-world variables that may affect either a clinician's ability to conduct a treatment effectively or clients' preferences for it. This section includes elements such as the level of training required for a clinician, the amount of time the treatment requires (both in terms of daily intervention or practice sessions and its expected duration), and cost. Required equipment and other materials are also described in this section.

In **Key Components of the Approach**, the ways in which treatment goals are addressed, the individuals involved in working with the client (e.g., the clinician, parents, teachers, and/or friends), and the general stages that might be expected to characterize the intervention are explained in some detail. This section also includes descriptions of any procedures used for follow-up after the end of formal treatment or for dealing with relapse after a formal follow-up period has ended. Procedures used by the clinician, sequences of specific goals, and activities during which treatment is pursued are also described.

The information provided in the preceding sections may allow clinicians to determine the extent to which a treatment described in this book may be appropriate for a particular client—a critical step in evidence-based practice (Sackett et al., 2000). There are several questions that clinicians must ask in taking this step. "Is my client similar to participants in studies of this treatment's effectiveness?" "Will the outcome of this treatment meet my client's hopes and expectations?" "Is the cost of this treatment in time and money commensurate with what my client wants to spend?" A discussion of these questions with the client or family may be the most appropriate way to uncover the answers. Such a discussion, coupled with the clinician's thorough understanding of the treatment, may lead to using the treatment in question, but with reasonable adaptations. For example, a treatment designed for parents to use with their children may be adaptable so that grandparents or other caregivers can use it. On the other hand, the discussion of the above questions may lead to finding alternative treatments to offer a client.

In addition to finding out whether the treatment can be suited to a client, clinicians will need to ask themselves whether *they* are suited to deliver the treatment. Do they have the training, time, and temperament to carry it out? In some cases, a treatment may be inappropriate not because it does not fit the client, but because it does not fit the clinician. If an equally well-grounded intervention that is within the scope of the clinician cannot be found, the client should be referred to a more appropriate clinician.

Assessment Methods to Support Ongoing Decision Making is the section in which authors describe the outcomes used to decide when goals have been achieved or when procedures should be altered. Although at times these methods will be those used in published research on the intervention, sometimes authors may suggest more efficient methods for clinical use. We call readers' attention to Chapter 3 by Richels and Conture. Unlike the majority of other chapters in this book, which focus on individual treatments or evaluations of treatments, their chapter provides a detailed description of a comprehensive approach to assessment that is firmly grounded in what is known about the nature of stuttering. In addition, it reports brand-new information about what factors may predict long- and short-term outcomes for young children in treatment and presents hypotheses held by an established group of researchers

about factors contributing to the onset and development of stuttering.

Tailoring the Treatment to the Individual Client guides readers in their thoughts about modifications related to cultural and personal factors. Because social roles and interaction patterns differ across cultural subgroups and individuals, clinicians need to anticipate modifications that can be both consonant with the principles of the treatment and beneficial to the individual client.

Application of the Treatment to an Individual Who Stutters allows authors to illustrate the decisions leading to the use of their intervention through an example describing a specific person who stutters, as well as the course of the intervention and outcomes associated with it. This element of the template is intended to help readers understand the intervention at a more compelling, personal level.

In **Future Directions**, authors outline the research they believe is needed for the continued development of their intervention and the evidence base supporting its use. For interventions in earlier stages of development, the evidence base may include studies of efficacy. These are "laboratory" studies demonstrating that the variables to be manipulated in the intervention do indeed produce desired effects. For interventions that have already been more extensively evaluated, this evidence may include studies of effectiveness. These are studies conducted under "real-world" conditions designed to indicate that similar effects are achievable in less controlled circumstances. The research paths that authors outline in this section may be ones that they themselves plan to undertake. Alternatively, authors may point the way for others whose independent inquiry and perspectives can only enhance the quality of empirical support available for an intervention.

In the section **Suggested Readings**, readers are directed to readings that provide critical background knowledge or more detailed accounts of the intervention's evidence base or application.

A set of one or more video clips on the publisher's textbook website ThePoint forms the final element of each treatment's description. Specific information on accessing this website is contained at the end of the book. It allows readers to gain an intimate experience of each intervention that even the best prose description cannot convey. Thus, it may help clinicians, clients, and families come to their conclusions about the extent to which the intervention seems likely to meet their needs.

HOW TREATMENTS ARE ORGANIZED: A MODEL OF TREATMENT STRUCTURE

In this section, we propose a structural model to make it easier for readers to compare interventions and incorporate them into their ongoing practice. By understanding the model, readers may more thoughtfully do what clinicians often do—be eclectic in their use and adaptation of interventions. In particular, they may better appreciate that any adaptation weakens the generalizability of previous research to their particular client. This may cause some readers to abandon the practice of adaptation and others to proceed more cautiously and be judicious in their modifications. Understanding the link between modifications and the constellation of support for an intervention may be of greatest value to those who will be willing to pursue their clinical adaptations through systematic research.

Understanding the structure of treatment can help in clinical practice as well as in treatment research. For practitioners, it can improve clinical practice by increasing their awareness of elements that may have escaped attention, thus allowing them to adjust elements that were making a client's treatment less productive. Similarly, understanding the structure of treatment may highlight elements that can be modified to address individual needs of specific clients, thereby improving their outcomes. Such an understanding is potentially instructive for clinical research because it may highlight vital ingredients of a treatment warranting additional study. Take the case of several different treatments with similar outcomes. A grasp of how treatments are structured may guide clinical researchers to identify either shared key ingredients that may not have previously been apparent or different ingredients that lead to similar positive outcomes but through different mechanisms.

Three examples can further illustrate how attending to treatment structure can improve clinical and research problem solving.

- Mike, an adult who stutters, had learned to manage his stutters using "pull-outs" (a technique for reducing tension) while conversing with the clinician in the therapy room. He and the clinician decided that a logical next step would be for Mike to use pull-outs while telling a rehearsed joke to a good friend. Much to their chagrin, the attempt was unsuccessful and undermined Mike's emerging confidence.

- Esperanza, age 8, is learning to use easy onsets when she expects to stutter on a word. She comes into treatment one day, excited about winning her event at the school track meet. As she is talking, the clinician repeatedly interrupts her to remind her to use easy onsets. Soon, Esperanza is talking less and less, and finally, she asks if she can go back to class.

- Joan is a speech-language pathologist who has been treating preschoolers who stutter by training their parents to use a facilitating style of communicative interaction. Her colleague Bob announces one day that he has adopted a much more effective approach that relies on teaching parents to use behavior shaping to help their children. They get into a disagreement that strains their friendship and changes neither of their minds.

As you read the description of the model that follows, keep these examples in mind.

Treatment can be conceived of as an ongoing process in time, with a beginning and an end, undertaken to meet one or more **basic goals** (Fig. 2.1A). Note in the figure that the basic goals persist throughout the entire course of treatment. Such basic goals will necessarily reflect the clinicians' philosophy of treatment and their views of stuttering, but should also reflect the clients' (or families') desired outcomes and preferences. For example, for a preschool child, the therapy would probably focus on fluency as a basic goal. For an adolescent or older adult, basic goals might include some combination of fluency, communicative effectiveness, and satisfaction in interpersonal communication.

To reach the basic goal(s), **intermediate goals** need to be established (Fig. 2.1B). Intermediate goals consist of those skills, abilities, and cognitions in important relevant contexts that enable the client to achieve the basic goal(s). Whereas treatments may sometimes focus on a single basic goal, they almost always postulate

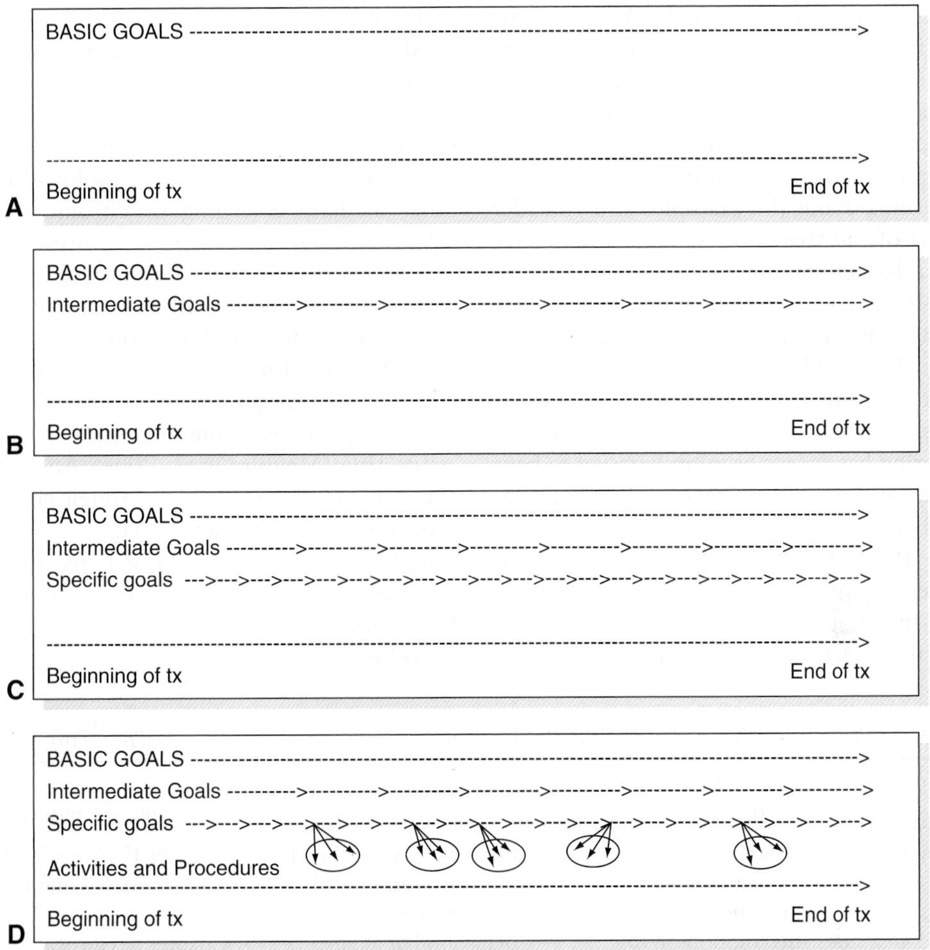

Figure 2.1. **(A)** Basic goals on timeline from beginning to end of therapy. **(B)** Basic and intermediate goals on timeline. **(C)** Basic, intermediate, and specific goals on timeline. **(D)** Basic, intermediate, and specific goals with arrows indicating that activities and procedures come from each specific goal.

numerous intermediate goals. Using the example of the preschooler for whom fluency is a basic goal, one intermediate goal might be fluent speech in conversation. On the other hand, an intermediate goal associated with a basic goal of improved communicative effectiveness for an adolescent or adult might be increasing participation in speaking situations.

Each intermediate goal also needs to be broken down into specific goals. Specific goals guide the most obvious aspects of a treatment plan because they have the most immediate effects on the choice of **activities** and **procedures** used in treatment sessions. In the example of the preschool child, the intermediate goal of fluency in conversation might be addressed using specific goals of more fluent productions in conversations of decreasing structure. For the adult who has an intermediate goal of increasing participation in speaking situations, a specific goal might be role playing a feared situation.

Specific goals are worked on via activities and procedures that occur on the treatment timeline. **Procedures** are the actions performed by the clinician or parent to move the client toward specific goals. **Activities**, on the other hand, are the ongoing communication contexts in which procedures are implemented. For example, in certain treatments for a preschool child with the specific goal of fluency in conversational situations of decreasing structure, the procedures might be having the parent provide verbal contingencies for fluency and stuttering, and the activity might be engaging the child in a conversation during a car ride. Alternatively, for a different method of treatment with the same specific goal, the clinician might have a mother adopt the procedure of slowing her rate in conversation with the child during the activity of a quiet conversation at home.

Now think about the examples and consider what part of the treatment structure may have been overlooked in each example, leading to the less-than-ideal outcome. For instance, are there cases in which basic and intermediate goals may be at odds with one another or where different procedures might lead to similar outcomes?

Stuttering has always been understood to have a widespread impact on the speech, communication, and quality of life of those who experience it (Curlee, 1993; Yaruss, 1998). More recently, researchers have probed beneath stuttering's physical manifestations in speech behaviors to examine the underlying brain structures and neu-

ral events that are associated with it (Ingham, 2003). One powerful way in which treatments can be categorized is according to the level of effects that they target (Table 2.3).

At the most basic level, interventions might aim at changing the neurophysiologic correlates that mediate emerging or chronic stuttering. Pharmacologic interventions represent current strategies of this sort. To date, pharmacologic interventions range from tranquilizers that decrease anxiety and tension (e.g., meprobamate) (Kent, 1963; Kent & Williams, 1959) to drugs that target specific neurotransmitters (e.g., dopamines) thought to be associated with stuttering (Maguire et al., 2004). Another intervention targeting neurophysiologic correlates of stuttering is transcranial magnetic stimulation (Ingham et al., 2000). In this book, Chapter 17 by Maguire and colleagues reviews a pharmacologic intervention that they are in the process of developing.

Table 2.3. *Interventions Discussed in This Book by the Level of Treatment Effects They Target*

Level of Treatment Effects	Description	Associated Treatments	Chapters in This Book That Discuss the Treatments
Neurophysiology	Differences in brain structure and/or function	Pharmacologic intervention or transcranial magnetic stimulation	Chapter 17 (Maguire, Riley, Franklin, & Gumusaneli)
Speech	Interruptions in the ongoing production of speech	Behavioral or augmentative/assistive techniques focused on speech production	Chapter 6 (Gottwald), Chapter 7 (Harrison & Onslow), Chapter 9 (Harrison, Bruce, Shenker, & Koushik), Chapter 10 (Runyan & Runyan), Chapter 11 (Craig), Chapter 14 (O'Brian, Packman, & Onslow), Chapter 15 (Kroll & Scott-Sulski), Chapter 16 (Ramig, Ellis, & Ryan)
Communication	Reductions in quality and quantity of communication because of the speaker's manner of stuttering (core and secondary behaviors, feelings and attitudes) interacting with listener's responses	Parent counseling with an emphasis on parent-child interaction; integrated approaches to stuttering intervention	Chapter 3 (Richels & Conture), Chapter 5 (Botterill & Kelman), Chapter 6 (Gottwald), Chapter 12 (Yaruss, Pelczarski, & Quesal), Chapter 15 (Kroll & Scott-Sulski)
Quality of life	Social, academic, and occupational limitations placed on speaker by self and others	Creating supportive environment; support or self-help groups; psychotherapy	Chapter 12 (Yaruss, Pelczarsky, & Quesal)

The speech correlates of stuttering probably constitute the most obvious level of effects targeted by treatments. Treatments that target this level are primarily concerned with the reduction of disfluencies among clients who stutter or, in adults, a reduction in the degree to which disruptions in speech fluency call attention to themselves. Clinicians who use such interventions may do so with the strong belief that broader effects on communication and quality of life will change naturally and without direct attention as fluency is improved. Because these interventions are most numerous, it is not surprising that 5 of the 13 treatment chapters in this book describe interventions with this focus.

Interventions that involve treatment procedures designed to directly affect a client's communication skills and attitudes toward speaking may be associated with two somewhat different beliefs. First, these treatments may be pursued in the belief that improvements in communication skills and attitudes toward speaking are needed in order for natural recovery to have an opportunity to occur or for gains to be achieved in fluency. This perspective is more commonly taken in treatments for children. Alternatively, such treatments may be pursued from the belief that, regardless of changes in fluency, improved communication skills and attitudes toward speaking are an independent goal well worth pursuing. This perspective is more commonly taken in treatments for older children and adults. Five interventions target effects at this level.

Improved quality of life is probably an implicitly desired outcome of every intervention.

Historically, as a direct effect, it has probably been most obviously pursued in psychotherapeutic interventions, such as those advocated by Travis (1957). However, it is an important component of a contemporary and grossly understudied intervention strategy—that is, support or self-help groups. Such groups reflect the self-healing impulses of people who stutter. In addition, speech-language pathologists often recommend such groups to help their clients maintain improved fluency. Chapter 12 makes such a recommendation for children and adolescents.

CONCLUDING REMARKS

We will return to the themes of evidence-based practice, treatment structure, and treatment efficacy in the four other chapters we have written for this book. Three of these will take the form of overview chapters at the beginning of the main sections, and one will be the final chapter. This final chapter will summarize the current state of evidence-based practice in stuttering and delineate research needs. Through these chapters, we hope to help readers look beyond differences in procedures and activities to see underlying similarities in basic goals, as well as the ways in which these goals may change for clients of different ages.

Thus, at the most immediate level, we hope that when readers finish this book, they will be able to adopt and implement treatments that best fit their clients and their own styles. At a higher level, we hope readers will have gained an appreciation of how treatments are structured, how they have been shown to work up to this point in time, and how they might be improved.

CHAPTER 3

Indirect Treatment of Childhood Stuttering: Diagnostic Predictors of Treatment Outcome

CORRIN G. RICHELS AND EDWARD G. CONTURE

CHAPTER OUTLINE

INTRODUCTION

The purpose of this chapter is to discuss the role of assessment as a means of diagnosing childhood stuttering as well as informing clinicians about the course and outcome of treatment. Because there are typically more males than females who stutter in childhood—the ratio being at least 2 boys for 1 girl (Ambrose, Cox & Yairi, 1997)—we will use the pronoun "him" to refer to the children in this chapter. We will focus on the assessment of preschool (ages 2.5 to 5 years) and young school-

age (ages 5 years to 6 years 11 months) children who stutter (hereafter referred to as child or children). This age range was selected because it brackets the time period during which the onset of stuttering is most likely to occur (Maansson, 2007; Yairi & Ambrose, 2005; Yaruss, 1999; Yaruss, LaSalle, & Conture, 1998). Additionally, the preschool and early school-age years involve the time period during which the differential diagnosis of children with incipient stuttering versus transient disfluency is most challenging (Curlee, 1993; Finn, Ingham, Ambrose, & Yairi, 1997).

To begin, we discuss the theoretical underpinnings that guide our assessment procedures as well as the empirical support for our means of assessing children known or thought to be stuttering. Following this discussion, the chapter presents the rationale, strategies, and outcome data regarding the present authors' approach to assessment as it relates to successfully implementing treatment for children who stutter.

The chapter concludes with a summary of what we believe to be the essential aspects of assessing children as well as areas in need of future exploration and modification. It is hoped that the reader of this chapter will better understand the importance of the initial assessment of children and families in the treatment of young children who stutter. Additionally, we believe that clinicians should then be able to appropriately modify our approach to best fit various service delivery settings as well as the individual needs of young clients and their families.

THEORETICAL BASIS FOR ASSESSMENT AND TREATMENT

In our opinion, the primary purposes of assessment of childhood stuttering are, first, to accurately, objectively, and reliably determine whether a child is indeed stuttering; and second, to address subsequent treatment-related decisions. These issues include the degree of risk for continued stuttering, the appropriateness of speech-language therapy, and the nature, duration, and means of delivery of treatment (e.g., individual, group, or both individual and group). Another equally important purpose for the assessment is to *orient* the child's family to the clinician's approach to the nature of the problem. At the time of the diagnostic session, therefore, families also should come to better understand the nature, duration, and probable success of treatment.

The methods used by a clinician in the assessment (and treatment) of childhood stuttering should be related to the clinician's theoretical and experiential perspective regarding childhood stuttering. The theoretical framework for the current chapter is based on the cumulative results of several descriptive studies (Anderson, Pellowski, & Conture, 2005; Pellowski & Conture, 2002; Karrass et al., 2006), as well as experimental studies of childhood stuttering (Anderson & Conture, 2004;

Arnold, Conture, & Ohde, 2005; Byrd, Conture, & Ohde, 2007; Hartfield & Conture, 2006; Melnick, Conture, & Ohde, 2003; Pellowski & Conture, 2005).

The findings from the descriptive and experimental studies cited above have recently been used to provide empirical support for a theoretical model (Conture et al., 2006) that we refer to as the "Communication-Emotional" (C-E) model of stuttering. This model asserts that the disorder of stuttering is a multifactorial phenomenon (Smith & Kelly, 1997), resulting from a complex interaction of several factors. These factors are communicative, linguistic, emotional, and motor variables (Fig. 3.1). The present chapter seeks to link elements of the C-E model (for further details, see Conture et al., 2006) to procedures we are developing to comprehensively assess childhood stuttering and help us better understand and predict treatment outcomes.

One of the major assumptions of the C-E model is that stuttering results from many factors, some of which are regarded as being relatively "distant" to instances of stuttering (i.e., distal) and some of which are hypothesized to be relatively "close" to instances of stuttering (i.e., proximal). In other words, "distal" variables (e.g., genetics, environment) are seen as general sources of or contributors to "proximal" factors (e.g., temperament) that indirectly or directly contribute to instances of stuttering. We also assume that viable models of stuttering must attempt to account for the forms that stuttering takes (e.g., sound-syllable repetitions, sound prolongations, etc.). Working from the top of the model toward overt instances of stuttering, we find the distal contributors of environment and genetics. We believe that these contributors may act individually or jointly, that they more than likely co-occur, and that the contributions of environment and genetics vary among individuals as suggested by Smith and Kelly (1997). These distal contributors lead to proximal contributors, such as speech-language planning and production, and to a greater or lesser degree involve the child's experience(s) with communication and related events (e.g., a child's experiences and then comes to expect that a parent will frequently interrupt his or her utterances). The model suggests that stuttering may be exacerbated by a person's experiences as well as emotional reactivity and regulation, both trait

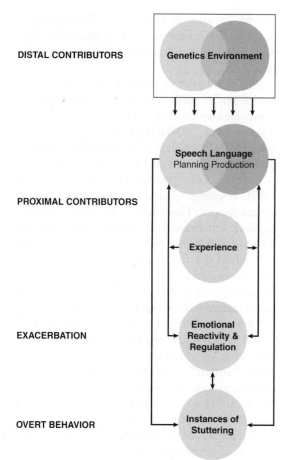

DISTAL CONTRIBUTORS

Genetics Environment

PROXIMAL CONTRIBUTORS

Speech Language
Planning Production

Experience

EXACERBATION

Emotional
Reactivity &
Regulation

OVERT BEHAVIOR

Instances of
Stuttering

Figure 3.1. Communication-Emotional model of childhood stuttering (after Conture et al., 2006). Within the context of this model, two levels of contributors to stuttering are posited: (1) distal, interactive contributors of genetics and environment and (2) proximal, interactive contributors of disruptions of speech and language planning and production, with (1) leading to (2) and (2) ultimately leading to instances of stuttering. Through experience, however, emotional reactivity and regulation are thought to exacerbate, interact with, and maintain instances of stuttering caused by (2).

(dispositional) as well as state (situational) elements of temperament (for an excellent review of temperament in children, see Goldsmith et al., 1987).

C-E MODEL: DISTAL CONTRIBUTORS TO STUTTERING

As mentioned earlier, the foundational or "top" distal contributors to instances of stuttering, as described in the C-E model, are genetics and environment (for more general discussion of genetic contributions, see Yairi & Ambrose, 2002;

Yairi, Ambrose, & Cox, 1996; for more general discussion of possible environmental contributors, see Adams, 1993; Yairi, 1997b). It is posited that these two variables—genetics and environment—can singularly or jointly, but essentially indirectly, influence stuttering. For example, a person's *genetic* propensities for relatively inefficient speech-language planning and processing in conversational speech can co-occur with a social, communicative, or emotional *environment* that expects or demands quick, mature and elaborately spoken communication. Indeed, we believe that these distal contributors are the most likely initial sources for any inherent predisposition (sometimes referred to as a "diathesis") to stutter and are proclivities that can interact with or be exacerbated by a host of stressors, for example, consistent parental encouragement to speak far more rapidly than typical (see Morgan & Simons, 1991, for detailed discussion of *diathesis-stressor* models).

In essence, the genetic and environmental aspects of the model attempt to account for the indirect contributions of both an individual's nature as well as the environment that nurtures him. This part of the model suggests that an individual's genetic makeup determines his or her minimum and maximum capacities for a many aspects of life (e.g., height, weight, intelligence). However, the individual's environment influences his or her ability to meet the maximum of his or her genetic potential, an ability that changes between and within days, weeks, and longer intervals, depending on a host of variables (e.g., fatigue, attention). Genetic potential and environmental facilitation, inhibition, and influences serve as essential building blocks for the proximal and exacerbating contributors speculated about in our model.

C-E MODEL: PROXIMAL CONTRIBUTORS TO STUTTERING

The proximal contributors to instances of stuttering are speech-language planning and production as well as, to some degree, experience. For the purposes of this chapter and for the C-E model, the term "experience" is meant to encompass what each individual encounters and takes away from his or her interactions with the world and includes but is not restricted to learning processes—for example, behavior shaped by response-contingent rewards and punishments.

The model (Conture et al., 2006, Fig. 2-1, p. 19) shows speech-language planning and production both as separate and overlapping phenomena. This reflects our belief that processes of speech-language planning and production, especially during conversational speech, occur *incrementally*. By incrementally, we mean that each point in planning and processing is necessary to move forward in time to the next point in planning and processing. Indeed, we believe that when the incrementality of speech-language planning and processing overlaps in time with attentional and emotional processes, stuttering is most apt to occur (see Bosshardt, 2006, for further discussion of the potential importance of incrementality of speech-language planning and production to stuttering). For example, from this aspect of our model, we would predict that a child will have more difficulty when relating a story he heard yesterday to his mother if his younger sister is persistently interrupting and requiring attentional resources of the child.

Many of our assumptions regarding speech-language planning and processing relate to Levelt's (1989) model of speech-language planning and production (for further review of this model, supporting evidence, and related speculation, see Indefrey & Levelt, 2000, 2004; Levelt, Roelofs, & Meyer, 1999). Hartfield and Conture (2006) briefly describe the model as follows:

> This model divides the complex process of speech-language planning and production into three inter-related subsystems or processing components: (1) the conceptualizer, (2) the formulator and (3) the articulator. Briefly, the *conceptualizer*, among various tasks, conceives the speaker's intention and selects the necessary information needed to be expressed to realize the speaker's intention. The output of this processing component is described by Levelt as the "preverbal message." The preverbal message, in turn, serves as input to the next processing component, that is, the *formulator*, which receives elements or fragments of the preverbal message, with the output of the formulator described as the phonetic or articulatory plan. This plan, in turn, serves as input to the *articulator*. The articulator's role is to execute the phonetic plan by means of the coordinated activities of the respiratory, laryngeal and supralaryngeal systems. (p. 304)

This temporal overlap, often referred to as *incremental processing* (or sometimes as "time sharing" among cognitive, formulative, and articulatory components) is thought to allow for speedy, efficient processing. Put another way, incrementality refers to the notion that when "once a piece of information (during language production) at a level of processing becomes available, it triggers activity at the next level down the production system" (Ferreira & Swets, 2002, p. 58) (again, for more on "incremental processing" and stuttering, see Bosshardt, 2006). Such processing, it is believed, is particularly salient during conversational speech when it is not possible to precisely plan, in advance, what we want to say and when we must plan and produce speech-language "on-the-fly."

Incremental Processing: An Example

To better appreciate how incrementality of speech-language production works and, in turn, may not work at times for children who stutter, we would like to consider how the speech-language planning and processing system might function to conceptualize, formulate, and then articulate the idea or thought "The dog ate it" in conversational speech (Fig. 3.2). To do this, the speaker "must" proceed from the covert preverbal message through overt articulation. To begin, the *message* or conceptualizer sends "thought element A—'The dog'" to the language formulation component. And while the *formulator* is planning "The dog," the *conceptualizer* moves on to "thought element B—'ate.'" While that is occurring, the formulator sends "The dog" on to the *articulator*. Thus, while the conceptualizer is processing "thought element C—'it,'" the formulator is processing "ate" (element B), and the articulator is processing "The dog" (element A).

It should be noted that about the time the speaker is overtly initiating the utterance, several other covert activities are "still in play," making the overt initiation of speech-language a potentially challenging cotemporaneous event, one that simultaneously involves cognitive, linguistic, and motoric processes. In our opinion, it is little wonder, therefore, that this "point" in the utterance—that is, the beginning of the utterance—attracts so many instances of

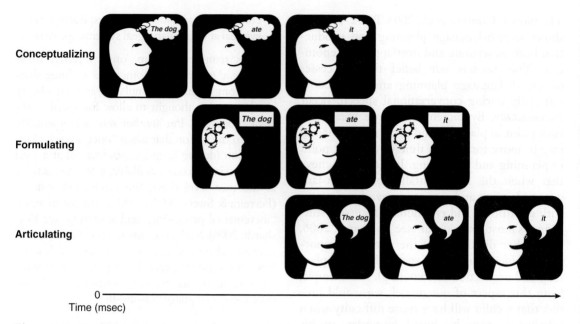

Figure 3.2. Graphic example of incremental processing of the utterance "The dog ate it," from conceptualization through articulation (after Levelt, 1989).

stuttering, especially for individuals whose underlying abilities to quickly and efficiently implement these various processes, much less coordinate them all, may be less than ideal (e.g., Bloodstein & Grossman, 1981; Richels, Buhr, Ntourou, & Conture, 2009). Be that as it may, and as mentioned earlier, this temporal overlap is thought to allow for speedy, efficient processing, particularly during conversational speech, where time demands and topic shifts are the most unpredictable. For an individual, the efficiency of each speech-language planning and processing component is thought to result from genetic influence. On the other hand, how the individual copes with possible discoordinations in processing that may occur during communication is likely due to the effects of his or her experiences in different communication environments.

EXPERIENTIAL CONTRIBUTIONS

As mentioned earlier, we believe that genetic influences predispose an individual to certain levels of skills and abilities for thinking, formulating, and articulating, as well as coordinating and integrating among these related but differing skills and abilities. These skills and abilities are more or less facilitated or inhibited by the individual's external and internal environment. We believe that these interactions between genetically endowed skills and abilities, as well as environmental facilitation and/or inhibitions, impact the accuracy, speed, and efficiency with which the child's speech-language planning and production occur. Genetics (nature) and environment (nurture) also influence, we believe, how "insulated" speech-language planning and production may be from contemporaneous demands for attentional, cognitive, and emotional resources. Experience, which in many ways is influenced by the accumulated as well as continuing interactions of nature and nurture, also plays a significant role in the development of speech-language planning and production. For example, some children may frequently experience someone in their environment who interrupts them; provides inappropriately rapid, overly complex communication models; talks for them; corrects their less-than-mature speech and language; frequently and critically concerns themselves with the child's speech-language imperfections; and so forth. If these experiences are consistent and frequent enough, we conjecture, they could "encourage" the child to avoid, modify, or reduce communication or try to rush the initiation as well as the ongoing speech-language planning and production in order to achieve communicative intent before being corrected. Whereas some children may adjust to such environmental diversions and attentional demands, it is quite possible that other children may not and, consequently, may find it difficult—in such a communicative environment—to fluently initiate or continue ongoing speech-language planning and production. Although presently we are unclear about what might distinguish these two groups of children, we speculate that for some children, exacerbating experiences such as these are aided and abetted by other exacerbating factors—the threshold and level/intensity of their emotional reactivity and the presence and effectiveness of their emotional regulation.

EMOTIONAL CONTRIBUTIONS

The terms *emotional reactivity and emotion regulation* (see Eisenberg & Fabes, 1992, for review) are fairly new to the literature on childhood stuttering (although the possible role that autonomic arousal/activation plays in stuttering has long been considered, e.g., Brutten & Shoemaker, 1967; Weber & Smith, 1990). Therefore, some definition and clarification seem appropriate (interestingly, empirical attempts to study variables related to arousability/reactivity have begun to appear in the literature on stuttering, e.g., Alm & Risberg, 2007; Guitar, 2003).

Emotional reactivity refers to the tendency for some individuals to experience frequent and intense emotional arousal and their ability to respond to that experience. Both the ease with which individuals become emotionally aroused and the intensity of emotional experiences are aspects of emotional reactivity. *Emotional regulation* involves the process of controlling the occurrence, intensity, or duration of internal feelings and emotion-related physiologic processes (Thompson, 1994). Emotional regulation is generally defined in terms of modulating internal (emotional) reactivity (Ahadi & Rothbart, 1994). We believe that these two aspects of emotions—*emotional reactivity* and *emotional regulation*—have potential for contributing to the frequency, duration, type, and severity of instances of stuttering.

Although our description so far of the C-E model emphasizes "top-down" influences on instances of stuttering, the proximal and exacerbating contributors of experience, emotional reactivity, and regulation may also act in "bottom-up" fashion to impact on initiation as well as ongoing speech-language planning and production. "Top-down" in this case is used to describe instances of stuttering as a result of factors moving from the "top" of the model (e.g., environment and genetics) toward the "bottom" of the model (e.g., experience, temperament, etc.). Therefore, "bottom-up" movement would suggest that instances of stuttering also impact on temperament, experience, and speech-language planning and processing. This bidirectional interaction is critical to understanding the role of emotions and the experience of stuttering in the exacerbation of the instances of stuttering themselves.

Referring back to the previous example of a child's experience of being interrupted while trying to communicate, we conjecture that emotional reactivity and emotion regulation may also determine the nature or quality of the child's response. For example, the child with *low* emotional reactivity and *high* emotion regulation may not experience undue disruption or interference in ongoing behavior due to, for example, interruptions by his or her listener. He or she will likely just "talk over" the interruption. However, the child who typically experiences *high* emotional reactivity and *high* emotion regulation may be more likely to be the one who shuts down or ceases to talk at all in the presence of such interruption. *High* emotional reactivity means that the child will quickly experience a fairly intense emotional reaction to being interrupted (e.g., frustration, attentional refocusing, etc.). However, this child's concomitant *high* emotion regulation means that the child will likely show no overt expression of the emotion; rather, he or she will internalize the intense emotion being felt with a resulting increase in anxiety and frustration. We further conjecture that a child who experiences *high* emotional reactivity but *low* emotion regulation will more likely start to rush to talk faster, yell, have a tantrum, or attempt to "shush" everyone who interrupts him. These are, of course, all empirical questions awaiting future investigations.

To date, of course, we know little about how interactions between emotional reactivity and regulation affect childhood stuttering. We would like to suggest, however, that the various reactivity and regulation scenarios described earlier have the potential for influencing how different children experience and react to stuttering. Specifically, each of these different "combinations" (e.g., high reactivity, low regulation) may influence how children attempt to cope with, modify, or even avoid experiences associated with communication, stuttering, and related events—for example, one-on-one versus small group conversations. The descriptions of the different combinations of reactivity and regulation are meant to help illustrate how beginning with a child's environment, the occurrence of one event—for example, communicative interruption—flows through the model and back. It also highlights the potentially infinite combinations between reactivity and regulation, combinations that may shift or change with changing circumstances or environments.

EMPIRICAL BASIS FOR ASSESSMENT AND INTERVENTION

Not surprisingly, the empirical support for our model of assessment and the C-E model itself is based not only on our own work, but also on the many contributions of others (e.g., Adams, 1991; Conture, 1997, 2001; Conture & Caruso, 1987; Conture & Yaruss, 1993; Culatta & Goldberg, 1995; Forsnot, 1992; Gordon & Luper, 1992; Gregory & Hill, 1992, 1999; Hayes & Pindzola, 2004; Peters & Guitar, 1991; Pindzola, 1986; Pindzola & White, 1986; Wall & Myers, 1995; Yaruss, LaSalle, & Conture, 1998; Zebrowski, 1994). Here we will organize discussion of that empirical support for elements of our assessments by beginning at the "top" of the model with genetics and environment and moving toward the "bottom," or the actual instances of stuttering.

GENETIC EVIDENCE

Our assessment methods include obtaining information about genetics because of a wide range of evidence that stuttering may result from genetic components. In a 1996 review, Yairi, Ambrose, and Cox reported that 20% to 74% of people who stutter report having at least one other relative who also stutters. Similarly, Graham and Conture's (2005) parent-report–based study found that families of preschool children who stutter (CWS) (n = 57) were significantly more likely to report at least one other family member with a history of stuttering than were families of preschool children who do not stutter (CWNS) (n = 57). Specifically, results indicated that 70% of the families of children who stutter reported at least one other family member who also stuttered. Interestingly, Graham and Conture found that the families of preschool CWS, when compared to those of preschool CWNS, were also more likely to report having a family member with attention deficit hyperactivity disorder (ADHD; Alm & Risberg, 2007; Healey & Reid, 2003), a topic seemingly in need of further empirical study.

Studies that attempt to link genetic transmission to stuttering are divided into essentially two models of transmission: (1) single-gene or major gene transmission, and (2) multigene or polygenic explanations. In a segregation analysis study, Ambrose, Cox, and Yairi (1993) posited that transmission by a single major gene was the most likely avenue of transmission of stuttering. More recently, Shugart et al. (2004) linked stuttering to a large group of genes on chromosome 18. These researchers' (Shugart et al., 2004) findings of an identifiable group of genes on chromosome 18 add to the existing literature that stuttering may be a result of a polygenic explanation of the heritability of stuttering. Polygenic transmission is thought to be more mutable to the influence of environment because expression of multiple genes is more environmentally dependent (Felsenfeld, 1996). In single-gene transmission theories, the odds of a particular behavior being expressed require fewer environmental triggers or contributors. However, in polygenic transmission, it is posited that more environmental factors are necessary for the expression of the phenotype (i.e., in this case, stuttering).

ENVIRONMENTAL EVIDENCE

Despite the strong possibility of genetic influence as a contributor to instances of stuttering, the influence of environment is also considered a co-occurring and contributing agent (Yairi, Ambrose, & Cox, 1996). As with genetics, our assessment methods include obtaining information about the child's environment because of our belief that childhood stuttering can be influenced by environmental variables. Most importantly, it should be noted that these variables do not have to reach the level of pathologic (e.g., child abuse) to be pertinent to the child's problem (e.g., a perfectionistic father who routinely comments on and corrects many of the child's speech-language, social, athletic, etc., mistakes). As one example of the influence of environment on childhood speech-language and possibly stuttering, Graham and Hartfield (2006) reported that the scores of CWS (n = 166) on norm-based, standardized tests of speech-language were strongly influenced by the socioeconomic status (SES) of their families and the education levels of both of their parents. Interestingly, scores on norm-based standardized tests of speech-language for CWNS (n = 130) were less influenced by SES and paternal education but were definitely influenced by maternal education. Although one could argue that these findings are not devoid of genetic influences, they do seem to indicate that the speech-language (and possibly speech fluency) of children who stutter is more susceptible to differences in SES as well as education levels of both parents when compared with their nonstuttering peers. Results could be interpreted to further suggest that children who stutter, at least in terms of their speech-language, are more sensitized or more reactive to environmental influences than children who do not stutter (and/or their environments are more reactive to children experiencing fluency issues). Further evidence of possible combined influences of genetics and environment can be seen in research evidence related to differences in speech-language planning and production characteristics of children.

SPEECH-LANGUAGE PLANNING AND/OR PRODUCTION EVIDEN

Aspects of speech-language planning and production should be included in assessment as part of the thorough collection of data on factors that may be contributing to a child's stuttering. When we examine descriptive studies in this area, we find a mixed bag. In a survey of 2,628 children, Blood et al. (2003) reported that 62.8% of the children surveyed also had other co-occurring speech disorders, language disorders, or non-speech disorders (which was a finding consistent with an earlier survey by Arndt & Healey, 2001).

Homzie et al. (1988) surveyed 190 adults who stutter and adults who do not stutter. Results indicated that adults who stutter reported significantly more histories of delayed language, disordered articulation, and written language problems. Likewise, Yaruss, LaSalle, and Conture (1998) reported that 40% of children who stutter also have articulation problems. In summary, results of these and related studies (e.g., see Bloodstein, 1995, Table 18) suggest that stuttering is associated with less than typical speech and language characteristics that may contribute not only to the manifestation of stuttering, but also to subtle and not so subtle disturbances in other aspects of speech-language skills. However, others (e.g., Watkins & Yairi, 1997; Watkins, Yairi, & Ambrose, 1999) have reported, "...no evidence of pervasive expressive language difficulty in young children who stutter" (Yairi & Ambrose, 2005, p. 241). These rather equivocal descriptive findings neither fully support nor refute the notion that CWS differ from CWNS in terms of speech-language abilities and development; however, these findings may indicate that at least a subgroup of children who stutter is less efficient and developed in terms of their speech-language planning and production.

When we examine more experimental work in this area, however, the picture becomes a bit sharper. Developing empirical evidence based on experimental studies suggests that stuttering is, at least in part, associated with less rapid, efficient syntactic, lexical, and/or phonologic processing, even when children who stutter do not exhibit a clinical significant disorder (Anderson & Conture, 2004; Arnold, Conture, & Ohde, 2005; Au-Yeung & Howell, 1998; Byrd, Conture, & Ohde, 2007; Cuadrado & Weber-Fox, 2003; Hartfield & Conture, 2006; Melnick, Conture, & Ohde, 2003; Pellowski & Conture, 2002; Weber-Fox et al., 2004). Empirical investigation of numerous speech-language factors (see Hall, Wagovich, & Bernstein Ratner, 2007, for a review) has implicated the following as being associated with stuttering: word frequency (e.g., Hubbard & Prins, 1994), word type (i.e., function versus content words, e.g., Howell, Au-Yeung, & Sackin, 1999), sentence and clause boundaries (e.g., Bernstein Ratner, 1997; Howell & Au-Yeung, 1995; Wall, Starkweather, & Cairns, 1981), word position in the sentence

(Buhr & Zebrowski, 2007), and utterance length and complexity (e.g., Bernstein Ratner, 1995; Bernstein Ratner & Sih, 1987; Logan & Conture, 1995, 1997; Melnick & Conture, 2000; Silverman & Ratner, 1997; Yaruss, 1999; Zackheim & Conture, 2003). Part of the differences between descriptive and experimental work in this area, we would submit, has to do with the nature of the data (e.g., standard scores on a standardized test of language versus speech reaction time associated with picture naming) *and* the notion that differences in speech-language must be *clinically significant* to be *significant clinically*. That is, a standardized test of language is designed to identify large dissimilarities between children's broader speech-language skills when compared to their same-aged peers (i.e., the larger population). The dissimilarity between populations is what we deem clinically significant differences. Alternately, experimental manipulation is designed to isolate subtle differences in very specific skills that may not be detectable at the larger clinically significant level. However, the subtle differences in speech-language processing skills found in experimental manipulation may truly be significant clinically.

One developing line of empirical investigation, related to this discussion, involves the study of *dissociations* between speech-language planning and production skills in children who stutter. For present purposes, dissociations in speech-language planning/production are defined as occurring when one subcomponent might be dissociated in some children from other aspects of linguistic formulation. An example of a dissociation is when phonologic processing is found to be considerably less well developed or less efficient than other subcomponents of linguistic formulation processes, such as lexical retrieval, morphosyntactic construction, etc. (Anderson, Pellowski, & Conture, 2005). Encouraged by earlier findings/speculation in this area (Anderson & Conture, 2000; Hall, 1996, 2004; Hall & Burgess, 2000), Anderson, Pellowski, and Conture (2005) employed inferential statistical methodology developed by Bates et al. (2003) to investigate such dissociations.

Anderson et al. reported that children who stutter (n = 45) were three times more likely than children who do not stutter (n = 45) to exhibit dissociations (i.e., clinically and statistically sig-

nificant differences) between speech, vocabulary, and language skills as evidenced by their performance on standardized measures. For example, a child who exhibits expressive vocabulary 1.5 standard deviations *above* the mean concurrently with articulatory abilities 1.75 standard deviations *below* the mean could be described as showing a dissociation between expressive vocabulary skills and articulation skills. It is important to note that these between-group differences in dissociations were found even when CWS and CWNS were equated for overall language abilities (a replication of Anderson et al., i.e., Coulter, Anderson, & Conture, 2009, resulted in similar findings). Similar observations were made by Hall, Yamashita, and Aram (1993), who investigated the relationship between fluency and language in 60 children with language disorders and found that "highly disfluent" children (n = 10; 8.04% or higher total disfluencies) had significantly greater semantic than morphosyntactic capacities. Although the identification of similarly depressed performance in language subcomponents is of obvious clinical importance, overt dissociations among speech-language skills may reflect planning or covert dissociations within and between the conceptualizer, formulator, and articulator levels of processing (see Postma & Kolk, 1993, for review of covert repair hypothesis). Consequently, dissociations may point the way to a different set of treatment planning considerations than the simple injunction to "consider treating both areas" that could follow from similarly poor performances in several areas. In addition, such dissociations may be of particular theoretical interest to researchers.

EVIDENCE OF EFFECTS OF EXPERIENCE

Conture et al. (2006) describe the experience portion of the C-E model as being one bridge between the distal and proximal contributors to stuttering. For example, how an individual experiences instances of stuttering is going to be influenced by either his or her speech-language planning and processing skills as well as behavioral, dispositional (temperamental), and situational aspects of emotional reactivity and regulation. For example, in a quasi-experimental study of CWS (n = 13) and CWNS (n=14),

Schwenk, Conture, and Walden (2007) reported that, during conversational interactions with their mothers, preschool CWS are significantly more likely than preschool CWNS to attend to noise disruptions in their immediate environment and less likely to habituate to that noise disruption. It was felt that the children's repeated attention to the environmental distraction and relative inability to disregard or disengage from it offers some possible insight into how they may experience and react to (non) routine environmental disruptions, both endogenous (e.g., hunger, anxiety, thirst) as well as exogenous (e.g., noisy camera moving, parental interruptions) in origin.

We might relate this finding, by analogy, to the situation of giving a presentation where the LCD projector periodically looses power and the screen goes blank. In this case, the speaker is presenting when, intermittently, suddenly, and unpredictably, his or her slides disappear from the projection screen. Depending on the level and nature of the speaker's reactivity to the intermittent disappearance of the slides, many of the speaker's attentional as well as cognitive resources could be drawn away from his or her actual presentation to attend to the sudden disappearance of the slides. The initial reactivity to these "intermittent disappearances" would directly influence the speaker's speech-language planning and processing as would his ability to adapt to this set of circumstances. In essence, the nature and rapidity with which the presenter reacted and adapted to this situation would have a large influence on the quality and fluidity of the presentation.

Little, if anything, is known about how such micro-momentary environmental events influence the speech-language planning and production of young children, especially those who stutter. However, it seems quite reasonable to suggest that they do have some degree of influence and that they warrant further empirical study. The possible influence of attention on the exacerbation of stuttering is also an important factor during assessment. For some children, the novelty of the assessment environment may unduly call on their attentional reserves at a point in time when the assessment tasks themselves require complete concentration; for example, the child may frequently ask whether his or her response was correct, and rather than focusing on the task at hand, the child is focused on the perceived "correctness" or level of achievement.

EVIDENCE FOR EMOTIONAL REACTIVITY AND EMOTION REGULATION

Emotional processes can be viewed from the perspective that *emotion* is intimately involved with attention, as well as cognition (e.g., Damasio, 1994; Immordino-Yang & Damasio, 2007). For example, when a person is experiencing a heightened emotional state (e.g., fear, excitement, joy), his or her ability to attend to, concentrate on, or perform any behavior that requires attainment of a goal (e.g., finishing homework) may be impacted (Dolcas & McCarthy, 2006). This perspective seems fruitful to consider relative to the rapidity with which changes in both attention and stuttering frequency occur in a typical conversational interaction. That is, a person's attention to a particular task can be very transient, which is also how most parents and people who stutter describe the behavior of stuttering. To provide some conceptual framework for the possible influences of emotional processes on childhood stuttering, we have employed the notion of Cole, Martin, and Dennis (2004, p. 319) that emotion be viewed as a "a process, a constant, vigilant process" that is continuously operating. However, this conceptualization of emotion also allows for emotion to be viewed as "a transitory state change (i.e., moment-to-moment adjustments)" (Cole, Martin, & Dennis, 2004, p. 317). Together, these statements appear contradictory. However, the first statement is asserting that processing emotion is a continuous phenomenon, and the second statement allows for the ever-changing nature and intensity of emotion being experienced. The concept of emotion as ever present but also ever changing in quantity and quality seems to better map changes in emotions onto changes in stuttering than do approaches where "emotion" is considered a relatively "fixed" trait or behavior that is stable over time, such as in the concept of temperament (Anderson et al., 2003; Embrechts et al., 1998; Kagan, 1994; Rothbart & Bates, 1998). We believe it is particularly important to consider variables that change as rapidly as stuttering given the well-known within- and between-situation variability of stuttering (e.g., Johnson, Conture, Karrass, & Walden, 2009; Yaruss, 1997). In essence, we suggest that situational changes in emotional states, particularly those changes that divert attentional as well as cognitive resources, should have the ability, at least for some children, to influence the initiation as well as the maintenance of speech-language planning and production and possibly contribute to disturbances in the fluency of such planning/production.

EVIDENCE FOR METHODS OF MEASURING INSTANCES OF STUTTERING

Defining "instances of stuttering" provides a foundation for how we determine whether the client under examination does or does not stutter and how we document change during treatment. First, we define speech disfluency as any disruption in the forward flow of speech-language production (Conture, 1990; Conture, 2001; Wingate, 1964). Then we dichotomize speech disfluencies into stuttering-like disfluencies and non–stuttering-like or other disfluencies (after Yairi, 1997a). Stuttering-like disfluencies include sound-syllable repetitions (e.g., b-b-b-b-but), single-syllable whole-word repetitions (e.g., and-and-and-and-and), audible sound prolongations (e.g., aaaaaaand), and inaudible sound prolongations (e.g., b———-ut). Other or non–stuttering-like disfluencies—sometimes called normal disfluencies—include phrase repetitions (e.g., I went-I went-I went to the store), interjections (e.g., um, er, uh, well, like), and revisions (e.g., I went, I will go).

The actual visual and auditory appearance of instances of stuttering and disfluency varies, to greater or lesser degrees, across the population of people who stutter. Nevertheless, stuttering and disfluency categories possess enough distinguishing characteristics in terms of appearance that clinicians, with practice and experience, can come to identify instances of each relatively efficiently and reliably. This is not to say that within- and between-clinician errors in, for example, tabulation of frequency of stuttering do not occur (for greater discussion on this topic and meaningful attempts to mitigate such concerns, see Einarsdóttir, 2009; Ingham, Cordes, & Finn, 1993). However, much the same could be said about phonetic transcription, calculation of mean length of utterance (MLU), or administration of standardized tests. The question is not whether errors occur. Rather, the question is whether such errors introduce a difference that is diagnostically and therapeutically significant. Such errors would seem to have their least impact when measuring the stuttering of someone who frequently stutters (i.e., "more room for error") than they would for someone whose stuttering is right on the cusp between stuttering and nonstuttering speech-language production (i.e., "little room for error"). The variability in identifying stuttering for therapeutic and diagnostic purposes is one reason why clinicians should not base diagnosis on just one observation or speech sample (e.g., child talking with the parents; cf. Johnson et al., 2009). The clinician should attempt to assess all parameters of the client's speech-language, especially stuttering, during as many tests, tasks, and situations as possible before determining whether someone does or does not stutter (see Ingham, & Riley, 1998, for further discussion of repetitive and varied sampling of stuttering in children).

PRACTICAL REQUIREMENTS

For some children, the frequency of stuttering can change dramatically because of many different factors. Therefore, the thorough assessment of a child who is known or thought to be stuttering should also include the measurement of varying aspects of stuttering (i.e., frequency, duration, most common type of disfluency, severity, and chronicity) across as many tasks and situations as possible (e.g., telling a narrative, conversation with parents, conversation with clinician, responding to open-ended questions with and without time pressure, etc.). In our clinic, an assessment of stuttering takes between 2.5 and 4 hours. However, we realize that some clinicians and/or clinical settings are less able to devote that amount of time for assessment.

Given that reality, we suggest that clinicians who are unable to use more than 1 to 2 hours per examination period extend the assessment over the first several treatment periods (e.g., use several 1- to 2-hour "diagnostic therapy" sessions over the span of 2 to 4 weeks). Typically, the assessment itself unfolds into four interrelated parts: (1) observation of speech-language behavior in conversation, narrative, etc.; (2)

standardized speech-language assessment of the child; (3) interview of family or caregivers; and (4) sharing of results and recommendations with the child's parents. The following sections will detail the materials, time, and training necessary to achieve a reasonably thorough and accurate assessment of stuttering based on considerations just listed. For the purposes of this chapter, we use the term "parent" to encompass all caregivers or family members who might be in attendance at the evaluation.

OBSERVATION OF SPEECH BEHAVIOR IN CONVERSATION

Ideally, the observation of the parent-child interaction should take place with the clinician out of the room—for example, through audiovisual observation from an adjoining room. Having the clinician out of the room makes it easier for both parent and child to interact without the relatively awkward presence of a stranger busily taking notes, pressing a stopwatch, flipping through the intake folder, etc. Attempting to minimize emotional discomfort of both the child and parent during this interaction is reasonable given findings that children tend to be more reactive to their environment (Karrass et al., 2006; Schwenk, Conture, & Walden, 2007). We feel that having the parent(s) and child involved in the conversation keeps the interaction as natural as possible. Our goal is to avoid artificially inflating the child's stuttering or risking shutting the child down by having a team of strangers in the room. The total time for the conversational sample varies depending on the emotional, communicative, and social dynamics of the parent(s) and the child. However, in general, the conversational

sample will take between 20 and 40 minutes. Details of the measures taken during this time frame will be discussed in the later section titled "Key Components."

As with all children evaluated for speech-language concerns, clinicians will need to be trained to carry out language sampling efficiently while also conducting a disfluency count, timing utterances for speech rate, timing duration of stuttering, and noting any salient nonspeech behaviors and age-(in)appropriate speech sound errors exhibited by the child. Conducting these contemporaneous measures may sound a little overwhelming. However, like many other skills required of the speech-language pathologist, this is basically a matter of practice over time to master each of the various tasks. Each clinician will find his or her own system for doing things, but the following "plan of attack" detailed in Table 3.1 has worked well for the first author. If the clinician can arrange to have more than one clinician involved in the assessment, the next two components can be conducted simultaneously.

STANDARDIZED SPEECH-LANGUAGE TESTING

Unfortunately, too few children who "stutter" receive a comprehensive assessment of speech-language development. This is quite problematic given the frequency with which stuttering is comorbid with other speech-language concerns, particularly articulation/phonologic disorders (e.g., Blood et al., 2003) and the real need, for many of these children, to prioritize the delivery of services when two or more problems coexist within one child (cf., Rousseau et al., 2007).

Table 3.1. *Suggested "Plan of Attack" or Sequence of Events (1 to 6) and Corresponding Rationales for Their Order in a Diagnostic Session Involving a Child Who Stutters and His or Her Family*

Measure	Rationale for Order
(1) Disfluency count	The disfluency count is first in order to avoid the adaptation effect (Wingate, 1988)
(2) Stuttering duration	Duration may also be amenable to adaptation
(3) Speech rate	Done close to the beginning before family can think about and/or concentrate on reducing speaking rate
(4) Language sampling	Language sampling is thought to be more accurate after a period of "warm up" (Miller, 1981)
(5) Observing associated nonspeech behaviors	Observing behaviors throughout the clinician-child conversation is appropriate
(6) Noting speech sound errors	Noting errors throughout the clinician-child conversation is appropriate

If there is only one clinician conducting the evaluation, completing standardized testing is seemingly more efficacious when children's fatigue is minimized by their not having to wait for parents to finish talking with the examiner. In other words, testing the child prior to the parent-clinician interview would be the wisest course of action. And, if time restraints require, the "conversational sample" and "standardized testing" could occur during the first testing session, with the second testing session involving the parent interview and then providing the parents with results and recommendations. While perhaps obvious, the duration of standardized testing is highly variable between children. Many factors, including the child's ability level, attention span, fatigue, and separation anxiety, as well as the examiner's proficiency, can contribute to the time needed to complete standardized testing. In general, however, testing generally takes a minimum of 1 hour and a maximum of 2 hours.

Again, as with all speech-language disorders, speech-language pathologists should be trained in the proper and standard administration of the measures to maximize appropriate scoring and interpretation of results. Clinicians must also be trained to adapt administration without unduly violating the standardization protocol in order to keep the child engaged. For example, the Peabody Picture Vocabulary Test (Dunn & Dunn, 1981; 1997; 2006) can be given on the floor, under a table, with the book on a windowsill, or with pictures being identified via "dinosaur puppet pointing." In short, the clinician must be flexible enough to be able to focus on the needs of the child in front of them instead of wondering which picture, subtest, etc., comes next. One important procedural variable to consider, however, is that the clinician should assiduously avoid praising, rewarding, or reinforcing the child's correct responses to the standardized tests. If such praising or rewarding for correct performance takes place, the child can come to realize, when the clinician's praising stops as the test gets harder and the child begins to fail, that they are not doing as well. This realization, for more than a few children, can reduce motivation, cooperation, and attention to the task at hand. Instead, to help motivate the child and maintain the child's attention, the clinician, can reward or praise the child's test-taking behavior;

for example, "That's real good pointing.... I like the way you try.... You are really listening well."

PARENT INTERVIEW

The parent interview is where the clinician can truly begin to weave together the entire tapestry of variables that may be causally contributing to, as well as manifest in, the child's instances of stuttering. One basic purpose of the parent interview is to ascertain the degree and kind of impact the environment may be having on the child's stuttering. Ideally, the parent interview will take place in a separate room while the child is being administered standardized tests; however, as stated earlier, it may be conducted on a separate day. Parents are much more likely to be forthright about their child's behavior and stuttering when the child is not listening. In some settings, it may not be possible to have the parents present at the evaluation at all. Under those circumstances, parents should be interviewed at the minimum by phone. However, if it is not possible to do the parent interview without the child present, then having the child be as distracted as possible with games and toys is the only other option (see Boey et al., 2007 and Boey, 2008 for similar strategies for testing children and their parents). The total time for the parent interview also varies, depending on how loquacious the parent is, how many questions the parent has, how concerned the parent is that the clinician is going to determine that the parent "caused" the child's stuttering, and how complicated the family situation is (e.g., divorced parents, recent death in the family, economic hardship, abuse situations). However, in general, the parent interview can take a minimum of 30 to 45 minutes to a maximum of 2 hours. Details of the measures taken during this time frame will be discussed in the following section titled "Key Components."

Clinicians will need to be trained to efficiently determine the time since onset of the stuttering, obtain a family history of stuttering and related speech-language behavior, and complete the Temperament Characteristics Scale (Oyler, 1996a) and the "Reactions" section of the Stuttering Prediction Instrument (Riley, 1981). Clinicians should become comfortable with (re)directing parental conversation in order to accomplish these tasks. (For further details on the amount, nature, and sequence of questions used when interviewing parents, please see Conture, 2001, pp. 67-77.) There is a great deal of subtlety and finesse involved in encouraging a reticent parent to talk and, conversely, redirecting an emotionally discomforted parent who cannot stop talking. However, building a good rapport with parents—which such an interview can engender—is crucial to building the trust and respect necessary to carry out successful treatment and to orient the parents to what you think stuttering is about, what may cause it, and your approach to remediating it.

SHARING OF RESULTS AND RECOMMENDATIONS

As mentioned earlier, the relationship established at the time of assessment is vital for setting the stage for a good, long-term therapeutic relationship. Sharing results of testing and the recommendations for further action must be done in a thoughtful, respectful, and empathetic manner. It is quite possible that you, the clinician, are the first person to report to a particular family that there is actually something clinically "wrong" with this child. For some parents, the news that their child truly is or is not stuttering is an affirmation of the beliefs they brought with them to the evaluation. However, for some families (especially those expecting perfection in themselves and their children), the news that their child has a diagnosable disorder can be as seemingly devastating as being informed of a serious or terminal illness. Consequently, the time required to share the results and recommendations can be anywhere from 15 minutes to 1 hour.

For sharing with the parents diagnostic results and recommendations, the materials needed by the clinician include at least a summary of (1) the measures taken during the observation, (2) the standard scores and percentile ranks for the standardized tests completed, and (3) scores for related tests—for example, the Temperament Characteristics Scale and Stuttering Prediction Instrument. In addition, the clinician should have on hand relevant supporting literature that the parent can take home after the evaluation (e.g., see the Stuttering Foundation of America website—http://www.stutteringhelp.org—for a variety of useful literature

and videos for parents). Likewise, the clinician should develop a one-page summary form to hand to the parent at the end of the evaluation as well as place in the child's file prior to the development of a complete diagnostic report (see Fig. 3.3 for an example of a diagnostic summary form). If treatment is recommended, this sharing time with the parents is also an opportunity to clearly and patiently orient the parent to the treatment that will be used, provide the name of the treating clinician if it is different from the diagnostic clinician, and answer any questions the parents might have about the diagnostic and/or prescribed treatment.

KEY COMPONENTS

Having discussed the practical requirements of time, training, and materials, the following discussion will relate the practical to the theoretical. The purpose of this section is to discuss the details of the parts of the diagnostic in terms of (1) where each piece fits in the C-E model, (2) who participates in each part, and (3) the general procedures for administration of each measure. Table 3.2 provides this information in a more concise format.

ASSESSING THE ENVIRONMENT

To achieve a realistic assessment of the communicative, emotional, and social environment in which the child is functioning, we try to assess: (1) selected aspects of the parent interview questionnaire; (2) speaking rate/turn-taking skills (of parents and child); (3) the family history of stuttering and related disorders; and (4) medical and developmental history. Therefore, the primary participants in this part of the assessment are the clinician and parent. The parent interview helps the clinician ascertain, among other things, the nature of the parents' attitudes or beliefs regarding when, how, and why their child's stuttering began.

Parent Interview

The clinician uses the parent interview as an opportunity to better understand parental beliefs about "how" the stuttering has changed or "how" it currently sounds and looks. Parents may report that the child was repeating words and syllables

CLIENT_____Winston Churchill_____ BIRTHDATE____04/25/00____

PARENT/S_____Lori Churchill_____

ADDRESS___15 Jolly Old, Englang, OH_____

PHONE___hm: (615) 555-1212_____FUNDING____VHP_____

DATE OF EVALUATION_____05/12/04_____AGE AT EVALUATION____4;0____

DIAGNOSIS: Winston exhibits a severe stuttering disorder that may be, in part compounded and/or exacerbated by a very rapid rate of speech as well as below normal limits receptive vocabulary and language skills. Additionally, there is a significant gap or disparity between his expressive and receptive vocabulary and language scores. This gap or disparity may suggest different ability levels in Winston's efficient retrieval and use of his language. Such as difference in skill levels may contribute to and/or exacerbate his stuttering.

STANDARD TEST RESULTS:
CWS = Children who stutter

Test/Measure	Standard Score	Score/Percentage/ Percentile Rank	Clinical Significance/Rating
Disfluency Count			
Total Disfluencies/Total words:		20.5	*Typical of CWS*
Total Stutter-like Disfluencies/Total Words		18.8	*Typical of CWS*
Total Stutter-like Disfluencies/Total Disfluencies		91	*Typical of CWS*
Most Common disfluency type		Sound-syllable repetitions	*Typical of CWS*
Stuttering Severity Instrument-3 (SSI-3)		29	*Severe*
Stocker Probe		64%	*Typical of CWS*
Stuttering Prediction Instrument		22	*Moderate risk*
Temperament Characteristics Scale		20	*Typical of CWS*
Kiddy-CAT		8	Not typical of CWS
Goldman Fristoe Test of Articulation	112	79	Within normal limits
Speech rate (child): Typical range (140-160)		535 wpm (range: 345-667)	*Very rapid rate*
Speech rate (mother): Typical range (160-180)		635 wpm (range 484-909)	*Very rapid rate*
Peabody Picture Vocabulary Test (PPVT-IIIB):	78	7	*Below Normal Limits*
Expressive Vocabulary Test (EVT)	97	42	Within normal limits
Mean Length of Utterance (MLU) expected for his age: 4.39 range 3.45-5.33	4.46 z = +0.07	53%	Within normal limits
Test of Early Language Development - 3			
Expressive Language Score	72		*Below normal limits*
Receptive Language Score	86		Marginally within normal limits
Total Language Score	75		*Below normal limits*

Figure 3.3. Example of Vanderbilt University's recommendation and referral form for sharing results following a diagnostic evaluation.

or that the child simply "couldn't get the words out" around the onset of the stuttering. Some parents indicate that the stuttering has changed over time, whereas others indicate that it has been essentially the same since onset. It is particularly instructive for clinicians to probe the parents' beliefs about "why" people start to stutter and

specifically "why" they think their child is stuttering. Frequently, the clinician's dispelling of erroneous parental beliefs constitutes the essence of the initial therapy sessions!

It is also instructive to ask the parent to demonstrate or imitate their child's stuttering. The parent should actually demonstrate, not tell, the

Table 3.2. *A Relatively Concise Overview of the Essential Parts of the Communication-Emotional (C-E) Model*[a,b]

Corresponding Part of the Model	Measure	Participants	Data Obtained
Environment	Parent Interview	Parents and clinician	Parent attitudes about stuttering; child's stuttering frequency across contexts and speaking tasks
Environment	Speech Rate of Parent(s)	Parent and child	The length, complexity, and speed of communication in the child's environment
Environment	Stuttering Prediction Instrument	Parent and clinician	The possible chronicity of the stuttering without intervention
Genetics	Family History	Parent and clinician	Information regarding familial incidence of stuttering and other speech-language disorders and psycho-social adjustment issues in the family
Speech-Language Planning and Production	Speech-Rate of Parents and Child	Parent and child	How fast speech-language planning and processing for the initiation and maintenance of communication typically occur for the child, with or without the parent
Speech-Language Planning and Production	Parent Interview	Parent and clinician	Where in the word, phrase, or utterance the child tends to stutter
Speech-Language Planning and Production	Standardized Testing	Child and clinician	Point-in-time information regarding performance on standardized speech-language tests when compared to same chronologic-age peers
Speech-Language Planning and Production	Stocker Probe Test of Communicative Responsibility	Child and clinician	Whether frequency of stuttering changes with increased linguistic demand
Experience	Parent Interview	Parent and clinician	Whether the child has been teased about his or her speech or other personal attributes; whether the child is aware of his speech difficulties; whether the child avoids speaking; where, when, and with whom the child experiences more or less stuttering
Experience	Time since Onset of Stuttering	Parent and clinician	A bracketing procedure done by the clinician with the parents to approximate how long the stuttering has been present
Experience	Kiddy-CAT	Child and clinician	Estimates of awareness and concern exhibited by the child
Emotional Reactivity and Emotion Regulation	Parent Interview	Parent and clinician	What the child's attitudes about making mistakes are; how the child reacts to discipline, conflict, and siblings; what a typical day is like for the family; how the child handles/reacts to mistakes, criticism, and frustration in the home, at school, and during speech
Emotional Reactivity and Emotion Regulation	Temperament Characteristics Scale (TCS)	Parent and clinician	Seven-question 5-point Likert scale that rates separation skill, fears, reactivity to novelty, etc.
Instances of Stuttering	Stuttering Severity Instrument (SSI)	Clinician	A measure of severity based on frequency, duration, and nonspeech behavior
Instances of Stuttering	Disfluency Count	Clinician	Actual frequency of stuttering and disfluency

[a] Examples are provided of corresponding measures and participants involved with each part/measure and data obtained.

[b] Relative to various diagnostic measures, participants involved and data obtained from measures/participants.

clinician what the child does that the parent is concerned about—that is, what the parent believes to be the child's stuttering. Although some parents quickly seem to understand the request to demonstrate their child's stuttering and readily show the clinician what their child's stuttering sounds or looks like, others are much less inclined to do so. Such parents may quickly and repeatedly tell, but not show, what their child does when he or she is stuttering. It is our clinical experience that the more such parents resist demonstrating their child's stuttering, the greater their concern about or aversion to their child's stuttering and the more challenging therapeutic progress will be until these parents develop a more appropriate degree of acceptance or tolerance of their child's speech disfluencies/stuttering (this informal clinical observation awaits, of course, support or refutation by means of objective empirical study). Indeed, we have had such parents repeatedly insist that their child is still stuttering—"at alarming levels"—after several contiguous treatment sessions where the child produces instances of stuttering well within normal limits (e.g., 0-2 stutterings/100 words). Some of this insistence, of course, relates to the fact that these parents may "see" a different child at home, fluency-wise, than we do in the clinic; however, some of this insistence may be also based on zero tolerance for speech disfluencies of any kind. These parents' strong aversion, dislike, or shame about the presence of even one very brief stutter floating on a deep and wide sea of communicative fluency is something the clinician wants to explore at the time of the diagnostic and address during treatment.

In terms of events related to the onset of stuttering, some parents are able to identify a particular event that "caused" the stuttering. Others report that they think the child was simply having a growth spurt or some other developmental event. The parents' explanation can offer important insight into what levels of guilt parents have regarding their role in the cause of their child's stuttering as well as provide an idea of how (im)mutable the parents believe the problem is to their or the clinician's influence. A parent who believes that he or she contributes to the child's stuttering is more easily empowered to help change the home environment than a parent who believes that the family is the passive victim of the child's problem, that the child's stuttering was "visited on" the family, and that there is little they can do to help.

Speech Rate of Parent(s) and Child

Another means of assessing the linguistic environment that the child is experiencing is by sampling the speech rate of both the parents and the child. Research suggests that the speech rates of mothers and fathers may affect the severity and rate of a child's stuttering (Kelly, 1993; 1994; Kelly & Conture, 1991). Additionally, Yaruss and Conture (1995) found that the greater the *differences* are between the speaking rates of mothers and their children, the greater the child's stuttering severity. Clinical manipulation of speech rate has also suggested that decreasing speech rate results in a reduction of stuttering frequency in preschool and young children who stutter (Guitar et al., 1992; Ryan, 2000; Stephenson-Opsal & Bernstein Ratner, 1988; Wood & Ryan, 2000). To be able to change parental speaking rate—either directly or indirectly—the clinician should obtain a baseline rate for each interactional partner during conversational speech. By obtaining these baseline rates, the clinician is better able to determine whether large discrepancies between the parents' and child's speaking rates exist and whether such discrepancies should be tracked over the course of treatment.

Family History

Using the form in Figure 3.4, the clinician asks the parent(s) to identify all members of the family with any (1) communication disorders, (2) attention deficit hyperactivity disorder, and (3) psychosocial adjustment disorders. When asking families to identify communication and related disorders, we describe them as (1) speech disorders (e.g., stuttering, pronunciation), (2) language deficits (e.g., late to talk, immature grammar), (3) voice disorders (e.g., polyps, nodules, oral and laryngeal cancer), and (4) learning disabilities (e.g., dyslexia, dysgraphia). In the case of attention deficit or attention deficit hyperactivity disorder, we ask the parents whether they believe or have been told by a healthcare provider that it is primarily hyperactivity, impulsivity, or inattention, or some

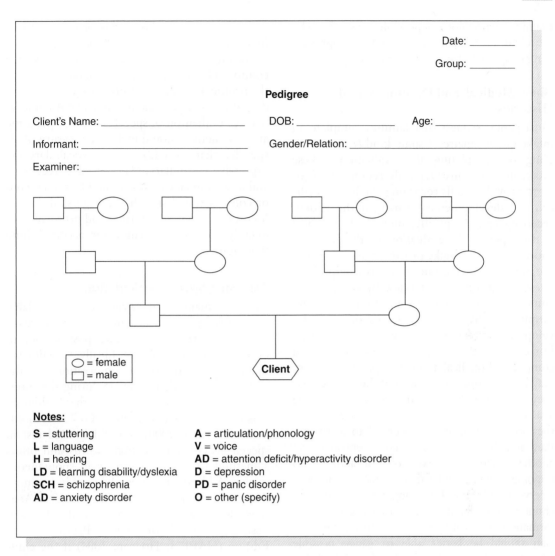

Figure 3.4. Example of a form used to record family history of speech-language, voice, hearing, attention deficit hyperactivity disorder, psychosocial, and learning disabilities.

combination of the three. To help the parents determine the presence of psychosocial adjustment issues in their family, the clinician can describe psychosocial adjustment problems as involving such concerns as depression, panic disorders, and the like. For a relative to be positively identified with a history of one of these issues, the parent needs to indicate that the relative (1) has been involved with or received therapy, (2) has received a professional diagnosis, or (3) was prescribed medication for treatment. It is not sufficient for the family member to simply describe Aunt Lucy as the "strange woman who doesn't talk right" or as "someone who *should*

have been diagnosed as depressed." Information obtained during the family history interview is relevant not only in tracking the possible familial course of stuttering, but also in providing the clinician with additional information regarding family dynamics. For instance, a family with a long history of concomitant speech-language problems may be more familiar with the therapy process than a family without such a history. Likewise, if the child seems to receive less than adequate benefit from treatment, besides adjusting treatment, the clinician can consider the child's possible inattentiveness to therapy or parental psychosocial issues (for example, depression) as possible causes for why the child and/or parents are not appropriately "engaging" with the therapeutic process.

Birth, Medical, and Developmental Histories

Most clinics request that families complete an intake questionnaire of some kind *before* scheduling or completing the evaluation. These intake questionnaires typically require the family to provide details regarding the birth, medical, and developmental history of the patient receiving care. Typically, individuals involved in this aspect of the evaluation are the person(s) coordinating the intake process, the parent, and the clinician. Intake questionnaires help direct questions during the interview by allowing the clinician to ask follow-up questions regarding hospitalizations, medications, and or other developmental treatments the child has received. For example, the parents of a child who has a complicated medical and developmental history may be more open to the idea of therapy because they may have already had experience with the assessment/treatment process. On the other hand, they may become very concerned to learn that they and their child may need to enroll in yet another form of intervention, in addition to ongoing medical, educational, or psychosocial interventions of the child being evaluated or other children in the family. In either case, with the information provided by the intake form, the clinician should be better able to gauge possible advantages or obstacles the family might bring with them to the therapy process.

ASSESSING SPEECH-LANGUAGE PLANNING AND PRODUCTION

To obtain sufficient information about the child's speech-language planning and production, a combination of norm-referenced, criterion-referenced, and clinician-generated observations are necessary. For this portion of the evaluation, the child and the clinician are the principal participants. Depending on the child's chronologic age and developmental age (not to mention adaptability to novelty and change, such as separation from parents), the child's parents may need to be in the room. Needless to say, this is the less than optimum option but, as mentioned

earlier, some have shown this procedure to be functional (e.g., Boey et al., 2007).

Ideally, the clinician and child are seated comfortably at a child-friendly table with all of the protocols and test materials required to conduct the evaluation readily available. A comprehensive evaluation of speech-language planning and production should include a measure of (1) speech articulation; (2) receptive vocabulary and expressive vocabulary; (3) expressive, receptive, and total language abilities; and (4) spontaneous or conversational speech-language skills. What follows is a suggested format and protocols frequently used in our clinic for accomplishing these four tasks.

Assessing Speech Articulation

There are many standardized measures available for assessing speech articulation and language skills, so here we offer one possible set of options, not a prescription. Ideally, the clinician fits the protocol to the observations of the child's speech-language made during the spontaneous sample. For example, the Goldman-Fristoe Test of Articulation–2 (GFTA-2; Goldman & Fristoe, 2000) is a widely used test of speech articulation in single words and offers a method for eliciting targets in spontaneous speech. Additionally, it can be used in conjunction with the Khan-Lewis Phonological Analysis (Khan & Lewis, 2002) or the Hodson Assessment of Phonological Patterns–Third Edition (HAPP-3; Hodson, 2004) if the clinician suspects that many process errors are present in the child's speech.

The importance of considering articulation/phonology when assessing and/or treating children who stutter can be supported on several grounds:

1. Children who stutter appear to be at somewhat greater risk than normally fluent children of exhibiting articulation/phonologic difficulties (e.g., Arndt & Healey, 2001; Blood et al., 2003; Cantwell & Baker, 1985; for reviews, see Bloodstein, 1995, Table 18; Byrd, Wolk, & Davis, 2007; Louko, Edwards, & Conture, 1999; cf. Nippold, 1990; 2002).

2. Children who stutter appear to differ from children who do not stutter in terms articulation/phonology abilities, even when both talker

groups exhibit articulation and phonology within normal limits (Pellowski et al., 2001).

3. Children who stutter, when compared to children who do not stutter, appear delayed in making the developmental shift from holistic (i.e., word-level) to incremental (i.e., sound-level) processing of phonologic representations, a phonologic skill that may affect reading skills (Byrd, Conture, & Ohde, 2007).

4. Children whose stuttering persists exhibit slower phonologic development than children who eventually recover (although this finding should not be taken to mean that phonologic delays predict persistence/recovery of stuttering; Yairi & Ambrose, 2005).

Thus, the presence or absence of a concomitant articulation/phonologic problem may influence the nature and length of treatment, but at the very least, it will influence recommendations made for additional or concomitant services (for one data-based, experimental approach to simultaneous treatment of stuttering and phonologic concerns, see Conture, Louko, & Edwards, 1993).

Expressive and Receptive Vocabulary Skills

Vocabulary skills are related to the storage and retrieval of individual words from a language. Therefore, assessing vocabulary provides necessary information on how well the child is learning the words used in his or her environment. Additionally, results from Anderson, Pellowski, and Conture (2005) suggest that children who stutter may have disassociations in their abilities to learn and access single words efficiently, relative to their articulatory and/or syntactic abilities.

To be precise, an experimental dissociation "...refers to the absence of a positive association between dependent variables on two different tasks" (Tulving, 1983, p. 73). For example, in the field of stuttering, during an experimental therapy session, a person who stutters might decrease stuttering when reading in relation to a pretreatment baseline but, in conversation, might show little change or even increases in stuttering in relation to a pretreatment baseline. The one dependent measure—stuttering—would perform differently or be dissociated on two different tasks—that is, reading versus speaking.

Our study of dissociations in young children's performances on several standardized tests of speech-language performance, which should be roughly similarly developed across tests (as it is for most children we tested), did not involve experimental manipulations. Instead, we described children's performances on several different tests but were not interested in children who performed relatively low or relatively high across all such tests. Rather, we were interested in those children whose scores were "dissociated"— statistically determined—from one another between two or more tests—for example, when a child would perform high on expressive vocabulary but low on receptive vocabulary (for similar considerations regarding fluency and language, see Hall, 1996; Hall, Yamashita, & Aram, 1993; for similar considerations relative to childhood stuttering, see Hall, 2004; Hall & Burgess, 2000).

To measure vocabulary skills, the Peabody Picture Vocabulary Test (PPVT) (Dunn & Dunn, 1981; 1997; 2006) and the co-normed Expressive Vocabulary Test (EVT) (William, 1997; 2006) are routinely administered (the EVT provides norms for determining whether differences between the EVT and PPVT are significant). As mentioned previously, disassociations in skills may reflect inefficient or discordant speech-language processing. Although we are still in an incipient stage of understanding how such disassociations impact stuttering, (Coulter, Anderson, & Conture, 2009)—in a follow-up study to Anderson, Pellowski, and Conture (2005)—found that within 85 preschool-age children who stutter, 24 of them exhibited one or more statistically significant disassociation between standardized tests of speech-language. Preschool-age children who stutter and exhibited dissociations were significantly more likely to exhibit interjections or revisions as their most common disfluency type. Thus, a larger difference between dissociated scores tends to be associated with a greater frequency of total disfluencies and stuttering-like disfluencies. Thus, at least for children with apparent speech-language dissociations, speech disfluencies seem to be impacted, a finding that suggests that, for these children, such disassociations may need to be considered or targeted indirectly during the course of therapy.

Expressive, Receptive, and Total Language Abilities

Unlike a test of vocabulary, a comprehensive measure of expressive and receptive language abilities provides a clinician with information on a child's ability to apply the rules of language. Many measures are available to accomplish this. However, the Clinical Evaluation of Language Fundamentals–Preschool 2 (Hresko, Reid, & Hamill, 1991; 1999) and the Clinical Evaluation of Language Fundamentals–4 (Semel, Wiig, & Secord, 2003; 2004) provide several subtests and many opportunities for a child to demonstrate areas of strength or weakness. However, if the clinician is evaluating a very young or immature client, the Preschool Language Scale–3 (Zimmerman, Steiner, & Pond, 1997) is normed on children from birth through 6 years 11 months old and offers a variety of manipulative objects that can be engaging to young children. Identifying a child's strengths, weaknesses, or areas of deficit in expressive, receptive, and total language skills is an important component in establishing goals for treatment and informing parents of possible obstacles to a speedy therapy process.

Spontaneous Language

Standardized, norm-referenced tests are necessary to identify specific areas of strength and weakness in speech, vocabulary, and language skills. However, equally necessary is a qualitative measure of what the child actually uses, in terms of speech and language, while trying to communicate. Therefore, during the spontaneous speech portion of the evaluation, the clinician will want to complete an intelligibility count and obtain a conversational sample of at least 50 utterances to estimate the child's mean length of utterance (MLU).

An intelligibility count can be done using a form similar to a disfluency count that has a grid divided into 100 word blocks. Clinicians can use plus and minus signs to differentiate intelligible words from unintelligible words. This is a simple quantitative way to measure the qualitative phenomena of speech intelligibility in a known context with an unfamiliar listener.

MLU can also be done on a form that provides 50 numbered lines and an area to put identifying information and calculations (Figure 3.5). A spontaneous language sample is an important indicator of grammatical and syntactical complexity. Several studies have shown that increases in length and complexity of a child's utterances lead to increases in disfluency (e.g., Bernstein Ratner & Sih, 1987; Gaines, Runyan, & Myers, 1991; Logan & Conture, 1995; 1997; Logan & LaSalle, 1999; Richels et al., 2009; Zackheim & Conture, 2003). Therefore, information regarding the child's MLU at the time of evaluation is critical in determining what targets or goals there should be for treatment. An average length of a child's utterance may also provide insight into how hard the child is pushing his or her linguistic system. That is, a child whose standard scores on all other measures of speech, vocabulary, and language are in the low average to average range but whose MLU is twice what would be expected for his or her chronologic age is likely trying to put together more words than his or her speech-language production processes can efficiently handle (see Yairi & Ambrose, 2005, Chapter 7, for related discussion). On the other hand, a child whose standard scores on the other measures are average to above average and whose MLU is half of what would be expected for his or her chronologic age may be minimizing talking to avoid stuttering (for discussion of MLU and age, see Klee et al., 1989). Either scenario provides the clinician with insight into what linguistic factors the child will bring into the therapy session.

Besides using the traditional conversational sample to assess spontaneous language in children, the clinician may want to consider using a narrative, for example, having the child tell a story based on a wordless picture book like Mercer Mayer's *Frog Where Are You?* (see Berman & Slobin, 1994, for overview of research pertaining to this story and resulting empirical findings). Use of such narratives during speech-language sampling for children who stutter provides a degree of standardization within and between children. It is strongly recommended as a relatively easy to obtain but important addition to clinical data collection.

Another method for determining the relative effect of increases in utterance length and complexity is the Stocker Probe Technique (Stocker, 1977). The Stocker Probe Technique is a systematic way to move a speaker from the

Child's Name: _____

Child's Age: _____

DOB: _____

Date: _____

SPONTANEOUS LANGUAGE SAMPLE (MLU)
The spontaneous language sample can be obtained by writing down anything said by the child freely or in conversation/play with the clinician but not in response to closed questions. Obtain at least 50 utterances. Record the length of the utterance in terms of morphemes in the right hand column.

Total Number of Morphemes: _____ Computation of MLU (MLU = number of morphemes / number of utterances, e.g., 100 / 25 = 4

Length of   Utterance

1._____   _____
2._____   _____
3._____   _____
4._____   _____
5._____   _____
6._____   _____
7._____   _____
8._____   _____
9._____   _____
10._____   _____
11._____   _____
12._____   _____
13._____   _____
14._____   _____
15._____   _____
16._____   _____
17._____   _____
18._____   _____
19._____   _____
20._____   _____
21._____   _____
22._____   _____
23._____   _____
24._____   _____
25._____   _____
26._____   _____
27._____   _____
28._____   _____
29._____   _____
30._____   _____
31._____   _____
32._____   _____

Figure 3.5. Example of a form used to collect a 50-utterance mean length of utterance (MLU) value.

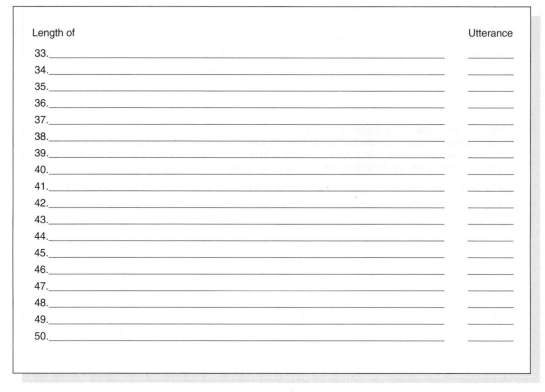

Figure 3.5. (Continued).

linguistically simple task of one-word answers to the linguistically complex task of organizing and telling a story. The child is presented with an object and then asked a series of five questions that move from the least complex at level I (e.g., "Is this real or a toy?") to the most complex at level V (e.g., "Tell me your own story about it."). Because there are five questions per object, the clinician can elicit a large amount of speech in a short amount of time. The Stocker Probe Technique is fairly easy to administer and score. Because it systematically moves the client through varying levels of linguistic demand, the clinician has an opportunity to observe at what level of complexity the child may or may not be fluent. Knowing what level of linguistic complexity the child can tolerate provides the clinician with helpful insights regarding what level questions to ask the child during therapy to enhance fluency.

ASSESSING EXPERIENCE

Information regarding the child and families' experiences with the problem of stuttering and related matters (e.g., possible impact on social interactions) should be ascertained during the parent interview. Therefore, the parent and clinician are the principal participants in this portion of an evaluation. The clinician should ask questions that are geared to finding out what the child's and parents' experiences have been. As much as possible, the clinician should remain open to the individual client's issues rather than assuming "group tendencies." As mentioned earlier, pivotal questions include those addressing when, where, with whom, and for how long the stuttering has taken place.

Parent Interview

Several "themes" should be addressed during the parent interview, including the following: (1) *awareness*—for example, is the child aware that he or she stutters or "can't get words out"? If so, what is the basis for the parents' assessment of "awareness"?; (2) *reactions*—for example, does the child avoid speaking? Does the child let or encourage others to talk for him?; (3) *teasing*—for example, has the child been teased? If so, by whom and how often? What was the child's and the parents' reaction to the teasing?; and (4) *situational variations in stuttering*—for example, where, when, and with whom does the child experience more or less stuttering? We submit that little is known about the role that implicit (procedural, relatively unconscious) and explicit (declarative/episodic, relatively conscious) memory plays in these "themes," particularly the first (awareness) and second (reactions). For instance, we do not know whether the onset of "concern" on the part of the child about his or her stuttering reflects or rests on the emergence of his or her explicit or declarative/episodic memory—a conscious, autobiographical memory comparing past to present personal experiences (for further discussion of the development of implicit and explicit memory, see Rovee-Collier, Hayne, & Colombo, 2001). Until we better understand such cognitive-emotional processes and their relation to the onset and development of stuttering, our understanding of why some children recover and some persist with their stuttering will remain incomplete.

Each of these themes provides different perspectives on the child's stuttering as well as child/parent reactions. One of these themes, situational variability, offers important insight into changes, or the lack thereof, that the child experiences with his or her stuttering throughout a day or week. It is fair to say that one of the more frustrating aspects of stuttering for parents is the variability with which it occurs. Parents often report that they do not understand why the stuttering seems to come and go (for example, stuttering being better in the clinic than at home). To the parent, these comings and goings of stuttering seem random and mysterious—or even willful. These seemingly unpredictable occurrences of stuttering can be frustrating for both the parents and the child who stutters. Thus, it is the clinician's job to find the regularity among the variation to help the parents better understand stuttering and its vagaries. For example, some parents may report that their child is typically more disfluent at home in the evenings, especially during dinner time. This information suggests to the clinician that the child may have more difficulty remaining fluent when he or she is tired at the end of the day or during family mealtime conversations in which "anything goes" communicatively speaking. Information about who, where, and when the stuttering occurs also provides the clinician with examples of situations to probe for fluency as

the course of treatment unfolds. However, recent findings (Johnson et al. 2009) suggest that although stuttering frequency does vary among preschoolers who stutter with changes in conversational partner (parent versus clinician), situation (home versus clinic), and task (conversation versus narrative), these differences do not necessarily make a difference diagnostically. That is, a clinician is just as apt to diagnose that a child stutters based on observing the child in the home talking to his or her mother as in the clinic talking to a clinician, even though stuttering frequency may change somewhat between these situations.

Time Since Onset of Stuttering

One critical component of experience is how long and how often the stuttering occurs. To date, some of the best information regarding this has been provided by Yairi and Ambrose (2005). Furthermore, recent findings by Maansson (2007) add to our factual understanding of this puzzling but important problem: What does the duration since onset of stuttering tell us about how likely a child will recover without treatment?

Although children who stutter can recover without treatment for several years after onset (Yairi & Ambrose, 2005), it seems that by 4 years after onset, 74% of children who will recover have recovered; thus, a child who has been stuttering for 4 or more years is unlikely to recover naturally (note that this is a statement of probability rather than certainty). Clinicians, however, cannot typically wait 4 years to determine whether a child will recover before beginning treatment. Although the Yairi and Ambrose (2005) data are a treasure for clinician and researchers alike, what appears most helpful from their findings, relative to the present discussion, is the fact that beginning in the latter part of the first 12 months after onset, the rate of stuttering and/or stuttering severity of those children who will recover begins to decrease, whereas it remains stable or increases in children whose stuttering will persist. Thus, waiting for 6 to 12 months after onset, perhaps monitoring the child every 3 to 6 months, and observing the "developmental trajectory" of the child's stuttering frequency can provide the clinician with support for initiating or further delaying treatment.

Unfortunately, by the time most children come to clinicians, they have been stuttering for many months. Thus, the clinician should begin by trying to assess how long the parents have noticed the problem. To determine when the approximate onset of the child's stuttering occurred, the clinician may use a bracketing technique (Anderson et al., 2003; Yairi & Ambrose, 1992) to determine when the approximate onset of the stuttering occurred. The bracketing technique involves asking the parent how old the child was when they first noticed the stuttering and then using that number to work toward an exact month in a specific year. Essentially, the clinician will ask the parents to remember if the child was stuttering at various points in time using relatively well-remembered events, for example, birthdays, major holidays, and vacations, as mnemonic "hooks" or benchmarks to aid in recollection (Ambrose & Yairi, 1999; Anderson & Conture 2004; Richels & Conture, 2007).

Kiddy-CAT

A measure to determine the child's level of awareness and concern should be included in assessment. Recently, a measure to ascertain the awareness and concern about stuttering for young children has been developed by Vanryckeghem and Brutten (2006) and is called the Kiddy-CAT. (This test is a preschool/early elementary school version of the "older" children's Communication Attitude Test [CAT] instrument developed by DeNil & Brutten [1991].) The authors have experience using prototypes of this test. To administer it, the clinician asks the child 12 yes-or-no questions designed to allow the child the opportunity to express any concerns about his or her speaking. The clinician uses the carrier phrase, "Do you think that…" prior to each question, and the child responds either yes or no. Any response that is indicative of concern or awareness of stuttering is given 1 point. Higher scores suggest greater awareness and or concern, whereas lower scores indicate lesser awareness or concern.

One challenge to this test, or any other such test, is the fact that children under 4 years of age can get into a "response set" whereby they answer yes or no for *all* questions. If this happens, the experienced clinician should be able to readily detect this "tendency" and either redirect the child or determine that this test is not appropriate for the child. Another challenge to the test, particularly for children 4 years and younger, is the

rate and level of development of the child's declarative/episodic memory, a form of memory that this test would appear to be tapping when asking the child to respond to what are, in essence, autobiographical questions involving, at least in part, comparisons of past to present experience. These issues aside, this is one of the best norm-based tests regarding awareness in preschool-age children available at present. It deserves serious consideration by clinicians desiring the development of a comprehensive assessment/intervention approach. The state or situational aspects of emotions—emotional reactivity and emotion regulation—that each member of the family brings to the experience of stuttering is the next area to evaluate.

EMOTIONAL REACTIVITY AND EMOTION REGULATION

The parent interview and clinician observation again represent the best means of obtaining information regarding the situational aspects of emotions, emotional reactivity, and emotion regulation. There are also several quantitative measures that provide excellent information on these temperamentally related variables. In our clinic, we most frequently use two parent questionnaires: the Temperament Characteristics Scale (Oyler, 1996a; 1996b) and the Behavioral Styles Questionnaire (BSQ) (Carey, McDevitt, & Associates, 1995). Our mention of these tests is meant to be suggestive, not prescriptive, given that other tests are also available, for example, the Children's Behavior Questionnaire (CBQ) (Rothbart et al., 2001). Details regarding information obtained during the parent interview and from the Temperament Characteristics Scale and BSQ follow.

Parent Interview

During the parent interview, the clinician will want to ask questions that resemble the following: (1) What are the child's apparent or expressed attitudes about making mistakes, not just when speaking but during all activities—for example, coloring pictures, cutting out shapes/pictures from paper, drawing, learning a new skill, etc.? (2) How does the child (non)verbally react to discipline, conflict, and siblings? (3) What is a typical day like for the family? In other words, are the child's daily life activities consistently structured by the parents, or is it more "go with the flow" with little structure (e.g., sleep/wake times that are inconsistent from day to day, breakfast/lunch/dinner served at variable hours)? All of these questions help the clinician determine the child's dispositional/situational reaction and adaptation to his or her environment (especially environmental changes). In addition, they provide information about how the environment is structured and shaped by the parents to guide the child through daily life activities and events.

A parent might respond to Question 1 by indicating that the child consistently reacts strongly and negatively to making mistakes of any kind and will tantrum or abandon a task when it may seem "too hard" or is not going perfectly. We can speculate that this "perfectly-perfect-or-bust" child may have similar reactions to routine disruptions in his or her speech-language planning and production (more than a few times, we have found that this "all right or all wrong" perfectionistic approach on the part of the child is associated with parents, as we discussed earlier, who are reluctant or unable to actually demonstrate to us or show us what their child does when he or she stutters). Likewise, in response to Question 2, the clinician may learn that the child consistently reacts to discipline with similar behaviors—for example, screaming, biting, or flopping on the ground. Or in answer to Question 2, the parents might say that the child simply shuts down and stops talking or interacting with the family at the slightest hint of parental criticism. Such information, we believe, has important ramifications for the course of treatment. A child who consistently exhibits strong, relatively volatile responses to his or her daily environment—particularly changes, differences, or novel occurrences in that environment—may also exhibit similarly strong, volatile responses to the changing demands of treatment, no matter how appropriate and benign such changes may be. Such volatility, we suspect, can even be reflected in up-and-down patterns in his or her stuttering frequency. Put differently, during the course of therapy, such children may not exhibit a relatively smooth, downward trend in stuttering but a pattern of stuttering seemingly little influenced by treatment as the child's stuttering increases, decreases, increases, etc., from one

week to the next. Conversely, a child who tends to shut down at the slightest sense of emotional upheaval or uncertainty may (1) take weeks or even months to begin talking sufficiently in treatment to allow us to measure and note real change or (2) take a similarly long time to engage enough in the treatment session to gain benefit. Suffice it to say, that at the time of the diagnostic evaluation, parental observations and reports regarding these types of behavior are invaluable in tailoring treatment to the individual needs of the child.

Parent Report Questionnaires

As mentioned earlier, some quantitative ways to capture emotional reactivity and emotion regulation involve the administration of the Temperament Characteristics Scale (Oyler, 1996a; 1996b) and BSQ (Carey, McDevitt, & Associates, 1995). The Temperament Characteristics Scale entails the clinician asking seven questions that have parents rate their child's separation skill, fears, and reactivity to new environments and people. Each question has a 5-point scale that attempts to encompass the extremes of certain aspects of young children's behavior. On this scale, low scores on an item (i.e., 1 to 2) indicate more reactivity/more inhibited tendencies, and high scores (i.e., 4 to 5) indicate less reactivity/greater expressive tendencies. Temperament Characteristics Scale scores are on a continuum from 7 (very behaviorally inhibited) to 35 (very behaviorally expressive). For example, the first question asks the parent to rate how the child approaches people and objects, with a rating of 1 being "usually retreats" and a rating of 5 being "approaches easily." Ratings of 3 are considered average or typical for most children. The Temperament Characteristics Scale is very easy to administer and score. Oyler's data (1996a; 1996b) indicate that children who do not stutter score an average of 24.60 (standard deviation = 3.75), whereas children who stutter score an average of 19.72 (standard deviation = 3.46).

Our considerable experience with the Temperament Characteristics Scale to date suggests that scores of 18 or less are indicative of a more inhibited/higher reactivity child, whereas scores of 23 or greater suggest a less reactive/more expressive child. In our experience, behaviorally inhibited children (i.e., lower Temperament Characteristics Scale scores) tend to exhibit and/or experience more difficulty separating from parents and dealing with change, novelty, and differences; have strong fears; are more reactive; and may be more poorly regulated than children who are behaviorally expressive. Again, the Temperament Characteristics Scale is a simple, short test to complete and represents just one data point or observation relative to children's emotional, social, and behavioral characteristics. Nonetheless, it provides a nice overview of the child's dispositional/situational reactivity and the parents' perception of it. If the clinician desires a more thorough overview of the child's behavior, the BSQ (Carey, McDevitt, & Associates, 1997) is one of the measures available for assessing temperament in young children.

The BSQ has 110 questions that take, on average, 20 minutes for the parent(s) to answer. As noted in the Anderson et al. (2005, p. 1225) article, "the BSQ assesses the parent reported temperamental characteristics of children from 3 to 7 years of age along nine dimensions: activity level, adaptability, approach-withdrawal, mood, intensity, distractibility, attention span/persistence, sensory threshold, and Rhythmicity." The BSQ can be scored either by hand or by using software purchased from the publisher (Behavioral-Developmental Initiatives; http://www.b-di.com). Although, similar to the Temperament Characteristics Scale, the BSQ provides the clinician with more detailed information regarding the child's temperament that may assist in decision making during treatment. Correlating results from the three BSQ subtests developed by Karrass et al. (2006)—emotional reactivity, emotion regulation, and attention regulation—we have found that the Temperament Characteristics Scale significantly correlates with emotional reactivity ($r = -.39, p < .01$), emotion regulation ($r = .46, p < .01$), and attention regulation ($r = .20, p < .05$). For example, if the data obtained from the Temperament Characteristics Scale and/or BSQ indicate that the child is slow to warm-up to new people, does not handle environmental change easily, or has difficulty separating from his or her parent, then the clinician can be relatively confident that the first few (and as many as the first eight) sessions of treatment are going to involve helping the child adjust to the people, activities, and setting involved with treatment (some of these children, we have experienced, take 2 or more months to warm-up to treatment, essentially being off-task, e.g., crying, refusing to enter the treatment room, or throwing tantrums, for several minutes during the beginning of each treatment session).

INSTANCES OF STUTTERING

One of the most traditional ways of obtaining information about instances of stuttering, which still possesses a great deal of face validity, is through direct observation by the clinician. Therefore, the primary participants of this aspect of the diagnostic session are the clinician observing the parents and the child who stutters during spontaneous speech. The observational measures will provide quantitative and qualitative information regarding the actual stuttering in terms of severity and frequency. Details regarding the Stuttering Severity Instrument–3 (SSI-3) (Riley, 1994) and the disfluency count follow.

Stuttering Severity

Perhaps one of the most widely used measures to assess stuttering severity is the SSI-3 (Riley, 1994). The SSI-3 is comprised of three weighted sections: (1) frequency, (2) duration, and (3) physical concomitants. The frequency section is divided into a readers and a nonreaders section. The clinician is instructed to use either of the sections but not both. The frequency term relates to the actual frequency of stuttering, not to overall disfluency. The duration section of the SSI-3 is obtained by timing the duration of at least 10 instances using a stopwatch to the nearest tenth of a second. From the 10 durations obtained, an average of the longest three is used to obtain the scale score for this section. The last section of the SSI-3 is the physical concomitants section. This section requires the clinician to rate the person who stutters on the nonspeech behaviors of (1) distracting sounds, (2) facial grimaces, (3) head movements, and (4) movements of the extremities (for a further, detailed description of nonspeech behaviors associated with childhood stuttering, see Conture & Kelly, 1991). Examples of specific behaviors are described on the form. The clinician rates each observed behavior on a 5-point scale ranging from 0, or none observed, to 5, which indicates that observed behaviors are "painful looking." The scores from the three subsections are totaled to create an overall score. On the back of the form are three tables that provide severity equivalents and severity ratings for the total overall scores. The clinician uses this information to provide the family with an index of the child's stuttering severity at the time of the evaluation. The clinician's ability to quickly and correctly tabulate stuttering frequency and severity at the time of the evaluation can be influenced by many factors discussed previously (e.g., the child's dispositional/situational reactivity, the conversational length, complexity and style of the person[s] conversing with the child, etc.).

Disfluency Count

The purpose of the disfluency count is to obtain an estimate of the number of disfluencies and stutters produced during conversational speech. Figure 3.6 is an example of a disfluency count performed during a diagnostic with a child who was a severe stutterer. As Figure 3.6 shows, there are three sections, with each section consisting of 100 word units. Each disfluency or stutter is noted with an accompanying abbreviation indicating type of stutter, and each fluent word is noted with a dash (e.g., SSR, sound/syllable repetitions; ASP, audible sound prolongation; for further definition of such acronyms, see Figure 3.6 caption). At the end of the disfluency count, the clinician is able to calculate percentages of total disfluency for the total number of words, total stuttering for the total number of words, and the ratio of stutters to the total number of disfluencies. The percentage of stutters per total words is the number used to find the stuttering frequency on both the Stuttering Prediction Instrument and the SSI-3. Additionally, empirical evidence suggests that the ratio of stutters to the total number of disfluencies discriminates not only between children who do versus do not stutter (Pellowski & Conture, 2002), but also between persistent stuttering and transient stuttering (Yairi et al., 1996). Our clinical experience to date suggests that children whose stuttering-like disfluency/total disfluency ratio is 70% or greater are at risk for persistent stuttering, whereas children whose stuttering-like disfluency/total disfluency ratio is 40% or less are at far less risk for stuttering. In the following section, how the disfluency count is used to track progress in therapy will be discussed.

ASSESSMENT METHODS TO SUPPORT ONGOING DECISION MAKING

One of the primary purposes of a thorough assessment is to ensure that clinicians are identifying children who stutter as well as discriminating between those children who truly need treatment and those who do not. Once that determination has been made and a child is scheduled for treatment, at least some of the diagnostic information should help provide insight into the length, nature, and relative success of any prescribed therapy. Therefore, it important to consider both (1) the components of the diagnostic evaluation most predictive of treatment outcome and (2) the frequency and means by which stuttering and related behaviors are measured on an ongoing basis during treatment to determine outcome. To provide such prediction, we have examined the various components of the diagnostic evaluation as well as clinician-friendly measures of changes in stuttering (i.e., "change scores," to be described later).

PREDICTIVE MEASURES

What follows is a discussion of an empirical study demonstrating how well diagnostic data predict both short-term outcomes (data taken from the first 12 sessions of treatment) and long-term outcomes (data taken from a minimum of 12 sessions through the end of treatment). The indirect, family-centered treatment sessions (e.g., Richels & Conture, 2007) each child participated in consisted of 50 minutes of treatment, conducted once per week.

Short-Term Predictors

To begin our examination of the relationship between diagnostic measures and treatment outcome, we identified theoretically relevant diagnostic variables seemingly useful for predicting short-term improvement in stuttering—that is, improvement in stuttering near the *beginning* of speech therapy. Participants for this study of short-term predictors were 3 to 7 years old (n = 42; mean age = 52.7 months; SD = 11.3 months; 83.3% male). These children were just beginning speech therapy, and all had participated from their first through their 12th weekly therapy session. Using the diagnostic measures

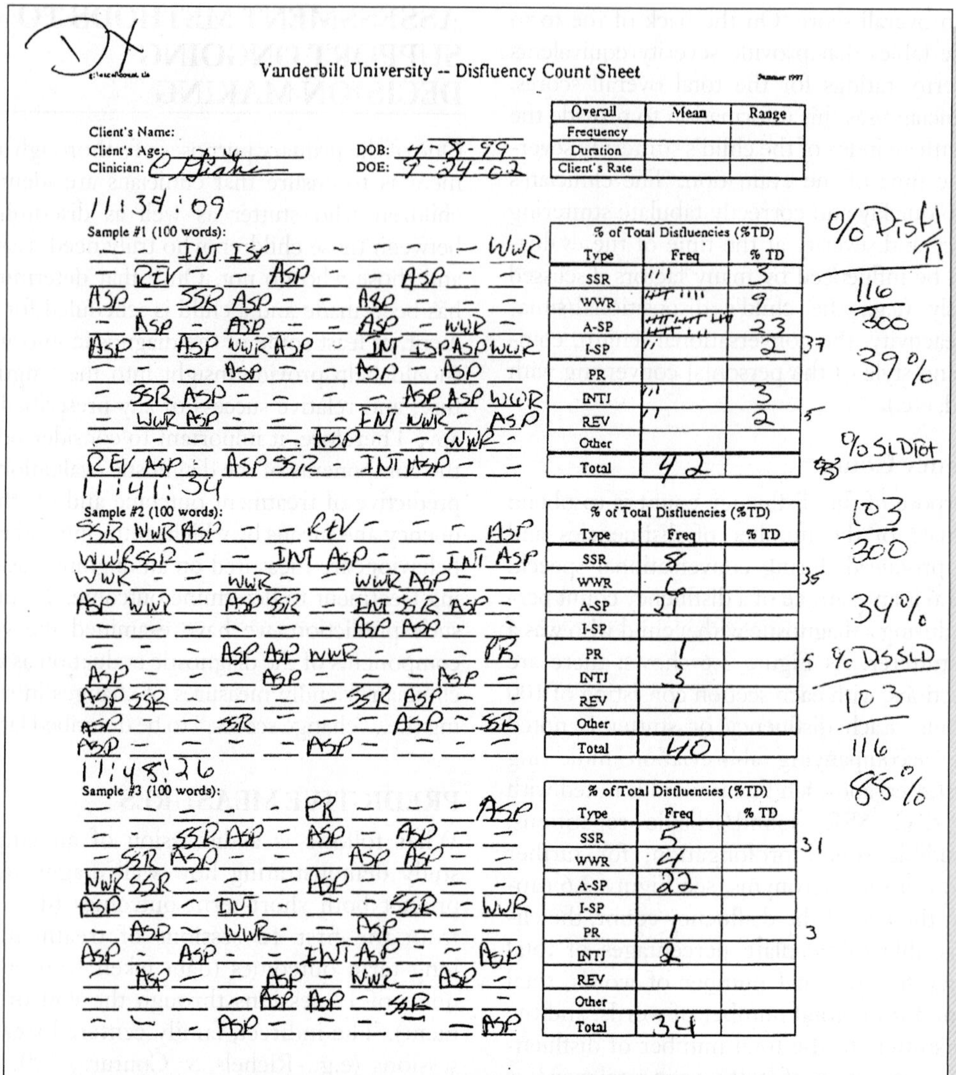

Vanderbilt University -- Disfluency Count Sheet

Client's Name:
Client's Age:
Clinician:
DOB: 4-8-99
DOE: 9-24-02

Overall	Mean	Range
Frequency		
Duration		
Client's Rate		

11:34:09

Sample #1 (100 words):

% of Total Disfluencies (%TD)		
Type	Freq	% TD
SSR		3
WWR		9
A-SP		23
I-SP		2
PR		
INTJ		3
REV		2
Other		
Total	42	

11:41:34

Sample #2 (100 words):

% of Total Disfluencies (%TD)		
Type	Freq	% TD
SSR	8	
WWR	6	
A-SP	21	
I-SP		
PR	1	
INTJ	3	
REV	1	
Other		
Total	40	

11:48:26

Sample #3 (100 words):

% of Total Disfluencies (%TD)		
Type	Freq	% TD
SSR	5	
WWR	4	
A-SP	22	
I-SP		
PR	1	
INTJ	2	
REV		
Other		
Total	34	

Speech Rate	Child	Mother	Father	Duration
Mean				
Range				

Rank order of Disfluency Types						
Type	1	2	3	Mean	Range	Rank
SSR	3	8	5			
WWR	9	6	4			
A-SP	23	21	22			
I-SP	2	0	0			
PR	0	1	1			
INTJ	3	3	2			
REV	2	1	0			
Other	0	0	0			
Total	42	40	34			

Total = 116

%DisFl/TT: 116/300 = 39%

%SLD/Tot: 103/300 = 34%

% DSSLD: 103/116 = 88%

Notes: (do not count disfluencies, pauses, hesitations, etc.)
(use back of form to calculate speaking rates and stuttering duration)

Figure 3.6. Example of a disfluency count form obtained during a diagnostic assessment. Horizontal dashes are fluent words, and acronyms correspond to disfluent word. Abbreviations: **SSR**, sound-syllable repetition; **WWR**, whole-word repetition; **ASP**, audible-sound prolongation; **ISP**, inaudible-sound prolongation; **INT**, interjection; **REV**, revision; **PR**, phrase repetition.

and methods described earlier, the children's chronologic age and time since onset at the initial diagnostic were obtained. Besides these measures, we determined, at the time of the initial diagnostic evaluation and at each weekly treatment session, the frequency of total, stuttered, and other (normally fluent) disfluencies. Likewise, we measured the ratio of stuttered to total disfluencies (Pellowski & Conture, 2002) at the initial assessment as well as at each weekly therapy session.

During the initial diagnostic session of these same participants, emotional reactivity was measured through parent report on the seven-item Temperament Characteristics Scale (Oyler, 1996). (As mentioned earlier, we have found that the Temperament Characteristics Scale significantly correlates with the emotional reactivity and regulation subscales of the BSQ [Carey, McDevitt, & Associates, 1995], with significant $r = .20$ and .46, reported by Karrass et al. [2006].) Also at the time of the initial diagnostic evaluation, the following speech-language behaviors were measured: receptive and expressive language (Test of Early Language Development–Third Edition), receptive vocabulary (PPVT-III), expressive vocabulary (EVT-II), and articulation (sounds and syllables

subtest from GFTA-2). A language difference score was created by subtracting the child's lowest standard language score from the child's highest score, consistent with calculations to detect dissociations used by Anderson et al. (2005). MLU was calculated from a clinician-child conversation.

Prior to final data analysis, stuttering and related disfluency data from the children's first 12 sessions of participation in indirect treatment were grouped using a statistical procedure, Proc Traj. Proc Traj groups longitudinal data into distinct trajectories (Jones & Nagin, 2006; Jones, Nagin, & Roeder, 2001). Figure 3.7 shows a three-group solution, which was the best fit to the data (BIC = –2945.98), resulting in Improved (n = 19), No Change (n = 10), and Worsened (n = 13) groups (see Fig. 3.6 and see Table 3.3 for descriptive data). In terms of client dropout, our records for this sample are similar to our research studies with this age population (i.e., approximately one to two children per 10 who are diagnosed as stuttering leave treatment prior to completion for numerous reasons, e.g., financial reasons, move out of town, find clinical approach not suited to their needs, schedule conflicts, etc.).

Descriptively, the percent stuttering-like disfluencies of the Improved group decreased

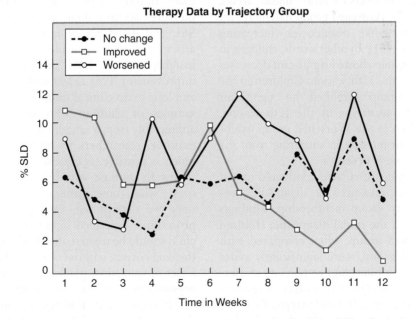

Figure 3.7. Short-term (first 12 sessions) treatment outcome trajectories. Preschool-age children beginning speech therapy were grouped based on their trajectories of changes in percent stuttering-like disfluencies for 12 weeks. The *No Change* group had a flat trajectory (i.e., no significant change), the *Improved* group experienced a significant decrease in percent stuttering-like disfluencies over time, and the *Worsened* group experienced a significant increase in percent stuttering-like disfluencies over time.

Table 3.3. *Central Tendency and Dispersion of Scores for Each Speech, Language, Fluency, and Related Variables Measured[a]*

Variable	No.	Mean	Standard Deviation
Time Since Onset at Initial Assessment (months)	46	17.54	10.50
% Total Disfluencies at Initial Assessment	44	14.38	8.25
% Stuttering-Like Disfluency (SLD) at Initial Assessment	44	11.35	7.30
% Ratio of SLD to Total Disfluency at Initial Assessment	44	76.11	15.76
Most Common Disfluency Type (median)	44	23	Sound-Syllable Repetition
Stuttering Severity Instrument–3	42	22.71	7.57
Temperament Characteristics Scale	43	21.41	5.29
% Rank Goldman-Fristoe Test of Articulation–2	45	59.78	27.03
% Rank Peabody Picture Vocabulary Test–III	47	57.17	28.81
% Rank Expressive Vocabulary Test	45	60.24	27.87
% Rank Mean Length of Utterance	38	55.34	29.28
% Rank Receptive Language	42	57.02	31.83
% Rank Expressive Language	41	44.94	32.08
% Rank Total Language Composite	41	52.31	32.08
% Change in Stuttering (SLD)	48	35.04	31.07
% Change in Other Disfluencies	48	−3.39	43.52
% Change in Total Disfluencies (TD)	48	22.09	28.97
% Change in SLD/TD	48	15.70	23.20
Number of Sessions	48	36.08	16.26

[a]Measures were not available for all participants (e.g., if a child became fatigued or produced considerable off-task behavior during testing), thus the number (No.) of available participants for each variable is also indicated. Note that 23 (52%) of 44 participants exhibited sound-syllable repetitions as their most common disfluency type.

across the 12 sessions (downward linear trend, $p < .05$); the No Change group had stable % stuttering-like disfluencies (no linear trend, $p = .16$), and the Worsened group had increased percent stuttering-like disfluencies (increasing linear trend, $p < .001$). In other words, children in the Improved group showed significant decreases in stuttering by the 12th session. Children in the No Change group exhibited no significant change in their stuttering by the 12th session. Finally, children in the Worsened group exhibited a significant increase in stuttering from the first session to the 12th session.

Paired-sample t-tests were conducted to test which variables measured at diagnostic predicted trajectory group membership. Findings indicated that at the initial diagnostic, children in the Improved group, when compared with the Worsened group, were significantly older ($p < .01$) and exhibited higher percent stuttering-like disfluencies ($p < .05$), with consequently higher SSI scores ($p < .01$) and marginally lower articulation scores ($p < .10$). Therefore, the data for the short-term outcomes (i.e., children within the first 12 sessions) suggest that older children show more improvement more quickly

despite having higher percentages of stuttering at the beginning of treatment. In other words, these findings suggest that initial diagnostic measures of chronologic age, percent stuttering, SSI, and standardized tests of speech sound articulation may provide the clinician with insights into at least short-time change or improvement. One *caveat* with both our short- and long-term clinical studies is that our clinical samples of children who stutter may differ appreciably from a random research sample. For example, researchers try to assess children, as much as possible, as close to onset of their stuttering. In contrast, with this clinical sample, we took "what came through the door"; that is, once we determined, through the diagnostic procedures described in this chapter, that the child should be treated, the child was included in the data corpus, without regard to time since the onset of stuttering, gender, amount and type of previous treatment, socioeconomic status, etc.

Although these findings are interesting, as shown in Conture (2001) and Richels and Conture (2007), the time course of our treatment of childhood stuttering from beginning through maintenance through termination is typically longer than 12 weeks. Thus, we thought it would be appropriate to conduct a more long-term study of the relationship of diagnostic predictors of treatment outcome. To do this, analyses were conducted to determine which variables taken at the initial diagnostic were predictive of improvement during indirect therapy over a longer course of therapy.

Long-Term Predictors

For these analyses, data from the 48 preschool and young school-aged children who stutter and who were included in the previous study (80% males) were examined to determine which measures taken during the diagnostic assessment were predictive of more long-term treatment outcome. Because there were more data points available for the analysis, grouping by trajectory was not calculated. Data taken at the time of the initial diagnostic were correlated with change scores derived from the average number of stuttering-like disfluencies, nonstuttering/other disfluencies, and total disfluencies observed during weekly treatment sessions. Change scores for each of the 48 preschooler children who stutter were calculated by averaging the number of stuttering-like disfluencies, nonstuttering/other disfluencies, and total disfluencies for the first four treatment sessions (T1) and the last four treatment sessions (T2) (after Conture, 2001; Richels & Conture, 2007; Zackheim et al., 2003). The averaged data were converted into a change score using the following formula: % change = $(T2 - T1/T1 + T2) \times 100$.

Correlations between change scores and disfluency measures at the time of the diagnostic were computed to determine which variables were significantly related to more long-term treatment change measures and therefore should be included in the analyses. Interestingly, unlike the case with short-term outcomes, none of the initial diagnostic disfluency counts at diagnostic were significantly related to any of the long-term disfluency change scores. Pearson product moment correlations were between $r = .06$ and $r = .12$. Similarly, stuttering severity at the time of the diagnostic was not significantly related to any of the change measures; Pearson product moment correlations were between $r = .01$ and $r = .16$. Finally, correlations of change scores with socioeconomic status, age, and gender were computed. The only significant correlations was between gender and change

in total disfluencies ($r = .34$). Therefore, gender was included in all models predicting change in total disfluencies to control for its effect. Specifically, the females in this particular sample (n = 10) had a greater average improvement over the course of treatment than the males. This finding may be an artifact of this particular sample and may or may not generalize to other samples.

Given that initial diagnostic measures of speech disfluency were not particularly predictive of long-term treatment change in stuttering, we attempted to use "emotional" and "speech-language" variables to predict long-term change in stuttering. Because of the relatively large number of speech-language variables relative to the sample size, to do this, a Principal Components Analysis (see Dunteman, 1989) was conducted to reduce the speech-language variables to one factor. This factor, which we will refer to as the Language Composite, explained 51.9% of the variance in language scores. Subsequently, two independent variables—the Temperament (Temperament Characteristics Scale) score and the Language Composite—were further used to predict long-term therapy change from diagnostic data.

Four regression analyses were conducted, predicting Change in Stuttering-Like Disfluencies (C-SLD), Change in Total Disfluencies (C-TD), Change in Non–Stuttering-Like Disfluencies (C-NSLD), and Change in Stuttering-Like Disfluencies Divided by Total Disfluencies (C-SLD/TD). The F values for the four regression equations and the standardized betas for the individual predictors are presented in Table 3.4. The regression equation predicting C-SLD from initial treatment and Language Composite was statistically significant, with Expressive Temperament as the only significant predictor. In essence, stuttering-like disfluencies of children, as a result of treatment, showed a larger decrease when their temperament scores were higher. Readers will recall that higher temperament scores indicate lower levels of inhibition (i.e., more behaviorally expressive). In addition, the regression equation predicting C-TD was statistically significant, and again, children with more expressive temperaments had a greater decrease in total disfluencies in therapy. The equation predicting C-NSLD was not statistically significant, and the C-SLD/TD was marginally significant, with a marginally

Table 3.4. *Regression Statistics Predicting Change Scores from Temperament and the Language Composite (F = analysis of variance; β = beta weight)*

Predictors	C-SLD		C-TD		C-NSLD		C-SLD/TD	
	F	β	F	β	F	β	F	β
Overall Model	6.29[a]		4.17[b]		1.13		2.95[c]	
Temperament		.40[b]		.36[b]		.23		.19
Language Composite		−.22		.03		.08		−.27[c]

Note: df = (2, 40). Abbreviations: **C-SLD**, Change in Stuttering-Like Disfluencies; **C-TD**, Change in Total Disfluencies; **C-NSLD**, Change in Non–Stuttering-Like Disfluencies; **C-SLD/TD**, Change in Stuttering-Like Disfluencies Divided by Total Disfluencies.
[a] $p < .01$.
[b] $p < .05$.
[c] $p < .10$.

significant relation to Language Composite, such that children who changed more in therapy (in terms of stutterings per total disfluencies) began treatment with lower language abilities.

The latter finding (i.e., that children with the greatest changes in stuttering had lower speech-language abilities) was taken to suggest that children whose language abilities/usage are furthest away from mean or maximum language abilities and usage exhibit the greatest change in stuttering during therapy. It is unclear whether this finding means that treatment (in)directly assisted or facilitated their language development, which in turn assisted their stuttering, or whether there was a natural or spontaneous improvement of language (due to maturation) during the time course of treatment that therapy neither targeted nor impacted. Obviously, these findings suggest that when predicting/planning long-term change in childhood stuttering, researchers should give careful consideration to variables other than those related solely to measurement of speech disfluency (for related discussion, see Rousseau et al., 2007; Zebrowski, 2007; Zebrowski & Conture, 1992).

Summary of Predictive Measures

Short-term changes in stuttering can be predicted by initial diagnostic measures of stuttering, but long-term changes in stuttering appear more readily predicted based on emotional and speech-language measures at the time of initial diagnostic assessment (i.e., before beginning therapy). This may suggest that relatively quick changes in stuttering during treatment are related to the frequency, nature, and severity of initial stuttering (e.g., if a child stutters a lot initially, he or she has

a lot of "room" to change and change quickly) but that long-term changes in stuttering are more related to developmental changes—whether natural, therapy facilitated, or both—in emotional and speech-language variables. Of course, these possibilities are based on results of just two relatively small studies from one clinic and must await replication by the current authors as well as independent investigators.

One of the more interesting findings, we think, is that children with the most expressive (i.e., least inhibited) temperaments exhibited the greatest decrease in stuttering over a relatively long-term course of therapy. These essentially longitudinal data indicate that emotional and speech-language variables have potential to discriminate children whose stuttering persists versus children who recover from stuttering and to predict the time course of changes in stuttering frequency associated with treatment. Furthermore, the trajectories or patterns of change displayed in Figure 3.6 may indicate the presence of *subgroups* within children (for further study of subgroups and stuttering, see Schwartz & Conture, 1988; Yairi, 2007). Again, if these findings are replicated in another sample by the present or other researchers, they would seemingly have considerable implications for how to tailor treatment to the individuals experiencing the treatment as well as how to assess whether the client is making progress on a daily, weekly, and monthly basis.

ONGOING ASSESSMENT DURING TREATMENT

A disfluency count is taken at the beginning of every treatment session based on conversational interaction between child and clinician. It is important to assess stuttering at the *beginning* of the session to avoid possible inflation of fluency data if assessed at the end of the therapy session. By the end of the session, the child has had a chance to adapt to the setting, clinician, and activity and has also received the immediate benefit of treatment. Conversely, obtaining the data at the beginning of a treatment session, after several days or even weeks (for those in the maintenance phase of treatment), seems likely to provide a better estimate of the carryover of improvement in the child's stuttering.

To collect such a sample, at the beginning of each treatment session, the clinician and child engage in a spontaneous conversation during which the clinician takes a disfluency count on the first 100 words uttered for each child. The disfluency count data are then entered into an Excel spreadsheet containing previous session data, graphed (see Fig. 3.6 and Richels & Conture, 2007, Fig. 5-4), and displayed on a computer monitor for the clinician and parent to study. Using the data collected and graphed at each treatment session, the clinician can assess performance over the entire course of treatment (i.e., from the daily session data to performance since the beginning of treatment). "No shows" are specifically included in the graphs by inserting "0" or no information for all measurements of speech (dis)fluency for the date of the scheduled session. In this way, if parents comment on lack of progress, we can show them that "regular change requires regular attendance," something they may not have been doing according to the graph. This visual reminder helps some parents understand the importance of regular attendance.

The disfluency count for every session and the cumulative graph are used by the clinician to make ongoing judgments about the success of treatment, the need to modify procedures, and the child's readiness for maintenance (e.g., attending every other week rather than every week). Each week, the clinician pairs the session data with the parent report given during the parent session to determine whether the session data reflect the child's disfluency or are unique to the treatment session itself (for details, see Richels & Conture, 2007). Comparing and contrasting the data from each session and parent report enable the clinician to make changes needed to maximize each child's meaningful, timely progress.

One exception to the rule of counting stuttering at the beginning of the treatment session has to do with the child who the clinician believes is improving but the parents do not. Sometimes this is related to high parental expectations for rapid change in stuttering, parental zero tolerance for any and all mistakes/speech disfluencies in their child's speech, less than ideal parental observational skills, etc. Whatever the case, with these children and their parents, it can help to show the parent the the child's individual session's initial "stuttering count" versus the same treatment session's final "stuttering count." This comparison helps to show the parent that the child is indeed making change in treatment during each and every session. What constitutes "real" change when comparing treatment session initial count to treatment session final count? There are no fast and firm rules here, but our experience suggests that a 25% or greater change (decrease) in stuttering within a treatment session is not random fluctuation and that a 50% or greater change (decrease) in stuttering within a treatment session indicates real change more than likely related to the treatment session.

TAILORING THE TREATMENT TO THE INDIVIDUAL CLIENT

As we have discussed throughout this chapter, and as most experienced clinicians come to appreciate, it is important to keep the needs of each client at the forefront during assessment and treatment. As we have tried to show, a comprehensive assessment is one important cornerstone for building successful treatment. Not only do initial speech-language characteristics, including stuttering frequency, predict success (at least in the short term) in treatment, but nonspeech characteristics (e.g., emotional disposition, temperament, speech-language characteristics) also seem to contribute significantly to how the child verbally and behaviorally reacts to daily life activities and, by extension, treatment. Therefore, the clinician needs to continually consider various aspects of child and parental behavior, not just speech disfluencies and speech-language scores, but also related behavioral characteristics such as attention regulation. Indeed, some of these characteristics may be shared by both child and parent. For example, a child who exhibits difficulty maintaining attention during the child-group portion of treatment may have a parent who is also having trouble maintaining attention in the parent portion of the treatment or during the sharing of the results and recommendations portion of the assessment (Rettew et al., 2006).

Likewise, both child and parent may have difficulty adapting to new situations and need more time to warm up to the therapy environment (as many as four to eight sessions or perhaps even longer). The clinician should be prepared for the possibility that it may take multiple sessions for some parents to understand and interpret the data graphs (careful, slow, and repeated explanations of what the graphs do and do not mean may be required for several weeks for some parents). In fact, in this case, redundancy is probably a virtue.

As clinicians, it is sometimes difficult to separate our perceptions of our own performance during therapy from that of the client in front of us. This is not to suggest that clinicians have minimal influence on the performance of their clients; on the contrary, they can have profound influence on the child's success in treatment. However, as clinicians, we must strive to see the bigger picture, for example, the role of the parent, the characteristics the child brings to treatment, the family dynamics (e.g., intense sibling rivalry between the client and an older sister), and so on. As a result, we can better use the information we gain from the assessment to guide us during treatment. We have tried to empha-

size throughout this chapter the critical importance of giving each and every family the opportunity to be unique participants in the assessment process, particularly through the parent interview and the other described measures. Full participation of families, children, and each clinician helps to ensure the most successful future for all participants.

CASE STUDY

The purpose of this section is to describe a particular individual through the assessment and into ongoing treatment. Table 3.5 displays the descriptive data taken at the time of assessment, and Figure 3.8 shows the ongoing data taken during treatment. The child we describe is a 6-year-old boy who reportedly had been stuttering since he was approximately 3 years old. When first seen, his time since onset was 36 months—a timeframe that, although not out of the realm of possibility for "natural recovery," did not make natural recovery particularly probable (see Yairi & Ambrose, 2005).

ENVIRONMENT

The boy's parents did not seek treatment at the onset of his stuttering because they believed that it was "developmental." The boy began receiving treatment through his local school system initially for a suspected articulation disorder at the age of 3.5 years. Although he received services twice a week for 30 minutes, his parents

Table 3.5. *Descriptive/Demographic Data for Case Study of 6-Year-Old Boy*

Variable	Value
Time Since Onset at Initial Assessment	36 months
% Total Disfluencies at Initial Assessment	18
% Stuttering-Like Disfluency (SLD) at Initial Assessment	15.3
% Ratio of SLD to Total Disfluency at Initial Assessment	85
Most Common Disfluency Type	Sound-Syllable Repetition
Stuttering Severity Instrument–3	27 (moderate-severe)
Temperament Characteristics Scale	12 (inhibited)
% Rank Goldman-Fristoe Test of Articulation–2	30
% Rank Peabody Picture Vocabulary Test–III	73
% Rank Expressive Vocabulary Test	87
% Change in Stuttering (SLD)	2.70
% Change in Other Disfluencies	0
% Change in Total Disfluencies (TD)	1.64
% Change in SLD/TD	1.06
Number of Sessions	25

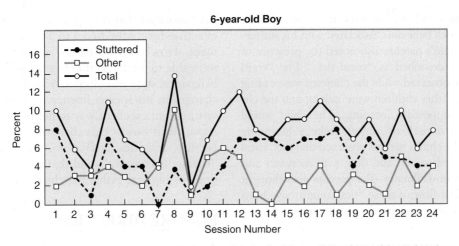

Figure 3.8. Example of a treatment se ssion graph (developed through a Microsoft Excel spreadsheet) that charts disfluency measures calculated from a 100-word disfluency count taken during weekly treatment sessions. Open circles represent the percent of total disfluency. Filled circles represent the percent of stuttering-like disfluency, and squares represent the percent of other/non-stuttering-like/normal disfluency for the same. *Note:* This graph depicts the speech disfluency data of a fairly slow-to-warm-up child, one who took 8 or more treatment sessions to adapt/adjust to clinician, therapy setting, etc. before he provided truly adequate speech-language samples.

indicated that they had not noticed significant improvement in his stuttering behavior. Both the parents' and the child's speech rates exceeded the "ideal" rate, with the father's rate being the most rapid in the family. Family history was positive for the father having a mild developmental stuttering disorder as a child. The parents reported that the child's birth, medical, and developmental histories did not include any unusual or significant events.

SPEECH-LANGUAGE PLANNING AND PRODUCTION

Results of articulation testing indicated skills within the broad range of normal limits. Errors noted included substitutions of /d/ for initial voiced "th" and /f/ for medial voiceless "th." Receptive and expressive vocabulary testing yielded results within to above normal limits. Additionally, the child passed a criterion-referenced language screening. Spontaneous language indicated appropriate syntactic and grammatical development. However, consistent with the findings of Anderson et al. (2005), the difference between this child's percentile ranks for the articulation (lower) and vocabulary (higher) measures indicated a significant dissociation between the two speech-language skills. In essence, the child's speech sound articulation was significantly less well advanced than his performance on the vocabulary measures.

EXPERIENCE

Parental report indicated that at onset, the child's stuttering was characterized by repetition of the first sound of sentence-initial words. As the time since the onset of the stuttering increased, his parents observed sound prolongations and "blocking" behavior accompanied by the nonspeech behavior of stomping his foot. The child's parents reported that he began using "starter words" at the beginning of phrases (e.g., "hey," "and," "so") and that he repeated the entire word before getting to the content of what he would like to say. Although he did not seem to withdraw from speaking situations, parents noted that he would say "You tell them" as a way of having someone else talk for him.

EMOTIONAL REACTIVITY AND EMOTION REGULATION

The child reportedly did well, fluency-wise, during the academic portion of his day but had increased difficulty with the social and emotional aspects of kindergarten. The parents noted that he had a very difficult time separating from them and had episodes of crying related to different activities of the school day (e.g., gym class, cafeteria). His mother noted that he did not like any change in routine (e.g., he got very upset when she put a different thermos in his lunchbox). His mother also indicated that he was very difficult to redirect "when he gets his mind (set) on something." In addition to nonspeech behaviors associated with his stuttering, the child's parents also noted the presence of what they described as "vocal tics." The "vocal tics" were observed while the clinician was reading and when other children were talking and the client was supposedly listening. The child would mutter to himself or almost make a humming sound. The child's parents observed that the "vocal tics" seemed to ebb and flow with increases and decreases in disfluency (the parents also thought the ebb and flow of these "tics" might have been seasonal and/or associated with allergies).

INSTANCES OF STUTTERING

Other nonspeech behaviors noted during instances of disfluency included physical tension in facial muscles. The child's parents reported that he used "starter words" at the beginning of utterances almost like he was warming up for speaking the rest of the sentence. Consequently, whole-word repetitions were noted as the second most common disfluency type.

ONGOING DECISION MAKING

Three months after the initial evaluation, the child began treatment in one of the Parent-Child Stuttering (Indirect) Treatment Groups described by Richels and Conture (2007). Looking at Figure 3.8, it appears that the boy's stuttering had actually improved between the evaluation and the beginning of treatment and then got worse as treatment continued. In actuality, he took nearly 12 sessions (3 months) to sufficiently adjust to the therapy environment to begin talking as he usually would (behavior that paralleled the child's difficulties starting the new school year). The graph reflects the increase in the quality and quantity of conversational speech as an increase in stuttering (i.e., more complex utterances produced, more stuttering exhibited, e.g., Zackheim & Conture, 2003). The child finally began to actively engage in the therapy process and make gains in fluency beginning at session 19 (nearly 5 months into the treatment process). If the clinician had not been aware of the extent to which the child exhibited inhibited/nonexpressive behavioral characteristics as well as how resistant to change the child was, both parents and clinician would

have assumed that therapy was simply not very effective during the first 3 to 5 months of treatment. However, the parent and the clinician were able to work together to support the child's behavioral style and ultimately facilitate positive changes in his speech fluency. Indeed, a group setting is an excellent way to help such children learn, albeit slowly, that changes in group membership, activities, and so on, are typical; that "change is constant"; and that change is something to adjust to rather than be afraid of.

FUTURE DIRECTIONS

Applied and basic research is warranted to behaviorally and psychophysiologically investigate children's dispositional and situational emotional reactivity and regulation, the interaction of these variables with speech-language variables, and their combined contributions to instances of stuttering. As our data suggest, these variables, singularly and in combination, seem to contribute to treatment outcome.

Additional empirical study of the contribution of dispositional/situational aspects of parental emotional reactivity and regulation also seem like a promising avenue of investigation. Work in progress from the Developmental Stuttering Lab at Vanderbilt University suggests that parent attitude and changes in the way parents structure their interactions and the environment during their child's treatment may have significant long-term effects on whether a child maintains fluent speech. Such a comprehensive approach—considering both speech-language and associated emotional variables for both children and parents—should help clinicians and researchers comprehensively view the causal and aggravating contributors to childhood stuttering through a lens possessing the widest conceptual and practical depth of field possible.

CHAPTER SUMMARY

- Whenever possible, assessment and treatment should be supported by a strong theoretical rationale and evidence base.
- Comprehensive, effective, and thorough assessment is essential to comprehensive, effective, and thorough treatment.

- Diagnostic information should be based on interviews, observation of spontaneous speech, and administration of standardized measures of speech and language.
- The key components of a comprehensive assessment of childhood stuttering include assessing the following:
  - Parental interview (environment)
  - Speech-language planning and production (child)
  - Experience (parent and child)
  - Emotional reactivity and emotion regulation (child and, if possible, parent)
  - Instances of stuttering and related aspects—for example, stuttering severity (child)
- Decision making during treatment should be based on data collected at every treatment session, the aggregate of data across sessions, and data provided by parents. Such data should be graphed and shared with the child's caregivers on a routine, if not weekly, basis.
- Although our understanding of how dispositional/situational aspects of emotional reactivity and regulation impact childhood stuttering is still far from complete, we should be mindful of how these variables may influence the rate, amount, and quality of change the child will make in treatment.
- Although similarities exist among children who stutter and their families, every child and family are unique (i.e., we typically study stuttering in groups, but groups do not enter our treatment centers, individuals do). Therefore, treatment should be continuously monitored and viewed through the unique lenses of the lives of each child and family.

SUGGESTED READINGS

COMMUNICATION-EMOTIONAL MODEL

Conture, E., Walden, T., Arnold, H., Graham, C., Karrass, J., & Hartfield, K. (2006). Communication-emotional model of stuttering. In N. Bernstein Ratner & J. Tetnowski (Eds.), *Current Issues in Stuttering Research and Practice* (pp. 17–46). Mahwah, NJ: Lawrence Erlbaum Associates.

INDIRECT TREATMENT OF CHILDHOOD STUTTERING

Conture, E. G. (2001). *Stuttering: Its Nature, Diagnosis, and Treatment* (pp. 167–177). Boston: Allyn and Bacon.

Melnick, K., & Conture, E. (1999). Parent-child group approach to stuttering in preschool and school-age children. In M. Onslow & A. Packman (Eds.), *Early Stuttering: A Handbook of Intervention Strategies* (pp. 17–51). San Diego, CA: Singular Publishing.

Richels, C. G., & Conture, E. G. (2007). An indirect treatment approach for early intervention for childhood stuttering. In E. Conture & R. Curlee (Eds.), *Stuttering and Related Disorders of Fluency* (3rd ed., pp. 77–99). New York: Thieme Publishers.

EMOTIONAL REACTIVITY, REGULATION, TEMPERAMENT, AND CHILDHOOD STUTTERING

Anderson, J., Pellowski, M., Conture, E., & Kelly, E. (2003). Temperamental characteristics of young children who stutter. *Journal of Speech, Language and Hearing Research, 46*, 1221–1223.

Guitar, B. (1997). Therapy for children's stuttering and emotions. In R. F. Curlee & G. M. Siegel (Eds.), *Nature and Treatment of Stuttering* (2nd ed., pp. 280–291). Needham Heights, MA: Allyn & Bacon.

Karrass, J., Walden, T., Conture, E., Graham, C., Arnold, H., Hartfield, K., & Schwenk, K. (2006). Relation of emotional reactivity and regulation to childhood stuttering. *Journal of Communication Disorders, 39*, 402–423.

Johnson, K., Conture, E., Karrass, J. and Walden, T. (2009). Influence of variations in stuttering frequency on talker group classification. *Journal of Communication Disorders, 42*, 195–210.

AUTHOR NOTE

We sincerely thank Dr. Janis Karrass for her assistance with data analysis but stress that any errors in the conduct or reporting of these analyses are totally our responsibility. We would also like to thank the many children and their families we have assessed and treated for childhood stuttering at Vanderbilt University. We have learned far more from these children and families than they have ever learned from us.

Correspondence concerning this chapter can be addressed to both authors (cgrichels@aol.com; edward.g.conture@vanderbilt.edu). Development of this chapter was made possible in part by grants from NIH/NIDCD (3R01DC000523-14; 1R01EC006477-01A2) to Vanderbilt University.

CHAPTER 4

An Overview of Treatments for Preschool Stuttering

BARRY E. GUITAR AND REBECCA J. MCCAULEY

INTRODUCTION

The three treatments featured in this section are all designed to help preschool children become normally fluent. Each, however, takes a different approach to achieving this goal. A major point of contrast is the degree to which the child's speech behaviors are dealt with directly, as opposed to indirectly, through working with the family to make the child's environment more fluency facilitating.

As you read the overview of each approach, note that we are using terms introduced when we discussed the structure of treatments in Chapter 2 to facilitate our comparison of the three treatments in this section. Specifically, we have delineated basic and intermediate goals, activities, and procedures that the clinician uses with the child and family and the contexts in which the activities and procedures take place. Additionally, because this is a text with considerable focus on theoretical foundations and evidence-based practice, we have also described the theoretical perspective behind each approach and the research evidence that supports it.

PALIN PARENT–CHILD INTERACTION

This approach is aimed at children up to 7 years of age who stutter. For their research studies, the Palin Centre clinicians include only children who have been stuttering for 12 months or more, but their usual clinical practice is to treat children who have been stuttering for less time

if such factors as family history, a worsening of stuttering since onset, and increasing parent concerns indicate a high level of risk for continued stuttering.

The basic goals of this approach are (1) to increase parents' abilities to manage stuttering, (2) to reduce family anxiety about stuttering, and (3) to decrease children's stuttering to within normal limits (<3% syllables stuttered). Intermediate goals are (1) to have parents identify and then change interaction patterns so that they become as fluency-facilitative as possible; (2) to have parents increase their confidence and reduce their concerns regarding the child's stuttering, as reflected in their questionnaires, homework sheets, and verbal responses; and (3) to gradually decrease the child's stuttering, as reflected in the clinician's measures and the parents' rating sheets. The major activities and procedures used to achieve these goals are video recording and playback of parent–child interactions in the clinic, discussions between the parents and clinician to increase the parents' facilitative interactions with the child, parents' work at home on fluency-facilitative interactions, and completion of the related homework sheets recounting the work done. The contexts in which these facilitative interactions are practiced range from in the clinic to "special times" at home to other situations throughout the day.

The Palin Parent–Child Interaction approach is based on a multifactorial theoretical perspective, which suggests that stuttering arises from many factors, including inherited or acquired neurophysiologic factors affecting speech motor and linguistic skills as well as temperamental vulnerability. The environment is hypothesized to interact with these constitutional factors, potentially stressing the child via conversational and social pressures. Treatment is aimed at reducing these pressures through parent training.

Evidence supporting the effectiveness of the Palin approach has been gathered for a number of years. Matthews, Williams, and Pring (1997) reported a case study showing significant reduction in stuttering in a 4-year-old child undergoing therapy with the Palin approach. This was followed by another single-case study by Crichton-Smith (2002), who showed that a 4-year-old child who was administered the Palin treatment achieved normal fluency. Using the strongest treatment design for this approach, Millard, Nicholas, and Cook (2008) used a replicated single-subject design to study the effect of Palin treatment on six children between the ages of 3 years and 4 years 11 months who had been stuttering for more than 12 months before treatment. Assessed a year after treatment, the children reduced stuttering from a mean of 8.4% syllables stuttered to a mean of 2.7%. Careful analysis of the frequency and variability of stuttering during baseline and after treatment indicated that four of the six children reduced stuttering significantly with both parents. Of the two other children, one child reduced stuttering with one parent only, and the other needed direct therapy before significant progress was made.

Other aspects of the Palin treatment in addition to effectiveness have also been explored. Nicholas, Millard, and Cook (2003) demonstrated that children's language continued to develop at normal rates during Palin treatment, a reassurance that the changes parents were making did not negatively affect language. This group also demonstrated that certain parent behaviors, such as length of speaking turn and types of utterances, were changed (in a way that was hypothesized to facilitate fluency) by the Palin approach. The clinician-researchers at the Palin Centre continue to expand the numbers of subjects they follow after treatment, so more data will eventually provide evidence about the approach. Although they do not intend to compare their approach with a no-treatment control group, it may be hoped that they will compare it with other available approaches for this age

level. It would also be desirable for the authors to gather data on how many of the children who they treat are regarded as nonstutterers when they are followed up long term. Typical fluency for the child's age is a basic goal for this approach, as well as for the two other preschool interventions described in this section.

STUTTERING PREVENTION AND EARLY INTERVENTION

Gottwald's approach to treatment targets children 2 to 6 years old who are unlikely to recover from stuttering without intervention. Gottwald's approach defines these children as children who (1) show signs of physical struggle and other reactions to their stuttering, (2) have some of the risk factors thought to predict chronic stuttering such as a family history of the disorder or increasing severity of stuttering, or (3) have both of the previous criteria.

The basic goal of this treatment is to help these children achieve normal fluency. Intermediate goals vary from child to child and family to family. In general, one set of intermediate goals is to reduce stress on the child; these goals include demands that may lie within the child himself or herself, such as perfectionism, or that may occur in the child's environment, such as the predominance of a rapid conversational speech pattern in the home. A second set of intermediate goals consists of helping the child enhance his or her capacity for fluency; these goals may include increasing aspects of language production ability or motor coordination. Activities and procedures for the family include clinician guidance in identifying family interaction patterns that may put stress on the child, changing these patterns through the clinician's counseling, and modeling of new behaviors, for example, by having the family watch video playback of their own interactions to identify targets for change and practicing new interaction patterns at home. Activities and procedures focused on the child include teaching the child a slower, more relaxed way of talking and, for a child with more struggle behaviors, helping the child learn to stutter in an easier fashion.

The contexts for the family's changes are in the clinic as well as in the home. Contexts for the child learning a slow and relaxed speaking style and/or a looser, easier way of stuttering are (1) in structured situations in the clinic, (2) in less structured situations in the clinic that have more demand attached to them, and (3) in the home with the families.

Gottwald's approach is based on a theoretical perspective that as children grow, they develop capacities or skills in areas related to speech and language production. These include linguistic and motor skills, among others. At the same time, the children's environments place on them many demands or expectations for performance in speech, language, social, and emotional domains. When demands exceed capacities, stuttering arises in some children. The treatment that derives naturally from this theoretical perspective is to help children who stutter to increase their underlying capacities for fluency and to help families decrease demands that stress their children's fluency.

Evidence for the effectiveness of this approach has been presented in several publications. Starkweather, Gottwald, and Halfond (1990) reported on a pre- and posttreatment study of 39 children who stuttered. Seven children dropped out of treatment and three were still in treatment at the time of the report; however, the remaining 29 children achieved normal fluency and retained it for 2 years after treatment. Children who dropped out did so because families moved or decided that the treatment was not right for them. Gottwald and Starkweather (1999) reported on an additional 15 children who were treated by Gottwald using the approach detailed in this chapter. One child withdrew from treatment, but the remaining 14 children achieved normal levels of fluency and maintained fluency for 1 year after treatment. In her chapter in this volume, Gottwald presents evidence that a further 27 children have completed the program, with 26 found to have retained normal fluency for 1 year after treatment. The average number of treatment sessions for these 26 children was 13.5, with a range of five to 31 sessions.

As with the Palin Centre treatment, additional studies using controls, comparisons to one or more other treatments, and random assignment to groups would strengthen claims of effectiveness advanced for this intervention. Given objections to withholding treatment that might effectively prevent a future of lifelong stuttering, it is understandable that a control group might not be used; however, in its absence, it is unclear to what extent positive outcomes in study participants do not simply reflect the very high recovery typically seen in youngsters who stutter.

LIDCOMBE PROGRAM OF EARLY STUTTERING INTERVENTION

The Lidcombe Program was designed to treat children up to 6 years old who stutter. The major criteria for admittance to the program are that the child is definitely stuttering and that adequate time has passed prior to treatment to allow for natural recovery (i.e., 1 year as a rule), as long as treatment is begun before age 6. The clinician's judgment must be used to determine whether other factors suggest treatment sooner than 1 year after onset. One such factor is the parents' severity ratings of the child's speech over time. If several weeks or months pass when the daily parent ratings of severity do not show a steady decline, then treatment is usually begun. Other factors affecting the clinician's decision to begin treatment include the level of the child's and family's distress and known risk factors for continued stuttering, such as the child's sex and family history of persistent stuttering.

The Lidcombe approach uses two measures of stuttering to determine progress in the program. The first is the severity rating, which is a 1-to-10 scale that the parent uses, after clinician training, to give daily assessments of the child's speech. A rating of 1 indicates normal fluency, and a rating of 10 indicates the worst the child's stuttering has ever been. The second measure is percent syllables stuttered (%SS), which the clinician measures at the beginning of each weekly session with the parent and child.

The basic goal of the Lidcombe Program is stutter-free speech or nearly stutter-free speech that is shown to endure 1 year or more after it is achieved. The first intermediate goal requires achievement of two benchmarks of fluency: (1) daily severity ratings by parents that average less than a score of 2 (with at least 4 days of scores of 1) for 3 weeks in a row, and (2) clinician ratings of the child's speech in the weekly session of less than 1% SS for the same 3 weeks. The second intermediate goal is to maintain those benchmarks as clinician contact is gradually faded from once-weekly meetings to meetings that occur 2, 2, 4, 4, 8, 8, and then finally 16 weeks apart.

Activities and procedures include (1) weekly meetings with the clinician in which the clinician assesses the child's speech and then guides and supports the parent to conduct treatment at home, (2) daily structured conversations between parent and child in which the parent uses verbal contingencies for stutter-free and stuttered speech, and (3) gradual replacement of structured conversations by unstructured conversations in which the parent continues to use verbal contingencies but now in more commonplace daily activities. Contexts begin with a one-on-one speaking situation in which the parent constrains the child's verbal output (e.g., by setting up a set of questions to be followed by predictable answers) and uses verbal contingencies to promote fluency. Once the child is approximately 90% fluent in this situation, the parent lets the child talk more freely in a natural conversation and continues the verbal contingencies to maintain fluency. The context gradually changes to unstructured situations, in which the child may be talking to the parent in the car, in the grocery store, or around the house. Other speakers, such as the other parent or a grandparent, are then trained to use verbal contingencies during unstructured conversations.

The developers of the Lidcombe Program hypothesize that there are deficits in the speech production patterns of children who begin to stutter. These deficits make it difficult for these children to produce the patterns of stressed and unstressed syllables of their language. Treatment, therefore, stimulates the children to adjust their speech production patterns at an age when they are flexible. Treatment is able to do this because stuttering can be changed via verbal consequences delivered by parents. Specifically, positive consequences for fluency (praise) and negative consequences for stuttering (acknowledgement or request for correction) are the active ingredients of Lidcombe treatment.

A series of studies has been conducted with the Lidcombe Program to demonstrate its efficacy. Onslow, Costa, and Rue (1990) first studied the effect of the treatment with four preschool children, who responded positively to the intervention and maintained fluency for 9 months after treatment. Lincoln and Onslow (1997) studied 42 children treated by the Lidcombe Program and demonstrated that they maintained essentially fluent speech 4 to 7 years after treatment. In a study of 250 children successfully treated by the Lidcombe program, it was shown that the median treatment time—to the point where children meet the two benchmarks of fluency—was 11 sessions (Jones et al., 2000). Several studies have shown the Lidcombe Program to be more effective than no treatment, but the most recent such study was a randomized control trial that showed greater improvement in Lidcombe-treated children (n = 29) versus children who were not treated (n = 25) (p = .003). The effect size of the treatment was 2.3% SS (Jones et al., 2005); this is a very large effect size for a clinical trial (Cohen, 1988).

DIFFERENCES AND SIMILARITIES AMONG APPROACHES

As can be seen in Table 4.1, the most obvious difference among the three approaches is the one described at the beginning of the chapter—the degree to which the treatment works directly on the child's speech. The Palin Parent–Child Interaction is the most indirect approach—changing parent behavior to influence the child's speech. Video feedback of parent–child interactions and parent counseling are used to help parents discover and change elements in the interaction that appear to be the most relevant to the child's fluency. The child's stuttering is not directly addressed but is monitored to ensure that as parents change the child's environment, stuttering gradually diminishes to normal levels of fluency.

Gottwald's approach of stuttering prevention and early intervention incorporates approaches that are both indirect (changing parent behavior) and direct (changing child behavior). More indirect aspects of this approach include educating parents about stuttering and helping parents identify and change factors that make fluency more difficult for the child. Direct work with the child, which begins at the same time as indirect work with the parents, involves teaching

Table 4.1. *Characteristics of Interventions for Preschoolers Who Stutter*

Parent–Child Interaction Prevention and Early Intervention of Early Stuttering Intervention

VARIABLE	TREATMENT		
	Chapter 5: Palin Parent–Child Interaction	Chapter 6: Stuttering Prevention and Early Intervention	Chapter 7: Lidcombe Program
Nature of Goals	Increase parents' abilities to manage stuttering; reduce family anxiety about stuttering; decrease child's stuttering to within normal limits	Normal fluency	Stutter-free or nearly stutter-free speech that is shown to endure for more than a year after it is established
Client Population	Children up to age 7 years who stutter	Children, age 2 to 6 years, who are unlikely to recover without intervention	Children up to age 6 years who stutter
Intervention Agents	Parents, guided by clinician	For environmental changes: parents, guided by clinician; for child's speech changes: clinician, assisted by parents	Parents, guided by the clinician
Nature of Session	Individual sessions; parent counseling, supplemented by video feedback to parents	Individual sessions; for environmental changes: parent counseling; for child's speech changes: instruction and modeling by clinician and practice by child	Individual sessions; clinician guides parent by modeling, feedback about conduct of home treatment, and discussion of child's progress
Demands for Technology	Video recording and playback equipment	Limited use of video recording and playback equipment	Device for assessing %SS online is helpful
Frequency of Sessions	1 hour per week for 6 weeks, then weekly 10-minute telephone contact for 6 weeks, then 1-hour consolidation session, then checkup every 3 months for 1 year, with total contact time of 8 hours	1 hour per week plus parent "special times" at home with child	1 hour per week with clinician, plus 15 minutes of daily treatment by parent at home during stage 1, plus intermittent daily treatment at home during first part of stage 2
Overall Duration of Treatment	12 weeks, followed by 1 year of monitoring	Average of 12 weekly sessions, but some children need as many as 30 weekly sessions	Median is 11 weekly sessions to achieve fluency, but some children need much more; 1 year of gradually faded contact after fluency is achieved
General Characterization of Methods	Clinician works with family to decrease stress on child, especially in communicative interactions; method involves modeling and coaching family and then having family practice on their own, with video feedback to family	Clinician works with family to decrease demands on child and increase support for child; clinician also works directly on child's speech if necessary	Clinician trains parent to administer praise and corrections in structured and unstructured daily situations; clinician discusses child's progress as measured by parent's daily severity ratings and clinician's assessment of child's %SS in clinic

the child to talk more slowly and, if needed, to reduce tension and struggle in moments of stuttering.

The Lidcombe Program uses only direct treatment of the child's speech. The parents, however, are highly involved in the treatment. They administer praise for fluent speech and acknowledgement of stuttering and requests for corrections (i.e., fluent repetitions). If the child's communicative environment changes (as it does in indirect treatments), it is assumed that this occurs only in the daily structured conversations that are designed to maximize fluency and the daily unstructured conversations during which the parent rewards the child's fluency or highlights stuttering.

Despite the differences in these three approaches, there are impressive similarities among them. For example, all three approaches appear to increase the amount of one-on-one time parents spend with their child. The Palin Parent–Child Interaction approach does this through "special time"—the home practice sessions that are conducted three to five times a week. Gottwald's stuttering prevention and early intervention approach asks families to set up daily speech play times during which parents help children practice new skills, model appropriate communication behaviors, and reinforce changes the child is making. The Lidcombe Program begins with daily structured one-on-one conversations between parent and child that are focused on increasing fluency and decreasing stuttering. Later, the parent conducts daily unstructured conversations with the same aim. In all three approaches, the predictable time each day that a child has alone with the parent focusing on him or her will undoubtedly improve the child's sense of well-being and may by itself improve fluency—although this idea is as yet untested.

Another similarity across these three treatments is the extent to which the child receives praise and support from parents. The Palin Parent–Child Interaction encourages parents to praise their child for desirable general behavior each day and provides log sheets on which parents can record the praises they administer. Gottwald's stuttering prevention and early intervention approach considers giving support to their children a major role parents play in treatment. This approach suggests that parents both praise the child's new speech skills and let the child know how much they enjoy listening to him or her. The Lidcombe Program uses praise very specifically contingent on the child's fluency, but it probably increases the child's confidence, as does the praise used in the other approaches. Again, the child's overall sense of being positively regarded and successful may engender increased confidence, which may help increase the child's fluency.

A third similarity is the fact that all three treatments provide a system through which parents assess the child's stuttering week by week and discuss the child's progress or lack thereof with the clinician. The Palin program asks parents to fill out rating scales assessing the child's severity of stuttering (as well as their own level of concern). Parents in the Gottwald stuttering prevention approach complete fluency charts or journals that are shared with the clinician. The Lidcombe Program uses severity rating scales filled out daily and brought in to the weekly sessions for discussion. This common element may cause parents to develop clearer pictures of their children's need for support that may prove facilitative to the child's development of more fluent speech.

The fourth similarity is the ubiquity of support for parents given by all three approaches. The Palin Parent–Child Interaction puts a great deal of emphasis on affirming and empowering parents. The developers of this approach espouse a philosophy that, rather than instructing parents about how best to interact with their children, helps parents realize that they are already doing many things that help the child's fluency and that, with some discussion and insight, they can discover ways to further facilitate their child's fluency. The stuttering prevention and early intervention approach focuses in part on the feelings of family members and helps them deal with feelings, such as guilt, that may interfere with therapy. In addition, Gottwald emphasizes that families take the lead in identifying elements of the environment that may impede fluency; families work as a team with the clinician to brainstorm ways in which the environment can be made more facilitating to the child's speech. The Lidcombe Program supports parents by guiding them to be the principal therapist for their child, thus giving them the experience of being the agent of change for the child's speech. The clinic sessions are focused primarily on helping and supporting the parent, rather than working with the child. For all of these approaches, parent support appears to be an ingredient in the therapeutic mix, whether acknowledged or not.

A final similarity of these interventions, although not captured in Table 4.1, is the time demands they place on parents of preschoolers who stutter. First, these interventions are similar in the time demands associated with the number and length of formal sessions with the clinician. All three approaches require approximately 12 contacts with the clinician during the intensive phase of treatment. These face-to-face or telephone meetings may be challenging for families with several children and/or limited resources, but doubtlessly even more demanding will be the parents' daily sessions with the child and daily record keeping across the course of active treatment.

SUMMARY

The interventions presented in Chapters 5, 6, and 7 are just three of the many approaches used with preschool children around the world. They were chosen, in part, because their developers have taken care to assess their effectiveness after the first blush of success has appeared and has had time to either fade or endure.

Of the three, the Lidcombe Program has the most extensive research support, beginning with the publication of Onslow, Costa, and Rue (1990) and continuing through more than two dozen publications. Interestingly, in the very same year as the first publication on the Lidcombe Program, the first evidence for the effectiveness of stuttering prevention and early intervention was published (Starkweather, Gottwald, & Halfond, 1990). The Palin Parent–Child Interaction was developed in the 1980s (e.g., Rustin, 1987) but has only recently been carefully assessed for long-term outcome (Millard, Nicholas, & Cook, 2008).

It is interesting that the developers of each approach seem to use their approach for all children who are deemed to need treatment. It may be that future research will identify some children who need a more indirect approach and other children who need a more direct approach. Further study is also needed to discover what the critical elements of each approach are. As we indicated in our comparison of approaches, some elements are common to all three approaches— one-on-one time, praise and support of the child by parents, systematic assessment of progress, and support for parents. Studies might be done to evaluate the importance of these elements compared with other elements that are different from one intervention to another.

Bloodstein (1995) has written eloquently about the need for evaluation of treatment effectiveness. In his handbook, he pointed out that a treatment must be shown to "be effective in the hands of essentially any qualified clinician… when [the treatment] is no longer new and the initial wave of enthusiasm over it has died away" (p. 445). Thus for all of these approaches, their real-world utility must await evidence that they can have as equally effective outcomes in the hands of "any qualified clinician" as they have when administered by their developers.

CHAPTER 5

Palin Parent–Child Interaction

WILLIE BOTTERILL AND ELAINE KELMAN

CHAPTER OUTLINE

KEY TERMS

Palin Parent–Child Interaction: therapy program using video feedback to help parents develop styles of interaction to facilitate their child's fluency.

Multifactorial perspective: a number of different factors may be relevant in the onset, development, and persistence of a stuttering problem and are therefore also considered in its treatment.

Special Time: 5-minute, play-based sessions for the parent and child to practice specific fluency-facilitating targets in the home.

INTRODUCTION

Palin Parent–Child Interaction (Palin PCI) (Kelman & Nicholas, 2008) is a therapy program conducted at the Michael Palin Centre (Palin Centre) for children up to 7 years of age that uses play-based sessions with parent–child pairs, video feedback, and facilitated discussions to help parents support and increase their child's natural fluency. It is often the first and only intervention for young children at the Palin Centre. It differs from other approaches to modifying parent–child interaction in the following ways:

- It is a facilitative rather than an instructive approach: parents' instinctive expertise is elicited, reinforced, and developed.
- Parents use video feedback to set their own targets and reinforce progress.

There are some children who also benefit from other interventions such as language therapy or speech sound work, as indicated, once Palin PCI has been completed.

PRINCIPLES OF TREATMENT: UNDERSTANDING THE CHILD'S NEEDS

Palin PCI is based on the therapist's and parents' shared understanding of the child's particular profile of speech motor and linguistic strengths and vulnerabilities. These are identified during the assessment and provide the context for exploring what the child needs in order to plan, organize, and deliver a message fluently.

PRINCIPLES OF TREATMENT: PARENTS ARE ALREADY HELPING

A key principle is that parents of children who stutter are already interacting with their children in ways that support natural fluency. The young children seen at the Palin Centre are fluent much more often than they stutter. Parents seek help because they are worried about the development of persistent stuttering, and they feel ill equipped to help their child. Palin PCI provides the means by which parents become increasingly knowledgeable about their child's communication skills and helps them to identify what they do that supports the development of fluency. Palin PCI aims to empower and reinforce parents' ability to interact in ways that match the child's fluency needs and focus on increasing these interactions in the home environment.

PRINCIPLES OF TREATMENT: PARENTS (OR KEY CAREGIVERS) ARE INVOLVED IN DIRECTING AND DELIVERING THERAPY IN THE HOME

Palin PCI is based on the principle that parent involvement in therapy is essential to reduce stuttering in the young child. Where appropriate, both parents attend the initial assessment and all therapy sessions, carry out homework tasks with their child, and provide feedback on progress. Central to this approach is the establishment of a collaborative therapeutic relationship in which the parents' and the therapist's knowledge and perceptions are shared and in which parents are encouraged to make their own observations, draw their own conclusions, set their own goals, and reflect on their progress each week. Within this relationship, the therapist's role is to facilitate and affirm, rather than instruct, advise, or model.

PRINCIPLES OF TREATMENT: STUTTERING IS DISCUSSED OPENLY

Parents are encouraged to acknowledge stuttering openly; they are helped to identify their fears about acknowledging stuttering and are encouraged to use age-appropriate, child-centered terminology. Normalizing the problem from the beginning can substantially reduce the anxiety and fear associated with stuttering for parents and for children. Although anxiety does not cause stuttering, stuttering causes anxiety.

GOALS OF TREATMENT

The primary goal of Palin PCI is to establish a foundation of parental understanding, knowledge, skill, and confidence in managing stuttering, which will support and augment the child's fluency during each stage of therapy. Another goal is to reduce the family's anxiety about stuttering and ultimately reduce the instances of stuttering in young children to within normal limits.

THEORETICAL BASIS FOR TREATMENT APPROACH

It is our view that any therapeutic approach to early stuttering must not only account for the many factors that may be contributing to the onset and development of stuttering in the individual child, but also acknowledge and harness the strengths and resources that the child and family bring to the clinical setting. This understanding of the nature of each child's difficulties as well as their strengths informs the therapy process from the beginning.

A **multifactorial perspective** (Smith & Kelly, 1997; Starkweather & Gottwald, 1990; Wall & Meyers, 1995) is supported by growing evidence that there are factors that may account for the child's underlying vulnerability to stuttering and its onset; factors that contribute to the development of the problem and, in some cases, its persistence; and factors that contribute to the moment of stuttering.

FACTORS THAT MAY CONTRIBUTE TO THE ONSET OF STUTTERING

Genetics

The underlying vulnerabilities to stuttering are highly complex and continue to be the focus of extensive research. It seems incontrovertible that genetic factors play a role in the onset of stuttering, and linkage studies are getting closer to finding the specific genes that predispose children to the disorder (Cox et al., 2000; Drayna, 1997; Shugart et al., 2004; Suresh et al., 2006). However, it is important to note that genes alone do not produce or determine behavior, especially one as complex and variable as stuttering; they only increase the probability that it will occur (Starkweather, 2002). It is acknowledged that a wide range of factors influences the extent to which a behavior trait such as stuttering finds expression (Starkweather, 2002). The complexity of the genetic predisposition was also discussed by Ambrose, Cox, and Yairi (1997), who suggested that an other factor—such as rapid rate of speech, low tolerance for frustration, slow reaction time, word retrieval or sentence formulation skills, chronic or excessive muscle tension, or any combination of these—may be the inherited variable that results in stuttered speech.

In addition to whether or not stuttering is likely to occur, Ambrose, Cox, and Yairi (1997) and Suresh et al. (2006) both report data that suggest the predisposition to recover or persist in stuttering is also inherited.

Neurophysiologic Factors

While the nature of the genetic transmission is still being investigated, parallel areas of research suggest that the onset of stuttering may be related to some underlying structural and or functional differences in the brain (Foundas et al., 2000; Fox et al., 2000; Sommer et al., 2002).

Findings from brain imaging and brain function studies have not yet been replicated in children, so it is not possible to determine whether any identified differences are responsible for the onset of stuttering or are a response to it. However, it has been suggested that an underlying neurologic dysfunction may be disrupting the complex two-way interaction between language planning and motor processing in children who stutter (Caruso, Max, & McClowry, 1999; Ingham & Cordes, 1998; Peters, Hulstijn, & Van Lieshout, 2000).

Speech Motor Skills

Stuttering presents as a breakdown in speech motor control, and as a result, there has been considerable research related to this area over the years, particularly in adults. The results are sometimes conflicting but suggest that there are differences in the speech production processes of adults who stutter compared with adults who are typically fluent. Although there has been less research on speech motor skills in children than in adults, there are indications of some subtle deficits in children (see review by Conture, 1991). In particular, studies have suggested that children who stutter have reduced oromotor skills (Riley & Riley, 1980), slower vocal and manual response times (Bishop, Williams, & Cooper, 1991), and difficulty stabilizing and controlling laryngeal movements, even during perceptually fluent speech (Conture, Rothenberg, & Molitor, 1986).

The Communication Environment: Interaction Styles

Considerable research has been carried out concerning the role that the communication environment and interaction styles may have in the onset of stuttering. The results suggest that there is no evidence that the interaction styles of parents of children who stutter and children who do not stutter are different (for a review, see Nippold & Rudzinski, 1995) or have a role in the onset of stuttering. Miles and Bernstein Ratner (2001), however, suggested that although the input of parents of children who stutter is parallel to that of parents of children who do not stutter, children who stutter might have more difficulties assimilating or responding to this input as a result of their underlying linguistic and or temperamental vulnerabilities. Perhaps the underlying vulnerabilities that predispose children to stutter also make it more difficult for them to be fluent in the context of typical adult-child interactions.

Summary

Many researchers agree that, for most children, the onset of stuttering will be shown to have a physiologic base that affects the delicate and complex balance of the child's developing linguistic and motor skills.

FACTORS THAT CONTRIBUTE TO THE DEVELOPMENT OF STUTTERING AND RISK OF PERSISTENCE

There is considerable agreement that it is the interplay between the child's underlying vulnerabilities and his or her temperament and linguistic and social environment that contributes to the development of stuttering and the risk of persistence (Yairi & Ambrose, 2005).

Linguistic Factors

Thus far, research suggests that there are no differences in the overall linguistic abilities of children who stutter (see Kloth et al., 1999; Watkins & Yairi, 1997; and Yairi et al., 2001 for a discussion). However, in a recent study, Anderson, Pellowski, and Conture (2005) assessed the expressive and receptive language and phonologic skills of children who stutter and children who do not stutter and looked at the dissociations or mismatches within or between components of these skills. They found that children who stutter are three times more likely to exhibit these mismatches than their fluent peers. The fact that

there were children who exhibited dissociations but who did not stutter and there were children who stuttered but who did not exhibit dissociations means that linguistic dissociations on their own cannot account for stuttering onset but may be relevant in combination with other factors or in relation to persistence.

The role of phonologic skills has also been well researched, with high proportions of children who stutter also having speech sound impairments (Yaruss, Lasalle, & Conture, 1998). In addition, an association has been found between reduced phonologic skills and persistence of stuttering (Paden, Yairi, & Ambrose, 1999).

Gender

Research seems to indicate that more boys than girls persist in stuttering (Yairi & Ambrose, 2005). The ratio of boys to girls who stutter is reported to be as low as 1:1 (Yairi, 1983) close to onset and increases with age to about 6:1 (Bloodstein, 1995).

Time since Onset

For the majority of children, recovery occurs within the first 12 months (Yairi & Ambrose, 1992; Yairi et al., 1996) to 18 months (Johannsen, 2000) after stuttering begins. Although some children will still achieve fluency after this (Yairi & Ambrose, 1999), the probability of recovery decreases with age (Seider, Gladstien, & Kidd, 1983) and length of time stuttering (Yairi et al., 1996). These studies also identified that children who persist in stuttering demonstrate a relatively stable level of stuttering over time. In contrast, children who recover show a marked reduction in the amount of stuttering during the first year after onset, and this pattern of improvement continues over time.

Psychological-Emotional Factors

Significant research continues to investigate the role of psychological factors, particularly temperament, in contributing to the development of persistent stuttering. Researchers such as Conture (2001) and Guitar (2006) suggest that temperament traits, such as sensitivity, inhibition, and reactivity, among others, may maintain or exacerbate stuttering. The research suggests that children who stutter are more sensitive and inhibited (Anderson et al., 2003; Embrechts et al., 2000). It is suggested that children who stutter may be intolerant of disruptions in their speech and react in ways that exacerbate the problem rather than ameliorate it. Recent research findings by Conture's research team at Vanderbilt University have suggested that "the relatively greater emotional reactivity experienced by preschool children who stutter, together with their relative inability to flexibly control their attention and regulate the emotions they experience, may contribute to the difficulties these children have establishing reasonably fluent speech and language" (Karrass et al., 2006, p. 402).

Within the clinical environment at the Palin Centre, parents frequently describe their child who stutters as being "highly sensitive," "easily upset," and "a bit of a worrier." In addition, parents say their children who stutter seem to "set themselves high standards," "be perfectionists," and "like to get things right" and are often "anxious to please." It has also been proposed that a child's temperament may influence how he or she responds to different parental interaction styles (Felsenfeld, 1997), and there is a growing body of research that seems to support the idea that the temperament of the child has an important role to play in the development and possibly the persistence of stuttering. Therefore, temperament may be an important variable to consider in therapy.

The Communication Environment: Interaction Styles

Although there is no evidence that parents' interaction styles have a role in the onset of stuttering, Kloth et al. (1998) provide evidence from their longitudinal study that mothers made changes in their interactions in response to the stuttering of their children. This study showed that after the onset of stuttering in their children, mothers tended to be more intervening, take more turns, use shorter pauses, make more requests for information, and use more affirmatives than they had used before onset. Rommel (2000) was also looking at factors that affect the development of stuttering and found that the more complex the mother's language and the greater the discrepancy between mother and child linguistic variables were, the higher the chances of persistence.

Summary

Anderson et al. (2005) concur red with Hall (2004) by suggesting that "it is the child's attempt to reconcile or manage dissociations in speech and language that contributes to disruptions in their speech and language production, which in combination with a genetic predisposition towards stuttering or, perhaps a temperamental disposition that is relatively intolerant of any such disruptions, that results in the emergence of persistent stuttering" (p. 242).

FACTORS THAT CONTRIBUTE TO THE MOMENT OF STUTTERING

Linguistic Factors

There are a number of research studies that have looked more closely at the relationship between length and complexity of utterances and stuttering frequency. These have shown that children are more likely to stutter when using longer, more complex sentences (Logan & Conture, 1995; 1997; Logan & LaSalle, 1999; Melnick & Conture, 2000). However, Yaruss (1999) pointed out that this was true of only some children in his study.

Other studies have looked at factors that influence the location of stuttering and demonstrated that it tends to occur at the beginning of an utterance (Howell & Au-Yeung, 1995), on function rather than content words (Howell, Au-Yeung, & Sackin, 1999), and on longer words (Rommel, 2000).

The Communication Environment: Interaction Styles

Parents and their children live in a socially interactive environment. Children's social, emotional, and behavioral development is influenced by the way their parents "parent." Furthermore, the way in which children respond and develop affects their parents. It is a dynamic, constantly evolving relationship that is unique to each child and family.

Many early intervention approaches have been based on helping parents make changes in the communication environment of the child in the belief that this will reduce the amount of stuttering. There is at least some evidence that parental interaction styles can be modified (Nicholas, Millard, & Cook, 2003), and stuttering has been shown to decrease when parents slow down their rate of speech (Guitar et al., 1992), when they increase pause time and response latency time (Newman & Smit, 1989), and when they put in place structured turn taking (Winslow & Guitar, 1994). Interestingly, closer inspection of the results indicates that the impact of the changes made by parents seems to have been somewhat idiosyncratic (Zebrowski et al., 1996), with the frequency of stuttering reducing in some children but not in others.

Not only is there some evidence that modifications in a parent's interaction style can reduce the frequency of stuttering, but there is also evidence that stuttering influences parent interaction style (Meyers & Freeman, 1985a; 1985b; Zenner et al., 1978). These studies showed that mothers of both children who stutter and children who do not stutter use a faster rate of speech (Meyers & Freeman, 1985b), interrupt more frequently (Meyers & Freeman, 1985a), and are more anxious (Zenner et al., 1978) when interacting with children who stutter compared with children who do not stutter. Several authors emphasized the important role played by the family and family dynamics in the therapy process (Cook & Botterill, 2005; Kelly & Conture, 1992; Manning, 2001; Wall & Myers, 1995). Shapiro (1999) concluded, "stuttering, and other communication disorders exist and must be addressed within a family context" (p. 125).

Summary

There are important linguistic considerations and interaction styles that influence the moment of stuttering during communication. These are unique to each child and family and are important to take into account when planning and delivering therapy.

THE MICHAEL PALIN CENTRE MULTIFACTORIAL FRAMEWORK

The multifactorial framework depicted in Figure 5.1 interprets the previously outlined research as suggesting that predisposing physiologic and linguistic factors may be significant in the onset and development of stuttering. Furthermore, the interaction of these factors with emotional and environmental aspects is thought to contribute to the severity and persistence of the disorder and the impact it has on a child and

the family. For each child, there is a unique combination of these factors that contributes to the onset and subsequent development of stuttering toward either recovery or persistence.

ASSESSMENT AND THERAPY

Because of the relationships described earlier, it is essential to conduct a comprehensive, multifactorial assessment to identify the factors that are pertinent to each child's difficulties. Assessment of the child's speech, language, and fluency skills, as well as information from structured interviews with children and their parents or caregivers, provides the basis for identifying children at risk of persistence. It also provides the information necessary to make recommendations and tailor therapy to meet the needs of individual children.

PROFILE OF VULNERABILITY

It is not yet possible to predict precisely the level of risk or the "weighting" of those factors that make one child more vulnerable than another. Furthermore, it is still not possible to predict with any accuracy what the eventual outcome is for any individual child, either with or without therapy (Bernstein Ratner, 1997). However, research has been able to isolate factors that are most likely to help identify children who are at some risk of stuttering (Kloth et al., 1999; Yairi & Ambrose, 1999). On the basis of current research and clinical expertise, therapists at the Palin Centre select children for therapy according to their vulnerability to persistence. This is based on information about family history, time since onset, the changes in stuttering since onset, and the child's or parents' concern about the problem. Children who are involved in the research program are only selected if they have been stuttering for more than 12 months. Routinely, treatment is offered to children who have been stuttering for less time if the levels of concern are high.

THERAPY – PALIN PCI

Palin PCI is based on the premise that the underlying vulnerabilities that predispose children to stuttering may also make it more difficult for them to be fluent in the context of typical adult-child interactions.

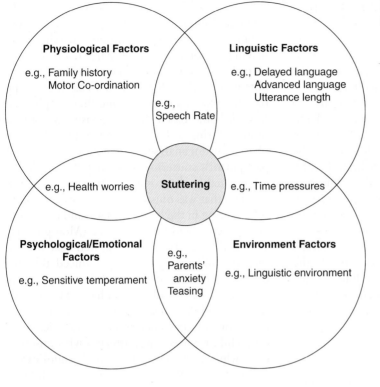

Figure 5.1. The Palin Centre Multi-factorial Framework.

The main focus of Palin PCI is the child, his or her profile of skills, and facilitating further development of the naturally occurring fluency within the environment. It also aims to build on parents' or caregivers' knowledge and confidence in what helps and enhances existing behaviors that support fluency.

The intention of therapy is to establish strategies that support the child's natural fluency and minimize the impact of the stuttering on both the child and the family through:

1. Interaction strategies: These may include, for example, changes in rate, length, and complexity of utterances; turn taking; use of pausing; comments; and following the child's lead.
2. Family strategies: These can include strategies such as managing anxiety about stuttering, coping with highly sensitive children, confidence building, behavior management, and turn taking.
3. Child strategies: These are included for some children as appropriate. They may include direct speech modification, fluency-enhancing strategies, language therapy, or speech sound therapy.

EMPIRICAL BASIS FOR TREATMENT

The previous section has provided the rationale for the Palin Centre conceptualization of stuttering and some of the evidence that supports this view.

Palin PCI was developed at the Palin Centre in the early 1980s (Rustin, Botterill, & Kelman, 1996). Since then, it has drawn on the experience of expert clinicians and the families that they have worked with, and it has been influenced and shaped by the work of academic researchers and respected authorities in the field.

Evidence-based practice is now an essential component of ethical working within the field of speech and language therapy. Sackett et al. (2000) emphasize the multidimensional nature of evidence-based practice and describe it as the "integration of best research evidence with clinical expertise and patient values" (p. 1). The clinical work at the Palin Centre is informed by a wide range of theoretical perspectives from the field of psychology as well as speech and language therapy, providing a broad evidence base to support our practices. In addition, the Palin Centre is committed to continuing professional development, updating the Centre's research knowledge, and maintaining an active clinical research program that consistently seeks the opinions of the children and parents who use the services.

This section provides a description of the clinical research framework that the Palin Centre is using to explore the effectiveness of Palin PCI. The framework is based on the model proposed by Robey and Schultz (1998), which Pring (2005, p. 245) applied to stuttering research. The model advocates a progression from treatment efficacy research, where therapy is investigated under optimal conditions, to treatment effectiveness research, where therapy is investigated under clinical conditions. As the process develops, the factors that influence outcome are isolated and investigated. There are five phases of research described in a logical series but that are not discrete.

PHASE 1

In phase 1, clinical reports, small group studies, and single-case studies are used to demonstrate potential therapeutic effects. Clinical reports detailing the positive impact of Palin PCI for individual clients, such as the case reported in this chapter, have been available for a number of years (Rustin, Botterill, & Kelman, 1996). Matthews, Williams, and Pring (1997) presented a single case study reporting stuttering frequency data relating to Palin PCI. In this study, the progress of a 4-year-old boy was monitored for 6 weeks before therapy, 6 weeks during therapy, and 6 weeks after therapy. The percentage of words stuttered was calculated from speech samples obtained while the child played with each parent in the clinic for a period of 20 minutes once a week. The therapy resulted in a significant reduction in the frequency of the child's stuttering during therapy that was maintained during the posttherapy phase.

The design and methods employed by Matthews, Williams, and Pring (1997) were adapted and improved by Millard, Nicholas, and Cook (2008) to include increased participant numbers, nonclinic measures, and long-term follow-up data. Millard, Nicholas, and Cook used a single-subject methodology to investigate fluency development in six children, less than 5 years of age, who had been stuttering in excess of 12 months. Stuttering frequency measures were obtained from video recordings of the child playing at home with each parent. From these recordings, stuttering frequency data were obtained weekly during a 6-week pretherapy baseline phase, a 6-week clinic therapy phase, a 6-week home-based therapy phase, and once a month during a 1-year posttherapy follow-up phase. Cusum analyses were conducted on each participant's stuttering frequency data to determine whether there was a systematic change in the data that was outside the range of variability of stuttering in the baseline phase and that could not be accounted for by chance (Montgomery, 1997). The analyses demonstrated that four of the six children significantly reduced the frequency of their stuttering with both parents by the end of the consolidation phase. Therapy for these four children focused on the development of interaction and management strategies only. One child reduced his stuttering with one parent, while the remaining child significantly reduced her stuttering by the end of the follow-up period. Both of these children went on to receive direct therapy input during the 1-year posttherapy follow-up phase.

There are a number of advantages to using single-subject designs with children who stutter. The use of repeated measures prior to the introduction of therapy allows the detection of any signs of pretreatment recovery. It also enables observation of each child's individual variability and provides a more representative picture of a child's overall fluency skills (Ingham & Riley, 1998). The child's progress can then be measured against his or her normal variability in fluency, which eliminates the problem of withholding therapy. It is also argued that it is a more clinically relevant design, particularly for heterogeneous disorders, because it can be used within the context of regular clinical work (Pring, 2005).

PHASE 2

In phase 2 research, studies are designed to show how the therapy works, which clients are suitable for a particular program, the amount of therapy needed, and the method of delivery.

Consideration of the information from phase 1 clinical reports and single-subject data, along with evidence from other researchers in the field, led to the development of hypotheses about why and how Palin PCI might work. Exploration of the mechanisms of change would constitute phase 2 in the research framework.

Because Palin PCI places a strong emphasis on modifications to parent interaction style, it might be assumed that this would change as part of the therapy process. Using the recordings collected as part of the Millard, Nicholas, and Cook (2008) study, preliminary data reported by Nicholas, Millard, and Cook (2003) suggested that parents are able to make changes during Palin PCI and that these changes can be maintained over time. Nicholas et al. found that fathers significantly reduced the proportion of utterances that were requests for information and reduced the length of their turn, whereas mothers significantly reduced the number of their utterances that were instructions. There is evidence, therefore, that this line of inquiry should be extended in a larger study involving the analysis of longer term data and increased subject numbers.

Millard, Edwards, and Cook (2009) observed a relative reduction in the expressive language scores of five children who began therapy with above-average scores. Each of these children did not maintain the above-average scores 6 months after therapy but achieved scores that were within the normal range. Since their receptive skills maintained the advanced developmental trajectory, Millard et al. concluded that the observed relative reduction could not be explained by a linguistic environment that was inadequate to maintain language growth, as has been proposed in the past (Miles & Bernstein Ratner, 2001). They suggested that the data adds further support to the possibility of a fluency-language trade-off (Miles & Bernstein Ratner, 2001).

Phase 2 also seeks to identify the appropriate outcome measures for use in effectiveness studies. We consider that outcome measures should reflect not only stuttering frequency, but also the multidimensional nature of stuttering, the impact that it may have on both children and parents, and the expectations and needs of the client.

Frequency of stuttering represented as a percentage of syllables stuttered is usually cited as the only evidence of success in therapy for young children who stutter. Although this is clearly an essential measure, it provides a somewhat one-dimensional perspective of stuttering behavior. It is well known that stuttering in young children varies considerably from day to day and situation to situation, and it is common for children to be much more fluent in clinic than at home, or vice versa. Obtaining a single measure of stuttering frequency from one speech sample is unlikely to be representative of a child's overall fluency. Although use of multiple measures and contexts partly addresses this issue (Ingham & Riley, 1998), other important aspects of the problem are not reflected. The aims of Palin PCI are much broader than singularly reducing stuttering frequency and include developing parents' knowledge about stuttering, reducing their worries about their child's speech, and increasing their knowledge and confidence about strategies for managing their child's stuttering more effectively. Because parents/caregivers are an integral part of the therapy process, it is essential that they are involved in providing additional clinical outcome data. However, there are few assessment tools that adequately evaluate these broader issues.

Parents' Ratings of Outcome

In an attempt to address the need for parental input, Millard (2002) conducted a qualitative study to find out what parents consider to be the most important outcomes in therapy and to develop an outcome measurement tool for parents who receive Palin PCI. The design of the study followed the principles of the Delphi approach. This is a structured methodology that aims to obtain a group's opinion or judgment on a topic (Goodman, 1987) and to arrive at consensus through a specified procedure (Mosley & Mead, 2001). In this instance, the "group" consisted of parents who had attended the Palin Centre for therapy with their children during the previous year. The resulting rating scales contained a wide range of themes that reflected the broad nature of the therapy they had received. In addition to reductions in stuttering frequency and severity, the parents considered reductions in the child's anxiety, frustration, and concern about speech and increases in the child's confidence in speaking and turn-taking skills to be important indicators of improvement. The parents also considered positive changes in their own level of concern and confidence in managing the stuttering effectively, along with the impact on the family as a whole, to be important outcomes of the therapy program. The resulting questionnaire consists of a series of visual analog scales that allows a numerical value to be obtained before therapy and at intervals throughout the therapy process so that change can be evaluated. This rating scale is used routinely at the Palin Centre, in conjunction with fluency and language measures and is available in Millard, Edwards, and Cook (2009).

PHASE 3

Phase 3 of the research framework relates to large-scale efficacy research. Although randomized controlled trials (RCTs) are generally viewed as the "gold standard" methodology for treatment efficacy research (Jones et al., 2001), they are not without their limitations.

The strength of large-scale RCTs is that the results can be generalized to a wider population than the participants studied. The limitation is that group studies do not capture individual responses to therapy and group findings cannot be used to predict how an individual will respond to a given therapy. The need for large subject numbers can restrict the range of dependent variables that can be monitored, which could result in potentially informative findings or new discoveries being missed (Schwartz & Conture, 1988; Watkins & Yairi, 1997). On a practical level, the large subject numbers that are required to account for the heterogeneity of stuttering and individuality of therapy have significant implications for recruitment and resources. There are also ethical considerations in withholding treatment from a "no treatment" control group and methodologic limitations in substituting a best practice control group (Pring, 2005). In our attempts to conduct an RCT to investigate Palin PCI with young children who are at risk of persistent stuttering, we have encountered all of these difficulties. Like Onslow, Andrews, and Lincoln (1994), we found that the practical and ethical difficulties of maintaining a no treatment control group resulted in a design that was impractical and inappropriate and that had to be abandoned

The emphasis in single-subject studies is to incorporate controls to obtain high internal validity—that is, that the findings can be justifiably applied to the individual studied. The external

validity of single-subject studies is low—that is, the findings cannot be generalized to the population as a whole and it is this that is important in a phase 3 study. However, replicating findings across individuals helps to increase external validity (Pring, 2005), and there is an argument that appropriately designed and well-controlled single-subject experimental designs that are replicated can be considered to be strong sources of evidence alongside RCTs (Kully & Langevin, 2005). Because of the advantages of using single-subject studies to investigate therapy with this client group and because of the difficulties inherent in conducting an RCT, we have decided to continue and advance our research program through the implementation of replicated single-subject studies.

In addition to the children reported by Millard, Nicholas, and Cook (2008), results from a further six children who received Palin PCI were described by Millard, Edwards, and Cook (2009). Once again, stuttering frequency data were obtained from video recordings made at home while the child played with a parent. These were made once a week for 6 weeks prior to therapy, 6 weeks during clinic therapy, and 6 weeks during the home-based therapy period. The follow-up phase took place 6 weeks prior to the 6-month review appointment and again involved once-weekly video recordings. All six children showed a reduction in stuttering by the end of the study, according to the cusum analyses, and we can be confident that this was associated with the therapy in four cases because the data reached significance in the therapy phases. None of the participants received direct therapy focusing on the development of child strategies. In addition to a reduction in stuttering frequency, the parent rating scales indicated that parents perceived the child's fluency to have improved; they felt more knowledgeable and confident about managing the stuttering and were less worried and anxious about it 6 months after receiving therapy than they had been before.

The combined findings of both the Millard, Nicholas, and Cook (2008) and Millard, Edwards, and Cook (2009) studies indicate that Palin PCI can be effective in reducing stuttering in young children who are at risk of persistent stuttering. The results seem to indicate that approximately two-thirds of children will show a reduction in stuttering during the clinic therapy or home-based therapy (consolidation) periods and require only the indirect components of Palin PCI. This is similar to outcomes reported by Conture and Melnick (1999). There are also indications that stuttering may be reduced over a longer term in children who have received Palin PCI, although it is not possible within the current designs and methods to attribute this directly to the therapy.

PHASE 4

Within phase 4, researchers continue to define those clients who benefit, and variations to treatment and delivery are explored. Importantly, the research emphasis shifts towards the investigation of treatment effectiveness. Thus, having demonstrated that Palin PCI is effective under optimal conditions, which include being implemented by speech and language therapists who are expert in the approach within a well-resourced, specialist environment, it is necessary to establish whether the approach is effective when implemented in other settings with different subgroups of the clinical population of children who stutter. The Matthews, Williams, and Pring (1997) study described earlier could be considered to be phase 4 research because a nonspecialist clinician in a nonspecialized clinical context conducted it. This single-case study was subsequently replicated by Crichton-Smith (2002), who demonstrated a reduction of stuttering to within normal with a 4-year-old child who received Palin PCI. Therefore, there is early evidence that Palin PCI can be successfully implemented by speech and language therapists who have received training in Palin PCI but who are not necessarily specialists in the approach.

PHASE 5

Phase 5 research focuses on the issues of cost effectiveness, client satisfaction, and the effect of therapy on quality of life. The parent rating scales already provide useful information related to these issues and are incorporated into the development of phase 2 and phase 3 research.

SUMMARY

The research at the Palin Centre has developed and advanced with increasing pace over the last 5 years. The framework adopted has helped to structure and prioritize research activities.

Careful consideration and experience with a range of methods have resulted in relevant and realistic research designs and protocols. The evidence indicates that Palin PCI can be effective with children who stutter, and this research evidence is used to inform the clinical decisions made within the Palin Centre. However, research evidence is not the only information considered. Expert experience and opinion are highly valued, and informal feedback from clients is regularly sought.

PRACTICAL REQUIREMENTS

TRAINING

As with all therapeutic methods that are not routinely taught within undergraduate or postgraduate education, additional training and supervision are necessary to ensure that Palin PCI is delivered ethically and appropriately. The Palin PCI training course is a workshop that lasts 3 days and is designed to provide trainees with the knowledge and skills they need to carry out Palin PCI in their clinics. The 3-day workshop includes:

- Review of current literature and evidence as it applies to this age range
- Theoretical perspective of the multifactorial nature of stuttering and implications for therapy
- Rationale for the case history and detailed child assessment
- Developing skills in the formal and informal measures of fluency, speech, language, and social communication skills
- Clinical decision making
- Rationale and practical clinical skills for delivering Palin PCI
- Clinical skills in working collaboratively with parents

The training course is an interactive workshop in which trainees are involved in practical and experiential exercises; in the viewing of videotapes of clinicians, parents, and children who stutter; and in role-play activities. The training is evaluated routinely using a standard questionnaire that is filled out before and after training and then 6 months later. The data collated from these questionnaires demonstrate that trainees gain knowledge, skills, and confidence in managing stuttering and that this has resulted in positive changes in their clinical practice (Botterill, Biggart, & Cook, 2006). Trainees are also encouraged to telephone or email and "troubleshoot" with the team at the Palin Centre.

A new manual (Kelman & Nicholas, 2008) has recently been published that provides a step-by-step guide to Palin PCI and incorporates recent research evidence. This manual, in conjunction with the practical training course described earlier, will equip therapists to carry out Palin PCI as it is conducted at the Palin Centre.

ASSESSMENT SKILLS

Clinicians are required to use formal and informal assessments to measure children's speech, language, and social skills. The ability to undertake a quantitative and qualitative analysis of stuttering using video or audio recording equipment is also necessary. The clinician is also required to take a case history from the parents and then process this information together with the rest of the assessment findings to develop a case summary, which is presented to the parents in clear and accessible terms.

THERAPEUTIC SKILLS

Central to the Palin PCI approach is the idea of collaboration and partnership between the clinician and the parent. This involves the therapists drawing on their core counseling skills and listening to and observing the parents carefully so that they can facilitate the parents' discovery of what they already know and are already doing to help their child. In this way, the therapist elicits and uses knowledge from the parents rather than imparting information, teaching, or offering advice.

TECHNICAL EQUIPMENT AND SKILLS

A video camera and television monitor are integral to Palin PCI. A tripod is also useful. A level of competence and confidence is required to operate this equipment.

ACCOMMODATION

The therapy room will need to have a range of play materials appropriate to the child's age and with space for the child to play on the floor or at a table. The room should be sufficiently large for video recordings to be made and viewed. A separate viewing room from which the play can be remotely video recorded can be a useful option.

ADMINISTRATION

The following paperwork is required:

- Consent forms for treatment and video recording
- Assessment record forms, including detailed case history form
- Special Time instruction sheet and homework sheet; this records the details of this home-based task and facilitates a discussion at the beginning of each therapy session
- Praise logs to record the specific praise that the parents are encouraged to give to their children each day
- Treatment record forms

Parents are also encouraged to read *How to Talk So Kids Will Listen and Listen So Kids Will Talk* (Faber & Mazlish, 1980). This is a parenting book that is easily accessible and that most parents find helpful in a variety of ways. The chapter on dealing with feelings is especially relevant for parents who describe their children as very sensitive. The chapter on praise offers parents a way of praising their children that specifically describes the child's actions and then provides the child with a positive attribute/adjective that describes the behavior. An example is: "Thank you for putting your clothes on the chair (description) that was very helpful/thoughtful/responsible (attribute) of you." Parents are often aware of the effect confidence has on their child's fluency and are pleased to notice the difference when they add these details to the praise they already give to their children.

TIME REQUIREMENTS

Palin PCI involves more assessment time than other approaches; however, less time is usually required in the treatment phase. The child assessment and analysis takes approximately 90 minutes, and the parent interview takes an additional 90 minutes. These 3 hours ensure an individually tailored approach to the child's and family's specific needs.

Treatment then involves six 1-hour therapy sessions (including 5 minutes for record keeping) during the first 6-week phase, followed by six 10-minute contacts (by telephone, letter, or email) during the consolidation phase. A 1-hour review session follows the consolidation period. Thus a total of 8 hours is required to deliver a program of Palin PCI over a course of 3 months.

Following this, the child is monitored every 3 months for 1 year. Some children require further direct fluency input, which can be delivered in up to six once-weekly therapy sessions. Children who present with concomitant speech or language problems may receive further therapy targeting these specific difficulties.

KEY COMPONENTS

OVERVIEW

The main focus of the Palin PCI approach is the child and his or her profile of skills. The aim is to facilitate natural fluency within the child's usual social environment by building on the parents' knowledge of what helps fluency and augmenting behaviors that are already in evidence. The approach is based on the belief that parents can and do influence their child's communication skills and confidence and that, in the case of young children, they are pivotal to the process of change (Kelman & Nicholas, 2008).

The approach is flexible and adapted according to each child's individual and changing needs. For most children, the goal of Palin PCI is to achieve fluency within normal limits (<3% SS) or until the parents are no longer concerned. For children with more complex needs, the intention is to establish family strategies that support the child's natural fluency and develop the child's confidence. For the small proportion of children who continue to stutter despite intervention, the approach aims to minimize the impact of the stuttering on both the child and the family.

During Palin PCI sessions, parents view video recordings made while they are playing with their child in the clinic. Drawing on the shared understanding of their child's needs, parents are guided through a process of identifying and augmenting those interaction and communication styles that they judge will promote their child's fluency. Parents are also introduced to ideas and strategies that build

confidence and self-esteem. In addition, when parents raise concerns about the impact of other issues such as tiredness and lack of routines on the child's fluency, these are addressed as part of therapy.

After the multifactorial assessment, Palin PCI is implemented in three distinct stages. The first stage consists of six once-weekly, clinic-based sessions that both parents (as appropriate) attend with their child. In the second stage, the Consolidation Period, parents continue to implement Palin PCI for a further 6 weeks in structured home-based practice sessions that are closely monitored by both parents and the therapist. The third stage starts with a Review Session in which further clinical decisions are made based on progress reports from parents and formal reassessments in the clinic. In some cases, supplementary clinic-based therapy sessions may be offered for further Palin PCI, language or phonology therapy, or direct fluency therapy, as appropriate. All children are monitored for at least 1 year after therapy.

MULTIFACTORIAL ASSESSMENT

The multifactorial assessment comprises a thorough evaluation of the child's strengths and underlying vulnerabilities within the context of the family, including the child's receptive and expressive language, articulation, speech rate, social communication skills, and general presentation. Detailed case history information is gathered from both parents to identify developmental, familial, psychosocial, health, and personality factors that they consider to be influencing their child's stuttering, and the parents complete the parent rating scales.

At the end of the assessment, parents are given a formulation or summary of the assessment findings. This formulation aims to provide parents with a clear understanding of the multifactorial nature of stuttering with particular reference to the factors that are relevant to their child's current difficulties. It provides the rationale for the recommendations that are made and the therapy that is considered most appropriate for the child's difficulties. Throughout the process, great emphasis is placed on developing the client-clinician relationship and helping parents make the best use of their own problem-solving and management skills.

STAGE 1: WITHIN CLINIC SESSIONS
Initial Session: Introducing and Setting Up Palin PCI

The goal of the initial session is to establish an open dialogue about stuttering and fluency, to develop mutual responsibilities in the therapy program, to review the assessment findings and clarify any questions, to set up Special Time contracts, and to ensure that parents have a clear understanding of what therapy will involve.

Video and treatment consent forms are signed, and an initial 5-minute video recording is made of each parent playing with their child within the clinic setting. It is important to explain that the video will be used as a basis for exploring ways in which the parents can build on and enhance their child's fluency in future sessions. Parents' initial self-consciousness about the video camera is quickly offset by their child's naturalness and curiosity about new toys and activities. Between the sessions, the therapist will view the video and identify examples of interactions that facilitate fluency. The parents will watch the video at the beginning of the next session.

Next, parents are introduced to the concept of Special Time. These are designated home practice sessions with their child that continue throughout the therapy program. They consist of a fixed 5-minute playtime that each parent completes individually with the child. Parents are asked to agree to a set number of Special Times per week, with a minimum of three and a maximum of five. During the week after the first session, parents establish the routine of Special Times for the agreed number of sessions.

The aim of Special Time is to provide parents with a designated time to practice implementing an interaction target in a relaxed, one-on-one, play setting. Following Special Time, parents/caregivers complete a homework sheet, which helps them to reflect on their target in a structured way. The therapist uses this record sheet to monitor how the parents are implementing the targeted change.

Second Session

The initial task in this session is to make sure that the Special Time routine has been successfully established. When, from time to time, parents discover that they have committed themselves to more than they can manage, their contract is adjusted appropriately. If parents have been unable to do Special Time, this is discussed constructively to discover what is getting in the way and to problem solve how this can be resolved. The Palin PCI program only starts when the minimum number of Special Times is established because they are the "vehicle of change" within the home environment.

The therapist and parents then revisit the assessment summary to focus on the factors that seemed to be affecting the child's fluency and review what the parents already know that seems to help the child. For example, the assessment may reveal that the child has well-developed language skills but his speech sound skills are still developing, that he stutters most when he is competing with his siblings to speak, and that it seems to help when he can "take his own time." The first two video clips on the publisher's website for the book (thePoint) illustrate this process with parents.

See Video Clip 1, Evan's mother and father are discussing the factors that they think have contributed to Evan's current difficulties as revealed in the assessment completed 2 weeks previously. This is followed by a discussion about what they think Evan needs in light of this to help him with his fluency.

See Video Clip 2, Elaine asks Jayneequa's mother what her instincts tell her that Jayneequa might need to help with her fluency.

The next step in this session is to use the videotape made in the clinic the previous week to begin to identify interaction styles that support the child's fluency by looking at examples from the tape where parents are already doing things to help. These might include helping the child to take his time by following his lead in the play, by encouraging pauses, or by having an unhurried manner. The next clip on the DVD shows a clinician helping a mother identify a fluency-facilitating behavior that she is already engaging in.

See Video Clip 3, Jayneequa's mother has just watched the first video of her playing with Jayneequa. Elaine asks her what she noticed that seemed to be helping. She notices that she is patient and gives Jayneequa time. Elaine then asks her how this helps Jayneequa's fluency.

Each parent observes their own section of the interaction video, and the therapist asks them individually to comment on aspects of their interaction with which they were pleased. Starting with this encouraging approach is reassuring and sets the stage for a positive experience. Initially their observations might be quite general, for example: "We both seemed to be enjoying the game" or "We were doing lots of laughing!" The therapist's role is then to guide the parents to notice the behaviors that they are already engaged in that support the child's fluency needs and to reinforce these observations. Some parents find it difficult to see what is going well and focus instead on more negative aspects. Watch the next video clip to see how a clinician can help a reluctant parent find something quite helpful he is already doing.

Video Clip 4 demonstrates how to turn this around for a parent. Dylan's father is finding watching the video hard and is describing how nervous and unnatural he felt. Elaine asks what was going well, and he finds this question difficult to answer. She selects a piece of the video and helps him to look again and focus on something positive. They work it out together until he can see how following Dylan's leads helps to slow down the pace of the interaction to suit Dylan. They then set this as a target for Special Times.

In addition, the therapist may prompt the parents when necessary by highlighting key moments during the video—for example, by drawing attention to pauses in the interaction when no one is talking:

Therapist: "What is happening here?"
Parent: "Nothing, no one is talking."
Therapist: "With your child's needs in mind, how will pauses like that be useful?"
Parent: "It helps calm things down."
Therapist: "What difference does that make?"
Parent: "It slows us both down and lets him know there is no hurry. He can respond or not in his own time."
Therapist: "And how does that help?"
Parent: "Well…he's usually more fluent when that happens."

Parents often find it easier to be critical of themselves when they watch the video than to see what is working well. Therefore, it is important for therapists to develop ways to help

parents focus on the things they are doing that support the child's fluency.

Parent: "I can see that I'm busy doing it all for him."
Therapist: "And when you are not doing it for him, what is happening?"
Parent: "I am watching and waiting for him to do it."
Therapist: "And how does that help?
Parent: "Well, he gets to do it for himself."
Therapist: "And what difference does that make?"
Parent: "He finds out he can do it himself and that helps his confidence."
Therapist: "And when he's more confident?"
Parent: "He's often more fluent."
Therapist: "So let's look for the times when that is happening."

General questions such as "What are you doing that seems to help?" or "What is working well here?" provide a general orientation and can be effective in eliciting observations from some parents. For others, the therapist will provide more specific guidance and orientation by referring to particular moments captured on the video. The therapist uses carefully focused questions to help parents notice supportive behaviors that are already present, no matter how brief they might be. Pausing or replaying sections of the video and using questions (such as "What did you do there that worked well?" "What happened when you did that?" "What difference does that make?" or "How does that help his/her fluency?") help parents to observe their interaction in a positive way that links it specifically to their child's needs.

As explained earlier, the process of watching the video, discussing observations, and setting goals is done on an individual basis with each parent. Parents quickly learn to observe their videos objectively. While each parent is party to their partner's discussion with the therapist, they are not invited to comment on each other's videos. However, if they wish to do so, they are reminded that their comments should be positive and constructive.

The therapist uses facilitative questions to elicit ideas or thoughts from the parents about *why* these particular interactions might support their child's fluency. For example, having observed a noticeable pause before responding to the child, a question such as "How is that pause helping?" makes parents consider the positive consequences of their behavior and ensures that a clear rationale is established for encouraging this particular interaction style. Each parent then individually selects an interaction style that he or she would like to try to perform more often; this is briefly practiced in a video-recorded play session with the child and then played back on the video. When each parent is confident that they know what they are targeting and why, the identified parent behavior becomes a goal for practice during Special Time at home for the coming week.

The interaction style that parents notice most often as helpful in increasing fluency seems to be related to the child leading the play and setting the pace of an interaction. Once a parent notices this and waits for the child to take the lead more often, the child then sets the play agenda, the language level, and the pace of the interaction. The more the child takes the lead, the more the parent needs to observe and listen in order to follow the child and the easier it is to match their own level of language and pace to that of the child. Parents also begin to notice that making a change in one aspect of their interaction style often has an effect on another aspect, for example, resulting in changes in patterns of turn taking or in the balance of turns or the number of pauses that occur.

As parents identify target behaviors that they think are helpful and would like to do more often, they also explore with the therapist how increasing these targets might also support the child's language skills, phonology, general confidence, and autonomy. It is important to note that parents rarely have more than three targets throughout the therapy because change in one target area usually involves shifts in another; for example, targeting an increase in the use of pauses often results in shorter, simpler sentences and an overall reduction in rate.

Once parents are satisfied that the targets they are working on are having the desired effect (i.e., a reduction in the type or frequency of disfluencies within the Special Times), they are encouraged to begin to identify other key times during the day when they can interact with the child in ways that they know facilitate the child's fluency, for example, on the walk home from school, in the car, or at mealtimes. These are in addition to their regular Special Times and can also be logged on the homework sheets along with Special Time. (See Figs. 5.2 and 5.3 for an example of how these sheets might be organized and completed.) Parents continue to make comments about the effect that this intervention has and gradually increase the occasions when they monitor their interactions until it becomes routine and natural.

Parents/caregivers leave every session with a homework sheet that identifies their targets and the number of sessions of Special Times they have agreed to undertake. They fill in their homework sheet at the end of each Special Time and return to the next session with homework completed and comments made about their experience of putting the targets into practice.

Structure of Sessions 2 to 6

Each treatment session includes the following components. First, the therapist checks the feedback from the parents' homework sheets and answers any queries about Special Time targets and their impact. Then, a new video is made of each parent playing for 5 minutes with their child, putting into practice their interaction targets. The therapist and the parents watch the new interaction video and have a discussion about the video that focuses on the positive changes that will support their child's communication needs. Questions are asked, such as "What is going well?" Follow-up questions are also asked, such as "What else can you see that is helping?" and "What difference does that make?" Parents then identify a new goal for their Special Time and take away a homework sheet to complete. The next video clip illustrates what this scenario might look like.

See Video Clip 5, Evan's parents are in session 3. They talk about the targets they set for themselves and discuss what they have learned from the exercise. Evan's father was trying to match Evan's rate of talking and to pause more often. He talks about realizing that Evan's natural rate of speech is very slow.

SPECIAL TIME TASK SHEET

NAME OF PARENT: _____   NAME OF CHILD: _____

NUMBER OF SPECIAL TIMES: _____

TARGETS FOR SPECIAL TIME: _____

_____

DATE	ACTIVITY	COMMENTS ABOUT THE TARGETS

IN ONE SENTENCE, WRITE DOWN WHAT YOU HAVE LEARNED FROM THIS WEEK'S ACTIVITIES:

Figure 5.2. Sample of sheet used to record observations made about Special Time activities conducted as part of treatment homework and a completed example showing how the sheet is used.

The mother's targets were leaving gaps in the interaction and not feeling the need to fill in the pauses. The parents then watch the video. Willie asks them what they saw that was going well. She reinforces their ideas and continues with "What else?" and "How does that help?" or "What difference does that make?" Finally, Willie helps both parents identify a target for the coming week.

SPECIAL TIME TASK SHEET

NAME OF PARENT: _____Mary_____   **NAME OF CHILD:** _____Jo_____

NUMBER OF SPECIAL TIMES: _____4_____

TARGETS FOR SPECIAL TIME: _____follow Jo's lead, use more pauses_____

_____

DATE	ACTIVITY	COMMENTS ABOUT THE TARGETS
22/01/08	Played shops	I waited and watched for a bit so I could follow what Jo was doing rather than doing my own thing. It was hard pausing more as I love to talk but I think I managed it a bit more than usual, I felt more relaxed.
24/01/08	Played with her dolls	She loves to play dolls and got quite bossy with me telling me what to do! I did as I was told and she loved it!
26/01/08	Played tummy ache game	Jo showed me how to play it and I joined in. I think I am better at leaving pauses and now find it easier and it all feels a bit more like there is more time which is good.
IN ONE SENTENCE, WRITE DOWN WHAT YOU HAVE LEARNED FROM THIS WEEK'S ACTIVITIES:		

Figure 5.3. Sample of completed Special Time task sheet.

Other Components of Palin PCI

In addition to the major components described earlier, sessions 2 to 6 routinely incorporate topics such as openly acknowledging stuttering, building confidence, turn taking, dealing with feelings/emotions, and managing problem behavior. The discussion of these topics is facilitated by referring to specific chapters in the book by Faber and Mazlish (1980) in which parenting skills are described in a clear and accessible style. The parents then record examples of praise that they give the child on a daily basis and note the child's response on a praise log, which is returned weekly along with the homework sheets.

If, during the assessment, parents highlighted concerns related to child management or the establishment of routines (e.g., bedtime routines) that they feel are affecting the child's fluency, additional strategies are discussed and included in the 6-week program. Therapists typically talk through the situation and then help the parents problem solve alternative ways to manage the problem. These may include negotiating some family rules (e.g., for bedtimes or turn taking), using praise and/or a reward system, setting clear boundaries, and being consistent.

STAGE 2: THE HOME-BASED CONSOLIDATION PERIOD

Session 6 of Palin PCI begins with the same format as previous sessions followed by a discussion about the next 6 weeks, which is referred to as the home-based consolidation period. During these 6 weeks, the parents continue to do Special Time with their child at home, implementing their targets and completing the homework sheets. They also continue to incorporate activities for developing the child's confidence, for promoting turn taking within the family, and for any other relevant management issues. Although the family does not attend the clinic during the consolidation period, they continue to send in their homework sheets so that the therapist is able to monitor progress and respond by letter, telephone, or email. If there is any deterioration in the child's fluency during this time or if other problems arise, the parents agree to telephone the therapist as soon as possible. It is also agreed that if the therapist does not receive the homework sheets, contact will be made with the family. A review session is held at the end of the 6-week consolidation period.

STAGE 3: THE REVIEW SESSION AND CLINICAL DECISION MAKING

In the Review Session, parents complete rating scales and discuss the Special Times and any other matters that may have arisen during the consolidation period. They also have an opportunity to share their observations of the changes they have made and the effects of these changes on the child's fluency and communication skills. A formal fluency analysis is made from a tape-recorded speech sample, and a parent–child interaction video is made and viewed with both parents. This provides objective evidence of progress and gives the parents an opportunity to consider the impact of the changes they have made over the 6 weeks. The therapist reinforces the progress and invites a discussion about the factors that the parents consider to be particularly important in increasing the child's fluency and confidence and how they will continue to make progress.

The results of the assessment, the parents' questionnaires, and the feedback from the weekly homework sheets will help the parents and the therapist decide whether they are ready to go on to the Monitoring Only phase. The criteria for moving to Monitoring Only are a combination of factors, such as a noticeable increase in fluency and a decrease in the amount and/or severity of the stuttering, an increase in parental confidence, and a reduction in parental concern. At this point, we expect that two-thirds of children will go on to Monitoring Only, and the parents will continue regular Special Times and complete homework sheets that they will continue to send in. They will be reviewed again at intervals negotiated with the family, usually 6 to 12 weeks, and for a period of at least 1 year after therapy.

Children who are not improving sufficiently or who have reached a plateau and whose parents continue to be concerned will start sessions of direct fluency work within the clinic, which will be supported by parents during home practice sessions in addition to their Special Time. In the section on the theoretical basis of Palin PCI, we indicated that we believe some children have a greater vulnerability to stuttering. It may be that these children have a greater physiologic "weighting" for persistent stuttering and need support to manage their speech motor control systems more efficiently. Alternatively, it may be necessary to address any identified mismatches in their speech, language, and/or motor systems by working directly on those domains.

ADVANTAGES OF PALIN PCI

There are a number of advantages to Palin PCI. First, it can be implemented with children for whom direct therapy would not be indicated. For instance, it can be used with very young children and is not reliant on a child having well-developed attention, listening, cognitive, meta-linguistic, or self-monitoring skills.

Second, although the approach encourages parents to acknowledge their child's stuttering, the main focus of the initial stages of the program is not on the child's speech. This focus has the advantage that it can be used with children whose temperament is described as highly sensitive and who may interpret direct therapy as suggesting that stuttering behavior is unacceptable.

Third, Palin PCI lays the foundations for those children for whom the direct therapy component of the program is also recommended. The insight, knowledge, and skills gained by parents during the assessment and therapy process play an important role in helping the child to transfer the speech management skills learned during the direct therapy stage of the program.

SUMMARY

The key component of the Palin PCI approach is the use of video feedback to help parents develop strategies to facilitate their child's fluency, based on their unique profile of skills. These strategies are practiced at home in structured Special Time sessions, and then generalized and combined with other strategies, such as turn taking and confidence building. The family attends six clinic sessions and then continues the program in a 6-week home-based Consolidation Period, followed by a review and further direct input or other therapies as necessary or by moving into a Monitoring Only stage.

ASSESSMENT METHODS TO SUPPORT ONGOING DECISION MAKING

INITIAL ASSESSMENT TO SUPPORT DECISION MAKING REGARDING INTERVENTION

The assessment protocol encompasses the cognitive, linguistic, social, emotional, and physiologic components of the child's stuttering. The information is collected during a comprehensive child assessment and a detailed interview with both parents.

The assessment protocol includes the following:

- Formal and informal measures of the speech, language, and social communication skills of the child.
- A recorded speech sample is transcribed and used to calculate a percentage of syllables stuttered (%SS) and to make comments about the type and duration of stuttered moments.
- An interview to gauge the level of the child's concern and his or her perception of the problem.
- A video recording of each parent/caregiver playing with the child. This provides a naturalistic sample of the child's speech while interacting with each parent/caregiver and allows further insight into the child's skills. It also provides an initial record of the parent–child interaction style.
- A detailed case history from both parents (as appropriate) to explore the history and development of the stuttering and other pertinent issues within the family (e.g., difficulties managing family routines such as bedtimes, getting to school in the morning, or sibling rivalry).
- Parent rating scales provide an insight into their level of knowledge, concern, and confidence in managing the child's difficulties (Millard, 2002).

This detailed assessment procedure ensures that a profile of the child's strengths and needs within the context of the family can be obtained. The information from all these sources provides the basis for the formulation. This is a summary of the assessment findings and the factors that we have identified that seem to be relevant to the onset and development of their child's stuttering. This summary is discussed with the parents and explained within the context of the multifactorial framework of stuttering. This is important in establishing a shared understanding of the problem and encouraging the collaborative relationship that is fundamental to Palin PCI. Parents and children are also encouraged to acknowledge and discuss stuttering openly from the beginning with an implicit rationale that talking about difficulties reduces anxiety and makes them easier to manage.

Once it has been established that intervention is appropriate, the information from the assessment indicates which areas should be addressed in the therapy program.

Palin PCI routinely involves parents in considering their interaction and behavior management strategies. It also involves the child in developing speech-related strategies. Although the delivery of Palin PCI will be similar across families in terms of number of sessions and session plan, the content of the sessions will vary, depending on the individual needs of the child and the family. These are determined in consultation with the parents and in response to individual needs identified in the assessment.

ONGOING ASSESSMENT TO MONITOR TREATMENT EFFECTIVENESS

The program is delivered as a 6-week package of once-weekly sessions followed by a 6-week consolidation period during which the Special Times are continued by the parents at home. Progress is monitored throughout the 12 weeks through the parents' written and verbal reports of the child's fluency, confidence levels, and the family's progress with other strategies. Written homework sheets, which record the interaction targets identified by each parent during the therapy sessions, are completed by the parents each week and brought or sent to the therapist for monitoring and feedback. Parents are also encouraged to provide verbal feedback about their child's progress and their own perception of how the therapy is going. During the clinic sessions, a video recording is made, providing a sample of the child's fluency during play and a record of the changes in the parent–child interactions. The therapist also observes the child's fluency levels throughout the session. The combination of this verbal and written parental feedback, together with the therapist's observations, enables decision making about next steps in treatment and about the appropriateness and effectiveness of the intervention.

At the end of 12 weeks, the family returns to the clinic for a reassessment and review of the child's progress. As before, this includes a recorded speech sample from which an analysis of the fluency is made and another completion of the rating scales by parents. A further video recording is made of the parent and child interacting. Based on these reassessments and discussions with the parents, decisions are made regarding the need for further therapy and, if it is needed, what form it should take. The options include working with the child more directly on the stuttering or therapy directed at other areas of difficulty in the child's speech and language skills that were identified during the comprehensive assessment and that are not resolving (e.g., a phonologic problem).

Therapy sessions are no longer indicated when the level of stuttering is within normal limits (<3% SS) and/or the parents are no longer concerned, as recorded in the clinic measures, and the family is reporting a similar pattern at home. Parents would also be reporting reductions in their anxiety about the problem and higher levels of confidence in their ability to manage the stuttering, as indicated by their verbal feedback and the rating scales.

Most families reach this stage at the end of the 12 weeks and continue to be monitored and reviewed at regular intervals as agreed by the parents, usually every 6 to 12 weeks for up to 1 year. The same assessments are completed at the review sessions for at least 1 year. If the parents express concerns, a review appointment will be made earlier to determine if further action needs to be taken.

TAILORING THE TREATMENT TO THE INDIVIDUAL CLIENT

Therapy programs provide a useful structure for clinicians, guiding them through a series of steps and treatment stages. However, a one-size-fits-all approach is unlikely to meet the needs of all clients, and this is certainly true with children who stutter. Most researchers and clinicians agree that no two children who stutter are the same; therefore, each child will require treatment to be tailored to his or her specific needs.

As stated earlier, Palin PCI starts with a detailed assessment from which an individualized treatment program is devised. The child's needs, together with the family's circumstances, dictate the specific components of the therapy. This means that personal and cultural factors for the child and family are integral to the assessment and therapy process.

To ensure that children and families from diverse cultural and linguistic backgrounds have access to this approach, it is frequently necessary to arrange for advocates and/or interpreters to assist in assessment and therapy. At the Palin Centre, professional interpreters who have been appropriately trained are used, rather than family members, to ensure that interpersonal factors are not interfering with the information that is being exchanged. Interpreters can also be invaluable in providing the clinician with general information about a particular culture; for example, attitudes to disability, roles of mothers and fathers, and expectations of therapy. However, these generalizations about a culture must always be regarded as such, as each family will have its own unique set of attitudes and customs.

In a similar way, it is important that families have equal access to Palin PCI, whatever their personal circumstances may be. When there are two parents with the child at home, both are involved in the assessment and therapy program. When one parent is living away from home (e.g., working or studying abroad), therapy would proceed with the parent who is available, and then further input would be arranged when the other parent is at home. If parents have separated or divorced but are both caring for the child, they are asked whether they want to attend sessions together or separately. In the case of single-parent families, if there is a significant other caregiver (e.g., a new partner or a grandparent who the parent wishes to include), they are invited to participate in sessions. If another person cares for the child (e.g., foster parent, child minder, nanny, or grandparent), this person can be involved in assessment and therapy.

Other personal factors may have an impact on the timing and nature of therapy. Parents who are experiencing relationship issues or health, finance, or housing concerns may find it difficult to engage with the therapy process because these issues may be a greater priority for the family. Clinicians may be able to provide support, give practical guidance, or help parents to find support elsewhere. In circumstances like these, it is important to be realistic about expectations of what therapy can achieve. For parents, taking on new tasks as a part of therapy is always a challenge, and to try to do this in the context of other stresses requires sensitivity and flexibility to reach a successful conclusion.

As with all speech and language therapy, there are some cultural groups who find aspects of Palin PCI challenging. For example, there are some parents who may not be accustomed to the idea of playing with toys and do not usually engage in imaginative play with their preschool child. However, they may be encouraged to consider other activities they engage in at home that are also suitable for Special Times, such as a cooking activity or going to the park together. Furthermore, cultural differences may exist with regard to use of eye contact, taking turns to speak, or sleep regimens. However, these can usually be managed within the framework of Palin PCI because the fundamental principle of the therapy is to work with the family to identify what works for them and how this can be adapted to support the needs of the child who is stuttering.

One of the strengths of Palin PCI is that it is based on the premise that parents instinctively know what helps their children and are already acting on this knowledge much of the time. Palin PCI helps them to do more. Therefore, they are not being asked to stop doing something or to start using a new and different style. This means that whatever a parent's cultural or personal style may be of interacting with and managing their child, they will be developing the aspects of this that they understand to be most helpful to their stuttering child. In this way, Palin PCI has, at its core, the means to be sensitive to individual families' needs, both culturally and personally.

APPLICATION TO AN INDIVIDUAL CHILD

M and his parents came for a full assessment of his fluency when he was age 3 years 8 months. He started to stutter gradually at the age of 2.5 years. He was reported as talking late with a limited vocabulary compared with his peers, and his mother said that "he had never spoken clearly and his sounds weren't right." M was referred to the Palin Centre by his local speech and language therapist who had been offering advice and monitoring over an 18-month period. M's mother said that during that time, his fluency had been patchy and that each time stuttering re-emerged it stayed longer. She said that the stuttering had become increasingly severe over the last 6 months with no periods of remission, and she noticed that excitement and tiredness made the stuttering worse. She also reported that he had been a confident little boy but that this confidence had been decreasing over 6 months. At the time of the assessment, she noticed that he was hesitant in new situations and talking less and that other people were beginning to talk for him. M's mother described herself as becoming increasingly anxious as she watched him struggle to get the words out, and despite following all the advice she had been given, nothing she did seemed to help. She was also worried that he might get teased or bullied when he started school. His father had a more laid back approach to M's stuttering, believing it would get better in time.

There was a maternal family history of stuttering. M's grandfather stuttered throughout his life, and an uncle stuttered until he was a teenager but subsequently recovered.

During the initial assessment, a speech sample was video recorded and analyzed, identifying a rate of 6.4% syllables stuttered. There were repetitions of up to 12 times, prolongations that lasted up to 6 seconds, and blocks accompanied by facial tension.

When asked about his talking, M said that sometimes "it was hard for him to say things." His parents said he would refer to his "bad voice," and they had noticed times when he would give up or change words that were proving hard to get out. M's parents described his speech on the day of the assessment as being "in a good phase" and that his stuttering was often much more severe. On a rating scale of 0 to 7, where 0 is normal and 7 is very severe, both parents rated M's speech as 5 on the day of the assessment (in a good patch) and 7 at other times. In terms of their worry about the stuttering, they rated themselves as 6, where 0 is not worried at all and 7 is extremely worried.

During the assessment, The British Picture Vocabulary Scale (BPVS) (Dunn et al., 1997), a formal measure of M's receptive language skills, was administered and demonstrated that he had above-average scores for his age. The Renfrew Action Picture Test (Renfrew, 1997), an expressive language test, placed him above average for giving information but only average in his knowledge and use of grammatical skills. Furthermore, there was evidence of immaturities in his speech sound system. At age 3:8, he was still fronting sounds such as /k/ and /g/ and reducing blends such as "weet" for "sweet," which sometimes made his speech difficult for people to understand. M's attention span was observed to be short. In terms of temperament, M was described by his parents as a sensitive child who likes to get things right and is easily upset.

These assessment findings identified the factors that seemed most relevant in the development of M's stuttering and indicated his level of vulnerability to persistent stuttering.

M's level of vulnerability to persistent stuttering was judged to be moderate to high, based on the following indicators:

- History of delayed speech and language development
- Mismatch in speech and language skills
- Time since onset of stuttering
- Stuttering getting worse over time
- Family history of stuttering
- Parental anxiety
- Child's sensitivity and reactivity to errors

On the strength of this assessment, it was decided to offer the family a course of Palin PCI. M's age, his short concentration span, and his sensitivity to the breakdown in his fluency made this a more appropriate option than a more direct speech approach at this stage.

Palin PCI was tailored to M and his family's needs by focusing on the following areas:

- Establishing Special Time
- Building M's confidence
- Helping M manage his feelings more easily
- Monitoring tiredness and bedtime routines
- Interaction strategies aimed at helping M give himself sufficient time to think and plan what he is going to say

SESSION 1

Session 1 started with a reminder of the results of the assessments and M's particular needs, such as having complex things to say and needing more time to plan, structure, and produce them. M's parents were also concerned about his sensitivity and were wondering how best to handle his worries. They reported that after the assessment, they were already being more open about his struggles with words and they had noticed that they had all been more relaxed about it.

Special Time was introduced, and the number of sessions was negotiated with M's mother, who decided she could do six a week, and M's father, who agreed to do four. A video was made of each parent playing with M for 5 minutes in the clinic.

The parents were also interested in reading about children's feelings, and a chapter called "Helping Children Deal with Their Feelings" in the book by Faber and Mazlish (1980, pp. 1-47) was recommended.

SESSION 2

After checking that the homework had been completed, M's parents were invited to consider what M needed based on their understanding of his current skills in order to be more fluent. They said they thought that "his brain was going faster than his mouth" and he needed to give himself more time to plan and structure the complicated ideas he was often trying to express. They then watched the video made the previous week. They were encouraged to look at their communication with M and notice the things they were doing that seemed to help. M's father found this difficult at first, but once directed to look at a particular section, he noticed that the pace of the conversation was relaxed and unhurried and that there were often pauses when no one spoke. He also noticed that they each had an equal share of the turns. These observations were discussed in terms of how they might help support M's fluency. When asked to consider a target that he would like to concentrate on during his Special Times, M's father said that he thought comments worked better for M than questions, and so he would concentrate on making more comments. M's mother noticed that she was pausing at times, had good eye contact, and was sitting at his level and opposite him so she could see his face and he could see hers. She decided that it helped when she paused and followed M's leads in play, and she decided to work on following his leads more because this would help him dictate the pace and focus of the play. These

targets were also discussed in terms of M's identified needs and how they might help him with his fluency, his language, and also his confidence.

The chapter on helping children deal with their feelings from Faber and Mazlish (1980) was discussed with the parents, and they decided to implement some of the strategies suggested in the book, such as listening, acknowledging his feelings, and resisting the temptation to give advice.

The targets for the week included to follow M's leads for the mother and to make more comments instead of questions for the father.

SESSION 3

Both parents had completed their homework but were worried that they had not been able to implement their targets as well as they would have liked. However, once they had made a new video and looked at it, they realized they were doing much better than they thought. M's father noticed that he was making many more comments and pausing and pacing himself in a way that he could see was helpful to M. He thought that his new target could be to use shorter sentences that matched M's more often because he could see how that might help M keep his language simple and increase his fluency.

M's mother was pleased with her ability to follow his lead and also thought she was pausing more and matching his rate better. She had become aware that M's natural rate was slow and that he seemed to need the extra time.

M's parents were also keen to help build M's confidence, so the chapter on praise from Faber and Mazlish (1980) was recommended.

The targets for the week included matching M's rate of speech for the mother and matching M's sentence length for the father.

SESSION 4

Under normal circumstances, six consecutive sessions would be arranged. However, for M's family, the fourth session came after a short break because the family had been away. There had been an increase in stuttering for several days over this period. M's parents reported that they believed this increase was due to excitement, tiredness, and lack of the normal routines. They reported that they had managed the situation very differently this time because they knew what to do. They made efforts to restore the normal routines and get M to bed on time. As a result, when they came for the session, they felt that M's speech was beginning to get back on track. They made a video and were able to reinforce themselves for the changes they could now see in their communication styles. The mother was aware that her comments were more helpful than questions, and the father noticed that M responded well when he followed his leads in play.

The targets for the week included making more comments for the mother and following M's lead more often for the father.

SESSION 5

When asked to indicate what was going well concerning their son, both parents were pleased to report that they were noticing more fluency, especially in their Special Times. They said they were more relaxed about M's speech and feeling more confident about what they were doing. They also reported feeling more comfortable with the changes they were making and the impact these were having. Both parents had read the Faber and Mazlish (1980) praise chapter. Although they were aware of the importance of praise and felt they were quite good at praising generally, they could see the added value of the specific praise described in the chapter. They agreed to praise M once a day in this way and record it on the praise log. They made a new video and reinforced the strategies that were going well, of which there were many; they also commented that M was often more fluent during the

Special Times. Both parents decided that their current three targets were sufficient.

SESSION 6

This session followed the same format as before and included a discussion about how to continue working on their targets during the home-based Consolidation Period.

After 6 weeks, they returned for a reassessment of M's speech, and the parents again completed the parents' rating scales. M's fluency had increased, and both parents were pleased with the progress he was making. They were more confident in managing his fluency. In fact, they were sufficiently confident to want to continue on their own, sending in homework sheets with occasional monitoring over the next 3 months.

Figure 5.4 tracks M's stuttering over time. These measures were obtained from 10-minute video samples of M interacting with his mother at home in a play session. The tapes were collected at weekly intervals for (a) 6 weeks prior to therapy to establish a baseline, (b) 6 weeks during therapy, (c) 6 weeks during the home-based consolidation phase, and (d) 6 weeks after the consolidation. The next six occasions were collected at intervals of approximately 6 weeks. The increase in stuttering in phase (b) was associated with considerable excitement over a holiday break. The two increases in phase (d) were associated with starting nursery school and settling in. M took a little time to settle in, but his parents felt very comfortable about seeing him through this time without further help.

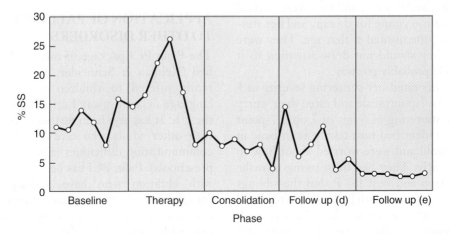

Figure 5.4. M's fluency in percent syllables stuttered (%SS) over the five phases of baseline, treatment, and follow-up.

CASE STUDY

P was 4 years 2 months old when the family was referred to the Palin Centre for an assessment. She had been stuttering for 18 months, and her parents were very concerned because it was not getting any better.

The child assessment indicated that P had above average verbal comprehension. However, her expressive language scores indicated that she had some difficulties with planning and organizing complex grammatical structures and had specific difficulties with word retrieval. She was aware of her stuttering and had no strategies for managing it. She said that sometimes it was "hard to get the words out" and that it made her feel "a bit upset."

The interaction video demonstrated that P's parents were supporting her fluency in a variety of ways, some of which could be built upon to address her particular difficulties, such as increasing the use of pauses, reducing the pace of interactions, and following P's leads more.

During the parent interview, P's parents said she had started talking later than her sisters and that her speech had never been very fluent. They said they were worried because the stuttering had changed and P was now getting stuck at times and screwing up her face in an effort to get the words out. They said that her speech was most fluent in one-to-one situations and when there was no time pressure. She had two articulate older sisters and a younger brother, and there was a strong family history of persistent stuttering on both sides of the family. She was described by her parents as sensitive, a worrier, and easily upset by little things. The family saw a therapist when P was 3, and they were advised that she was too young for therapy and her stuttering was quite normal at that age. They were told that they should not draw attention to it and it would probably go away.

P's parents rated her stuttering severity as 5 out of 7 on a 7-point scale and rated their worry about her stuttering as 6 out of 7 on a 7-point scale. They identified turn taking as an issue in the household and were worried about how to handle it fairly. They had been trying to make everyone stop and wait for P, but the siblings were not so accommodating. They also reported that P's speech was worse when she was tired, under pressure, or the center of attention. P's parents talked about the difficulties they had organizing routines such as getting the children to bed on time. They said that P needed her sleep and often went to bed later than they felt was good for her.

The parents said they wanted to understand what they could do to help and for P to get some help "so she doesn't struggle so hard to get the words out."

CASE STUDY QUESTIONS

1. What factors in the case history indicate that this child is at risk of persistence?
2. What role might parental anxiety play in the management of early stuttering?
3. How might following a child's lead influence the interaction between parent and child?
4. How is transfer managed in Palin PCI?
5. What factors should be considered in the timing and nature of more direct work on fluency?

FUTURE DIRECTIONS

TRAINING

The Palin Centre has a comprehensive training program and offers postgraduate training in Palin PCI across the United Kingdom (UK). As a result, Palin PCI is used extensively in speech and language therapy clinics throughout the UK as a standard package of care for early stuttering. This training program is being extended outside the UK into European countries and the United States.

APPLICATION OF PALIN PCI TO OTHER DISORDERS

The Palin PCI package of care has been modified (Kelman & Schneider, 1994) and is currently offered to children with speech and language delay in many Early Years Centres in the UK. It has also been further adapted for use with other adults who care for children with communication difficulties (e.g., in schools and preschools). Palin PCI has been used effectively with children who have additional and/or complex speech and language difficulties (e.g., children with autistic spectrum disorder, children with learning difficulties).

RESEARCH

Future research needs to focus on further developing hypotheses regarding which children are likely to respond to Palin PCI, which children may need additional direct fluency therapy, and which may need only direct fluency therapy. In addition, further research is needed to understand the mechanisms by which Palin PCI significantly reduces stuttering and which components of the program are essential in bringing about this change. It will be important to consider clinical effectiveness of Palin PCI in a wider range of nonspecialist settings, as well as measuring its effects as it is applied to other populations, such as other speech and language disorders or bilingual children.

SUMMARY

We expect that Palin PCI will continue to change and evolve over time. This is as it should be. Reflective practice, user feedback, and advances in research will continue to inform this process, and Palin PCI will develop accordingly.

CHAPTER SUMMARY

- Stuttering is viewed as multifactorial; predisposing physiologic and linguistic factors may be significant in the onset and development of stuttering, and the interaction of these with emotional and environmental aspects may contribute to the severity and persistence of the disorder and the impact it has on a child and the family.
- A detailed multifactorial assessment identifies those factors that may be contributing to the stuttering, as well as the child's level of vulnerability to persistence, and indicates areas for therapeutic intervention
- The main focus of Palin PCI is the child, his or her profile of skills, and facilitating further development of the naturally occurring fluency within the environment.
- Palin PCI is conducted over six once-weekly treatment sessions with Special Time as home practice, followed by a home-based consolidation period of 6 weeks, and then review and further input as appropriate.

Palin PCI achieves its effects by:

- Building on parents' or caregivers' knowledge and confidence in what helps and enhancing existing behaviors that support fluency.
- Developing with parents a shared understanding of the child's particular profile of speech and language strengths and vulnerabilities.
- Acknowledging that the underlying vulnerabilities that predispose children to stuttering may also make it more difficult for them to be fluent in the context of typical adult-child interactions.
- Using video feedback to help parents discover what they are already doing that supports their child's fluency, and reinforcing their ability to interact in ways that match the child's fluency needs.
- Collaborating with parents in setting their own targets and reinforcing themselves and their children as they make progress.
- Facilitating parents rather than telling them what to do; a parent's instinctive expertise is elicited, developed, and reinforced.
- Providing parents with a better understanding of the problem and confidence in their ability to use a number of strategies to manage the problem successfully.

CHAPTER REVIEW QUESTIONS

1. What factors might indicate that a child is at risk of more persistent stuttering?
2. What are the similarities and differences between this program and a direct therapy program for this age group, such as the Lidcombe Program?
3. When compared with other programs that involve parents, what is different about the way this program engages parents in therapy?
4. What are the key principles of Palin PCI?
5. How might you help parents identify targets to work on?
6. What skills might a therapist need to support parents in the therapy process?
7. What factors might explain variability in the outcome of therapy?
8. What factors would indicate that a child is appropriate for therapy?

9. How could this program be adapted to allow for cultural differences?
10. How might this program be applied to a stuttering child who also has significant delays in speech and language development?

SUGGESTED READINGS

Guitar, B. (2006). *Stuttering: An Integrated Approach to Its Nature and Treatment* (3rd ed.). Baltimore: Lippincott Williams & Wilkins.

Kelman, E., & Nicholas, A. (2008). *Practical Intervention for Early Childhood Stammering: Palin PCI.*

Milton Keynes, United Kingdom: Speechmark Publishing Limited.

Matthews, S., Williams, R., & Pring, T. (1997). Parent–child interaction therapy and dysfluency: a single-case study. *European Journal of Disorders of Communication, 32,* 346–357.

Millard, S., Nicholas, A., & Cook, F. (2008). Is parent–child interaction therapy effective in reducing stuttering? *Journal of Speech Hearing and Research, 51,* 636–650.

Millard, S.K., Edwards, S. & Cook, F. (2009) Parent–child interaction therapy: Adding to the evidence. *International Journal of Speech & Language Pathology,* Vol 11. Issue 1. pp 61–76.

CHAPTER 6

Stuttering Prevention and Early Intervention: A Multidimensional Approach

Sheryl R. Gottwald

CHAPTER OUTLINE

KEY TERMS

Capacities (for fluency): areas of skill that contribute to a person's ability to speak rapidly, smoothly, and with ease, including speech motor control, language formulation, social-emotional maturity, and cognitive skill.

Demands (on fluency): conditions that place stress on a child's ability to speak with normal fluency that originate from the child or may be imposed by the child's communication partners.

Regression: when stuttering reappears after a period of remission.

INTRODUCTION

PRINCIPLES OF THERAPY

The benefits of early intervention for stuttering have been heralded by numerous research efforts over the last 20 years (for example, see Gottwald & Starkweather, 1999; Onslow, Packman, & Harrison, 2003; Yaruss, Coleman, & Hammer, 2006). The early intervention stuttering treatment method described in this chapter is a multidimensional one. First, the child's fluency skills are strengthened through participation in direct therapy. At the same time, fluency stress in the child's environment is reduced to provide an optimal setting for the prevention of a lifelong stuttering problem.

NATURE OF INTENDED CLIENT

In this method, children between the ages of 2 and 6 years and their families are considered eligible for participation. Because a large number of preschool children who stutter will outgrow the problem without help (Ryan, 2001; Yairi & Ambrose, 1999), families are counseled to make decisions about participating in therapy based on several factors. Children who show signs of struggled stuttering, are reacting to their speech difficulties, and/or demonstrate a large number of risk factors, such as family history or a worsening of the stuttering problem (Ryan, 2001; Yairi et al., 1996), are encouraged to engage in therapy as soon as possible.

PRIMARY GOAL

The primary goal of this treatment approach is that of *secondary prevention* (Cole, 1986). By intervening early, young children who are at risk for persistent stuttering have the opportunity to learn to speak with normal fluency. The method is usually implemented over a relatively short period of time, although some families may take a much longer time for successful completion. The family is the primary unit for intervention, but the term is used flexibly. The child's parents, siblings, and any other significant person in the child's life (e.g., grandparents, other caregivers, teachers) may be invited to become active participants.

METHODS

Children and their families participate in an hour-long therapy session once per week. During this session, children may learn to speak in a slower, more relaxed way, use *normal disfluencies*, and/or replace stuttering with a less struggled production of the word. Their families will learn about fluency and stuttering, will identify factors that support fluency for their child, will learn how to modify their child's talking environments to include those fluency supports, and will learn how to talk about their child's speech with their child and with other significant people in the child's life.

THEORETICAL BASIS FOR THE TREATMENT APPROACH

VIEWS ON THE NATURE OF STUTTERING

Stuttering is a disorder in which the movements of speech may be poorly coordinated, not well planned, inappropriately timed, and/or slow (Starkweather, Gottwald, & Halfond, 1990). In addition, cognitive organization, speech-language formulation, temperament, and the pragmatic demands of interaction affect a speaker's ability to produce speech in a smooth, effortless, and rapid way. Difficulties organizing language ideas, retrieving words, responding flexibly, or initiating interactions may challenge the fluency of preschoolers who stutter (Starkweather & Givens-Ackerman, 1997).

The method described in this chapter is based on the "demands and capacities model" of stuttering development (Adams, 1990). Throughout early childhood, children are acquiring the **capacities** (skills) they need to speak fluently. These skills include speech motor control, language formulation, social-emotional maturity, and cognitive ability. At the same time, **demands** (expectations) placed on the child from listeners or from the child himself or herself are also growing. When skills and expectations develop concurrently, the child is able to speak with normal fluency. If, at any time, expectations exceed the child's skills, stuttering occurs. If the child's skills develop rapidly enough or if environmental expectations are minimized, stuttering remits.

As an example, consider Danny, a 4.5-year-old boy who had been stuttering for over a year before he and his family started therapy. Danny's mother and his two sisters spoke rapidly and often. Danny, on the other hand, spoke much more slowly than his family did. However, he attempted to participate in conversations with them at their fast-paced level. When Danny rushed to get a turn to express his opinion, stuttering was often apparent. In therapy, Danny learned to use a slower, more relaxed speech style when he conversed with his family. This adaptation facilitated speech motor coordination, allowing Danny to better manage normal fluency.

Danny's family learned to share conversational turn taking with Danny, to allow pause time between conversation turns, and to use a slower speech rate themselves. These environmental modifications decreased the time pressure demands that were associated with Danny's stuttering. By reducing these environmental demands and by supporting Danny's ability to better control his speech-motor system, Danny was able to speak with normal fluency.

CAPACITIES FOR FLUENT SPEECH PRODUCTION

To speak in a continuous, rapid, and effortless way, children develop competencies in several areas. The first area is that of speech motor control. This area includes the rate of syllable production and the coordination of speech movements independent of rate. Capacities such as reacting quickly to external and internal stimuli, moving muscle groups rapidly, and timing movements in a reciprocal fashion contribute to speech motor control (Starkweather, 1987).

Research suggests that a child's ability to speak quickly and continuously develops as the child grows (Kowal, O'Connell, & Sabin, 1975; Walker et al., 1992; Yairi, 1981). Two-year-old children speak more slowly (Amster, 1984) and use more discontinuities (Wexler & Mysak, 1982) than 5-year-old children do. Likewise, the child's ability to manage the rhythm, coordination, and timing of speech production also develops (Allen & Hawkins, 1980; Starkweather, 1987).

Capacities for fluency related to language include the ability to retrieve words, to formulate the grammar of sentences, to produce lengthy and complex utterances, to use language for a variety of purposes, and to interact. We know that when sentences increase in length, typical preschoolers increase their speech rate (Amster, 1984). In light of speech motor constraints, increasing speech rate may be disruptive to fluency for children who stutter.

Numerous studies have assessed the relationship between language capacity and stuttering. Children who stutter are often reported to have depressed language scores when compared to matched controls (Arndt & Healey, 2001; Kline & Starkweather, 1979). Research by Wilkenfeld and Curlee (1997) suggested that stuttering was more likely to occur in longer utterances. In another study, as language complexity increased, so did stuttering (Weiss & Zebrowski, 1992).

In this same study, when children were more assertive with language (e.g., when they made requests, statements, or performatives such as jokes), stuttering occurred more frequently than when the children answered questions ($\chi^2(1) = 28.66$, $p < .001$). When language formulation demands increased, the frequency of disfluencies also increased (Peterson & Gordon, 1982).

Cognitive and social-emotional capacities may promote fluent speech, but the literature is less clear about these relationships. There is some evidence that children who stutter are more sensitive and perfectionistic than their counterparts who do not stutter (Oyler & Ramig, 1995). Anderson et al. (2003) further demonstrated that the children who stuttered in their study were more hypervigilant ($F(1,60) = 7.45$, $p = .008$), slower to adapt ($F(1,60) = 6.14$, $p = .016$), and had more difficulty managing biologic functions such as toileting ($F(1,60) = 4.93$, $p = .03$) than their same-age peers who did not stutter. These authors suggested that these temperamental characteristics might conceivably contribute to increased stuttering.

DEMANDS ON FLUENCY

Environmental factors that encourage children to talk quickly with few pauses place motoric demands on the child's fluency system. For example, the speech-language behaviors of the significant people in the child's life may inadvertently increase motoric demand. If the child has to answer a more complex question, repeat a sentence because it was not clear, say a long sentence, talk in a rushed atmosphere, keep up with a fast-speaking parent, and/or give information while an adult is waiting, the child may feel increased time pressure (Starkweather & Givens-Ackerman, 1997). This need to speak quickly and continuously seems likely to precipitate stuttering for children whose speech motor systems work more effectively at a slower speed.

Research has demonstrated that children with more advanced stuttering had parents who talked much more quickly than the children (Kelly, 1994; Yaruss & Conture, 1995). Research has also shown that mothers of children who stuttered spoke faster than mothers of children who did not stutter (Meyers & Freeman, 1985a). In addition, Guitar et al. (1992) found that parent speech rate was significantly correlated with the child's stuttering in a single case study design. When the mother reduced her speech rate, the child's stuttering decreased ($r = .70, p < .01$).

When children interrupted others or were interrupted, their stuttering increased (Meyers & Freeman, 1985b). Likewise when one speaker began talking before the other one had finished, stuttering was more likely to occur (Kelly & Conture, 1992). Children may feel pressured to maintain the pace of conversation set up by their partner's rapid speech rate and turn-taking style. However, these children may not have the speech motor capacity to do so, and their fluency may therefore be compromised.

Language, cognitive, and personality demands may also stress fluency. When adults asked children questions requiring longer responses and/or more complex responses, the children's stuttering increased (length: $t(22) = 5.216; p < .001$; complexity: $t(22) = 5.21; p < .001$; Gaines, Runyan, & Meyers, 1991). In several studies, maternal language complexity was significantly related to whether or not stuttering persisted. Mothers who used more complex language (Kloth et al., 1999) or produced longer sentences and a larger number of different words (Rommel et al., 2000) were more likely to have children who continued to stutter after several years.

A child whose motor speech capacity is less well developed must put additional mental effort into talking. If the child must also formulate an answer to a more complex question, remember details about a story, or talk during an exciting or anxious experience, fluency will be stressed. As Levelt (1989) and others (Peters & Starkweather, 1990) have noted, demands on one performance area (e.g., cognitive, language, or social-emotional) may decrease functioning in other areas (e.g., speech motor skill).

RATIONALE FOR THERAPY APPROACH

It is widely believed that stuttering is likely caused by a combination of factors rather than a single etiology (Guitar, 2006). A child whose family history is positive for stuttering, who has a sensitive, hypervigilant personality, who interacts in a fast-paced household, and who uses more complex language may be at a higher risk for stuttering than a child demonstrating just one of these risk factors. This child's capacity

for fluency may be compromised by a weak speech motor system and by personality characteristics that are less tolerant of disruption. These capacities may be further stressed by demands to move faster and to speak in a more complex way that are covertly expressed by the child's environment.

The treatment plan that emanates from this model is a simple one conceptually but may sometimes be not so simple when applied to the individual clients. The speech-language pathologist identifies the child's capacities that are more susceptible to breakdown and then supports the development of those capacities through direct intervention. Simultaneously, the clinician and family identify demands that may be stressing the child's skill use and modify them to provide a more ideal environment for fluency growth.

It is important to keep in mind that capacities and demands will change as children and their families grow. Therefore, the "demands and capacities" model is not a static one. The child's fluency skills (capacities) will develop with time and practice, and the expectations (demands) placed on the child to use those skills will also change. It is essential that the child's treatment team adapt the treatment plan to meet the evolving nature of the child's fluency needs.

EMPIRICAL BASIS FOR THE TREATMENT APPROACH

A number of treatment programs have presented strategies to help young children improve their capacities for fluency (e.g., Ingham, 1999; Onslow & Packman, 1999; Pindzola, 1987; Riley & Riley, 1991; Runyan & Runyan, 1993). Likewise, many preschool treatment regimens have focused on helping parents decrease demands as they support their children's fluency (e.g., Guitar, 2006; Rustin & Cook, 1995; Yaruss, Coleman, & Hammer, 2006). Some programs address fluency skills and environmental demands concurrently (e.g., Conture, 2001; Fosnot & Woodford, 1992; Gottwald & Starkweather, 1995; Gregory, 1999). This chapter will first review the outcomes of a sampling of these programs since they provide support for the multidimensional treatment program described in this chapter. Next, it will review studies that have examined the impact on fluency of modifying one or more environmental demands. Finally, outcome data for the method described in this chapter will be reviewed.

OUTCOME DATA FOR PROGRAMS ADDRESSING CAPACITIES AND/OR DEMANDS

Conture and Melnick (1999) reported on a parent-child group approach to treat early stuttering. Groups met once a week in 12-week cycles. Parents learned how to speak slowly to their children while adjusting the length and complexity of their sentences. They also worked on talking with the child without interrupting. Parents were encouraged to focus on incorporating one skill at a time and to use group support to help in the change process.

In the children's group, youngsters also learned how to take appropriate conversation turns, how to wait for a turn to talk, and how to listen to others. If a more direct approach to therapy was indicated, children learned techniques to adjust the timing and the tension of their speech.

Treatment efficacy data shared by these authors indicated that of 200 youngsters who completed the program, 70% maintained near normal fluency ($\leq$3% stuttered syllables over an 8-week period) in 12 to 36 weeks from the time of treatment onset. Of the 30% who continued to stutter, approximately 10% recovered with a longer treatment time. The authors suggested that the remaining 20% may have achieved adequate fluency but required a different treatment approach. Since these youngsters and their families did not successfully complete the parent-child group therapy program, they were no longer followed by the authors of this study.

Yaruss, Coleman, and Hammer (2006) described a family-focused treatment approach that included both parent counseling and direct intervention for their children. The parent component, consisting of six to eight sessions scheduled once per week or every other week, was conducted prior to initiation of the child's direct treatment.

Parents learned ways to become involved in their children's treatment and implemented modifications in their interactions with their children that supported fluency. The program began by educating parents about stuttering and

fluency development. The speech-language pathologist then helped parents minimize aspects of their interaction that appeared to be fluency stressful such as rapid pace of conversation or use of demanding questions.

If the child was still stuttering following completion of the parent-focused part of the program, direct child therapy was initiated. The child-focused components of therapy incorporated an array of approaches depending on the child's needs, including speech modification, stuttering modification, and development of effective communication skills.

Yaruss, Coleman, and Hammer (2006) reported outcome data for 17 preschoolers at risk for persistent stuttering. The children demonstrated a significant reduction in the frequency of stuttered disfluencies in the clinical setting ($z = -3.517$; $p < .001$), with a pretreatment mean of 16.4% syllables stuttered (standard deviation [SD] = 6.6%) and a posttreatment mean of 3.2% syllables stuttered (SD = 2.0%). Whereas 11 children achieved normal fluency after the parent-focused component of therapy, six children also received child-focused intervention. After successful completion of treatment, all but one of the children used normal fluency during follow-up evaluations conducted between 1 and 3 years after treatment.

Eleven of the 17 families completed questionnaires rating their satisfaction with the treatment program. Ninety-one percent of the families (10 of 11 families) reported that they were very satisfied with the parent-focused treatment, whereas one family reported feeling moderately satisfied.

STUDIES EXAMINING THE IMPACT OF ENVIRONMENTAL MODIFICATIONS

Although additional research is needed, there is some evidence that when parents modify specific fluency demands, their children's fluency skills improve (Nipold & Rudzinski, 1995). For example, Langlois and Long (1988) reported on a case study examining the impact of turn taking on fluency. When an equal number of parent and child speaking turns were established in this family, the child's stuttering frequency decreased. Likewise, Winslow and Guitar (1994) reported that a preschool child's fluency skills improved when the family structured turn taking by instituting talking-time rules.

Much of this research has focused on how reductions in the mother's speech rate affected her preschool child's fluency performance. Stephenson-Opsal and Bernstein Ratner (1988) presented two case studies that showed significant correlations between reductions in the mother's speech rate and reductions in the preschool child's stuttering. In another study, Guitar and Marchinkoski (2001) found that when mothers reduced their speech rates, five of the six children in the study also showed significant reductions in their speech rates. In a single-case study, Guitar et al. (1992) found a strong correlation between reductions in the mother's speech rate and reductions in her preschooler's primary stuttering.

A pilot study conducted by Starkweather and Gottwald (1993) looked at the relationship between changes that occurred in the child's environment and changes in the child's fluency levels over the course of treatment. Environmental variables that were examined included parent speech rate, number of questions parents asked, and the number of times parents interrupted their children. Although all of these behaviors changed over the course of treatment, the variable that significantly correlated with reduction in the child's stuttering was reduction in the parent's speech rate ($r = .47$; $p < .05$; $N = 14$).

OUTCOME DATA FOR THE MULTIDIMENSIONAL METHOD DESCRIBED IN THIS CHAPTER

The method's effectiveness was first reported by Starkweather, Gottwald, and Halfond (1990). Of the initial 55 families who participated in the Stuttering Prevention Clinic at Temple University, 16 families received only brief parent counseling (one to three sessions) after a limited evaluation with no direct child therapy. Their children demonstrated close to normal fluency skills for their age and were not considered to be at high risk for persistent stuttering, and the parents expressed confidence in managing their children's fluency without direct intervention. All 16 children continued to demonstrate normal fluency according to parent report during follow-up telephone calls made for 2 years after the family was seen in the clinic.

Of the initial 55 families, 39 children and their families participated in comprehensive evaluations followed by treatment at the Stuttering Prevention Clinic. While the child participated in 1 hour per week of direct individual therapy conducted by a second-year graduate student, the child's family worked with a another graduate student to address the child's fluency environment. Seven families withdrew from the program before its completion. When those families were contacted prior to the 1990 report, four of the children continued to stutter.

Of the remaining 32 children, three children were still in therapy at the time of the report, and 29 children had successfully completed the program. Each family was monitored for up to 2 years after discharge from therapy. Their children continued to speak with normal fluency according to parent report. The average length of therapy was 12 sessions, but some children required up to 40 sessions before being dismissed from treatment.

Gottwald and Starkweather (1999) reported on an additional 15 families who were treated in southern New Hampshire by the first author from 1993 to 1996 using the method described in this chapter. One child withdrew from the program, and on follow-up phone calls, that child continued to stutter. The remaining 14 children achieved normal fluency ($\leq 1\%$ stuttering-like disfluencies) and continued to use normal fluency for at least 1 year after discharge according to parent report via telephone contact. The average duration of therapy was 14.5 sessions, including family counseling and direct therapy for the children.

From 1997 to 2006, an additional 30 families participated in this multidimensional treatment method. Families were enrolled in therapy if their children were at high risk for persistent stuttering (Ryan, 2001; Yaruss, Coleman, & Hammer, 2006). Specifically, children were considered at high risk when several of the following factors were present: (1) the family reported that the child's stuttering problems had become significantly more frequent and/or struggled over time, (2) there was a family history of stuttering, (3) the child was a boy, (4) the child's stuttering emerged after age 4 years, and (5) the child presented with other speech, language, or motor delays.

Chronologic age at initiation of services ranged from 2 years 10 months to 6 years 2 months, with an average age of 4 years 3 months. There were 23 boys and 7 girls. Time spent stuttering prior to therapy varied widely from 3.5 months to 24 months, with an average of 13 months elapsing before families sought help. Thirteen of the families (43%) reported a family history of stuttering, and 16 of the children (53%) had other speech and/or language problems in addition to stuttering.

At least three different speech samples were analyzed to compute percent syllables stuttered at the outset of intervention. Figures ranged from 3.5% to 19.8% syllables stuttered, with an average of 9.03% syllables stuttered for the group when therapy began. Three families continued in treatment at the time these results were reported. The 27 families who completed the program participated in an average of 13.7 sessions prior to discharge, with a range of 5 to 31 sessions. Percent syllables stuttered averaged over the last three therapy sessions ranged from no stuttering (0% syllables stuttered) to 3.5% syllables stuttered, with an average of 1.51% syllables stuttered at discharge for the 27 children. During follow-up telephone calls made to families no less than 1 year after discharge from therapy, parents reported that 26 of the 27 children (96%) continued to use normal fluency. One girl who moved out of state began stuttering again following the family's relocation. She required additional therapy for stuttering into her elementary school years and continued to present with a mild stutter.

PRACTICAL REQUIREMENTS

SETTING FOR INTERVENTION

Both family and direct child therapies should be conducted in a quiet play space equipped with developmentally appropriate toys. The environment should afford the family privacy as they share their feelings and work on developing a supportive fluency model. When those conditions can be achieved, this method can be effectively implemented in a variety of settings, including the family's home, a preschool or daycare, a hospital or university clinic, and a private practice.

MATERIALS AND EQUIPMENT

Direct therapy for the child is conducted through play. Therefore, developmentally appropriate play-based materials must be available. Depending on the child's skill level, toys may be needed to facilitate spontaneous speech, such as having a tea party with stuffed animals or building with Legos. Or the child may need more structured practice as skills are in the process of being learned. Table-top games such as Candyland or Go Fish may be more appropriate when greater structure is desirable.

Clinicians will also need a camcorder and playback equipment on hand during each session. Video recordings will assist in the collection of ongoing assessment data to verify progress and to identify areas of treatment that need change. By watching interactions on tape with the clinician, family members can identify those aspects of the interaction that are associated with the child's fluent and stuttered speech. In addition, family members can assess their own skill development. For example, parents might use the video recording to evaluate how well they have implemented a slower speech rate.

CLINICAL SKILLS

Clinicians implementing this early intervention method must have their Certificate of Clinical Competence from the American Speech, Language and Hearing Association and experience in working with preschool children or be directly supervised by a speech-language pathologist with these qualifications. Likewise, clinicians must be knowledgeable about fluency and stuttering development and signs of risk for continued stuttering. Professionals using this method must have experience with how to shape fluency (e.g., understand how to help children reduce speech rate, initiate phonation gently, blend words in a phrase, and produce speech sounds easily) and how to modify stuttering in young children (e.g., understand how to help children identify, evaluate, and change stutters). An understanding of the process of behavior change, the principles of learning, and the importance of reinforcement is also crucial to successfully using this method.

Since working with families is an integral component of this method, clinicians will need to feel comfortable and confident interacting not only with their child client but also the client's parents, siblings, teachers, extended family members, and any other significant person in the child's life. Although speech-language pathologists may have much experience working with children, they may have less experience, and thus may feel less secure, when working directly with the child's family. By spending time with families, using their strengths in therapy, and joining with families to help their children, the speech-language pathologist will gain the experience needed to effectively intervene at this level.

Clinicians wishing to help families support their preschool children who stutter will need to call upon counseling skills to effectively implement this method. Feelings and attitudes affect behavior. A parent who is consumed with guilt about having caused the child's stuttering will have little energy left to devote to therapy. Unless those feelings and attitudes are addressed, they have the potential to continue to sabotage intervention (Egan, 2002; Flasher & Fogle, 2004; Hill & O'Brien, 2000; Luterman, 2001; Murphy & Dillon, 2003).

TIME DEMANDS OF THE PROGRAM

The program is designed to be implemented in one 60-minute block per week with time devoted to a combination of direct child therapy and family counseling. The amount of time spent working directly with the child or counseling the family varies depending on need. At times, clinicians may devote the entire hour to family counseling. The child's parents may meet alone with the clinician for this hour to address feelings such as frustration or to grieve their child's imperfect speech. On the other hand, the hour might be devoted to teaching both the child and family how to speak in a slower more relaxed way. Typically, though, some of this hour-long session will address the child's speech skills or feelings while the remainder of the hour will be spent helping families.

Sessions where both child and family needs are met usually begin with a play period where the child, family, and clinician interact spontaneously around some preferred toys. This allows the clinician to observe the child's fluency as well as the family's use of previously learned interventions. The clinician will often videotape this play period so that the parents

and clinician can evaluate the factors that supported the child's fluency.

See Video Clip 1 for this chapter on thePoint for a sample of parent-child play recorded early in the child's treatment program. In this play segment, the child has several stuttering events. The mother uses a relatively slow speech rate but asks questions requiring longer, more complex answers. The mother does not seem to be sure how to respond when the child stutters.

Following this play, the parents and clinician can discuss the child's fluency patterns over the previous week, talk about the skills that the parents practiced, and identify issues to address in the current session (e.g., environmental factors that may benefit from change, such as the child's response to feeling rushed). The parents and clinician may brainstorm solutions for the identified issue, and the parents will select the solution that best fits their family. If the solution is a speech, language, or interaction skill that the clinician can demonstrate and that the parents can practice (e.g., using the 2-second pause to decrease time pressure), they can spend the next part of the session playing with the child and practicing the skill. If the solution is something the parent will implement at home (e.g., adjusting the daily schedule so there is more time for transitioning from one activity to the next), then the parents write the modification down on their home practice sheet to address later.

Next, the parents and clinician can play with the child as the child develops the skills that they feel will foster development of normal fluency. A child may learn how to speak more slowly and wait his or her turn to talk. In addition, the child may learn how to identify stutters and replace them with more relaxed and typical disfluencies. The family will leave with tasks to implement over the coming week that are based on the issues and skills addressed in the session.

KEY COMPONENTS OF THE PROGRAM

GOALS OF TREATMENT

Once a preschool child has been identified as being at risk for continuing to stutter and the family has expressed a desire to participate in this multidimensional treatment program, therapy is initiated. The goals of treatment are two-fold: (1) reduce the demands or stressors on the child's current fluency level, which may stem from the environment or the child, and (2) support the child's capacities for producing normally fluent speech. Treatment is individualized for each family and evolves as the child's and family's needs change.

Objectives of the Family Component of the Program

The significant people in the child's life will first learn about fluency and stuttering development so they have the information they need to make educated decisions for their family. Family members will next learn about things that stress fluency and how to alter those stressors to make it easier for the child to speak smoothly. Families may also learn how to speak in a different way to provide more appropriate fluency models for their children. They will learn how to practice with their children, when to reinforce their children's use of new skills, and how to support their children's sense of self-esteem.

Families will develop these skills through discussion with the clinician, by watching the clinician work with the child, by sharing ideas with other families, and by practicing skills under the guidance of the clinician. Families complete home practice activities designed to test the benefits of newly identified skills.

Families will also monitor their children's daily fluency levels as well as the environmental variables that impact fluency. Families will make note of easier and more difficult speaking times for their children. They will then identify the factors that appear to support and stress the child's fluency level. Finally, families will develop and implement modifications to reduce the stressors that they identified.

Objectives of Direct Child Therapy

Children will experience natural growth in each capacity area as they move through the preschool years (Starkweather & Givens-Ackerman, 1997). By communicating in a more appropriate environment where fluency demands have been reduced, children will gain the experience they need to support the growth of fluency capacities.

There are several things clinicians can teach young children to do that will also support capacity growth. Children may learn how to speak in a slower, more relaxed way and/or how to change struggled stuttering. Clinicians will use imagery, meaningful vocabulary, modeling, and praise to develop and establish these new skills. When children are ready, clinicians will gradually provide opportunities for use of the skills in more demanding environments. Activities are designed to slowly increase cognitive, language, speech motor, and pragmatic stressors. This may be accomplished in part by decreasing activity structure, increasing the number of communication partners, increasing the pace of conversation, and varying the kind of talking that takes place (e.g., answering complex questions, retelling, explaining).

Motivation is key to growth in therapy; it is essential that children have fun as they participate in therapy and that they experience success at each step of the treatment hierarchy. Children may still experience moments of struggled stuttering in and out of therapy as they learn new skills. It is vital that children have the opportunity to explore feelings related to their difficulties talking so that they continue to want to participate in therapy.

STRATEGIES AND PROCEDURES FOR WORKING WITH FAMILIES

Family Systems as the Focus in Therapy

It is important to keep in mind that children grow up in the context of a family system. For some children, the family consists of a mother, father, and siblings. For others, the family system includes not only nuclear family members but also grandparents, other extended family members, and people who are considered "family." When planning a change for one part of the system (e.g., the preschool child who stutters), all parts must be considered for the change to remain in place.

An example will help clarify this point. Children who learn to use a slower speaking rate will attempt to converse in that slower, more relaxed manner with family. Family members will react to the change in some way; they may slow down themselves, they may get frustrated, or they may speak faster in an attempt to make up time. If the family learns about the skill the child is developing and understands its usefulness, they will be better prepared to react in a more supportive way.

Families are the child's primary caregivers and partners. Their encouragement, acceptance, models, and unconditional love will make the path of change for their children that much easier to follow. In addition, stuttering is a speech disorder that affects the listener as well as the speaker. Families will have feelings about and reactions to their children's speech struggles. Consequently, children will observe those reactions and are likely to internalize those feelings. Families benefit from an opportunity to explore their feelings to help them react to their children's speech in a more supportive way.

The family system interacts with other systems that will be impacted by changes the family makes. These systems may include the extended family, the neighborhood, and the child's preschool. Families frequently ask me how to share information with relatives and neighbors without hurting their feelings when they unknowingly contradict what the child is taught in therapy (e.g., relatives may say to the child, "Take a deep breath; slow down"). Likewise, teachers have asked for guidance in structuring their classrooms to better support the child's fluency. If the child learns a skill, the family can also learn about the skill and how to support its use at home, in the neighborhood, with extended family, and so forth.

Roles Families Play in Therapy

Families can play many different roles in therapy as displayed in Table 6.1. The clinician can ask each family to choose how they would like to be involved. Families can help identify the objectives of therapy and the hierarchy in which they are addressed. One set of parents was especially concerned about their child's increased stuttering during large family gatherings. The extended family got together often, and they were reportedly a lively, fast-talking group. The parents wanted help to make these occasions more enjoyable for their child. We wrote this as an objective to be addressed early in the treatment process.

Another major role families can play is to simply support their children. If families understand the skills their children are learning, they can offer praise when the children use the skill (e.g., "Wow, that was great easy bouncing you just used!"). Families can also let their children know how much they enjoy listening to them regardless of fluency. They can reinforce their children's efforts, acknowledge how difficult talking can be at times, and provide encouragement by letting their children know that talking will get easier.

Families can be practice partners with their children outside of therapy. As children are learning new skills, they will need to practice them in order to use the skill easily. Families can set up speech playtimes on a daily basis and select fun activities that allow their children time to practice speech skills at a level at which they can be successful. Families will need to be able to model the skill themselves and know how to select a play activity that will allow their children to experience success. Other roles families can play include modifying their children's talking environments to reduce demands, learning new ways to talk to facilitate their children's fluency, and educating others about their children's fluency needs.

In sessions with families, the clinician can follow a structure that allows family members to identify the focus of the session and to develop solutions for the problems that are raised. This sequence of activities is displayed in Table 6.2. First, the clinician can review the family's experiences with their children's fluency since the last therapy session.

See Video Clips 2 and 3 for this chapter. In Video Clip 2 (Parents Debriefing), the parents share information about their experiences with their child's fluency over the preceding week. In Video Clip 3 (Parent Self-Evaluation), the mother describes how she feels her own speech rate is developing.

Families will share their fluency charts and/or journals, discuss notable talking experiences their children had, and evaluate how their home practice sessions went over the previous week.

Table 6.1. *Roles Families Can Play in Early Intervention for Stuttering*

1. Help develop goals
2. Provide the child with emotional support
3. Praise the child's use of skills
4. Practice skills with the child
5. Change the child's talking environment
6. Learn new ways to talk
7. Educate others

Table 6.2. *Components of Family Therapy Sessions*

1. Debrief the family's fluency experiences over past week
2. Identify areas for change with family
3. Ask family to select an area to focus on in the session
4. Brainstorm ways with the family to address the area
5. Ask family to select a preferred strategy
6. Family practices strategy with clinician and with child if appropriate
7. Family utilizes strategy outside of therapy
8. Family reports on strategy's effectiveness in next session

Next, the clinician can ask families to identify an area of focus for the current session by encouraging them to talk about problems they would like to explore, speech skills they would like to sharpen, or issues that they feel would benefit from discussion. There are times when families are not sure what they should focus on; the clinician can then provide them with suggestions based on my own observations of the families' interactions with their children.

See Video Clip 4 (Parents Exploring Issue) for this chapter for an example of how parents might begin to look at an issue that impacts their child's fluency skills.

After an area of focus is identified, the family and clinician may brainstorm solutions to problems, practice skills, or explore feelings through discussion. Open-ended questions (e.g., "So tell me more about what your family does during large family get-togethers."), rephrasing problems (e.g., "It sounds like your child stutters more when he is in a room with lots of people all talking at once. How might you provide him with opportunity to talk with a smaller number of people in a quieter place?"), and summarizing what families say (e.g., "These family get-togethers are important to you, and you would like to find a way to make them easier for your child.") may be helpful counseling strategies. By the end of the session, families may have a strategy or skill they can try out over the following week to foster growth in their children's fluency. The clinician can ask families to share with me the effectiveness of the skill when we meet again the following week.

See Video Clip 5 (Parents Brainstorming Solutions) for a sample of parents developing solutions for problems they have identified.

Table 6.3. *Helping Families Become Educated Consumers*

Issues for Discussion Include:

1. Cause of stuttering
2. Spontaneous recovery
3. Characteristics of normal fluency
4. Signs of stuttering risk
5. Things that maintain stuttering
6. The process of therapy
7. Regression
8. Behavior management
9. Talking about stuttering with the child
10. Educating others about stuttering

Helping Families Become Educated Consumers

The goal of this part of the program is to assist families in learning about fluency and stuttering development so that they will have the information they need to make well-supported decisions for their children. Although each family's need for information will vary, the areas listed in Table 6.3 are often addressed most frequently. One of the first things I ask families to do is to record their own speech while they talk with a friend either in person or on the telephone. When they listen to the recording, family members are often amazed to discover that they have many disfluencies in their speech as they talk spontaneously. We discuss the fact that normal disfluencies such as whole-word and phrase repetitions or use of filler words such as "um" and "ah" give speakers a bit more time to formulate and express their ideas. These disfluencies are a typical part of talking and are to be expected in their children's speech when therapy is completed.

Next, family members will benefit from learning about speech behaviors their children use that indicate stuttering is developing in severity. If they know that a rise in pitch accompanying a prolongation indicates increased tension, families can more readily identify and be able to address the demands that may have supported this behavior. Likewise, it is helpful for families to learn about various types of stutters and which types are associated with a more severe problem. With this information, families who see their children blocking will understand that the speech system is frozen in place, rather than assuming that the child is, "just thinking before he talks," as one parent commented. When children are in the maintenance phase of therapy, knowledge of signs of stuttering risk is once again helpful. If a parent notices an increase in part-word as opposed to whole-word repetitions or if the child begins to use a large number of filler words (e.g., um, ah), these behaviors may signal the need for more direct home management and/or active intervention.

Families will also benefit from learning about factors that may maintain stuttering such as time pressure, interruptions, and use of long, complex sentences. This may help families be better observers of their own children's fluency patterns at home. Another topic that may prove beneficial to address is **regression**. Fluency skills do not typically develop in a linear pattern. Children will acquire some skills, show growth in fluency, and then level out for a period of time during which additional fluency development is not noted. It is also not uncommon for children to make some gains but then revert back to more stuttering for a period of time. If families understand the process of fluency growth and are aware that regression may occur, they can be prepared to address the increased stuttering as soon as it appears.

When I talk with families about their behavior management techniques, they often report placing fewer expectations on their children who stutter for fear of putting undue stress on fluency. We talk about the importance of consistent behavior management and discuss ways to discipline without expecting (or allowing) children to talk at the time they are being reprimanded.

Families often express concern about whether they should talk about stuttering with their children and, if so, how they should talk about it. They worry that if they increase their children's awareness of speech difficulty, their children will become anxious and then stutter more. I tell families that even very young children who stutter are usually aware on some level that talking is hard at times. If parents do not address the topic or react with subtle disapproval, children will get the impression that stuttering is something they should avoid. The effort that children devote to trying not to stutter will most likely make the stuttering problem worse.

Families can acknowledge struggled stuttering using words that are meaningful to their children. It might be a neutral comment such as, "That was a tough word to say," followed by encouragement such as, "Words are hard to say sometimes, but it will get easier to talk as you get older." Or it may be an acknowledgement of the child's expressed or underlying feelings. After a particularly struggled stutter, one child told his mother that he was never going to talk again. It was important for this mother to let the child know that it must be frightening when you try but are unable to talk. I encourage parents to follow-up on discussions about difficulty talking by letting their children know that their family will listen no matter how long it takes for the children to express themselves and that the family is learning things to help the child speak more easily.

Modifying Speech and Language Skills of Family Members to Support Fluency

Increased time pressure for talking occurs in many ways (Starkweather & Givens-Ackerman, 1997). When children attempt to answer complex questions, time pressure may be evident. The person who asked the question is waiting for a response, but the child must spend time processing the question and formulating the answer. Likewise, when children attempt to communicate while the family is rushing somewhere, when older siblings are waiting for their turn to talk, and when children are speaking with an adult who is talking rapidly, time pressure is increased. If families can make adjustments in some of the factors that increase time pressure, such as those listed in Table 6.4, it will be easier for their children to speak without stuttering.

Research efforts have repeatedly shown that when families speak more slowly, children's fluency skills improve (Starkweather & Gottwald, 1993; Stephenson-Opsal & Bernstein Ratner, 1988). Therefore, it will be helpful to teach

Table 6.4. *Modifying the Speech and Language of Family Members*

1. Use a speech rate that more closely matches the child's
2. Pause between conversation turns
3. Eliminate questions requiring long, complex answers
4. Respond to the content of the child's message regardless of fluency
5. Acknowledge struggled stutters using meaningful words

adults who speak quickly to children who stutter how to slow down. Adults have learned to slow their speech rates by pausing more often and by slightly stretching continuant sounds. I have found that parents feel most comfortable using a slower speech rate after they have had a chance to listen to my models, to practice with me, and to evaluate their own use of slower speech rate while watching video-recorded interactions with their children.

While working on reducing speech rate, I also encourage families to slow the pace of conversation down. In a typical conversation, a respondent begins talking at the tail end of the first speaker's sentence. There is very little, if any, pause time between turns, placing a significant amount of time pressure on a young child. Also, research has shown that children tend to stutter more when interrupted and when interrupting others (Kelly & Conture, 1992; Meyers & Freeman, 1985b). In addition, research has suggested that when turn taking is established, fluency skills improve (Winslow & Guitar, 1994).

One suggestion I make to families is that they use the 2-second pause when interacting with the child who stutters. By pausing for a count of two before responding to the child or before saying another sentence, family members are allowing extra time between conversation turns and thus reducing time pressure associated with interaction. In addition, I ask families to talk about the importance of respecting the talking turns of others. Following this discussion, families may develop enjoyable ways to monitor turn taking at home. One family gave each person a cup of pennies at the dinner table. Family members then gave away pennies if they interrupted others and collected pennies if others interrupted them. Although this game did not extend over a long period of time, it helped to underscore the worthiness of waiting your turn to talk.

Answering questions in and of itself does not appear to be fluency disruptive for children who stutter (Wilkenfeld & Curlee, 1997). However, when children use longer, more complex sentences to answer questions, they are more likely to stutter (Gaines, Runyan, & Meyers, 1991). Parents can learn to ask yes or no questions or questions requiring a specific response (e.g., "Did you play on the swings or tricycles at recess today?"). They can also communicate with preschool teachers or daycare providers before talking with their children. In this way, parents will be able to talk about topics that are familiar to their children and will be able to share the communication load with their children more equally.

Helping Families Modify the Child's Talking Environment

Families can also decrease talking time pressure by adjusting environmental factors such as schedules and the pace of activities, as described in Table 6.5. One set of parents decided to get up a half-hour earlier so they would be ready to attend to their children in a more relaxed way when the children woke up. They reported that conversations around the breakfast table were more casual, that time pressure was reduced, and that the child's fluency improved. Another family realized that they had too many activities scheduled and were rushing from one thing to the next throughout the week. They decided to cancel several of these activities so they would have some time for relaxing together at home.

There are times in a family's daily life when the parents are occupied with household activities and cannot fully attend to conversation with the child. When parents are trying to fix supper with limited time, for example, it may be difficult for them to listen attentively to their preschooler. The child who stutters may feel that the parent has not heard them and may try harder to get and keep the parent's attention. With this increased effort, the child may stutter more. I suggest to parents that they consider

Table 6.5. *Modifying the Child's Talking Environment*

1. Institute turn-taking rules to eliminate interruptions
2. Allow ample time for activities and transitions
3. Show child ways to get a talking turn without stressing fluency
4. Eliminate talking at stressful times
5. Set up a special parent-child playtime each day
6. Maintain structure and routine where possible

setting up "quiet times" when they are not able to be effective listeners. The parent can help the child become involved in a nontalking activity until the parent is able to focus on the child once again. Activities such as having children watch a favorite movie, look at books, or play quietly with toys may be appropriate quiet time choices.

I also recommend that parents set up a special playtime each day for the child who stutters. Parents should select 15 to 20 minutes of time that they can devote their full attention to the child without interruptions from other family members, the telephone, or visitors. During this playtime, parents can help their child select a play activity that will allow the child to use normally fluent speech. Depending on the child's skill level, parents may offer more structured tabletop activities such as playing games (e.g., Candyland or Memory) or other less structured activities such as building with Legos.

The goal of the play activity is two fold: it is a time for children to practice speaking with normal fluency in a relaxed, nondemanding setting, and it is a time for parents to manipulate environmental variables to make it easy for their children to speak smoothly. Depending on the factors that are fluency supportive for individual children, parents may practice a slower speech rate, allow more silences as they play with their children, and refrain from asking their children to use long, complex language during this special playtime. Parents have reported looking forward to this playtime because it gave them an opportunity to successfully implement the strategies they were learning in therapy.

Parents have reported that during times of transition, such as getting ready to leave the house to go shopping, their children stutter more. The clinician may then talk about the stressors that may contribute to increased stuttering at these times. Parents have noted that they have many things to do during times of transition (e.g., making sure that the children have their jackets and snacks, that everyone has used the bathroom before leaving, that car seats are appropriately fastened). At the same time that the parents are focused on these tasks, their children are asking many questions about the upcoming activity. When parents identify the potential fluency stressors (e.g., a parent who may not be able to concentrate fully on the child's message, a child who is anxious or excited about the new activity), it is easier for them to develop a modification that decreases the demands. Some parents have set up no-talking rules during times of transition. They have told their children that it will be easier for the parent to listen once the activity is underway. Other parents have talked with their children before the transition about the schedule of activities once the change is made.

Helping Families Manage Feelings That Emanate from Stuttering

Families will first need to understand their own feelings before they are able to meet their children's emotional needs. There are many feelings that families have related to their children's stuttering. Families most often report feeling worried about their children's future if the stuttering should persist. This anxiety is expressed in many ways. Some parents told me that they got angry with their child when the child stuttered even though they knew that the child was not stuttering on purpose. Other parents said it was hard for them to even respond to the child because they were so worried by the child's stuttering. Still other parents reported turning away from the child or answering the child in a rushed way following a moment of stuttering.

Parents have also shared with me their feelings of guilt around their children's stuttering, believing that they must have done something wrong that caused this problem to develop.

They list such things as having used toilet training techniques that were too harsh or having gone on a vacation without the children as reasons why the child started stuttering. Parents have expressed sadness that their children have been confronted with such a difficult speech problem. If not addressed, all of these feelings can preoccupy parents, limiting the time and energy they will have available to devote to management of their children's fluency needs.

Therefore, it is essential to spend time helping families to share their feelings related to their children's fluency. By talking about their feelings, family members will understand them better and will not be so immobilized by them. For example, after expressing feelings of guilt in a supportive environment, families can then look more objectively at what were the more likely causes of the child's stuttering.

When families understand their own feelings better, they can then help their children. Families can be encouraged to put their children's feelings into words that are meaningful for the child. Young children are often puzzled when words are difficult to say and will ask their parents why they can't talk. Or, children may stamp their feet in an angry way when they have difficulty expressing themselves. Other children will stop talking altogether and will refuse to finish their message when stuttering has occurred.

I ask families to talk about how they think their child is feeling during difficult talking times and how the child is expressing those feelings. We then select words that the parents can say to help the child share his feelings. Usually something simple such as, "It makes you mad when words get stuck" or "It's a little scary when you try to say something and you can't," is enough. I encourage parents to let children know that they are still growing and that, as they get bigger, talking will get easier.

I also suggest that parents compare learning to talk with learning the many other skills their children are developing. If children understand that when they learned to ride a bike, they needed training wheels and that it was a little wobbly at first, it may be easier for them to respond in a less concerned way to their speech difficulties. If their parents respond to the stuttering in a neutral way, it will be easier for the children to do so as well.

Sometimes stuttering can become such a big issue in the eyes of the family that it is the only thing they think of when they consider the child. Feelings of anxiety and concern about the child's future can become all-encompassing, and the family may lose sight of all of the other aspects of the child's personality. So another focus of family therapy is to help the family once again value all of the child's strengths. I ask families to talk about their children, what they do well, and what makes them special in the family's eyes. Families then brainstorm ways to highlight these strengths. One family set up an elaborate gym in their backyard because they realized how skilled their youngster was on equipment such as parallel bars. The child soon became the gym champ of the neighborhood and took on the role of teaching the neighborhood children how to have fun on the gym set. The focus was directed to the child's strengths and away from his speech difficulty. When the child's confidence is increased, motor control and coordination overall seem to be enhanced.

It is often helpful for families to share experiences with other families whose preschool children stutter. Whenever numbers, meeting space, and staff permit, I supplement individual family therapy with group therapy. Group participation provides parents with the opportunity to learn how others are managing their children's fluency needs. It is also an opportunity for parents to share their feelings with, and receive support from, other parents who truly understand. With this chance to explore feelings in an accepting and supportive environment, parents are usually energized to more directly address their child's fluency needs. If group therapy is not possible, I encourage families to contact other families who have been or are currently participating in fluency services for their preschooler.

WORKING DIRECTLY WITH THE CHILD
Children Who Stutter with Minimal Struggle

These children typically use many whole-word and part-word repetitions. Although there may be two or more iterations of the unit and repetitions are often rapid, there is little struggle associated with the disfluency. Muscle tension is minimal, pitch is unaffected, and syllable structure remains unchanged.

The clinician will first set up a therapy environment that makes it as easy as possible for the child to speak with normal fluency. Since each child will have unique fluency profiles, clinicians will use information obtained during the assessment, as well as ongoing observation, to identify the environmental factors pertinent for each child. A fluency-enhancing setting might include some or all of the following components (Gottwald & Starkweather, 1999):

- Slow-normal speech rate
- Relaxed (less effortful) speech style
- Slow and relaxed conversation pace
- Numerous pauses and silences
- Reduced requests for nonspontaneous speech
- Use of disfluencies that are normal for the child's age
- Elimination of questions requiring long, complex answers

In addition, clinicians will allow ample time for completion of each activity so that the session remains relaxed and unhurried. Children will be invited to engage in activities that they enjoy and can be successful with. If children can effectively use fluency skills at the sentence level, clinicians will choose activities that allow practice at this level, such as barrier games with colorforms or using a recipe book to make a snack. As fluency skills improve, clinicians will increase fluency demands in the activities they offer children. At later stages in therapy, for example, children may be able to use fluency skills while they build with Legos or play a bean bag toss game. Both tasks include more spontaneous interactions with physical activity and increased emotional involvement.

Next, clinicians will help children use a slower and/or more relaxed speech style. First, clinicians will model a slower speech rate and will use longer pauses as they talk. To highlight the concept of "slow," clinicians will move in a slower way as well.

For children whose language skills are developed enough, it is often helpful to describe slow speech using words the child will understand. I suggest that clinicians provide possible labels but include the children in the search for the best name for slower, more relaxed speech. I frequently read an abridged version of the "Tortoise and Hare" fable. We talk about the slow and steady turtle who won the race and how talking slowly is helpful too. Following this introduction, some children choose the label "turtle talk" for the slower speech. Others have suggested labels such as "dinosaur speech," "sleepy time speech," or "snail speech." The children were able to easily connect the concept of "slow" with these animals with which they have had experience.

See Video Clip 6 (Labeling Turtle Talk) for a sample of this slower, more relaxed speech style.

Once the label has been selected, preschoolers enjoy moving their whole bodies around the therapy room like turtles or snails. I show the children how talking slowly is like moving slowly, and I model this reduced speech rate for them. It is also sometimes helpful to label the faster speech rate. I encourage children to choose fast-speech labels that are somewhat separate from the lives of small children such as "hare speech" or "fire engine speech." If children label faster talking as "race car speech" for example, they may want to emulate the race car that goes fast to win the race.

Some children are speaking at a rate that is appropriate for them but may have a higher level of muscle tension as they talk. For these children, it is helpful to focus on an easier speech style. I model a more relaxed speech style, label it "easy speech" or "soft speech" and compare that to "hard speech," which is tense and effortful. Children again choose labels for these different ways to talk. One label that preschoolers have preferred is "teddy bear speech." Most children have a beloved stuffed animal that is usually soft and cuddly. I compare easy talking with how their stuffed animals feel. We then contrast that with something hard such as a rock, and I model tight, tense talking that we might call "rock speech."

Children first use the new speech style in short, simple sentences, such as those used during a Go Fish card game. I provide much verbal praise for the child's use of slower speech. Children listen to their parents' and my use of the target rate as we play with them. Occasionally I will "forget" and use faster or tenser speech. Children have lots of fun catching me when I speak in the faster or tenser way. They can also listen for their family's use of slower speech at home. Preschoolers can have lots of fun handing out "speeding tickets" to family members who forget to speak slowly (Conture, 2001).

See Video Clip 7 (Practicing Turtle Talk 1) for a sample activity that allows parent and child to become comfortable with slower speech in a structured activity.

As children become more skilled with slow rate or gentle speech, fluency demands are increased. Depending on the child's profile, clinicians will select activities that require longer sentences and more spontaneous speech. In addition, pragmatic demands are increased along with the pace of conversation. Children may be required to use the new speech rate while interacting in a group, explaining an activity to a parent, or giving directions to a sibling. Cognitive demands are added such as engaging children in problem-solving tasks. Emotional demands are increased by incorporating excitement and tension into activities such as playing timed games or going on a field trip.

See Video Clips 8 and 9 (Practicing Turtle Talk 3 and Story Telling) for examples of how to extend use of slower speech to less structured activities.

Some children speak at the target rate in a relatively relaxed way but still stutter at the beginning of many of their sentences. I have found it helpful to teach these children to use a whole-word repetition at the beginning of some of their sentences to make getting started easier. We call them "easy bounces" or "bouncy words" and tell children that everyone uses this kind of talking at times. We practice using whole-word repetitions at the beginning of structured sentences, such as during a Memory Game (e.g., "I I got a _____."). These whole-word repetitions are slow, relaxed, and thoughtful in nature. The clinician models many whole-word repetitions at the beginning of sentences in spontaneous speech and comments on them (e.g., "That was my easy bounce."). When the

child uses a whole-word repetition spontaneously, the clinician points it out and praises the child for use of a "bouncy word." It is important that parents understand that whole-word repetitions are not necessarily stuttering and that preschoolers with normal fluency use many whole-word repetitions as they talk. If parents feel comfortable enough, they can learn to model whole-word repetitions in their own speech and praise the child for use of whole-word repetitions as well.

See Video Clips 10 and 11 (Teaching Easy Bounces and Secret Signal) for examples of how to help children use normal disfluencies and how to engage children in developing a signal they can use with their families to extend strategy use.

During direct child therapy, I also teach the concept of turn taking. I tell children that there is only one rule in my room and that is that only one person speaks at a time. I provide a way for children to let me know that they want a turn to talk. Some children have found it easy to put their hand on my arm when they have something to say or to raise their hand as they learned in preschool. It is important to keep in mind that for many of the young children I work with, conversational turn taking is a skill that is just beginning to emerge.

Some preschoolers will use volume in an attempt to manage fluency. If this is the case, I teach children about "indoor" and "outdoor" voices. We practice speaking in both ways and then identify the "indoor" voice as the preferred choice for the therapy room. By modeling the appropriate loudness level and praising the child's use of an "indoor voice," this secondary behavior is usually terminated without difficulty.

Since even very young children can understand on some level that talking is hard at times, I comment on this with all of the children I work with. I begin by telling children how much I enjoy playing and talking with them. I praise their storytelling abilities and display much interest in the things they share with me regardless of their fluency levels. As we play, I occasionally include a pseudo-stutter in my speech and comment in a neutral way on how sometimes it is hard for me to say words. I follow this comment by telling children that everyone has trouble talking sometimes, especially children, since they are still learning how to talk. I do not request that children participate in this exchange, but if they do, I acknowledge their comments.

Working with the Child Who Struggles to Talk

If children continue to stutter, it is likely that the stuttering will become tighter and tenser as they struggle to escape the unpleasant experience of stuttering (Gottwald & Starkweather, 1999). Preschoolers are often quite open in their attempts to stop stuttering. They may puff out their cheeks, push on their cheeks, stamp their feet, hit their legs, or jump up and down when they are stuck on words. One 5-year-old boy told me he was never going to talk again following a particularly struggled stutter. Clinicians will help these children learn how to decrease the struggle in their stuttering.

To change a behavior, children must know what the behavior is and when it occurs. Many of the preschool children I work with have not yet developed the metalinguistic skills necessary to think and talk about their speech. So it is helpful to talk about speech in terms that children will understand. I model a relaxed form of stuttering that the child typically uses and ask children to label that kind of talking. Some preferred labels children have offered are "bumpy," "sticky," and "slippery" speech. I help children find a label that describes the speech behavior underlying the stutter.

Once a label is chosen, the children and I play games to identify stuttering in each other's speech. We collect points each time we hear a stutter, and whoever gets the most points wins the game. In a matter-of-fact way, I label the kind of stuttering children identify (e.g., "Yes, that was bumpy speech!"), praise children for listening, and continue on with the game. Through this activity, children learn that stuttering is not something that needs to be avoided. When children start stuttering on purpose to get more points, I know that they feel more comfortable with stuttering and will be less likely to work hard to avoid it in the future.

Next I show children how to say the stuttered word differently. Depending on the child's needs and maturity, I may model one or more modification strategies. If children use many prolongations, I model "bouncy speech," where

the word or part of the word is repeated one time in a slow, rhythmic, and relaxed way (e.g., "s→o" becomes "so so"). If children use many repetitions, I model "stretchy speech," where the word is said in a slower way (e.g., "stre-stre-stretchy" becomes "streeetchy"). For children with blocks, I model "sliding speech" where the initial consonant is produced in a slower, gentler way (e.g., "→she" becomes "shhhhhe").

Sometimes it is enough to model the modified disfluency. Often children will imitate the easier disfluency without direct teaching. When this is not the case, I show children how to replace stuttering with the less tense disfluency. Children then are rewarded for replacing the stutter, first with my direction (e.g., "Can you say that word in a bouncy way?") and then independently. Preschoolers will often make the switch to easier, more typical disfluencies quickly, and struggled stutters then drop out.

It is important to continue to address the child's feelings throughout direct therapy. Earlier in this chapter, I talked about providing opportunities for children to express feelings in a nurturing environment as well as about providing them with reassurance that talking will get easier as they grow and learn. I recommend that clinicians provide children with the language they need to share their feelings. I plan activities around feeling expression and spend time examining with preschoolers what makes us mad, sad, confused, and embarrassed.

One procedure I have found useful in this regard is to read a fairy tale with the child. I select fairy tales that I think the child will like and in which feelings I would like the child to learn about are demonstrated. After reading, we may make puppets or paint pictures of the characters in the fairy tale. We then use those puppets or pictures to talk about and role play the feelings expressed by those characters. *Goldilocks and the Three Bears* gives us an opportunity to talk about being "scared," and we can role play the "mad" feelings expressed by the wolf in *The Three Little Pigs*. Likewise, I've used the *Cinderella* story and *Three Billy Goats Gruff* to begin discussions about feeling "sad."

One youngster related feelings to colors. When his mother was upset, she told him she was feeling "red." The family selected other colors for different feelings; for example, yellow was happy, while blue was sad. The mother told me that one morning her youngster greeted her with, "I woke up feeling red today, Mom." They then talked about things that made them feel upset and ended up giving each other a prolonged bear hug.

ASSESSMENT METHODS TO SUPPORT ONGOING DECISION MAKING

The purpose of assessment is to evaluate the child's capacities for speaking with normal fluency and to identify the demands that may be currently stressing those capacities. Assessment occurs with the first telephone contact and continues throughout the therapy program. Evaluations conducted at the beginning of each therapy session help clinicians continue to monitor how the child's fluency develops and responds to environmental change.

DIAGNOSING THE PROBLEM
Initial Contact with the Family

The initial telephone contact is an opportunity for family members to express their observations and concerns regarding their children's fluency. When families have a chance to share their worries with someone who is knowledgeable about the problem, their level of anxiety is often reduced. It is an opportune time, too, for clinicians to learn about the children's speech skills and possible environmental stressors. Clinicians will also begin to assess the likelihood that the children are stuttering and will continue to stutter. I answer the family's questions about stuttering and provide information about fluency and stuttering development.

While talking with the family on the telephone, I ask them questions to determine the presence of risk factors for persistent stuttering (Ryan, 2001; Yairi et al., 1996), such as gender, family history of stuttering, time since the onset of the problem, the development of the stuttering problem, and the presence of other speech-language or developmental difficulties. If there are a number of risk factors present or if the family expresses undue concern about the child's speech, I encourage the family to consider a formal evaluation to confirm the need for therapy. There are times when telephone counseling alone provides the family with the information and support they need to foster development of normal fluency for their children. When families feel comfortable managing their children's fluency on their own following the telephone contact, I suggest that we stay in touch over the next several months should their concerns about fluency once again escalate.

Interviewing the Family and Preschool Staff

The purpose of this part of formal assessment is to collect basic case history information, including detailed data about children's speech, language, and motor development and a history of the stuttering. The interview will also help us to identify environmental variables that may stress fluency, determine the kind of information families and teachers need to be educated consumers, and assess the level of emotional support these significant people require to participate actively in therapy.

One father I worked with felt that his child's stuttering was caused by a frenulum that was too short. Another mother felt sure that her child stuttered because she and her husband went on a vacation while leaving the children with their grandparents. It was clear during the interview that both families would benefit from information and emotional support to better understand the multiple factors that most likely contributed to the development of stuttering in their children.

Collecting Speech Samples for Analysis

I collect videotaped samples of the child interacting with family, teachers, and me to directly assess both capacities and demands. If possible, families also make a videotape of interactions with their children at home and at their preschools.

See Video Clip 12 (Initial Parent-Child Interaction) for a sample of the parent-child play session that was recorded in the family's home. You will observe the child's stuttering as well as the parents' interaction styles. The parents are involved in the child's play and praise the child's ideas. However, both parents ask many complex questions, speak quickly, and sometimes talk over the child.

The videotaped samples from at least three different contexts are transcribed, and a minimum of 25 utterances for each participant from the middle of each sample (providing 300 to 500 syllables per interaction) is used for examining the behaviors of both children and adults to aid in decision making.

Direct Assessment of Adult Speech

As noted earlier in this chapter, some aspects of adult speech may affect child fluency (Stark-weather & Gottwald, 1993). These variables may include speech rate, questions requiring long, complex responses, demands for speech, and interruptions. Thus, one component of assessment is to measure these speech variables in the people with whom the child spends considerable time interacting (e.g., parents, teachers, and siblings). I first listen to and then subjectively measure the speech rates of family and teachers as they interact with their children. If I observe that a family member or teacher appears to speak much more quickly than the child, I will collect a sample of the adult's speech on videotape, transcribe the sample orthographically, and measure speech rate in 10 consecutive utterances that are of relatively equal length.

When preschoolers who stutter use long, complex utterances, research has suggested that stuttering is more likely to occur (Weiss & Zebrowski, 1992; Wilkenfeld & Curlee, 1997). Thus, I also count the number of questions parents and teachers ask and identify which questions require longer, more complex responses from the child. For example, a question such as, "Are you done yet?" is much less demanding than, "Why did your teacher take your ball away today?" Likewise, if children who stutter are asked to perform verbally, such as, "Tell Daddy what happened at the park today," the stress of having to remember the details, organize the language, keep the adult's attention, and produce a longer more complex sentence may be enough to cause children to stutter. Therefore, I also examine the complexity of language tasks demanded of the child.

Research has also shown a possible relationship between interruptions and stuttering (e.g., Kelly & Conture, 1992; Winslow & Guitar, 1994). In that light, I count the number of times adults speak over their children. I also measure how much time adults spend talking compared with their children. If the adult monopolizes the conversation floor, children may feel pressed for time to express their own ideas. On the other hand, if the adult rarely contributes and children must take responsibility for the entire interaction, this added communication pressure may also prove to be fluency stressful.

In this phase of the assessment, clinicians will also examine how adults react to the child's stuttering. In one single-case study, Guitar et al. (1992) found that a mother's nonaccepting utterances were correlated significantly with her child's struggled stuttering. Verbal comments related to stuttering are noted, and nonverbal responses, such as facial expressions and body movements, are also recorded. In addition, I have found it helpful to count the number of positive and negative statements adults make to children who stutter. Shames and Florance (1980) provided a method for coding accepting and nonaccepting statements that I find useful in this regard. If children receive many negative comments and also struggle with their speech, feelings of self-worth may be jeopardized. If children feel badly about their abilities, their expectations to perform badly may be strengthened and then more easily played out.

Analyzing Children's Speech, Language, and Fluency Skills

To determine if a child is stuttering, I assess both the frequency and severity of the fluency problem. If 3% or more of the syllables produced by children are stuttered, they are considered to have a stuttering problem. However, the level of severity of the problem is based on a number of factors, including:

- Frequency of stutters
- Number of iterations per repetition
- Rate and rhythm of repetitions
- Schwa substitution for appropriate vowel
- Types of stutters (prolongations and blocks being more severe)
- Length of prolongations and blocks
- Presence of pitch rise, tremors, and/or loudness changes
- Presence of secondary behaviors
- Observable reactions to the stutter by child or family/teachers
- Difficulties in capacity areas that support fluency
- Response to trial therapy

First, I count the number of fluent syllables in the speech samples and evaluate the level of effort used to produce those syllables. I also count and record the types of normal disfluencies that are present. The child's rate of fluent speech is measured at this time.

Next, the number and kind of primary stutters are recorded. Stuttering types included in this count are (1) repetitions of some monosyllabic words, parts of words, and sounds; (2) prolongations with or without pitch rise; and (3) blocks before or in the middle of words. The frequency of occurrence per total syllables is determined (e.g., % syllables stuttered), and the frequency of occurrence of each stuttering type per total stutters is also determined. If a child uses a large number of blocks suggesting increased muscle tension, this may affect prognostic statements about length of therapy as well as therapy methods that are chosen. For example, a child with many repetitions and rapid speech rate may respond well to rate reduction therapy. On the other hand, a child with many blocks may already be speaking slowly and may benefit more from a program designed to help him or her replace the blocks with more normal disfluencies.

The average number of iterations per repetition for each type of repetitive speech is also computed. The rate and rhythm of these repetitions is assessed because fast, irregular repetitions may indicate a more advanced stuttering problem. Finally, the occurrence of pitch rise, vocal tremors, and alterations in volume in the vicinity of stuttering are noted because they are indicative of increased tension and a more advanced stuttering problem. In addition to these informal computations, a formal stuttering measurement device such as the Stuttering Severity Instrument, Third Edition (Riley, 1994) is administered to compare the child's stuttering with that of a representative group of children who stutter.

The number and kind of secondary behaviors are noted. Preschool children are often quite open about trying to avoid or escape from stuttering. Some young children I have worked with have stamped their feet on the floor, jumped up and down, and walked around in circles as they struggled to move through a difficult word.

Clinicians will also work directly with children to identify adult speech, language, and interaction behaviors that facilitate fluency. Clinicians will use a variety of fluency-enhancing strategies while playing with the child (Starkweather et al., 1990). These strategies will vary from child to child depending on the perceived demands observed in the family play session. For example, if the parents asked many demanding questions, in the clinical play session, I will avoid complex questions to see if that interaction change impacts the child's fluency.

It is also helpful to assess children's awareness of and reactions to stuttering as well as their willingness to address this topic. Even some very young children I have worked with have expressed concerns about their difficulties talking. Parents have reported that their children have asked, "Why can't I say that word, Mommy?" And children have said to me, "I don't talk right" and "I can't talk."

I begin assessing the children's awareness by pseudo-stuttering as we play, reflecting an unconcerned attitude, and commenting in a matter-of-fact way that sometimes my speech is bumpy/sticky. If the children do not noticeably react in some way to my pseudo-stuttering, I will once again pseudo-stutter, comment on it, and ask the children if they ever have bumpy/sticky speech. Children will frequently look up at me with wide eyes and say, "I have that kind of speech too!" This provides an opportunity for the clinician to talk with the child in a reassuring way using language that the child will understand.

Since fluency is supported by capacities in a number of areas, it is essential that those capacities be assessed during a diagnostic evaluation for stuttering. Clinicians will evaluate children's articulation, receptive and expressive language skills, and pragmatic skills using a variety of formal and informal measures. Cognitive skills, gross and fine motor skills, and social-emotional skills can be informally assessed through observation of the children's play, the children's interactions with others, and the children's response to evaluation procedures. If concerns arise following informal assessment, children should be referred to the appropriate disciplines for formal evaluation.

In the feedback session, I first provide families with information about their children's levels of growth in the speech motor, language, cognitive, and social-emotional capacity areas.

I then talk about specific environmental factors that seem to support and stress their children's fluency. I repeatedly tell families and teachers that the way they are interacting with their children now is not wrong and that their interaction styles did not cause the stuttering. In fact, I tell them that almost all families present with typical lifestyles that foster normal fluency growth for most children. The child who is stuttering is likely predisposed in some way. I tell parents that by altering environmental variables for a short period of time, families can better match this child's unique fluency needs.

Ongoing Assessment

The first 10 minutes of each therapy session are devoted to assessing (1) the children's current fluency levels and (2) potential fluency demands. The family plays together or children interact in their preschool classroom, depending on the setting for therapy. Clinicians observe the interaction and record the status of environmental variables that have been identified as demands in the past. Clinicians will also make note of other demands that may have arisen since the last therapy session. Using a data collection grid, clinicians will compute stuttering frequency for a 100-syllable corpus produced by the child during this interaction.

At the end of this 10-minute period, parents and/or teachers will share ratings they completed on a daily basis at home. Adults use a number scale to rate the overall level of fluency their children used throughout each day. This rating scale is based on one described by Onlsow, Packman, and Harrison (2003). Parents select a number from 1 to 10, with 1 suggesting that their children used normal fluency throughout the day and 10 correlating with the worst stuttering their children have ever demonstrated. Adults then use this graph to talk about their children's fluency variations and environmental variables that may have contributed to the changes in fluency levels.

Assessing Immediate and Long-Term Outcomes

As the frequency and severity of the child's stuttering decrease and the family learns how to modify the environment to support the child's developing fluency, treatment sessions are reduced to every other week for several months

and then once a month for the next few months. I feel comfortable discharging families when their children's frequency of stuttering is less than 3% syllables stuttered and struggled stuttering has been removed. In addition, families must feel comfortable managing their children's fluency on their own before they are discharged.

Families participate in decision making regarding when to reduce therapy sessions and how frequently therapy sessions should be scheduled. Some families feel confident enough to discontinue individual sessions sooner than others do. Once a family stops coming to therapy, they are encouraged to call the office any time they have questions about any aspect of their children's fluency, speech, or language functioning. I maintain telephone contact with families for 1 year after discharge. If families report that their children are continuing to demonstrate normal or close to normal fluency at the 1-year follow-up phone call, further contact is suspended unless families request input at a later date.

TAILORING THE TREATMENT TO THE INDIVIDUAL CLIENT

The multidimensional approach described in this chapter provides clinicians with a framework for developing individualized treatment for early stuttering. It is not designed to be a rigid set of instructions. Instead the program provides suggestions for intervention that clinicians can shape in an ongoing way to meet the individual needs of families. This flexibility in implementing the method is essential to its success.

Individuals react to change in different ways. It easier for some people to acknowledge differences in their behaviors and to embrace the change process than it is for others. I tell families that it is not necessary for each family member to be involved in all aspects of the program. I encourage family members to focus on treatment components with which they feel comfortable.

I once worked with a set of parents who both had high-powered business-related jobs. They were very concerned about their only child's stuttering problem, and both parents came to the initial assessment. As we talked about the treatment program, the father expressed reservations about his ability to slow his speech rate down and said he felt uncomfortable playing on the floor with his little boy. The mother on the other hand said she was interested in learning to talk in a more relaxed way and wanted to learn how to set up a fluency-supportive play environment at home. So the mother adjusted her communication style while the father supported the mother's efforts. The father also praised his son's developing speech skills. Both parents learned about fluency and stuttering. Given this family involvement, the child's fluency improved to normal levels by the 11th session, and the improvements were maintained over the following year.

When working with families with different cultural, linguistic, or socioeconomic backgrounds, it is fundamental that clinicians learn about the systems that are familiar to individual families. Clinicians can then alter this multidimensional treatment approach to best match the needs of the families they work with. When I worked in a Hispanic neighborhood in Philadelphia, I initially invited the parents of the child who stuttered to a meeting at the preschool to discuss their child's needs. I was viewed as the "professional," and it was difficult to get families actively involved in problem solving and planning. After discussion with the social worker on staff about cultural differences, I began setting up coffee hours during the day. I invited the family with the child who stuttered as well as relatives and friends. We had snacks and sat around talking about our lives and the lives of the children. The families in this neighborhood were more comfortable with this less formal, more community-based intervention format. In this way, the extended network learned about fluency and stuttering development and got involved in helping the child's mother reduce fluency demands.

Many of the families I have worked with have schedules that are packed with full-time work and numerous activities for their children. It has been difficult for some families to find the time to devote to weekly therapy sessions and daily speech playtime with their children. I have adapted my schedule to provide more opportunities for families to meet outside of work hours (e.g., early evening, lunch-hour appointments). I have also helped families brainstorm ways to incorporate speech playtime into an activity that is already a part of the daily schedule (e.g., bath time, story time).

A final challenge in implementing this method is related to the children. As research has suggested (Anderson et al., 2003; Olyer & Ramig, 1995), children who stutter may be more sensitive than their normally fluent peers. Some of the children I have worked with have been resistant to working directly on their stuttering. They appear to immediately interpret my suggestions to modify their stuttering as a criticism. It has taken considerably longer to help this group of children feel comfortable looking at, playing with, and ultimately changing stuttering. I have moved at the children's slower pace, providing a fun, safe place to explore and talk about stuttering. The children's families have learned how to talk about stuttering in an open, matter of fact way and how to reflect the feelings they suspected their children were dealing with.

APPLICATION TO AN INDIVIDUAL CLIENT: THE MERRILL FAMILY

EVALUATION

During an initial telephone conversation, Mrs. Merrill expressed significant concern about her 3.5-year-old son's persistent stuttering problem that had recently become even more noticeable. She said that Chris had been stuttering "since he began to talk around age 2" and that Chris had recently asked her why he couldn't say his words. Mrs. Merrill said she worried about her son's reactions to his speech difficulties and noted that she "wanted to take care of this problem as soon as I can."

Chris was 3 years 9 months old at the time of the initial evaluation. His mother, father, and 7-year-old brother, Kevin, accompanied him to the assessment session. In the first 20 minutes, the family played together while I videotaped the interaction for later analysis. Some of the characteristics of the family interaction that I felt were potential fluency disrupters included the following:

- Parents asked many questions, sometimes requesting complex language in the response.
- Parents did not talk at the child's level. They occasionally commented on the child's play but did not play along with Chris.

- Parents made frequent suggestions about how Chris could do things differently when he was playing, initiating suggestions with negatives (e.g., "No, Chris, do it this way.").
- Mother spoke much more quickly than Chris did with little pause time between sentences. Her sentences were usually long and complex. Dad used a slower, more relaxed interaction style.

During my case history interview with the parents, I learned that both parents were financial analysts in their own private practice. Chris attended preschool 5 days a week and was accompanied there before and after school by his older brother. The parents said that their days were usually rushed from morning until evening with work, extracurricular activities, and household tasks. The Merrills said they had an extended family support network and that the boys spent considerable time with their cousins.

While playing with his parents and brother, Chris stuttered on 6.42% of his syllables. Stutters included a large percentage of prolongations with some pitch rise. Following a stutter, Chris often became quiet, sometimes refusing to respond to a question asked by his parent. When I played with Chris and his brother, Chris stuttered on 5.4% of his syllables. Again, prolongations were the primary stuttering type, and they were sometimes accompanied by increased tension.

Chris scored in the high average range on tests of receptive and expressive language. Likewise, his articulation skills were appropriate for his age, and his speech was intelligible. He created complicated Lego structures during the evaluation, and his parents reported that Chris was at the top of his preschool class for mastery of preacademic skills.

Mr. and Mrs. Merrill said that Chris was a sensitive child who took a long time to warm up to new situations. Change was difficult for Chris, and he quickly became agitated when his expectations were not fulfilled. They also noted that Chris was generous and loyal once he felt comfortable with peers and adults.

THE INTERVENTION PROGRAM
Family Component

The first thing the family learned was to use a slower, more relaxed speech style. We labeled it "turtle talk" to provide an image that was mean-

ingful to the children as well as the adults. The model included not only a slower speech rate, but also a relaxed conversation pace. The family learned to pause before responding to each other. Whenever possible, all members of the family attended these family-focused sessions.

Chris enjoyed monitoring his family's use of slow speech at home. He gave out speeding tickets to his parents whenever he was able to catch them using faster speech. Each time he came to therapy, Chris proudly reported the number of tickets his parents received that week.

The next change the family implemented was to set aside a 15- to 20-minute period of time each day to play together in a relaxed way where fluency demands were minimized. The parents took turns conducting this speech playtime, and Chris's brother often participated as well. Following discussion in therapy, the parents learned to select activities and to structure interactions in a way that allowed Chris to be close to or normally fluent. As Chris's fluency skills improved, the family found ways to slowly increase demands and decrease structure.

The family completed a chart each day to rate Chris's fluency overall for the day and during the speech playtime specifically. We used those ratings and notes the family wrote on the chart to discuss other factors that impacted Chris's fluency. The parents discovered that fatigue appeared to be closely related to increases in stuttering. So Mr. and Mrs. Merrill implemented a structured bedtime routine that allowed the children to be in bed and asleep at a reasonable time each night.

Since Chris seemed to be stuttering more when talking with his mother than with his father, we talked about the differences in interaction style that may have been related to fluency. After watching several tapes of family interaction, Mrs. Merrill decided to reduce the number of questions she asked of Chris. As we played together with Chris, Mrs. Merrill practiced making statements instead of asking questions. When she felt comfortable with this in the therapy room, Mrs. Merrill transferred the skill to home. She said that there were many times that she caught herself beginning to ask Chris a question. She stopped and rephrased her idea into a comment instead.

Direct therapy for Chris revolved around using a relaxed speech style that we called "turtle talk." At first, Chris was not interested in using this new way of talking even when practice activities were play-based, fun, and involved a reward. However, when Chris had the opportunity to be the "police officer" and evaluate his family's use of slower speech, he was more invested in learning what "turtle talk" was all about. I praised Chris frequently for his use of slower, smoother speech and for his judgment of his parents' speech rates.

Chris also learned about the importance of turn taking. He was often the family member who interrupted others, especially his brother. We played games and collected points for appropriate turn taking in the office and then the family played those same games at home. When Chris wanted his parents' attention, the family decided that he should move close to them, put his hand on one of their arms, and wait until the family member looked at him before beginning his message.

In five sessions scheduled over 8 weeks, Chris developed the ability to use normal fluency (<1% syllables stuttered) in the clinic. Parent reports of fluency at home also improved considerably. Following a 4-week break from direct intervention, Chris's parents reported continued use of close to normal fluency at home. During phone calls made to the family's home over the next 6 months, Chris continued to demonstrate normal fluency with no stuttering according to parent report.

CASE STUDY

John is a 4.5-year-old boy who, along with members of his family, has participated in 19 30-minute treatment sessions over the past 7 months to address a moderately severe stuttering problem. During his initial evaluation, John stuttered on an average of 8.6% of his syllables in three different speaking contexts. His primary stutter was sound prolongation with occasional pitch rise. John began stuttering at 2 years of age, and his mother reported that the stuttering had increased in frequency and struggle since that time. John's articulation skills fell in the low average range, while his language skills tested in the 99th percentile, well above the average range. John had two older sisters who were quite verbal and a family history of stutter-

ing. John's father traveled frequently; he was not able to participate in therapy sessions because of work constraints.

During the first 3 months of therapy, John learned to use a slower, more relaxed speech style to replace stuttered (e.g., "sticky") speech. By the end of 3 months, John stuttered on an average of 3.7% of his syllables over the last three therapy sessions. His mother reported improved fluency at home as well.

John and his family subsequently took a month-long break from therapy in the summer and then returned for a follow-up visit. In this visit, John stuttered on an average of 3.2% of his syllables in three different speech samples. Stuttering consisted primarily of whole- and part-word repetitions. John's mother rated his overall daily fluency levels at home over the month as well. John averaged a rating of 2 over this period, with 1 representing normal fluency and 10 representing significant stuttering. Despite these promising fluency ratings, John's mother requested that occasional visits to my office continue since John was beginning preschool and his mother was not sure how this might impact John's fluency.

Over the next 3 months, John, his mother, and his sisters participated in one to two 30-minute treatment sessions per month. John's family learned how to take conversation turns and how to be sure that each family member got a turn to talk. In addition, John learned to use an indoor voice while at the same time maintaining his slower, more relaxed speech style. John's mother rated his speech at home primarily with a 1 and occasionally with a 2 over this time period. When we discussed the days that John's fluency was at the 2 level, his mother identified fatigue and unexpected interruptions in the daily schedule as possible contributors to the small amount of stuttering that occurred on those days. In therapy, John presented with normal fluency.

THE PROBLEM

At the end of this second 3-month period of therapy, John's mother and I talked again about taking an extended break from therapy given the consistently strong fluency skills John demonstrated over the past treatment period. When his mother discussed this option with John's father, he expressed concern that John still presented with some stuttering. John's father said he didn't always agree with the ratings that the mother gave John, suggesting that he felt John had slightly higher levels of stuttering.

1. How will you address John's father's concerns?
2. How will you determine if John is still stuttering at home as his father suggested?
3. How will you decide if John and his family should continue in regularly scheduled speech therapy sessions?
4. If you decide that additional speech therapy would be appropriate for John and his family, what objectives would you write for this next treatment period?
5. Given the father's extensive work schedule, will you include him in additional therapy, and if so, how will you do that?

FUTURE DIRECTIONS

This multidimensional method has been implemented successfully with preschool children from 2.5 to 6 years of age who are at risk for persistent stuttering. Each family has learned about ways to modify environmental factors to support fluency, and each child has participated in some form of direct fluency therapy. Additional research will help to answer the following questions:

- Can therapy be postponed for very young children who are stuttering and still have positive results? Would family supports be necessary during this waiting period, and if so, what would these supports consist of? Onslow, Packman, & Harrison (2003) recommended that the Lidcombe Program be initiated in the latter half of the preschool period and that postponing implementation of the program was not detrimental.
- Does each program need to include both direct child therapy and environmental modification from the outset? Can the least intrusive component be implemented first, followed by more direct intervention if necessary? Yaruss, Coleman, and Hammer (2006) presented data showing that 60% of the children they studied in an early intervention program for stuttering achieved and maintained normal fluency when environmental modifications alone had been implemented.
- Is this method effective when implemented with children who have other areas of need such as attention or intellectual deficits?
- Does it take longer for children with articulation or language disorders to achieve normal fluency using this method?

To continue to substantiate the effectiveness of this method, it is imperative that efficacy data be collected from a number of intervention sites. Treatment should be provided by a variety of appropriately trained clinicians who are not biased with regard to the treatment program. The third group of families described in the outcome section of this chapter was followed for one year after they were discharged from direct fluency therapy. It would be useful to follow families for longer periods of time to ensure that the children maintain normal fluency as their speech, language, and motor skills develop.

CHAPTER SUMMARY

- This multidimensional early intervention method for stuttering treatment helps most preschoolers develop normal fluency in a relatively short period of time. Over the last 10 years, this method has been implemented in two sites in southern New Hampshire. Of the children who were treated, 96% maintained normal fluency for up to 1 year after discharge.
- The method is appropriate for preschool children between the ages of 2 and 6 years who are at risk for persistent stuttering and for the significant people in their lives.
- The method is based on the Demands and Capacities Model of stuttering onset and development. It incorporates weekly, direct, and individual therapy for children to strengthen their fluency skills. In addition, weekly family therapy is conducted to help families develop an optimal environment for children in which they can practice fluency skills.
- Children may learn (1) to speak in a slower, more relaxed way; (2) how to use normal disfluencies; and/or (3) how to replace stuttering with a less struggled production of the word.
- Families will learn (1) about stuttering and fluency development; (2) how to modify their children's talking environments to support

fluency; and (3) how to talk about their children's speech needs with the children and with the other significant people in the children's lives.

- Treatment is completed when children demonstrate less than 3% stuttering-like disfluencies in a variety of contexts over time and when their families feel comfortable managing the child's fluency needs on their own. The average length of therapy for the families reported on in this chapter was 12 to 14 sessions.

CHAPTER REVIEW QUESTIONS

1. Who is this multidimensional treatment approach designed for?
2. How does the Demands and Capacities Model provide a framework for this multidimensional treatment approach?
3. Why is the family the focus of this intervention program and not the child alone?
4. What capacities support the development of normal fluency?
5. What environmental factors may be demanding of fluency for preschool children?
6. What research supports the link between parent speech variables and the fluency of preschool children who stutter?
7. How do clinicians help families with preschool children who stutter become educated consumers?
8. In this approach, direct therapy for the preschool child incorporates fluency shaping, stuttering modification, or a combination of both procedures. How would stuttering modification principles be implemented in this approach?
9. When is a family ready to be discharged from this multidimensional approach?
10. What is the predicted speech outcome for preschool children enrolled in this method?

SUGGESTED READINGS

Gottwald, S. R., & Starkweather, C. W. (1995). Fluency intervention for preschoolers and their families in the public schools. *Language, Speech and Hearing Services in Schools, 11,* 117–126. (This article describes the multidimensional method with a focus on its implementation from an educational perspective.)

Gottwald, S. R., & Starkweather, C. W. (1999). Stuttering prevention and early intervention: A multiprocess approach. In M. Onslow & A. Packman (Eds.), *The Handbook of Early Stuttering Intervention* (pp. 53–82). San Diego, CA: Singular Publishing Company. (The method is once again described in this chapter and includes follow-up data for an additional 15 families who were treated by the first author between 1993 and 1996 in southern New Hampshire.)

Starkweather, C. W., Gottwald, S. R., & Halfond, M. M. (1990). *Stuttering Prevention: A Clinical Method.* Englewood Cliffs, NJ: Prentice-Hall. (This text provides the first detailed description of this early intervention method as it was implemented at Temple University from 1983 through 1990.)

CHAPTER 7

The Lidcombe Program for Preschool Children Who Stutter

ELISABETH HARRISON AND MARK ONSLOW

CHAPTER OUTLINE

KEY TERMS

Percent syllables stuttered (%SS): a measure made by the clinician, describing the percentage of the child's spoken syllables that were unambiguously stuttered.

Severity rating (SR): a 10-point scale, where 1 = no stuttering, 2 = extremely mild stuttering, and 10 = extremely severe stuttering.

Stage 1: the part of the treatment in which the child is required to attain target speech performance for the LP.

Stage 2: the part of the treatment in which the child is required to maintain target speech performance for a clinically significant period.

Stutter: a moment of unambiguous stuttering judged by the parent and/or clinician while listening to the child's speech. Moments of stuttering that are judged to be ambiguous because they may be normal disfluencies are disregarded in the LP.

Stutter-free speech: a period of speech, judged by either or both the parent and/or clinician while listening to the child's speech, that contains no unambiguous moments of stuttering.

Verbal contingency: a comment made by the parent immediately after a stutter or stutter-free speech that is intended to serve as a mild punishment or reinforcement, respectively.

INTRODUCTION

NATURE OF INTENDED CLIENT

The Lidcombe Program (LP) was designed for young children who stutter, specifically preschoolers who are younger than 6 years. The program has been used with success with older children but was intended as an early intervention for stuttering (Onslow, 2003, p. 4). In Australia, the LP is the most widely used treatment for preschoolers who stutter (Packman et al., 2003). It is also used with preschool children whose case histories are complicated by medical problems and by communication disorders other than stuttering (Hewat, Harris, & Harrison, 2003).

PRINCIPLES OF TREATMENT

The LP is considered a direct intervention for early stuttering because its treatment components are focused on reducing the troublesome speech behaviors of young children who stutter to insignificant rates of occurrence. It is the specific targeting of child speech behaviors that distinguishes it from, for example, intervention based on the Demands and Capacities Model (see Gottwald, this volume, Chapter 6), where the focus also is on features of the child's living environment thought to be responsible for the disorder. The LP components reflect its origins in behavior therapy; they include attention to child responses and parental contingencies, consistent speech measurements, and performance-based progression between two stages. These program components are described in detail in the following sections.

The LP requires considerable parent involvement. Parents conduct the program during their everyday conversations with their stuttering children, and the role of clinicians is to train parents. In addition to learning to conduct treatment, parents also learn from the clinician how to measure the severity of their children's stuttering. Besides training parents in treatment and measurement, the clinician also ensures that children progress through the program in a timely manner.

Another principle of the LP is that children enjoy the treatment process. They are not expected to understand the treatment, monitor their speech, or modify their speech patterns in any way. They are expected only to participate in conversations with their parents and to have fun. The latter principle is so important that any sign of a child not enjoying the process is regarded as a guaranteed signal that something has gone wrong and that clinician and parents must make rapid changes to the way they are conducting treatment.

PRIMARY GOALS

The goal of Stage 1 of the LP is to reduce the frequency of children's stuttering to an insignificant level and to maintain this reduction for a clinically significant period. Expressed in speech measures, the goal is for children to attain the following criteria over 3 consecutive weeks: (1) weekly average severity ratings of less than 2, with at least four of the seven ratings being 1; and (2) less than 1% syllables stuttered in a conversation in the clinic that is a minimum of 300 syllables or 10 minutes in duration. (See the following section for definitions of severity ratings and percent syllables stuttered.) The primary goal of Stage 2 is for the child to continue to achieve the same speech criteria over many months. Children typically take between 10 and 12 months to complete Stage 2.

THEORETICAL BASIS FOR TREATMENT APPROACH

VIEWS ON NATURE OF STUTTERING

The development of the LP was not driven by a view of the nature and the cause of stuttering. The initial impetus for its development was a body of laboratory research driven by the theoretical perspective of stuttering as an operant, as described later. However, a subgroup of the developers of the LP has developed a theoretical perspective on the cause and nature of stuttering (Packman, Code, & Onslow, 2007) that is independent of the development of the LP. Nonetheless, this theoretical perspective, described in this section, is able to explain the growing body of evidence suggesting that the treatment is efficacious.

Linguistic stress, or emphasis, varies across syllables and is achieved by changing pitch, duration, and/or loudness by means of variations in motoric effort. Syllable Initiation (SI) theory (Packman, Code, & Onslow, 2007), which was based on the "Vmodel" (Packman et al., 1996), combines the findings of behavioral and brain research as well as theoretical models of stuttering to propose that stuttering involves difficulty in syllable initiation that is not experienced by nonstuttering speakers. This difficulty in syllable initiation is why stuttering often occurs on the first syllable of an utterance or in syllable transitions when syllables occur in sequence. Because of an unknown distal (not immediate) cause, stuttering occurs at syllable transitions when the difference in stress between syllables involving motoric effort is greatest. Therefore, SI theory locates the problem of stuttering at the interface of speech and language. This occurs when words are retrieved from the lexicon and syllabified at the phonologic word level. For example, when the words "fall out" are spoken as the syllables "fa-lout," the /l/ "straddles the lexical boundary" (Levelt & Wheeldon, 1994, p. 245). Therefore, this model predicts that stuttering would be likely to occur on the /l/ in such a word. According to SI theory, stuttering is neither a language problem nor a speech motor problem, but a problem at the interfacing of the two at the syllable.

Support for the view of stuttering as a difficulty that begins when children have to vary the stress on syllables comes from the fact that children do not stutter when they are babbling or when they are in the early stages of word production. SI theory posits that moving from single words with equal stress on each syllable to words with varied stress is the trigger for stuttering development. That is, children learn to de-stress syllables as they develop more adult-like speech production. For example, an early utterance might be "da-da," which later becomes "da-ddy" with stress on the first syllable. SI theory posits that stuttering appears when the motoric challenges increase to the point that they outstrip children's abilities as they learn to vary linguistic stress. Packman et al. (in press) claim that the SI theory, like any valid scientific theory, can be falsified. For example, the idea that stuttering involves syllable initiation would be wrong if stuttering occurred during extended vowel production, during which no syllabification occurs.

Packman, Code, and Onslow (2007) have proposed that the LP is efficacious because, in effect, it urges children to make some adjustment to their underlying neural processing patterns during a period when there are reasonable degrees of freedom in motor speech development remaining and before speech neural networks are firmly established. However, at present, there is no direct research evidence to support that proposition.

RATIONALE FOR TREATMENT APPROACH

In short, the theoretical perspectives of some of the developers of the LP do not provide a rationale for the LP treatment approach, and neither do any other theoretical perspectives on cause, development, and nature of stuttering. Instead, the rationale for the LP lies in an extensive body of literature showing the potential of operant methods to influence stuttered speech. Put simply, the theoretical perspective on which the LP rests is that events contingent on stuttered and stutter-free speech may influence it. More specifically, parental verbal contingencies on stuttered and stutter-free speech are the features of the LP intended to provide clinically useful influences on early stuttering.

The body of literature demonstrating the influence of operant methods on stuttering is extensive and sufficiently well known to not bear detailed description here. This literature has been reviewed in many places (e.g., Bloodstein & Ratner, 2008; Ingham, 1984; Nittrouer & Chaney, 1984; Onslow, 2003a; Prins & Hubbard, 1988), and the application of this literature to the treatment of stuttering children in the LP has been described (Onslow, 2003a)—"from laboratory to living room" (p. 21). However, in summary, the first generally recognized demonstration of operant methods with stuttering was a study by Flanagan, Goldiamond, and Azrin (1958) in which loud noise was presented contingent on stuttering. Subsequent to the initial work of Flanagan and colleagues, research into operant influences on stuttering was taken around the world, most prominently by Martin and colleagues at the University of Minnesota (e.g., Martin & Berndt, 1970; Martin & Haroldson, 1971; 1977; Martin & Siegel, 1966a; 1966b; Martin et al., 1975). These studies led to the famous time-out puppet study of Martin, Kuhl, and Haroldson (1972) with two preschoolers.

This study and the Reed and Godden (1977) study of the effects of the contingency "slow down" on the stuttering of two preschoolers were the direct forerunners to the idea of parents providing verbal contingencies to influence the stuttering of their preschool children.

EMPIRICAL BASIS FOR TREATMENT APPROACH

The empirical evidence in support of the LP has been outlined recently in several places (e.g., Harrison, Onslow, & Rousseau, 2007; Onslow, 2003a; 2004). For the purposes of this account, evidence is presented under the section headings "Clinical Trials Evidence" and "Treatment Process Research." The treatment process section describes research dealing with a range of topics not covered under the clinical trials section. Clinical trials are categorized within the loose phase I to III classification system (for an overview, see Robey, 2005). This classification is traditionally used in pharmaceutical trials but may be adapted for application to the speech pathology discipline. Table 7.1 summarizes how this might be done, based on Onslow et al. (2008). Onslow et al. (2008) also argue that the clinical trial is the fundamental interpretable unit of treatment efficacy research output, and for stuttering, they define a clinical trial as follows: "a prospective attempt to determine the outcome or outcomes of (1) at least one entire treatment with (2) at least one pre-treatment and one follow-up outcome of at least 3 months in the case of a reported positive outcome, and

(3) and where outcomes involve independent speech observations derived from recordings of conversational speech beyond the clinic." This definition is used to select studies for mention here.

CLINICAL TRIALS EVIDENCE
Phase I Clinical Trials

The first phase I clinical trial of the LP was published by Onslow, Costa, and Rue (1990), with three boys and one girl of preschool age. Within- and beyond-clinic assessments of percent syllables stuttered (%SS) and syllables per minute (SPM) were based on audiotape recordings of the children at pretreatment intervals of 2 months, 1 month, and 1 day and posttreatment intervals of 1 day, 1 month, 2 months, 4 months, 6 months, and 9 months. Covert assessment of the children was included. Results from this preliminary trial were encouraging, with some modest evidence from a limited number of participants that the treatment had beneficial effects.

Further phase I evidence for the LP occurred in two trials. The next clinical trial report of the LP (Harrison, Wilson, & Onslow, 1999) entailed its presentation in a telehealth format, where treatment occurred primarily by telephone contact, supplemented by mail transfer of materials or transfer by means of internet and cell phone technology. Materials so transferred included audio and video recordings of parents conducting the treatment and parent severity ratings. The authors presented a report of a 5-year 10-month old boy who could not access the treatment in his own country. Speech measures of %SS and SPM were

Table 7.1. *Summary of Phases of Clinical Trial Development as Applied to Stuttering Treatment Based on Onslow et al. (2008)*

Phase I	Preliminary investigations of new treatment
	Normally 1-10 participants
	Explores safety and viability
	Nonrandomized
Phase II	Continues to explore safety and viability
	Estimates proportion of treatment "responders"
	Normally greater than 10 participants
	Normally nonrandomized
Phase III	"Gold standard"
	Randomized
	Larger number of participants
	Allows mathematical estimates of treatment effect size

collected before treatment and at 12 months, 19 months, and 23 months after treatment using audio and audiovisual recordings of the participant conversing with his family members at home. Pre-treatment scores were high, in the range of 12% to 17% SS; scores in the posttreatment period had decreased to less than 1.0% SS in all assessments.

The second phase I trial of the LP in telehealth format was reported by Wilson, Onslow, and Lincoln (2004). As was the case in the original report (Harrison, Wilson, & Onslow, 1999), this trial was conducted in a "low-tech" format that did not involve internet or cell phone technology. Five preschool children—three girls and two boys—were assessed with 10-minute audio and audiovisual recordings in various situations beyond the clinic. One recording was collected covertly. Outcomes were %SS and SPM, and assessments were at 2 months, 1 month, and 1 week before treatment and 1 week, 1 month, 2 months, 4 months, 6 months, 8 months, and 12 months after treatment. These results provided some prospects that children who cannot access standard stuttering treatment services might eventually have a treatment option proven to be efficacious.

Phase II Clinical Trials

A phase II clinical trial of the LP was published by Onslow, Andrews, and Lincoln (1994). The trial did not succeed in maintaining a control group except for a few participants. Twelve children were studied at pretreatment intervals of 2 months, 1 month, and 1 week and posttreatment intervals of 1 week, 1 month, 2 months, 4 months, 6 months, 9 months, and 12 months. Outcomes were based on beyond clinic audio-tape recordings in a range of speaking situations, including one covert assessment. The primary outcome of %SS was reported for all children, but SPM was reported for only a few children as a result of reasons relating to data reliability. This trial, which included a substantial number of children, added to the credibility of the idea that the LP might be an efficacious treatment for early stuttering. Further phase II evidence was presented by Lincoln, Onslow, and Reed (1997), with long-term outcome data for 16 children in the Onslow et al. (1990; 1994) trials. An additional 27 children for whom pretreatment recordings were not available were followed up, but these retrospective data did not

meet the Onslow et al. (2008) criteria for a clinical trial. %SS scores were based on sets of audio recordings of children at yearly intervals for periods of between 1 and 7 years.

Additional phase II evidence for the LP was reported in the context of a study of predictors of treatment time in the LP (Rousseau et al., 2007; see following "Clinical Cohort Studies" section). For 29 preschoolers, the outcome measure of %SS was collected over two pre-treatment assessments and 6, 12, and 24 months after the children began Stage 2. A mix of within-clinic and beyond-clinic recordings was obtained, with some of the within-clinic recordings being audiovisual. At 24 months after completion of Stage 1, all children's %SS scores suggested that a large treatment effect might be present. The 29 children in this study roughly doubled the number of participants in phase II trials of the LP that had been published. The median time to complete Stage 1 reported by Rousseau et al. (2007a) was 16 sessions, which was higher than previously reported, for the reason that a recent change to the treatment manual (http://www.fhs.usyd.edu.au/asrc) required children to meet program criteria for 3 consecutive weeks to complete Stage 1 and begin Stage 2. The LP developers now use the rule of thumb that it takes around a median of 12 treatment sessions for children to attain speech that is sufficiently normal sounding to be a candidate to begin Stage 2 in subsequent weeks. The caveat to this rule of thumb is that it applies to a caseload in general, not to any individual child. Recovery plot studies (see following "Clinical Cohort Studies" section) show a large range of individual treatment times.

The first replication of positive results in a phase II clinical trial of the LP occurred in a report by Miller and Guitar (2009). Participants were 15 preschool children, 4 girls and 11 boys, who were treated by clinicians assisted by graduate students in a university clinic. Outcomes of %SS were collected from within- and beyond-clinic tape recordings, before treatment and at follow-up periods ranging from 12 to 58 months. The children required a median of 17 treatment sessions to reach Stage 2, showing a "large" treatment effect.

The phase I trials of telehealth adaptation of the LP were followed with a phase II randomized trial by Lewis et al. (2008). Nine children were randomized to the treatment group, and 13 were randomized to a no-treatment control group. (In randomized trials, it often occurs that when the trial stops recruiting participants, the randomization process results in different numbers in each group.) The primary outcome measure was %SS based on prerandomization and postrandomization conversational speech samples collected beyond the clinic. Using a definition of a "responder" as a child who decreased %SS scores by more than 80% at 9 months after randomization, Lewis et al. reported that six experimental children responded to the treatment, but only two control children were "responders" during natural recovery. The experimental group showed a significant response considering their prepretreatment to follow-up stuttering. However, adjusting for prerandomization %SS scores, gender, age, and family history, there was a 73% reduction in frequency of stuttering at 9 months after randomization in the treatment group compared with the control group. As occurred in the Wilson, Onslow, and Lincoln (2004) phase I trial, the telehealth format was not as cost efficient. Measures of treatment time showed that the telehealth version of the treatment requires approximately three times the clinician time resources than the standard version. However, for children isolated from standard clinical services, this appears to be far preferable to not receiving treatment in early childhood.

Phase III Clinical Trials

The essential differences between phase I and II clinical trials and phase III clinical trials are that greater participant numbers are normally involved and a true estimate of effect size is attained (see Table 7.1). This is because these trials eliminate bias because of randomization. It is well known that nonrandomized Phase I and Phase II trials overestimate the true effect size (Kunz & Oxman, 1998).

The first phase III evidence for the LP occurred in a randomized controlled trial (Jones et al., 2005) involving a group of children who received the treatment and a control group who received no treatment. This enabled a comprehensive assessment of the merits of the treatment in comparison to the effects of natural recovery and the first accurate assessment of

what the treatment effect might be for the treatment. Twenty-nine children were randomized to the LP group, and 25 were randomized to the control group. Outcomes were %SS scores collected from audiotape recordings of the children during everyday speaking situations. Speech samples were at least 300 syllables each. The children were assessed before randomization and at 9 months after randomization. There were two dropouts from the LP group and five from the control group. Differences found were large and statistically significant, with an odds ratio of 7.7. This means that a child who received the LP was 7.7 times more likely to have attained clinically minimal stuttering than a child who did not receive the LP.

Jones et al. (2008) provided long-term follow-up data on some of the children in the Jones et al. (2005) report when their mean age was 9 years (range, 7 to 12 years) at a mean of 5 years (range, 3.5 to 7 years) after randomization. In other words, the children in the treatment group were a mean of 5 years older than when they began their treatments. Long-term outcomes for 20 of the 29 children were obtained, 19 of whom had completed the treatment successfully in the original trial. Three of these children had relapsed at follow-up, providing a long-term success rate of 86%. Jones et al. (2007) noted that parents of half their sample reported some stuttering after the end of successful treatment, which was consistent with findings of the Lincoln, Onslow, and Reed (1997) trial. Hence, it was argued that it is important after Stage 2 for parents to continue to present verbal contingencies for stuttered speech and occasionally provide verbal contingencies for stutter-free speech. Table 7.2 summarizes the clinical trial research of the LP.

TREATMENT PROCESS RESEARCH
Clinical Cohort Studies

Two large cohort studies have used retrospective file audit methodologies to establish the shape of the recovery plot of a cohort of treated children and to establish whether there were any predictors of time required to complete Stage 1 of the treatment. Jones et al. (2000) studied a cohort of 261 children who began LP treatment in Sydney, of whom 250 completed Stage 1. These children were used to establish

Table 7.2. *Summary of Clinical Trials of the LP Using the Onslow et al. (2007) Definition of a Trial*

Phase I	Onslow, Costa, & Rue (1990)
	Harrison, Wilson, & Onslow (1999)
	Wilson et al. (2004)
Phase II	Onslow, Andrews, & Lincoln (1994)
	Lincoln et al. (1996)[a]
	Lincoln, Onslow, & Reed (1997)
	Rousseau et al. (2007a)
	Miller & Guitar (2009)
	Lewis et al. (2008)
Phase III	Jones et al. (2005)
	Jones et al. (2008)

[a] Participants were school-age children.

the shape of the recovery plot for this treatment. Additionally, logistical regression determined whether any case history variables predicted the time taken to complete Stage 1 and confirmed existing reports, albeit with smaller numbers, that the median number of clinic visits required to do so was 11. (An important caveat to this finding is that children in this cohort were treated with a version of the manual that did not specify that children were required to meet program criteria for 3 consecutive weeks in order to be admitted to Stage 2. Consequently, this estimate of median treatment time is likely to be low for the current version of the treatment specified in the manual. For this reason, as stated earlier, the LP developers suggest approximately 11 to 12 clinic visits for a child to attain speech that is sufficiently normal sounding for impending admission to Stage 2.) Consistent with a previous finding by Starkweather and Gottwald (1993), pretreatment stuttering severity predicted time to complete Stage 1. However, contrary to another finding by Starkweather and Gottwald (1993)—and contrary to general, intuitive expectations at the time—there was evidence that a shorter time since onset was associated with longer Stage 1 treatment times. In other words, the Jones et al. (2000) data suggest that, during the preschool years, longer periods since onset are associated with shorter treatment periods.

Kingston et al. (2003) replicated the Jones et al. (2000) study with a group of 66 British children younger than 6 years who were treated with the LP. Results confirmed the Jones et al. finding of a median of 11 clinic visits for Stage

1, based on the earlier version of the manual that did not specify 3 consecutive weeks at criterion speech performance in order to conclude Stage 1 (see previous paragraph). Furthermore, the Jones et al. finding confirmed that initial stuttering rate was a significant predictor of treatment time for Stage 1. The results of the two studies were pooled in a meta-analysis, which confirmed the result that children who had been stuttering for less than 12 months took significantly longer to complete Stage 1 than children who had been stuttering longer than 12 months during the preschool years. The Jones et al. and Kingston et al. studies have been primarily responsible for a recommended rule of thumb with the LP that treatment should not begin earlier than 6 months after onset of stuttering and that treatment should be timed to ensure that stuttering is under effective control by the time the child attends school at 6 years of age (Packman, Onslow, & Attanasio, 2003).

An intriguing addition to these regression studies of treatment time with the LP occurred with a prospective study by Rousseau et al. (2007a) of 29 successfully treated children. The prospective methodology allowed a study of phonology and language as predictors of Stage 1 treatment time. The previous findings of pretreatment severity predicting treatment time were replicated but with the interesting addition that stuttering severity combined with language (mean length of utterance [MLU]) and receptive language (Clinical Evaluation of Language Fundamentals [CELF]) scores predicted 35% to 45% of the variance in times to complete Stage 1. MLU was negatively correlated with treatment time, and CELF was positively correlated with treatment time. The former finding, which indicates that better language skills are associated with quicker outcomes, was thought to be intuitive and consistent with the Jones et al. (2000) and Kingston et al. (2003) results. However, Rousseau et al. found the receptive language component of this result unintuitive and difficult to explain; why would children with poorer receptive language respond to the treatment more quickly than children with better receptive language?

Koushik et al. (2007) studied 13 stuttering school-age children who were treated with the LP, strictly according to the manual, in a public clinic in Montreal. Outcomes of %SS were collected from routine pretreatment clinic recordings and at a mean follow-up period of 72 weeks (range, 9 to 187 weeks). Follow-up %SS scores were obtained from recordings of several telephone conversations with the children. For 12 of these children, mean %SS was 9.5% pretreatment and 1.8% at follow-up. A surprising feature of this report was that a median of 7.5 clinic visits was required for completion of Stage 1, which is far fewer than the median of 16 visits reported by Rousseau et al. (2007) for the LP with preschool children. The remaining child required a supplement to the LP comprising the traditional speech restructuring procedures of prolonged speech and did well with that clinical arrangement. This appeared to be necessary because of problems with parent compliance with the verbal contingencies of the treatment.

Measurement Procedures

The earliest treatment process research concerning measurement in the LP dealt with the 10-point scale of stuttering severity (SR) that is used during the treatment process. This SR scale is a convenient, covert, and inexpensive measure. Onslow, Costa, and Rue (1990) presented case studies of four stuttering preschoolers and their parents. For each child, 24 samples of 200 to 300 syllables were obtained. In the case of two parents, more than 90% of the speech samples were independently rated by parent and clinician with score differences of 0 and 1 scale values. With a third parent, approximately 70% of samples were rated with that agreement with the clinician, and a fourth parent was quite unreliable, indicating the need for

training during the clinical process for these parents. Onslow, Costa, and Rue (1990) also showed that the SR scale used by mothers was capable of rank ordering the severity of the samples in the same fashion as a clinician stuttering count measure, with Spearman correlations as high as .83 and .78. Subsequently, Eve et al. (1995) showed that three groups of listeners—stuttering specialist clinicians, generalist clinicians, and nonclinicians—were able to use the scale with adequate inter- and intrajudge reliability, as shown with high intraclass correlations. Hayhow, Kingston, and Ledzion (1998) reported a case study demonstrating the use of %SS and SR scores to guide management decisions during the LP treatment process. Harrison, Onslow, and Menzies (2004) randomized 38 children to receive a 4-week "dose" of the LP in an experimental design in which half of the children received treatment without any measurement procedures. Results suggested that the measurement procedures in the LP may not contribute to observed treatment effects, hence offsetting concerns that the treatment effects with the procedure may be attributed to increased attention to the children's speech.

Stuttering count measures are considered problematic from the viewpoint of reliability (e.g., Cordes & Ingham, 1994; Kully & Boberg, 1988). Additionally, in the case of preschool children, although diagnosis of stuttering generally is not a matter of debate (Onslow, Packman, & Payne, 2007), Bloodstein's (1970) "continuity hypothesis" suggests that it might be problematic to distinguish between some individual stuttered speech events and normal disfluencies. Indeed, there have been many reports suggesting an overlap in terms for speech behaviors between stuttering and nonstuttering preschoolers (e.g., Adams, 1977; 1984; Curlee, 1993; Johnson & Associates, 1959; Van Riper, 1971). Consequently, Lincoln, Onslow, and Reed (1997) sought to validate the use of the 1.0% SS criterion for acceptable speech performance in the LP. They did this by having experienced clinicians measure %SS in speech samples from children who had been successfully treated and control children. Results showed that preschool and school-age children treated with the LP received similar low values of %SS in comparison to control children with typical speech who were matched for age. In the second part of the study, experienced clinicians and unsophisticated listeners made judgements of "stuttering" or "not stuttering" on speech samples of preschool and school-age children successfully treated with the LP and made similar judgements on speech samples of control children matched for age.

A report by Onslow, Harrison, Jones, and Packman (2002) retrospectively studied 141 children treated with the LP. They demonstrated a strong correlation between parents' SR scores and the %SS measures made by clinicians at each clinic visit. An important finding was that 81% of the time, the two measures corresponded in terms of whether the children's speech was above or below the target speech criteria for ending Stage 1 of the treatment. This highlighted the important principle that both %SS and SR scores are needed during the treatment process to guide clinical decision making. Otherwise, on 19% of occasions, misleading information will be obtained; either a single %SS score or SR score will be misleading and the clinician will not be aware of this situation. However, if a clinician collects discrepant %SS and SR scores at one clinic visit, the problem can be solved either by checking the calibration of the parent's SR scores against clinician judgment or determining whether the parent is making misjudgments about what are and are not moments of stuttering. Additionally, Onslow, Harrison, Jones, and Packman (2002) showed that both sets of scores depicted a one-third reduction in children's stuttering severity during the first 2 to 5 weeks of treatment. The Onslow et al. data also showed that parental SR scores were as effective a predictor of treatment time as the clinicians' %SS scores that were examined as a predictor of treatment time by Jones et al. (2000) and Kingston et al. (2003).

Safety and Viability

Presumably because of the historic and extensive influence of Johnson's (1942) paradoxical theory that stuttering is caused by its diagnosis, the introduction and development of the LP was met with a guarded response (for an overview, see Onslow et al., 2004). The primary concern expressed was that the direct methods of the treatment—which in effect called attention to stuttered speech in preschoolers—were not safe (e.g., Cook & Rustin, 1997). This prompted a study of the psychological impact of the LP in eight successfully treated preschool children (Woods et al., 2002). Results showed that, according to the Child Behavior Checklist (Achenbach, 1988; 1991), there were no signs of anxiety in the children after treatment. In addition, there were no signs of negative change in the bond between parent and child after the treatment, as measured by the Attachment Q-Set. These findings seem to provide evidence that there is no reason to believe that the LP adversely affects preschool children.

EXPERIMENTAL STUDIES OF THE LP COMPONENTS

Three studies have presented a portion of the LP in the context of an experimental investigation of its viability. Harris et al. (2002) attempted to determine whether the treatment was capable of interrupting the developmental course of stuttering in preschoolers, above the effects of natural recovery. The rationale for the experiment was that the treatment would not be viable without evidence that it was capable of doing this. Harris et al. (2002) randomized 23 stuttering children to receive either a 12-week "dose" of the LP or no treatment. After this small "dose" of treatment, both groups improved, but the group that received the LP showed clinically and significantly greater improvement than the control group over the 12-week period of study. These data supplement the clinical trial findings of Jones et al. (2005) by showing that children are better off after receiving the LP in the short term as well as the longer term.

Franken et al. (2005) used a similar design to that used by Harris et al. (2002). Data were provided that were pertinent to LP viability by comparing the LP with a treatment based on the Demands and Capacities Model (see following "Underlying Mechanism" section) over a short period. Results showed no differences in the responses of the two groups after 12 weeks. However, these data are not as convincing as they might be had a control group been used to demonstrate that improvements were greater than those occurring with natural recovery; it could be that neither treatment was efficacious, and the study merely documented the effects of natural recovery. The Harrison, Onslow, and Menzies (2004) experiment, in addition to giving measurement procedures to half the participants (see earlier "Measurement Procedures" section), gave all the LP verbal contingencies to half the children and only verbal contingencies for stutter-free speech to the other half. This design tested the effect of verbal contingencies for stuttered speech. Results showed that the verbal contingencies for stuttered speech did make a contribution to treatment effects; all children reduced stuttering to the same extent after a 4-week "dose" of treatment, but 4 weeks later, the children who did not have the verbal contingences for stuttered speech began to lose their treatment effects.

UNDERLYING MECHANISM

At present, the mechanisms responsible for the LP's reported efficacy are not known. One mechanism might involve change in speech motor activity. Traditional behavioral treatments for adolescents and adults have involved speech restructuring, which is defined as any method requiring clients to learn a novel speech pattern that is incompatible with stuttering. Examples of speech restructuring tasks have included having clients learn to articulate with soft contacts or gentle onsets, prolonged vowel sounds, continuous airflow, and continuous voicing (for overviews, see Ingham, 1984; Packman, Onslow, & Menzies, 2000). A series of reports have shown clear and unsurprising evidence that these treatments are associated with increased durations of acoustic speech segments, reflecting the speech motor changes that seem to offset the disorder (Robb, Lybolt, & Price, 1985; Shenker & Finn, 1985; Webster, Morgan, & Cannon, 1987).

A preliminary report with two children (Packman, van Doorn, & Onslow, 1992) suggested that reduction in variability of acoustic speech segments is associated with the effects of the LP. Relying on the assumption that acoustic activity reflects speech motor activity, Onslow, Stocker, Packman, and McLeod (2002) followed up on this report and studied selected acoustic measures in eight children before and after their successful treatment with the LP in order to determine whether changes in motor speech activity might be associated with treatment effects. Results

showed no evidence that this was the case. However, considering that the signs of any speech motor adjustments that children might make in response to the LP are likely to be subtle, further research on this topic is needed to establish definitive conclusions. Such research methods would need to involve larger group studies or laboratory studies and would include kinematic speech analyses of children before and after treatment.

Somewhat more encouraging findings have emerged to advance the prospect that changes in parental language habits may be responsible for the apparent efficacy of the LP. In a general sense, the Demands and Capacities (DC) Model suggests that this might be the case. The DC Model has been developed predominantly by Starkweather and colleagues (Adams, 1990; Gottwald & Starkweather, 1995; Starkweather, 1987; Starkweather & Givens-Ackerman, 1997; Starkweather & Gottwald, 1990; Starkweather, Gottwald, & Halfond, 1990). The DC Model provides an explanation for stuttering during the preschool years, namely that stuttering occurs when a child's capacity for fluent speech is overshadowed by demands to produce fluent speech. The model posits that the capacity for fluency in childhood is influenced by developmental aspects of speech motor control, language development, social and emotional functioning, and cognitive development. Demands for fluency arise predominantly from the environment in which the child lives. These may include hurried and unpredictable lifestyle, time pressure, pressure to use complex language, factors that induce excitement and anxiety, and parental demands for improvement in a range of language-related functions such as cognition.

The DC Model suggests that language variables may contribute to the control of early stuttering, and there are some sources of evidence to suggest that this may be so. Stephenson-Opsal and Ratner (1988) showed that when mothers of stuttering children reduced their speech rate to the children, a decrease in stuttering occurred in the children with no corresponding change in speech rate. In a follow-up study, Ratner (1992) showed that when parents were instructed to slow down, they displayed a number of other changes, such as reduced length and complexity of utterance and increased interspeaker latencies. Taken together, these studies suggest that a slowing of parental speech rate may reduce a number of language variables, which may, in turn, alleviate children's stuttering.

Latterman, Shenker, and Thordardottir (2005) studied children's language after the LP in four preschool-age boys and found no evidence of changes in language function after the treatment. Similar results were obtained by Bonelli et al. (2000) with a larger group of nine children treated with the LP. There was no evidence in the data of a comprehensive and systematic alteration of language function after treatment. All children remained within normal developmental limits during the pre- and posttreatment period. More recently, Rousseau et al. (2007) reported a more comprehensive study of 29 children prior to the LP at the conclusion of Stage 1, when near-zero stuttering had been attained. Firm evidence was established by Rousseau et al. (2007) to confirm that there was no frank change in the children's language function after the treatment, either for the group or any individual children within the group. Taken together, the findings of Bonelli et al. (2000) and Rousseau et al. (2007) are all the more compelling because they were obtained *after* fluency had been established during Stage 1, not *during* the early stages of the treatments when any language variables that served to control stuttering might have been active. Interestingly, although the Bonelli et al. and Rousseau et al. studies found no change in language function after the treatment that might account for its mechanism, both studies reported some signs that when children receive the LP, their language development stalls for a short period. Rousseau et al. reported this with measures of MLU, number of different words, and developmental sentence scoring. Bonelli et al. argued that this effect is intuitive and consistent with "bucket" theory of language and phonologic development (Crystal, 1987).

Bonelli et al. (2000) suggested that it may also be the case that operant procedures, when they are found to influence stuttering in children, do so because contingencies for stuttered speech themselves directly induce language change in children. In the LP, for example, requests for correction of stuttered utterances and praise for stutter-free utterances may simply induce shorter utterances, utterances that are less likely to be stuttered than longer ones and are also likely to be less linguistically complex. Indeed, in a follow-up study, Onslow,

Ratner, and Packman (2001) showed that a boy whose stuttering was controlled with time-out in a laboratory showed corresponding reductions in lexical diversity, supporting the possibility suggested by Bonelli et al. Table 7.3 contains a summary of the treatment process research of the LP.

PRACTICAL REQUIREMENTS FOR THE TREATMENT

TIME DEMANDS

Parents and children typically attend weekly, 45- to 60-minute clinic visits with clinicians throughout Stage 1. During Stage 2, clinic visits are shorter, usually 30 minutes, and the frequency of visits decreases from every 2 weeks early in Stage 2 to a gap of 16 weeks between the final visits. Accounting for occasional missed clinic visits due to sickness and vacations, clinicians and parents can expect most children to take between 4 and 7 months (16 to 30 clinic visits) to complete Stage 1, and a further 10 to 12 months (7 to 10 clinic visits) to complete Stage 2.

Information about the time required to complete the program needs to be viewed with a great deal of caution. Empirical evidence reported in the previous section about median treatment time to complete Stage 1 was based on data collected from several clinics by clinicians in two continents. Some data came from specialist speech pathologists in public sector services, others came from a student clinic, and others were generated by a research clinician. So although the range of sites and specialization levels leads us to be confident about the robustness of the median treatment time data, there are still questions about treatment time to which we have no answers. For example, we do not know how long or how much experience it takes before an individual clinician can expect to meet those treatment time benchmarks. Perhaps clinicians need to have treated a certain number of clients and successfully guided them to complete the program. Perhaps it is not simply the number of successful "completions" that is important; perhaps it is more important to have had success with just one or two children who stuttered severely before treatment and to have worked through the problems that arose during the course of treatment. There is good reason then for clinicians to be cautious when telling parents about expected

Table 7.3. *Summary of the Treatment Process Research in the LP*

Clinical cohort studies	Jones et al. (2000)
	Kingston et al. (2003)
	Rousseau et al. (2007)
	Koushik et al. (2007)
Measurement procedures	Onslow, Costa, & Rue (1990)
	Eve et al. (1995)
	Hayhow, Onslow, & Menzies (1998)
	Onslow, Harrison, Jones, & Packman (2002)
	Harrison, Onslow, & Menzies (2004)
Safety and viability	Woods et al. (2002)
	Harris et al. (2002)
	Harrison, Onslow, & Menzies (2004)
	Franken, Kielstra-Van der Schalk, & Boelens (2005)
	Bonelli et al. (2000)
Underlying mechanism	Onslow, Ratner, & Packman (2001)
	Packman et al. (1992)
	Onslow, Stocker, Packman, & McLeod (2002)
	Lattermann, Euler, & Neumann (2008)
	Rousseau et al. (2007)

treatment times. We find that parents are reassured about the uncertainty of their particular child's treatment by also being told that the treatment process will continue whether or not the child meets the "median" treatment time or has a relatively long treatment time.

There is another perspective on the time demands of the LP that comes from considering the parents' point of view. Early in Stage 1, parents and children engage in treatment at home each day for between 10 and 15 minutes. Although this may not seem substantial at first glance, parents tell us that one of the most difficult aspects of treatment implementation is finding time each day for stuttering treatment (Packman, Hansen, & Herland, 2007). Part of the difficulty stems from the fact that the best times of day for treatment are when children are alert and cooperative, whereas the times to avoid are when they are tired or distracted. The result is that the best times for treatment are usually mornings or early afternoons. Parents tell us that they have to deliberately set aside time for treatment because these times are already filled with other events and activities.

After the first weeks of Stage 1, there is typically less need for 10 to 15 minutes of structured treatment conversations; instead, parents and children conduct treatment during their naturally occurring conversations. Although this change means that parents no longer need to set aside time for treatment exclusively, they still spend time—albeit less focused time—delivering treatment to their children each day.

TRAINING AND EXPERTISE REQUIRED OF CLINICIAN

There are several sources of information available for clinicians who wish to use the LP. These range from a comprehensive book (Onslow, Packman, & Harrison, 2003) to a professional education workshop that is provided through the LP Trainers Consortium (LPTC; http://www3.fhs.usyd.edu.au/asrcwww/index.html). At the time of writing, there are 13 LPTC members who are based in Australia, Canada, Denmark, Germany, New Zealand, the United Kingdom, and the United States. The LPTC is a not-for-profit group of researchers and clinicians who have professional speech-language pathology qualifications in their own countries. Although the training resources have been developed specifically with the aim of providing accessible clinician training, there is no licensing process for clinicians who want to use the program, nor is there any formal or informal process of registration or certification required to use it. Clinicians are not "required" to attend an LPTC workshop in order to use the LP. In fact, we know of many clinicians who first started to use the program after reading the treatment manual, or a brief description in a clinical research report, or a book chapter.

However, there is consistent feedback from clinicians who attend consortium workshops that they consider the training to have been invaluable. We strongly recommend that clinicians attend a workshop and, subsequently, continue to consult with the clinicians who presented it.

At the same time, attendance at an LPTC workshop is no guarantee that clinicians will use the program correctly. When parents ask for our recommendations about which clinicians to approach for LP treatment, we give parents written information about the program and suggest that they ask the clinicians if they have attended LPTC training workshops. The written information is a pamphlet that parents can download from the web (http://www.fhs.usyd.edu.au/asrcwww/ Downloads/index.htm; follow the link to "Lidcombe Program Brochures").

After completing training in the LP or at least gaining a thorough understanding of the program and its components from written sources, the other aspect of training that we recommend is the ongoing training and consultation with other clinicians who have more experience using the program. As a starting point, the members of the LPTC whose names are listed on our website (http://www3.fhs.usyd.edu.au/ asrcwww/index.html) know firsthand many local clinicians who are adept at using the LP and who are willing to consult with and advise clinicians. One hallmark of clinicians around the world who use the LP is their recognition of the value of seeking advice from and communicating with others when there is clinical problem solving to be done.

MATERIALS NEEDED

LP treatment is conducted in children's everyday environments, so the materials used by parents are simply those used in their everyday play and household routines with their children. The only unique addition will be to arrange a way for parents to note their daily measures of children's stuttering severity. There is a convenient form available for this on the web (http://www.fhs.usyd. edu.au/asrcwww/Downloads/LP_SR_Chart.pdf; see following "Frequency of Measures" section), but parents can report these measures to clinicians in other forms that may be more convenient. Examples of other methods include

PDA-based charts, voicemail or text messages to the clinician (Bennett & Harrison, 2005), and diary notes.

During clinic visits, clinicians and parents make use of the books, toys, play equipment, and stickers that are commonly found in pediatric speech-pathology settings. The following list is provided as an indication of equipment that clinicians generally find useful when using the LP, but it should not be regarded as a prescriptive list of essentials:

1. Information for parent. Before children begin Stage 1, parents should be given information about the LP so that they understand the nature of the program and have clear expectations about the roles to be filled by their children, themselves, and clinicians. One resource for that information is the DVD titled "Tom's Story" (available at http://www3.fhs.usyd. edu.au/asrcwww/), which includes a parent's point of view on the treatment process. A pamphlet about the LP has been written for parents and is available in several languages at the Australian Stuttering Research Centre website.

2. Equipment for speech measurement. The measure of stuttering rate that clinicians collect during clinic visits is percentage of syllables stuttered (%SS). This is calculated by dividing the total number of syllables spoken by the number of syllables that were unambiguous stutters and converting this to a percentage. A button press timing and counting device makes it viable for clinicians to collect valid %SS measures while engaging in conversation with children and parents. (Examples of button press timing and counting devices include handheld, battery-operated devices such as the TrueTalk [www.synelec.com. au] and the EasyRater [www.users.bigpond.com/ lunjef]. There are also computer programs, such as the Stuttering Counts CDROM [http:// www.latrobe.edu.au/hcs/resources.htm#stutter ing], and the Stuttering Management System [http://www.speech.ucsb.edu/allDownloads. php].)

3. Therapy materials for use during clinic visits. The typical materials that clinicians would use during LP clinic visits include age-appropriate therapy materials such as: (1) a range of picture books, including some with

minimal visual information per page and others with more complex pictures; (2) various toy sets that the child, parent, and clinician can play with together such as a train set with tracks and station; a farm set with animals, people, tractors, and farm buildings; and a tea set and kitchen equipment; and (3) several toys and games with many relatively small pieces, such as block sets, color and shape sorting kits, counters, or jigsaw puzzles.

KEY COMPONENTS

STAGES OF TREATMENT

The LP has two stages, called Stage 1 and Stage 2. The goal of Stage 1 is to reduce the frequency and severity of children's stuttering to criterion levels (see p. 133), and the goal of Stage 2 is for children to maintain these levels for around 12 months.

PARTICIPANTS

The roles of parents, children, and clinicians in Stage 1 and Stage 2 change to some extent as children's stuttering decreases. Weekly clinic visits by the parent and child are scheduled with the same clinician each week throughout Stage 1 and then less frequently during Stage 2.

In our experience, the child's mother typically fills the parent role in the program, although a father, grandparent, or even an older sibling can fulfill that role if circumstances permit. Sometimes both parents take on the role of being trained to conduct the LP; this often is the case when parents live separately and jointly share childcare responsibilities. Childcare staff or nursery school staff are rarely able to fill the parent role due to time constraints. Individual child carers such as nannies or family daycare parents may be able to take on the parent role in the program. In our experience, the critical factor when selecting a nonparent to take on the parent role is the amount of time that the person has available to spend on therapy activities on a daily basis.

Early in Stage 1 parents learn how to perform treatment and to measure the severity of their children's stuttering. They attend the clinic each week with their children and participate in clinic visits with the clinicians. Parents report their observations, impressions, and severity ratings and discuss the significance of these with the clinician. The most critical element to be learned by the parent is the effective delivery of verbal contingencies.

The role for children in this program is simple: they have fun. They are not required to monitor themselves or their speech or to produce either stutter-free speech or stuttered speech at particular times. They simply engage in conversations with their parents, and as described, parents deliver verbal contingencies to children's stutter-free and stuttered speech.

Clinicians primarily have the role of training parents, monitoring children's progress, and dealing with any issues that arise during the course of treatment. The clinician's role includes ensuring that progress is constant and that all program components are being used optimally for each child and parent. If progress stalls for more than a few weeks without a clear reason, then the clinician's responsibility is to consult with more experienced colleagues and to make changes that ensure progress continues.

ACTIVITIES AND PROCEDURES

The first program component that parents learn to use is SRs. These ratings are on a 10-point scale, with SR1 defined as "no stuttering," SR2 defined as "extremely mild stuttering," and SR10 defined as "extremely severe stuttering." Clinicians first establish the reliability of each parent's use of the SR scale. This is accomplished by asking the parent to rate the severity of his or her child's speech during a natural conversation in the clinic. If the parent's rating is within one scale value of the clinician's, then the clinician endorses the parent's use of the scale and requests the parents to collect SRs each day. In most cases, it is convenient for the parent to assign a single rating for the entire day. Alternatively, the parent can assign maximum and minimum SRs for each day. Another variation is for the parent to assign an SR to a 10-minute period each day. If this method is used, parents need to vary the times of day or speaking situations that they measure across each week so that a range of speech is sampled. For example, Monday ratings are at breakfast, Tuesday ratings are at early afternoon, Wednesday ratings are in the car on the way to childcare, and so on. In this way, SRs on particular days can be compared over several weeks. This third method is less desirable than the first two because direct comparisons can only be made from week to week. However, it is useful when parents find it difficult to assign SRs to whole days, as might be the case if they pick up their child after a long day at daycare and there is a short period until bedtime.

For an example of teaching the parent to use SRs, see Video Clip 1 for this chapter on thePoint.

Having learned how to measure and chart their child's severity ratings, the parent's next step is to learn how to conduct treatment in structured conversations. Early in Stage 1, these structured conversations are arranged so that most of the child's speech is free of stuttering. Commonly parents achieve this by eliciting short and linguistically simple responses. These child responses may be only one or two or three words, and the parent follows them with contingent comments, called "parental verbal contingencies." These contingencies vary according to whether the child's response was stutter-free or stuttered. They are summarized with examples in Table 7.4.

In the majority of cases, parents use each of the five contingencies from time to time, taking care to use contingencies for stutter-free speech many times more than contingencies for stuttering. The parent and clinician discuss the choice of contingencies at each clinic visit to ensure that the mix of contingency types and their frequency of use are optimal for each child. For example, if an individual child shows signs of not liking praise for stutter-free speech, that contingency is removed temporarily and reintroduced only when the child accepts it again as part of routine treatment in structured conversations. These discussions about treatment will typically take up one-third of each clinic visit.

Early in Stage 1, parent-conducted treatment sessions in structured conversations are usually conducted for 10 to 15 minutes each day, at a time when children are alert and most willing to cooperate. These structured conversations will often be about picture books, with children having the opportunity to choose several favorites to talk about on each occasion.

See Video Clip 4 for an example of a clinician teaching parent about structured conversations.

Initially, the clinician demonstrates treatment conversations using cues like binary choices (e.g., "Is this one red or blue?"), sentence completion or cloze tasks (e.g., "Jack and Jill ran up..."), and wh- questions (e.g., "Where's that koala hiding now?") to elicit short stutter-free responses. Following a few short responses from the child, the clinician might ask occasional open questions to elicit longer responses, before returning to more one-word tasks. Verbal contingencies are also demonstrated during these structured conversations, and the clinician ensures that the child is not overloaded with too many of them. After watching the demonstration, the parent continues the treatment conversation, thus allowing the clinician to observe the parent. This observation then leads naturally to the clinician giving the parent feedback, along with further discussion about daily treatment in the week ahead.

See Video Clips 2 and 3 for examples of a clinician and a parent demonstrating structured treatment conversations. See Video Clip 9 for an example of a clinician coaching the parent about structured conversations at home.

As children become accustomed to treatment in structured conversations and parents become comfortable conducting them, SRs often begin to show the first signs of response to treatment. Commonly, the first sign is a general decrease in severity, which is expected within the first 4 weeks of Stage 1 (Onslow, Harrison, Jones, & Packman, 2002). When a decrease in severity is noted, clinicians encourage parents to start using verbal contingencies in unstructured conversations that occur in everyday situations (see video Segment 8 for an example of verbal contingencies, and video segment 11 for an example of an unstructured treatment conversation). Parents continue to use more frequent contingencies for stutter-free speech than for stuttering and use contingency types that are acceptable to each individual child. This change means that treatment conversations are no longer confined to 10 to 15 minutes per day. Instead, verbal contingencies are used in many settings and at different times of each day. Subsequently, treatment conversations are conducted as structured 10-minute conversations

Table 7.4. *Types and Examples of Parental Verbal Contingencies in the LP*

Parental Verbal Contingencies for the Child's Stutter-Free Speech	
Acknowledgement	"That was smooth talking."
Praise	"Wow, great talking!"
Request for self-evaluation	"Did you say that smoothly?"
Parental Verbal Contingencies for Unambiguous Stuttering	
Acknowledgment	"That was a bump there."
Request for self-correction	"Can you say [stuttered word/ phrase] again?"

on some days and as less intensive unstructured conversations on other days.

See Video Clips 12 and 14.

Over time, as SRs continue to decrease, more and more treatment occurs in unstructured conversations, and the treatment in structured conversations is gradually dispensed with. After children reach Stage 2 criteria, nearly all treatment occurs in unstructured conversations.

The aim of Stage 2 is for children to maintain the same criterion speech performance that was used to determine their transition from Stage 1 and to sustain it over long periods. Parents continue to collect SRs throughout Stage 2 but only for 1 week before clinic visits. As the clinic visits decrease in frequency, parents gradually withdraw all verbal contingencies and manage any relapses that may occur. Discharge is determined when children complete this performance-contingent stage of the program.

CONTEXTS FOR INTERVENTION

Treatment in unstructured conversations in the LP can occur in any number of settings. Although most treatment naturally occurs at home, clinicians encourage parents to be flexible and to conduct treatment in many situations. This becomes easier to arrange when children are a few weeks down the track in Stage 1 and parents and children are comfortable with structured treatment. It is at this time that treatment occurs more often in unstructured conversations, such as when traveling together in the car, while playing in the local park, and so on.

At all clinic visits, clinicians and parents discuss the places and times that treatment was conducted in the previous week. In this way, clinicians are able to monitor the amount of treatment and the

variety of situations being used. Even within the home environment, parents are encouraged to vary the settings for treatment in unstructured conversations as much as they can right from the beginning of Stage 1.

ASSESSMENT METHODS TO SUPPORT ONGOING DECISION MAKING

MEASURES USED IN TREATMENT

There are two measures of stuttering severity used in the LP. The first is %SS. For validity and convenience, 300 syllables or 10-minute samples are commonly used; these are measured during a conversation between child and parent. Button press timing and counting devices, such as those described earlier, make the task of real-time measurement simpler.

The second measure is SR using a 10-point scale. There are only three descriptors on this scale: SR1 is "no stuttering," SR2 is "extremely mild stuttering," and SR10 is "extremely severe stuttering."

FREQUENCY OF MEASURES

Clinicians measure %SS of samples of children's speech at the start of all clinic visits. To do this, they engage the children in natural conversation with their parents, usually while playing with clinic toys or while talking about a topic of interest to the children. Sometimes children are curious about the counting device and like to press the buttons and look at the display. A short explanation by the clinician that it is being used to count their words invariably satisfies their interest.

See Video Clip 13 for an example of a clinician assessing %SS.

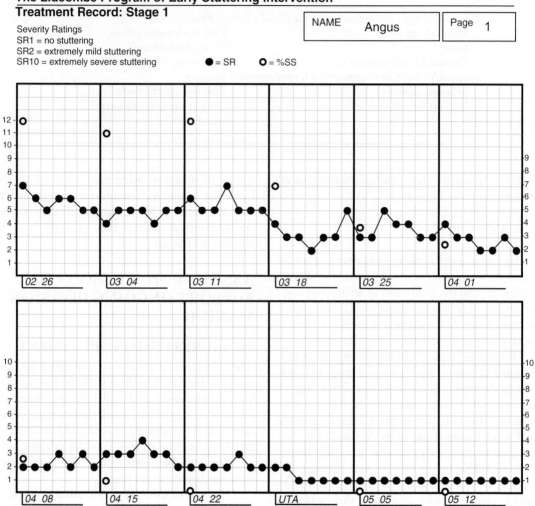

The Lidcombe Program of Early Stuttering Intervention
Treatment Record: Stage 1

Severity Ratings
SR1 = no stuttering
SR2 = extremely mild stuttering
SR10 = extremely severe stuttering   ● = SR   ○ = %SS

NAME   Angus   Page   1

Figure 7.1.   Example of a severity rating chart for a preschool-age child.

The %SS measures allow clinicians to monitor children's stuttering rates from week to week and provide the starting point for discussions with parents about changes in stuttering. The measures are entered onto children's clinic charts (see Fig. 7.1 for an example of one child's SR chart). On rare occasions when it is not possible to make %SS measures due to children's reticence, discussion with parents about beyond-clinic stuttering can still proceed and be based on SRs.

Parents assign SRs to their children's stuttering each day, chart them, and then report them during clinic visits each week

See Video Clip 5 for an example of a parent reporting SRs.

Clinicians train parents initially by asking them to assign ratings to clinic speech samples used for %SS measures. When first describing the scale to parents, the only information added to the descriptors is that SR10 is the most severe stuttering that the parent can imagine, rather than their own child's most severe stuttering.

Clinicians continue to check reliability of parents' SRs each week by asking them to assign SRs to within-clinic speech samples.

See Video Clips 6 and 10 for examples of a clinician checking reliability of a parent's SRs

Although it is uncommon, occasionally parents and clinicians have difficulty getting their SRs to match. In these cases, further information is needed about how both parties are identifying the child's stutters. It may be the case that the parent is unaware that what they have identified as simply a short pause in their child's speech is, in fact, an unambiguous stutter. Or commonly at the end of Stage 1, a parent may overreact to normal disfluency and score it more highly than the clinician. One useful method of resolving discrepancies is for the parent and clinician to listen together to an audio or video recording of the child. They can listen and watch together, identify normal disfluencies and unambiguous stutters, and thus increase their agreement.

Sometimes parents simply do not collect SRs and so have none to report at weekly clinic visits. LP treatment cannot proceed without these measures because clinicians rely on them when making decisions about treatment. Therefore, clinicians need to address the problem without delay and explore with parents the reasons why SRs were not collected. Something as simple as losing the SR chart can be the cause, or the parent may not have remembered when to do the ratings each day. It is also possible that the clinician's explanation of SRs and how to collect them was unclear or lacked detail. Whatever the cause, treatment should be delayed until the problem is identified and daily SRs are collected successfully.

FLOW CHART OF DECISIONS

See Figure 7.2 for a flowchart of decisions concerning LP treatment for preschool-age stuttering children.

TAILORING THE TREATMENT TO THE INDIVIDUAL CLIENT

There are many circumstances that affect the use of speech treatments with individual children and families. For clinicians, the ability to think creatively when applying treatments is a foundation skill. Their challenge when using a particular treatment—in this case the LP—is to maintain the program's integrity while taking into account those individual differences. Clinicians have used the LP successfully within many cultures and language groups, and we have written elsewhere about applying the LP to children whose personal circumstances had the potential to complicate

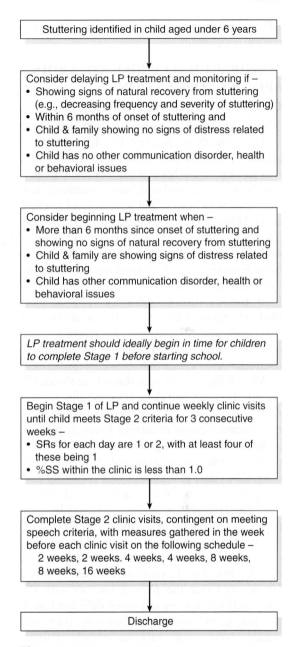

Figure 7.2. Flowchart of decisions concerning Lidcombe Program treatment for preschool-age stuttering children.

stuttering treatment. Hewat, Harris, and Harrison (2003) wrote about using the program with children who had other communication disorders or medical diagnoses, children from culturally and linguistically diverse backgrounds, sensitive or shy children, and children of working or busy parents. Rather than revisit those topics, the next section will deal with how clinicians can use the

LP within three other potentially challenging clinical populations.

POSSIBLE CHALLENGES REGARDING SPECIFIC POPULATIONS

Children with Separated Parents

There is no inherent reason for single parents to find it difficult to conduct the LP with their preschool-age children. After all, in families with two parents in the household, it is one parent—usually a mother—who delivers treatment, collects speech measures, and attends weekly clinic visits. Difficulties may arise because a single parent has less time available for treatment because of having sole responsibility for the entire household. Sometimes single parents are able to fit the extra commitment of stuttering therapy into their routine without difficulty. This is most likely to happen when there are few children in the family and making time for treatment and clinic visits requires only minor adjustment to routines.

More difficult is the situation where the child's parents live apart and share responsibility for and time with the child. Where there is already effective communication occurring between parents, cooperation concerning measurement and treatment activities can be arranged with little difficulty. The clinician establishes SR reliability with the parents during joint clinic visits and ensures that the treatment is being conducted by each parent in a manner that is optimal for the child. It is important to emphasize that this does not necessarily mean that the parents would need to conduct treatment in an identical manner. It would be expected that the parents interact with the child in different ways, talk about different topics, and play games differently; therefore, treatment conversations would vary accordingly. Parents might attend alternate clinic visits or vary the routine when one parent is unable to attend. The clinician can continue to monitor SRs and treatment at each clinic visit and thus ensure the child's progress.

The more challenging situation occurs when the separated parents are involved in the child's care and there is conflict between them. It can be useful to explain to the parents, albeit at different times, that the child's progress will be assisted by the parents agreeing to cooperate concerning treatment as negotiated with the clinician. If this agreement is achieved, then the clinician can proceed as usual, with each parent attending every second clinic visit. In the rare case in which there is no continuing communication between the parents and when each parent's training is being conducted every 2 weeks, the child's progress can be expected to be slow. It may also be necessary to defer the child's treatment until a more cooperative relationship is established between the parents.

Twins Who Both Stutter

Twins, like singleton siblings, are not likely to stutter in the same manner and with the same severity. Therefore, the parent's first step is to collect SRs for both children on a daily basis. If the parent finds this too difficult, then a better approach may be for the parent and clinician to begin SRs and treatment with one child and delay the second child's treatment until the first reaches Stage 2. Factors to consider when deciding which child should begin treatment may include severity of both children's stuttering (it may be easier for the parent to begin with the child whose stuttering is less severe), whether one child is more bothered by stuttering or is receiving negative peer reactions, or whether one child is generally more willing than the other to wait for his or her turn.

In cases where the decision is made to treat twins concurrently, SRs may be collected on alternate days for the two children if the parent finds this easier than daily ratings for both children. Structured treatment early in Stage 1 can easily be arranged so that the parent and both children participate together and the children take turns in the conversation and in choosing the topics or stimulus materials. However, as time goes on, it is likely that the children will progress at slightly different rates or respond best to different verbal contingencies. Parents will find it quite challenging to coordinate these slightly different aspects of treatment and will benefit from regular troubleshooting advice from the clinician.

Parents Who Stutters

Parents who stutter may initially be wary about their ability to conduct LP treatment with their children. Their concerns may stem from their awareness that they cannot always model stutter-free speech or from thinking that it would be unrealistic to encourage their children to speak with stutter-free speech when they cannot always do the same. Concerns such as these have been expressed to us in the past by parents who doubted that they would be able to help their children. Despite initial misgivings such as these, our experience is that parents who stutter certainly can use the LP successfully with their children.

Most young children who do the LP with stuttering parents will, at some point, comment on their parents' "bumpy words." It can be useful for clinicians to discuss this possibility with parents early in Stage 1 so that they are prepared to respond when it occurs. Appropriate responses that are consistent with the LP are those that both acknowledge children's comments and emphasize their stutter-free speech. An example of this would be, "You're right, but Daddy can't get rid of his stuck words like you can."

APPLICATION TO AN INDIVIDUAL CLIENT

DESCRIPTION OF MAJOR COMPONENTS OF INTERVENTION

Theo's mother Barbara referred him for an initial assessment at the speech pathology clinic when he was 3 years 8 months. They attended the assessment session with Theo's father Peter and younger sister Katelyn. Theo had started to stutter 9 months earlier, and his parents described the onset as sudden and severe, with his stuttering consisting of long strings of repeated syllables—15 repeats were common—and fixed postures with audible airflow. Barbara and Peter reported being alarmed by the severity of Theo's stuttering at first, even though they recognized what he was doing due to its similarity to his maternal grandmother's speech. After waiting a few weeks, during which the severity of Theo's stuttering decreased, Barbara sought advice from a local child health center. She was given general information about early stuttering and intervention services and advised to take Theo for speech pathology assessment if he was still stuttering at 3.5 years.

A sample of Theo's speech during a clinic conversation was measured as 6% SS and SR6. His stutters were multiple repetitions of sounds and syllables. Peter and Barbara agreed that this sample was typical of Theo's least severe stuttering and that he sometimes stuttered more frequently, although with the same types of stutters. The clinician recommended that Theo start the LP, and his parents agreed to put his name on the waiting list for treatment.

Two months later, when Theo was 3 years 10 months, he started Stage 1 of the LP. His stuttering had gradually become more severe after the assessment, and a speech sample during his first LP clinic visit was measured as 12% SS and SR8. Theo was reluctant to talk with the clinician, although he talked freely with his mother and seemed to enjoy playing with the clinic toys. The clinician explained SRs to Barbara and showed her how to chart her daily ratings during the week ahead. They discussed the range of severity of Theo's stuttering over the past weeks, and Barbara used the scale to describe the range as "minimum SR4 and maximum SR9." The clinician then described parental verbal contingencies for stutter-free speech and stuttering and recommended using only those for stutter-free speech for next week. Barbara agreed to do this and then, following the clinician's instructions, used praise and acknowledgment of stutter-free speech correctly in a short, structured treatment conversation with Theo.

In the second Stage 1 clinic visit, Barbara reported that Theo's SRs had varied between SR9 and SR6 over the previous week. They had played a "talking game"—as Theo described treatment in structured conversations—each day, and most of his responses had been stutter-free, short utterances of two to four words in length. A sample of his speech in the clinic was measured as 12% SS.

By the third clinic visit, Theo's SRs had decreased and were in the range of SR6 to SR3. A speech sample in the clinic was measured as 2% SS, and Barbara was using contingencies only for stutter-free speech during treatment in unstructured conversations.

Over the following 5 weeks, Theo and Barbara were unable to attend three clinic visits due to illness. It was clear from Theo's SR chart that his stuttering severity varied, and Barbara reported that they were able to do very few treatment conversations over these weeks. Apart from those weeks, Theo's Stage 1 treatment continued without any further substantial difficulties.

DESCRIPTION OF OUTCOME

Theo completed Stage 1 after 32 weeks, during which he attended 27 clinic visits. In the first 8 weeks of Stage 2, he failed to meet criterion speech measures on two occasions. Following discussion with the clinician, the strategy that Barbara used was to increase the rate of verbal contingencies for stutter-free speech during unstructured conversations, and Theo's SRs subsequently fell to SR1 again. Seven months after starting Stage 2, Theo successfully completed it and was discharged. By that time, he had consistently achieved ratings of SR1 for several months.

CASE STUDY

Claire lives with her father Tom, mother Rosemary, and two older siblings, Stephen (5 years) and Mason (7 years). She was initially assessed by a speech-language pathologist when she was age 3 years 9 months. Her parents reported a gradual onset of her stuttering approximately 14 months earlier. At first, they noticed occasional repetitions of sounds and words, usually two or three repeats each time. These repetitions became more frequent, and Claire started to prolong sounds. She became upset on a couple of occasions and said that her "tongue was stuck." A sample of her speech video recorded at home was measured as 9% SS and SR7, and her parents agreed that this was typical of her stuttering over recent weeks. The clinician outlined the LP and recommended it for Claire. Tom and Rosemary agreed, and Claire started Stage 1 a few weeks later.

In the first few clinic visits of Stage 1, the clinician introduced the SR scale and demonstrated structured treatment conversations using all of the verbal contingencies for stutter-free and stuttered speech. Rosemary demonstrated that she could use all contingencies correctly and reported being able to do daily treatment conversations and collect SRs regularly. The clinician and Rosemary established consistent agreement on SRs for Claire's speech samples in the clinic.

Claire seemed to enjoy the clinic visits, and Rosemary reported that she had no difficulty engaging her in treatment in structured conversations at home. She said that Claire stuttered very

little during these conversations, and Rosemary used all three contingencies for stutter-free speech.

Claire's SRs decreased over 3 weeks and then stabilized at SR3 and SR4 for several weeks. Her within-clinic speech samples, measured at the beginning of each clinic visit, also became stable and were consistently in the range 3% to 5% SS.

CLINICAL APPLICATION/CRITICAL THINKING QUESTIONS

1. What may be the reasons for the lack of decrease in Claire's SRs over several weeks?
2. What questions would you ask Rosemary about her SRs for Claire's speech at home?
3. Since Claire is enjoying treatment conversations at home and getting lots of stutter-free speech practice, is there any need to make changes?
4. When Rosemary and Claire do a treatment conversation during their next clinic visit, what will you look for in particular?
5. What is the most important change that you would like to introduce in Claire's treatment?

FUTURE DIRECTIONS

EXTENSION TO NEW POPULATIONS

Although the LP was designed and researched for children younger than 6 years, there has been one phase II clinical trial reported for a school-age group. Lincoln et al. (1996) explored the effects of the treatment with 11 children in the age range of 7 to 12 years. Measures of %SS and syllables per minute (SPM) were collected from audiotape recordings, including a covert assessment, at 2 months, 1 month, and 1 week before treatment and 1 week, 1 month, 2 months, 3 months, 4 months, 6 months, 9 months, and 12 months after treatment. In contrast to phase II clinical trials with preschoolers, Lincoln et al. (1996) reported an apparent "medium" effect size in beyond-clinic situations at 12 months after treatment. In addition, a recent retrospective (nonclinical trial) follow-up study of school-age children treated with the LP (Koushik et al., 2007) also reported a "medium" effect for this age group. (The Koushik et al. (2007) follow-up data are worth considering in the present context because they are based on beyond-clinic recordings and hence can be compared with the follow-up results of Lincoln et al. [1996].) The difference in apparent effects can be seen by comparing the last follow-up %SS scores in these reports with three phase II clinical trials of the LP. For school-age children, Lincoln et al. (1996) and Koushik et al. (2007) reported means of 1.0% SS and 1.8% SS, respectively, at the last follow-up. However, the mean 12-month posttreatment %SS scores in the Miller and Guitar (2009), Onslow, Andrews, and Lincoln (1994), and Rousseau et al. (2007) studies were much lower at 0.5% SS, 0.1% SS, and 0.8% SS, respectively. These data give the impression that school-age children are less responsive to the LP than preschool children. Such a prospect is certainly theoretically possible because it appears that children may have fewer degrees of freedom of speech motor activity during the school years compared with the preschool years (e.g., Wohlert & Smith, 2002) and hence may be less able to cope with stuttering rehabilitation. Additionally, the treatment recoveries of children during the preschool years are undoubtedly assisted by the natural recovery effect, and it is possible that this would explain why preschoolers appear to do better in clinical trials of the LP. However, without a phase III trial involving the LP, which would allow a trustworthy estimate of the true effect size (see earlier "Phase III Clinical Trials" section) with school-age children, this issue remains unresolved.

The clinical trials of the LP outlined previously dealt with the efficacy of the treatment and were conducted under carefully controlled scientific conditions. Although those conditions have mostly involved standard speech pathology service delivery in clinical settings, they have also involved specialist clinicians who are dedicated, for the period of the trial, to the treatment of the children in the trial and parents who have consented to be involved in research. An important issue in treatment development is the concept of treatment effectiveness. This refers to how well the treatment works when it is used by a population of nonresearcher, generalist clinicians who have received reasonable continuing education in the treatment method. At the time of writing, a study is being planned to determine the effectiveness of the LP when it is used by such a population of clinicians.

CONTINUING NEEDS FOR VALIDATION OF EVIDENCE

The bulk of evidence in support of the LP outlined in the preceding pages is reductionist in nature, involving dependent variables such as stuttering severity, time to recovery, anxiety, and acoustics. There is much that can be learned about the LP from constructivist or qualitative research paradigms that do not explore research issues in terms of dependent variables but that build information about issues using rich and detailed descriptions (for a comparison of reductionist and constructivist research paradigms in stuttering research, see Cheek, Onslow, & Cream, 2004). A good example of such research is a study that was in progress at the time of writing, with a purpose of establishing parents' experiences of the LP. It is intended that the output of this research will inform clinicians who train parents to perform the treatment and will inform those who provide instruction to students in the LP during professional preparation at universities.

The LP has been manualized. In other words, it has been described in great detail so as to allow any clinician to download the manual and conduct the treatment exactly as the clinicians did in published clinical trials. The manual specifies that the child and parent visit the clinician once per week during Stage 1. However, it is not necessarily the case that such a model is the most efficient. Two research projects are currently under way to explore different modes of service delivery of the LP. The first of these is a randomized trial designed to compare the standard, face-to-face format with a format in which children and parents visit the clinician in groups and in which those group sessions are supplemented by audiovisual instruction aids. The purpose of this study is to determine whether treatment efficiency gains can be obtained without the loss of any treatment efficacy. Another randomized trial in progress is designed to determine whether gains can be made in treatment efficiency by comparing the standard weekly treatment format with treatment formats where parents and children visit the clinic twice weekly and once every 2 weeks.

Additional studies are under way to understand how specific components of the LP affect treatment outcomes. At present, we and our colleagues are beginning a research project that is designed to further the results of the Harrison et al. (2002) study of the need for verbal contingencies. Parents and children who are receiving the LP will be studied to explore the number and type of verbal contingencies that parents actually present to their children. The study will also explore whether the number and range of verbal contingencies presented by parents predict treatment time. A much larger study is also under way that is designed to determine whether a variety of speech and nonspeech variables in children and parents have any predictive value.

CHAPTER SUMMARY

- The LP is a stuttering treatment program developed for children younger than 6 years.
- The LP reduces stuttering to near-zero levels in children.
- The LP is supported by replicated clinical trial evidence; a randomized controlled trial; large cohort recovery plot studies; psychological, linguistic, and acoustic assessments of outcome; social validity; and treatment process research.
- The aim of the LP is to reduce children's stuttering to a near-zero level (Stage 1) and to maintain that reduction for a clinically significant period (Stage 2).
- Parents conduct LP treatment during daily conversations with their children.
- Severity ratings (SRs) are used throughout the program and have the following definitions: SR1 = "no stuttering," SR2 = "extremely mild stuttering," and SR10 = "extremely severe stuttering."
- There are five parental verbal contingencies used in the LP, of which there are three contingencies for stutter-free speech and two for stuttered speech.
- Further research is planned or is already under way that aims to increase the efficiency of treatment and make the LP more easily accessible to families of young children who stutter.

CHAPTER REVIEW QUESTIONS

1. For what age group of stuttering children was the LP designed?
2. Are there any types of stuttering or characteristics of children, families, or clinicians that would rule out use of the LP?
3. The empirical evidence base of the LP is grouped in this chapter under two headings— "Clinical Trials Evidence" and "Treatment Process Research." What is the difference between these categories of research evidence?
4. What is the current rule of thumb for the median number of treatment sessions it takes for children to achieve the speech criteria to begin Stage 2?
5. What empirical evidence is available to support the recommendation that children should not begin the LP earlier than 6 months after onset of stuttering?
6. What are the scale value descriptions of SR1, SR2, and SR10?
7. Who collects SRs in the LP, and where and when do they collect them?
8. What steps would a clinician take to ensure correspondence of parent and clinician SRs?
9. What are the five parental verbal contingencies used in the LP?
10. Since parents deliver LP treatment with their children in conversations outside the clinic, what is the function of weekly clinic visits by the parent and child?
11. What are five differences between treatment in structured conversations and treatment in unstructured conversations?
12. What are the Stage 2 speech criteria?
13. If a clinician is unsure about how to solve a problem that arises during Stage 1, what sources of help or information could the clinician access?

SUGGESTED READINGS

Attanasio, J. (2003). Some observations and reflections. In M. Onslow, A. Packman, & E. Harrison (Eds.), *The LP of Early Stuttering Intervention* (pp. 207–214). Austin, TX: Pro-Ed.

Harrison, E., Ttofari, K., Rousseau, I., & Andrews, C. (2003). Troubleshooting. In M. Onslow, A. Packman, & E. Harrison (Eds.), *The LP of Early Stuttering Intervention* (pp. 91–99). Austin, TX: Pro-Ed.

Packman, A. (2003). Issues. In M. Onslow, A. Packman, & E. Harrison (Eds.), *The LP of Early Stuttering Intervention* (pp. 199–206). Austin, TX: Pro-Ed.

Packman, A., Code, C., & Onslow, M. (2007). On the cause of stuttering: Integrating theory with brain and behavioral research. *Journal of Neurolinguistics, 20*, 353–362.

CHAPTER 8

Overview of Treatments for School-Age Children Who Stutter

BARRY E. GUITAR AND REBECCA J. MCCAULEY

CHAPTER OUTLINE

INTRODUCTION

The treatments for preschool children who stutter described in the preceding section uniformly aim for complete fluency in their clients. Treatments for school-age children, on the other hand, are more varied in their goals and expectations, perhaps because stuttering in this age group is harder to completely eliminate. The four treatments for school-age children and adolescents presented here show a wide range of goals—from complete and normal-sounding fluency to effective communication despite residual stuttering. The first two treatments, the Lidcombe Program for School-Age Children and the Fluency Rules Program, are the most focused on fluent speech. The second two, Smooth Speech with Cognitive Behavior Therapy and Comprehensive Treatment, focus on communication attitudes and skills, as well as on improved fluency. As you read the descriptions, observe how the complexity of treatment goals influences the number of treatment elements. Also consider how each treatment deals with the fact that stuttering in school-age children and adolescents is often more complicated than stuttering in preschool children. We will compare and contrast the four approaches at the end of this chapter, after we have laid out their goals, procedures, theoretical bases, and supporting evidence.

LIDCOMBE PROGRAM FOR SCHOOL-AGE CHILDREN WHO STUTTER (CHAPTER 9 BY HARRISON, BRUCE, SHENKER, AND KOUSHIK)

This is an adaptation of the Lidcombe Program (LP) for preschool children. It has been used for school children between ages 6 to 12 years, especially those whose stuttering is relatively mild. Because it is administered with relatively few modifications from the preschool version, the description that follows is very similar to that of the original LP, presented in Chapter 7.

The basic goal of the treatment is stutter-free or nearly stutter-free speech that is shown to endure a year or more after it is achieved. The first intermediate goal is to achieve two benchmarks of fluency: (1) daily severity ratings by parents that average less than 2 (with at least 4 days of ratings of 1) for 3 weeks in a row, and (2) clinician ratings of the child's speech in the weekly session of less than 1% SS for the same 3 weeks. The second intermediate goal is to maintain those benchmarks as clinician contact is gradually faded from once-weekly meetings to meetings that occur 2, 2, 4, 4, 8, 8, and then finally 16 weeks apart. Evidence suggests that there is more variability in stuttering of school children compared with preschool children during this period when clinic meetings are gradually faded. In other words, school children are likely to show more ups and downs in their fluency as treatment is ending (Koushik et al., 2007; Lincoln et al., 1996).

As with the preschool LP, the school-age LP uses two measures of stuttering to determine progress in the program. The first is the severity rating (SR), a 1-to-10 scale that the parent uses, after training, to give daily assessments of the child's speech. A rating of 1 indicates normal fluency, and a rating of 10 indicates the worst the child's stuttering has ever been. One option for the LP with school-age children is to train the children themselves to use SRs and for the clinician to discuss both the parent's and child's weekly SRs during the clinic session. The second measure is child's percent syllables stuttered (%SS), which the clinician measures at the beginning of each weekly meeting with the parent and child.

Activities and procedures include (1) weekly sessions with the clinician in which the clinician assesses the child's speech then guides and supports the parent to conduct treatment at home, (2) daily structured conversations between parent and child in which the parent uses verbal contingencies for stutter-free and stuttered speech, and (3) gradual replacement of structured conversations by unstructured conversations in which the parent continues to use verbal contingencies but now in more commonplace daily activities. Contexts begin with a one-on-one speaking situation in which the parent constrains the child's verbal output (e.g., by setting up a set of questions to be followed by predictable answers) and uses verbal contingencies to promote fluency. Once the child is approximately 90% fluent in this situation, the parent lets the child talk more freely in a natural conversation and continues the verbal contingencies to maintain fluency. The context gradually changes to unstructured situations, in which the child may be talking to the parent in the car, in the grocery store, and around the house. Other speakers, such as the other parent or a grandparent, are then brought in to unstructured conversations to use verbal contingencies during unstructured conversations.

Although the main vehicle for changing the child's speech is the parent's praise of fluency and requests for correction of stuttering, the LP for school-age children may also incorporate tangible rewards to motivate the child. Another variation when the LP is used for school-age children is that if the parent is unavailable to deliver daily treatment, someone else from home or an older student or staff member at the child's school may take the traditional parent role in the LP treatment.

The theoretical basis of the LP for school-age children does not involve speculation about the cause of stuttering but simply asserts that stuttering has been shown to behave like an operant because it can be changed by response-contingent stimuli. In this intervention, the stimuli are verbal: parents' praise for fluency and parents' acknowledgement of their children's stuttering or their requests for children to correct their stuttering.

The evidence supporting the LP for school-age children is relatively modest compared with the evidence for the LP for preschool children. Two studies have been reported. Lincoln et al. (1996) published the first report on the LP for this age group, with a cohort of 11 children ages 7 to 12 years. Multiple pre- and posttreatment measures were made, showing that all children made substantial gains in fluency and that, for the most part, these gains continued during a 1-year maintenance program. This amount of progress by school-age children is impressive. However, the results of this early study must be interpreted with caution because 4 of the 11 children did not complete maintenance and no data were presented to establish that fluency gains continued after the maintenance program was over. Koushik et al. (2007) reported on 12 children between ages 6 and 11 treated by the LP. Mean %SS decreased from 9% (standard deviation [SD] = 7.5%) at the beginning of treatment to 1.8% (SD = 1.3%) at follow-up, measured from 9 weeks to 15 months (mean of 6 months) after stable fluency was achieved. At follow-up, 5 of the 12 children had %SS scores at or below 1.0% SS, 7 had scores below 2.0% SS, 9 had scores below 3.0% SS, and 12 had scores below 4.0% SS. In both reports, the school-age children's fluency was found to be more variable in the maintenance phase (Stage 2) than has been found for preschool children treated with the LP.

THE FLUENCY RULES PROGRAM (CHAPTER 10 BY RUNYAN AND RUNYAN)

This program was designed for preschool children and younger school-age children who stutter, but we will focus on the school-age children here. The authors of the program have used their approach primarily with children who stutter and who do not have other speech, language, learning, or cognitive problems. However, they have found it easy to adapt the program for use with children who have language problems, learning disabilities, cognitive challenges, or autism.

The program's basic goal is natural-sounding fluent speech. Intermediate goals are expressed in terms of various "rules" that children learn sequentially to become fluent. The first set of rules—thus, the first intermediate goals—are called Universal Rules because all children must learn and use some or all of them. The rules are as follows: (1) reduce speech rate, (2) eliminate the repetition of single-syllable words and/or part-words, and (3) eliminate prolongations. The second set of intermediate goals (rules) are called Primary Rules and are used with children who do not become entirely fluent after having learned the Universal Rules. These rules include learning to (4) breathe properly during speech rather than holding the breath during stuttering, (5) begin phonation gently rather than blocking at the larynx, and (6) touch articulators lightly rather than blocking at the tongue or lips. For children who persist in using accessory behaviors, such as eye blinks or head nods, after meeting appropriate earlier goals, a seventh goal (rule) is introduced: (7) use only speech helpers to talk rather than moving other structures when stuttering.

Activities and procedures for the Fluency Rules Program begin with an analysis of the child's stuttering to determine which rules apply. The clinician then teaches the appropriate Universal Rules to the child and uses conversational speech in games and other activities as the context in which the child can learn to use the rules. For example, the clinician models the child's type of stuttering in a "catch me" game to help the child learn to identify stutters; subsequently, the clinician rewards the child for identifying stutters in his own speech. Teaching Primary Rules begins with instruction in the fundamentals of speech production, including breath support, voicing, and articulator movement. The clinician then guides the child in practicing fluent speech production in a linguistic hierarchy, moving from isolated sounds to spontaneous speech. As the child makes progress towards fluent speech, several procedures are used to promote generalization. Early in therapy, words on which the child stutters outside of therapy are practiced in the therapy room. As therapy progresses, parents and teachers work with the clinician and child to develop visual cues to remind the child to use fluency rules in home and school environments. Toward the end of treatment, the clinician telephones the child at home with fading frequency to cue him or her to use fluency rules to retain fluency.

The authors have not attempted to develop their therapy on the basis of an etiologic model of stuttering, but rather have created therapy procedures based on their clinical observations of children who stutter. They surmise, for example, that these children do not have enough awareness of their stuttering to be able to correct it themselves. Thus, an early stage of treatment involves heightening awareness of stuttering without creating negative emotion. A second observation made in their theoretical basis section is that older children who stutter often have trouble coordinating the processes of speech production for fluent speech. Thus, an important component of Fluency Rules therapy for older children is learning about normal speech production and practicing a structured hierarchy focused on mindful use of the elements of fluent speech. In summary, like most treatments, the Fluency Rules Program did not emerge from a theory about deficits that cause stuttering that gave rise to a carefully considered set of procedures aimed at changing these deficits. Instead, it was constructed in a purely clinical spirit with components that seemed to make sense and work with this age group.

The evidence for the effectiveness of the Fluency Rules Program was reported in three book chapters. Runyan and Runyan (1991) reported on nine children between ages 3 and 7 years, treated in a public school setting. Follow-up for 1 to 2 years indicated that all children achieved and "maintained significant improvement in fluency, normal speaking rate and eliminated all secondary behaviors." However, the Runyans noted that all children still showed mild repetitions of one to two iterations. After making some modifications to the Fluency Rules Program, they reported on 14 children, age 3 to 11 years, treated in their private practice (Runyan & Runyan, 1993). At the time of the report, 10 of the 14 children had been dismissed with normal-sounding speech after an average of 9 months of therapy. The other four children were still in treatment. In 1999, Runyan and Runyan reported on another six children (two preschoolers and four school-age children). Five were dismissed from therapy with normal speech, and the sixth—a second grader with severe stuttering—was still in therapy at the time of the report.

SMOOTH SPEECH AND COGNITIVE BEHAVIOR THERAPY FOR THE TREATMENT OF OLDER CHILDREN AND ADOLESCENTS WHO STUTTER (CHAPTER 11 BY CRAIG)

This approach is recommended for children and young adolescents between 9 and 14 years who stutter. Recency of onset and severity of stuttering are not important considerations in determining which children are appropriate for this treatment.

The basic goals for this approach are to teach clients smooth speech and psychological skills to help them improve their ability to communicate and interact with others. Intermediate goals are as follows: (1) learn to speak without stuttering using smooth speech skills at slow and then progressively more normal speech rates in conversation; (2) complete a hierarchy of transfer activities designed to generalize speech with minimal stuttering to everyday life situations; (3) learn to use cognitive techniques to reduce fears and negative attitudes about speaking; and (4) develop a maintenance plan that involves client taking on more responsibility, including self-practice and self-evaluation, and that also involves family support.

Activities and procedures consist of the following nine stages. (1) Clinician assesses client's stuttering frequency, speech naturalness, anxieties, and communication attitudes. (2) Clinician teaches client smooth speech over 3 days, using gradually normalized speech rate in conversa-

tion. (3) Clinician videotapes client speaking at appropriate rate two times per day and plays back recording for evaluation. (4) Client practices smooth speech at home each evening with parent who has been attending sessions. (5) Once client has mastered stutter-free smooth speech in clinic and home, he or she completes transfer hierarchy to everyday situations, maintaining smooth speech with minimal stuttering. The client also records transfer assignments and evaluates them with the clinician's guidance. (6) During the transfer stage, the client learns, through instruction and discussion, about taking responsibility for his of her own progress. For example, the client sets his of her own goals and rewards himself or herself for achieving them. (7) Also during the transfer stage, the client learns cognitive behavioral techniques such as muscle relaxation and positive self-talk and applies these skills during transfer activities. (8) During the last 1 or 2 days of the intensive program, the client works on long-term maintenance strategies, including taking on more responsibility for evaluating his or her own speech and planning how to deal with relapse. (9) The client and the family meet with the clinician to engage the family in supporting the client as he or she works to maintain fluency. Over a period of a year, the client and family meet intermittently with the clinician to review progress and deal with maintenance issues.

The theoretical basis of this approach is twofold. First, it is assumed that stuttering arises from a neurophysiologic deficit that must be compensated for by the use of fluency skills, such as slow rate and gentle onset of phonation, that alter the entire pattern of speech. Inculcating these changes in children's speech enables them to make the complex coordinations for fluent speech that would otherwise be out of their reach. Second, it is assumed that stuttering in older children has an overlay of psychological factors, such as anxiety and avoidance, that have become associated with speech after years of stuttering. Thus, a variety of cognitive-behavioral techniques such as muscle relaxation and social skills training have been added to deal with these factors.

Evidence supporting the effectiveness of the Smooth Speech treatment comes primarily from two studies—Craig et al. (1996) and Hancock et al. (1998). These studies assessed the change in percent syllables stuttered from before treatment to (1) immediately after treatment, (2) 1 year after treatment, and (3) 5 years after treatment. Two different formats of treatment were used: clinic-based intensive treatment (5-day treatment in clinic) and home-based nonintensive treatment (1 clinic day for 5 weeks with parent providing treatment on the other days). Both types of treatment had a 1-year maintenance component. Results showed considerable change immediately after treatment, and much of these gains were maintained. Table 11.1 in the chapter by Craig (Chapter 11) presents results both in terms of percent change in frequency of stuttering and effect size. Data in the journal articles indicate that at both 12 months and 2 to 6 years after treatment, the mean %SS for both clinic-based and home-based treatments was approximately 3% SS. These data were relatively similar whether the measures were made in the clinic, on the telephone, or in the home. It should be noted, however, that standard deviations were approximately the size of the means, indicating a fairly large variability in outcome.

COMPREHENSIVE TREATMENT FOR SCHOOL-AGE CHILDREN WHO STUTTER (CHAPTER 12 BY YARUSS, PELCZARSKI, AND QUESAL)

This approach is designed to be used with children between age 7 and 17 years. The basic goal is for children who stutter to become effective communicators. For some children, this may mean that they still stutter but that their stuttering does not interfere with their freedom to achieve social, academic, and occupational goals. Intermediate goals include: (1) minimizing stuttering severity, (2) reducing the children's and others' negative reactions to stuttering, (3) improving children's ability to communicate in real-life situations, and (4) helping children generalize and maintain improvements in fluency and in communication.

The activities and procedures include: (1) learning a variety of techniques (e.g., slower speech rate, easy onsets) that lessen the severity of stuttering; (2) practicing the techniques in a hierarchy of easy to difficult situations; (3) exploring, with the clinician, what happens when stutters occur; (4) using voluntary stuttering to reduce fear and physical tension associated with stuttering;

(5) using voluntary stuttering in a hierarchy of easy to difficult situations; (6) discussing with the clinician the thoughts and fears associated with stuttering and developing new ways of thinking and feeling about stuttering; (7) meeting with others who stutter to share experiences and feelings; (8) educating others in the child's environment to increase acceptance of the child and his or her stuttering.

The theoretical basis underlying this approach is focused not on the cause of the stuttering but on how stuttering typically presents itself in school-age children. Specifically, in addition to core stuttering behaviors (repetitions, etc.), crucial aspects of stuttering are the children's behavioral, cognitive, and affective responses to stuttering. These responses, in turn, may lead to dysfunction in the children's communication effectiveness because of debilitating self-consciousness about speaking and widespread avoidance of speaking. Finally, the communication dysfunction often leads to reduced quality of life for school children who stutter because they may not participate fully and freely in academic, social, and occupational opportunities.

There is, as yet, no evidence for the effectiveness of the Comprehensive Treatment for school-age children who stutter. In place of data on outcome of their entire treatment package, the authors refer to published studies of some of the subcomponents of their approach, such as lessening severity of stuttering and changing negative reactions to stuttering. In considering future research on the effectiveness of their program, the authors describe the need to look beyond measures of stuttering frequency and severity, to measures of reactions to stuttering, communication function, and quality of life.

DIFFERENCES AND SIMILARITIES AMONG APPROACHES

Table 8.1 summarizes key characteristics of each approach.

The differences among the four approaches are many, but let us consider first their varied goals and methods to achieve them. **The Lidcombe Program for School-Age Children** focuses simply on helping children develop effortless, stutter-free speech in their normal

Table 8.1. *Characteristics of Interventions for School-Age Children Who Stutter*

	Treatment			
Variable	Lidcombe Program for School-Age Children	Fluency Rules Program	Smooth Speech and Cognitive Behavior Therapy	Comprehensive Treatment
Nature of Goals	Stutter-free or nearly stutter-free speech that is shown to endure for more than a year after it is established	Natural-sounding fluent speech	Managing stuttering and improveing communication and social interactions.	Effective communication and good quality of life
Client Population	Children 6 to 12 years old	School-age children who stutter; may be adopted for children with concomitant disorders	Older children and adolescents (roughly 9 to 14 years old)	School-age children from 7 to 17 years old
Intervention Agents	Parents, guided by clinician; when parent is unavailable, others, such as older sibling or teacher's aide, can substitute	Clinician is primary agent, but parents and teachers help child to remember to use his or her "rules" in home and school environments	Intensive version: clinician, although parent attends sessions and helps with transfer and maintenance; home version: parent, guided by clinician	Clinician works directly with child, but during treatment, others in child's environment become part of team
Nature of Session	Individual sessions; clinician guides parent by modeling, providing feedback about conduct of home treatment, and discussion of child's progress	As described, the treatment is administered individually, but the authors indicate that it works well in groups of children	Intensive version: may be group or individual; clinician teaches speech pattern and gives feedback; home version: individual, with parent guided by weekly visits with clinician	Treatment sessions can be individual or group depending on what suits child; for all children, meeting in group with others who stutter is encouraged
Demands for Technology	Device for counting stutters and syllables; parents may use audio or video recording equipment	No equipment needed, although a device is shown on a video clip that monitors a child's breathing	Device for counting stutters and syllables; audiovisual equipment for recording and playback; small digital or tape recorders	No special equipment is needed, although video recording and playback can be used to help child explore his or her stuttering
Frequency of Sessions	At home: daily for 10 to 15 minutes; in clinic: once per week	Although no details are given, it can be assumed that sessions are weekly	Intensive: 5 straight days; home program: 5 days in 5 weeks	May be once or twice weekly; may be beneficial to have more frequent sessions at beginning of therapy

Table 8.1. *Characteristics of Interventions for School-Age Children Who Stutter* (Continued)

	Treatment			
Overall Duration of Treatment	8 to 12 weeks to achieve fluency and then gradually faded contact for a year after fluency is obtained	The average duration is about 9 months, with a range of 2 to 20 months	One week (or 5 weeks) followed by a maintenance program managed by family with check-ups by clinician over a period of 1 year	Because of individual variability, duration of treatment is not easy to predict
General Characterization of Methods	Clinician trains parent to administer praise and corrections in structured and unstructured daily situations; clinician discusses child's progress as measured by parent's daily severity ratings and clinician's assessment of child's %SS in clinic	Clinician teaches child an individualized set of "rules" designed to change stuttering to fluent speech; once learned, these rules are used in conversation in various games and activities; clinician uses praise and correction to shape the child's speech output	Clinician uses behavioral techniques to train child in smooth speech pattern at gradually increasing rates while maintaining fluency; behavior shaping is also used to help client transfer and maintain fluency	A combination of behavioral, cognitive, and affective treatment is used; there is emphasis on making stuttering less severe and helping child communicate despite residual stuttering

environments. To achieve this, clinicians use verbal contingencies on fluent speech (praise) and on stuttered speech (request for correction), without any instructions to children as to how to achieve fluency. **The Fluency Rules Program** also aims to teach children natural-sounding fluent speech, but uses instructions, as well as rewards and corrections. Children are specifically taught to slow their speech rates, to say a word only once (rather than repeating), and to say words briefly (rather than prolonging sounds). More severely affected children are taught techniques—proper breathing, gentle onset of phonation, and light articulator contacts—to help them deal with moments of stuttering. The goals for **Smooth Speech with Cognitive Behavior Therapy** are a little broader than for the two previous therapies; they include controlling stuttering (rather than simply learning to speak fluently), but also improving social skills and communication attitudes. Control of stuttering is taught via a hierarchy of slow, prolonged speech that is gradually shaped to sound normal. Muscle relaxation is taught to help the clients contend with the muscle tension that accompanies more severe stuttering. Cognitive techniques such as positive self-talk are used to help clients improve communication and social skills and attitudes. It is important to note that the target population for this treatment is older children and adolescents. This age group is likely to have been stuttering for a longer time compared with the younger school-age children who are the target age for the Lidcombe and Fluency Rules Programs. As children contend with stuttering for many years, their stuttering patterns may become more ingrained and harder to eliminate, thus making "controlled stuttering" a more realistic goal rather than stutter-free speech. In addition, therapies for older school-age children need to deal with the fact that many of these children react to their stuttering with negative emotion about communication, leading to avoidance of speaking and social isolation (Bloodstein & Berstein Ratner, 2007). This change in the characteristics and consequences of stuttering as children grow older explains why the **Comprehensive Treatment** approach aims to help children become effective communicators rather than fluent speakers. Children are taught to modify stuttering by reducing speech rate and physical tension; they are desensitized to stimuli that previously elicited fear;

and they are helped to think differently about their past and future speaking experiences. This intervention has the broadest goals of any of the four approaches and may go the farthest toward meeting one of Bloodstein's famous criteria for effective treatment: "Treatment must remove not only stuttering, but also the fears, the anticipations, and the person's self-concept as a stutterer" (Bloodstein & Berstein Ratner, 2007). In summary, the four programs are presented sequentially in terms of how narrowly focused the goals are. The Lidcombe Program is the most narrowly focused on fluent speech; the Fluency Rules Program focuses on fluent speech, but employs some techniques to modify stuttering for children who do not respond to simpler treatment; Smooth Speech targets fluency but also communication attitudes; and Comprehensive Treatment does not choose fluency as a goal but, instead, aims for effective communication.

Despite differences in goals, activities, and age ranges targeted by these treatments, they have many similarities. By examining common elements, we may find important therapeutic principles for further study in treatments for school-age children who stutter. As we will see, even the similarities have differences, and these may be quite important. For example, all four treatments use reinforcement for behaviors the clinician wants to increase. Two of the approaches are systematic about reinforcing children for desired behavior. The Lidcombe Program is based on verbal contingencies (praise for fluency and requests for correction of stuttering), and the Smooth Speech approach employs financial incentives to children for completing many aspects of the program. Fluency Rules and the Comprehensive Treatment are far less systematic, but it is evident from the description of the programs and from the video clips that verbal praise and, for Fluency Rules, opportunities to take play breaks are used unsystematically to reinforce desired behavior. Whether stuttering treatment outcome is affected by how systematically reinforcement is delivered and how systematically it is faded is a question for future studies.

Another element common to the four treatments is the use of hierarchies in helping children learn and use new behaviors. Hierarchies are simply steps in therapy that go from an easy task or situation to a harder one. They are an almost universal principle of learning, and they are often used for two purposes—to help the child achieve mastery of a new behavior and to help the child generalize the use of the new behavior in situations outside the treatment room. Hierarchies are inherent in the Lidcombe Program's transitions from structured to unstructured conversations and from the regular weekly clinic session in Stage 1 to the gradually faded sessions of Stage 2. Within Stage 1, the child must be speaking in a situation and at a linguistic level that will elicit mostly fluent speech, but a carefully structured hierarchy is not called for. Hierarchies in the Fluency Rules, Smooth Speech, and Comprehensive Treatment programs are, on the other hand, more structured, especially in the latter two approaches, where they are used both in the initial learning of complex behaviors and in generalization of these behaviors to everyday situations. As you read about the hierarchies in all four treatments, pay attention to whether the hierarchies are developed by the clinician alone or whether the child takes an active part in creating them.

The final similarity to be discussed is the degree to which the child's family is involved in treatment. The family may be involved either from the beginning as active clinicians or later, once increased fluency is achieved, as part of the mechanism for generalization and maintenance of treatment effects. Both the Lidcombe Program and the home-based version of the Smooth Speech program require that a parent act as the child's clinician; in his chapter on the Smooth Speech program, Craig suggests that the home-based version may be slightly more effective because of the parent's role as clinician. This is particularly significant given that the children in the research on the home-based program had a mean age of 10.5 years (with a range of 9 to 14 years), indicating that even children as old as this can work effectively with a parent as their clinician. In the clinic-based Smooth Speech program, parents also take a very active role from the beginning, by sitting in on treatment sessions and then helping the child practice fluency skills at home. The Fluency Rules Program also involves parents and other family members, but this does not occur until after fluency skills are learned and the child begins to work on transfer of these skills to other environments. Throughout the transfer and maintenance phases of Fluency Rules treatment, parents are increasingly called on to cue the child to use fluency skills at home. Family involvement in the Comprehensive Treatment is somewhat different. Emphasis is placed on parents' understanding of the nature of stuttering and acceptance of the fact that the child may always stutter to some extent and that this is not a sign of failure. Rather than help the child practice fluency skills, parents of children in Comprehensive Treatment strive to create an environment in which stuttering is okay, thus freeing up the child to communicate openly. In addition to involving families in treatment, all four interventions also engage peers and classroom teachers. As you read each chapter, notice how different treatments accomplish this.

SUMMARY

The four treatments presented here are all aimed at school children who face the challenges of stuttering not only at home, but also in their school environment. Two of these approaches are applicable to the age range many regard as the most difficult to treat—older children and adolescents (Craig et al., 1996). Common among these approaches are the involvement of the family, the use of hierarchies to establish mastery of skills and to generalize the new behaviors, and the use of various kinds of reinforcement for changes in behavior. The goals for the first two approaches described—Lidcombe and Fluency Rules—are more optimistic than the goals of the latter two approaches—Smooth Speech and Comprehensive Treatment. That is, the first two aim for normal-sounding fluent speech, whereas the last two aim to help children reduce or control stuttering and improve their communicative effectiveness. This difference may be explained by the fact that the latter two approaches are designed for older children than the first two approaches.

CHAPTER 9

The Lidcombe Program with School-Age Children Who Stutter

Eᴌɪsᴀʙᴇᴛʜ Hᴀʀʀɪsᴏɴ, Mᴇᴌɪssᴀ Bʀᴜᴄᴇ, Rᴏsᴀᴌᴇᴇ Sʜᴇɴᴋᴇʀ, ᴀɴᴅ Sᴀʀɪᴛᴀ Kᴏᴜsʜɪᴋ

CHAPTER OUTLINE

KEY TERMS

Parent-implemented treatment: therapeutic intervention that is conducted by the parent or caregiver. The treatment program is guided by the speech-language pathologist but carried out by the caregiver.

Percent syllables stuttered (%SS): a calculation based on the number of stutters divided by the total number of syllables spoken.

Response-contingent stimulation: verbal or nonverbal feedback that is given immediately follows the behavior to be increased or decreased. Positive feedback is delivered contingent upon fluency to self-correct are given given contingent upon unambiguous stuttering.

Reinforcement: positive feedback delivered by the parent to the child contingent on the child's stutter-free speech. May be supplemented with tangible reinforcers or tokens.

Severity ratings: perceptual ratings assigned by the parent/caregiver and/or child that reflect the severity of the child's stuttering. A rating of 1 represents no stuttering, 2 reflects extremely mild stuttering, and 10 reflects extremely severe stuttering. This rating scale was researched and validaed by Eve et al. (1995). Severity ratings are useful as beyond-clinic measures to monitor changes in the child's stuttering over time.

INTRODUCTION

The Lidcombe Program (LP) of early stuttering intervention was originally developed for pre-school-age children, that is, those up to age 6 years (Onslow, 2003). However, the LP has also been used with some success with school-age children who stutter—those who are between 6 and 12 years of age. The aim of this chapter is to provide readers with an understanding of how the LP can be used with school-age children, outline research findings related to those applications, and describe how the program can be fine-tuned to be useful with older children.

BACKGROUND

The LP was initially designed for children less than 6 years old, and the earliest outcome studies were restricted to that age group (Onslow, Costa, & Rue, 1990; Onslow, Andrews, & Lincoln, 1994). For preschool-age children who stutter, the LP has been shown to be efficacious (Harris et al., 2002; Jones et al., 2008; Kingston et al., 2003), socially valid (Lincoln, Onslow, & Reed, 1997), and without harmful effects (Woods et al., 2002).

The LP (Onslow, Packman, & Harrison, 2003) was developed in Sydney, Australia in the early 1990s through collaboration between researchers at the University of Sydney and clinicians of the Stuttering Unit, located in the Bankstown Health Service, Sydney (see Onslow, 2003, for a summary). In the years since, the program procedures have been refined as the collaborators sought to optimize the program's effectiveness. Research continues to be conducted in an ongoing effort to answer questions that clinicians ask about the program when used with preschool-age children (see Chapter 7).

Use of the LP has expanded beyond its Australian origins. It is now used in other countries, including Denmark, Canada, Germany, the Netherlands, New Zealand, Singapore, South Africa, United Kingdom, and the United States. Therefore, there is continuing verification that the program can be implemented successfully by clinicians and families in many cultures (e.g., Hayhow, Kingston, & Ledzion, 2003; Jones, Blakeley, & Ormond, 2003; Shenker & Wilding, 2003; Wahlhaus, Girson, & Levy, 2003).

The program is influenced by the principles of behavior therapy (Packman, 2003). It has the goal of effortless, stutter-free speech that is established during Stage 1 of the program and maintained for an extended period during Stage 2. The program is implemented by parents, and treatment is focused on increasing children's stutter-free speech and eliminating stuttering in

their everyday conversations. Parents use verbal contingencies for stutter-free speech and stuttering during exchanges with their children throughout the day in many settings. In other words, parents occasionally comment on their children's speech, both stutter-free and stuttered. Clinicians ensure that they do this in ways that are helpful for children and are neither unpleasant nor invasive for them. Packman (2003, p. 204) explains the goal of the Lidcombe Program as follows: "Indeed, the goal of the Lidcombe Program is for children to speak without stuttering in their natural environment, despite the rough-and-tumble communicative demands of everyday life."

Parents measure their children's stuttering severity each day with a severity rating (SR) scale to monitor progress toward the program's goal. The LP is divided into two stages, and the goal of Stage 1 is for children to reduce stuttering to insignificant levels in their everyday speech. Expressed in terms of speech criteria, the goal of Stage 1 is for children to achieve the measures related to percent syllable stuttered (%SS) and stuttering severity for 3 consecutive weeks. The goal of Stage 2 is for children to maintain these speech criteria over subsequent months.

THEORETICAL BASIS

UNDERLYING ASSUMPTIONS

The authors make no assumptions regarding the nature of stuttering, given that the cause of stuttering remains under investigation (for a recent summary of theoretical models, see Packman & Attanasio, 2005). Indeed, Packman (2003, p. 203) has said that the "Lidcombe Program is a behavioral treatment and was developed empirically, rather than from a particular theoretical view of the nature or cause of stuttering." Assuming that the identification of a cause is not necessary in order to modify a resulting behavior, it could be said that the LP is based on the principles of learning that are documented in the psychology research literature. Therefore, one assumption that can be said to underlie the LP is that stuttering in young children behaves like an operant and is amenable to response-contingent stimulation. This assumption should not be confused with the notion that stuttering *is* an operant. In their review of behavioral research of stuttering, Martin and Ingham (1973, p. 126) concluded: "The empirical demonstration that stuttering frequency can be modified by response-contingent consequences does not necessarily mean that stuttering is an operant behavior. Nor does it mean that the onset and development of stuttering are best explained in terms of environmental consequences."

Although it is clear that there is no current consensus regarding the cause of stuttering, there is empirical evidence, summarized in the following section, that stuttering in young children responds to behavior therapy.

RATIONALE FOR THE LIDCOMBE PROGRAM

The LP uses well-established behavior therapy principles, specifically response-contingent stimulation (RCS), to increase the frequency of stutter-free speech and decrease the frequency of stuttered speech. The two child responses that are targeted in the LP are stutter-free speech and unambiguous stuttering. The contingencies that parents apply to these responses in the LP are verbal and, therefore, are parental verbal contingencies. Specifically, instances of children's stutter-free speech can be followed by parent's verbal praise (e.g., "Great smooth talking!"), acknowledgment of stutter-free speech (e.g., "That was smooth talking."), or a request to self-evaluate stutter-free speech (e.g., "Was that smooth?"). Instances of stuttered speech can be followed by requests to correct stuttering (e.g., "Can you try that again?") or acknowledgment of stuttering (e.g., "That one sounded bumpy."). Thus, different contingencies are applied to stutter-free speech and to instances of stuttering.

Operant principles of behavior learning are well established through empirical and scientific research conducted over several decades. More specifically, studies have established that fluency can be increased and stuttering reduced through the use of RCS in adults (Flanagan, Goldiamond & Azrin, 1958; Martin & Haroldson, 1977; Martin & Siegel, 1966a, 1966b; Martin et al., 1975). Martin, Kuhl, and Haroldson (1972) were the first to publish results from applying RCS to the stuttered speech of two preschool children. In a laboratory study, each child was individually engaged in conversation with a puppet that was illuminated in a box and controlled by a clinician.

After several 20-minute baseline conversations with the puppet, time-out was imposed contingent on the child's stuttering. This was achieved by extinguishing the light for a short time so that the puppet effectively disappeared and the interaction ceased. Then the light came back on, making the puppet reappear and allowing the conversation to resume. Stuttering was eliminated in both children, and the effect was generalized and maintained for a year after the end of the experiment. Subsequent efforts to replicate these results were unsuccessful (Onslow, 2003), but the possibility of using RCS to decrease stuttered speech in young children had been established. Consequently, developers of the LP modified the treatment, experimenting clinically until the emergence of the entire treatment package that is now recognized as the LP. Indeed, since this early exploration of this parent-implemented treatment methodology, positive results have been reported numerous times (Jones et al., 2000; 2005; Harris et al., 2002; Kingston et al., 2003; Lattermann, Euler, & Neumann, 2008; Shenker et al., 2005).

EMPIRICAL BASIS

There is some promising preliminary research supporting the use of the LP with school-age children. Specifically, two studies have examined the efficacy of the LP with this age group (Koushik et al., 2007; Lincoln et al., 1996). Lincoln et al. (1996) reported on 11 children between 7 and 12 years of age who were treated with the LP. They found that children completed Stage 1 in a median of twelve 1-hour clinic visits, with all children maintaining their reduced stuttering at the 12-month follow-up. Although all participants responded to the LP, there was a little more variability in their posttreatment speech measures compared to those of preschool-age children in an earlier study (Onslow, Andrews, & Lincoln, 1994). However, the parents of the children in the Lincoln et al. (1996) study reported being satisfied with their children's posttreatment speech.

Koushik et al. (2007) followed 12 school-aged children (nine boys and three girls) who were between 5 years 10 months and 10 years 8 months of age at the start of treatment. Most of the children were from culturally and linguistically diverse backgrounds. Eight children were introduced to a second language at 4 years of age or older and had English as their predominant language with a second language of French, Italian, Greek, or Portuguese. Four children were bilingual, with English as the predominant language and French, Hebrew, Vietnamese, or Italian introduced simultaneously from birth. English was the predominant language for all 12 children, and it was the language used during clinic visits. The blinded observer's mean %SS score was 9.0 (standard deviation [SD] = 7.5) before treatment and 1.8 (SD = 1.3) at follow-up. All children completed Stage 1 in a median of 7.5 weeks (range, 5 to 10 weeks). Four of the children were followed for less than 6 months after Stage 1, whereas the other eight children were followed for 38 to 187 weeks after Stage 1. At follow-up, seven children continued to meet Stage 2 criteria, whereas five children showed a mean of 2.1% to 3.8% SS at follow-up. Although Lincoln et al. (1996) suggested that school-age children may require longer periods of treatment to reach Stage 2, this was not the case for the children in the Koushik et al. (2007) study. However, the findings are consistent with the Lincoln et al. (1996) finding that school-age children's fluency can be more variable during Stage 2. Even so, these preliminary results are encouraging for clinicians who work with school-age clients who stutter. They suggest that the LP can be an effective treatment over clinically significant periods regardless of a child's age or linguistic background.

PRACTICAL REQUIREMENTS

RESOURCES

Clinicians who want to use the LP can access several sources of information about it, including a comprehensive text (Onslow, Packman, & Harrison, 2003), DVD (http://www3.fhs.usyd.edu.au/asrcwww/ASRC_shop/index.htm), treatment manual (http://www3.fhs.usyd.edu.au/asrcwww/Downloads/index.htm), and several book chapters (Harrison, Kingston, & Shenker, 2007; Harrison, Onslow, & Rousseau, 2007). There is a 2-day training workshop for speech-language pathologists offered in several countries by members of the international Lidcombe Program Trainers' Consortium (http://www3.fhs.usyd.edu.au/asrcwww/professional/index.htm). The workshop provides information and train-

ing through small and whole group discussions, short lectures, video demonstrations, and various training activities. Consequently, the workshop seems likely to lead participants to better learning outcomes than if they attempt to implement the program from written material alone.

TIME REQUIRED FOR LIDCOMBE PROGRAM TREATMENT

The time demands for the clinician and for the parent in implementing this program are comparable with clinic treatment times required by other interventions for stuttering. Nevertheless, time required for the program may present difficulties for some families. The parent, child, and clinician meet for weekly 1-hour clinic visits through Stage 1, with these visits becoming shorter and less frequent during Stage 2. Early in Stage 1, parents allocate 10 to 15 minutes per day to conduct treatment at home and devote a minute or so at the end of each day to record the child's severity rating (SR). Periodically, parents may video- or audio-record interactions with the child for later discussion with the clinician. The time demands for the parent, child, and clinician are such that noncompliance is uncommon. Later in the chapter, we address strategies that can be used if problems do arise.

EQUIPMENT

Since LP treatment activities are tailored to each individual child's interests and cognitive level, no special materials are required. The parent and clinician are guided by the child's own interests and the child's opinions when considering resources to be used during treatment conversations in the clinic and at home. Although school-age children's interests are often captured by the latest fad toys, we still find that more traditional games, toys, books, magazines, comics, and catalogs continue to be useful as stimulus materials.

The clinician collects a %SS measure during conversation between the child, clinician, and parent at the beginning of each clinic visit. Therefore, the clinician needs a means of counting syllables and instances of stuttering during approximately 10 minutes of conversation. One device that can be used for this task is the True-Talk (available from http://www.synelec.com.au/

synergy/home.html). Other options are the Palm Pilot counting application developed by Joseph Donaher at the Philadelphia Children's Hospital (http://www.chop.edu/consumer/jsp/division/generic.jsp?id=79351), the Stuttering Measurement System Training Program developed by Ingham et al. (2001), and the Computerized Scoring of Stuttering Severity developed by Bakker and Riley (1997).

CHARACTERISTICS OF SCHOOL-AGE CHILDREN

When considering practical requirements for working with school-age children, it is helpful to keep in mind some of their typical characteristics that may present challenges, independent of the treatment program. First, when compared with younger children, school-age children have different relationships with their parents and other adults. Adults typically become less directive with older children and consequently are more likely to ask children's opinions and consider their preferences. Shifts in adult-child relationships may lead to more negotiation in all areas of daily life, including treatment for stuttering. Second, the school years provide increased time constraints for children and parents because they have more frequent activities and engagements. Aside from time spent in school-related activities, children develop interests outside the home. Sports, hobbies, and friendships become increasingly important to them. Third, as children become older, they may start to form negative attitudes about differences between themselves and their peers. If such negative attitudes develop toward stuttering, children may be resistant to attending speech therapy and unwilling to engage in treatment activities. Fourth, bullying becomes more common during the school years. One result is that children become reluctant to stand out from the crowd and open themselves to the risk of being bullied. As a result, children who stutter may start to avoid such potential problems by changing the style of their conversational interactions so that their stuttering is less apparent.

There may be other common characteristics of school-age children that could be added here, but the point to highlight is that clinicians need to access existing knowledge spanning several related areas when applying treatment programs. In the case of stuttering treatment with school-age children, they plan and implement intervention that incorporates their knowledge of, for example, children, families, education, and stuttering. They combine this with knowledge about a particular treatment program—in this case, the Lidcombe Program—and apply it judiciously to specific children and families. Keeping this in mind, the following sections focus on the application of the LP with special emphasis on some of the typical characteristics of school-age children. Of course, illustrative examples cannot be comprehensive, but they are presented with the expectation that clinicians may find them useful when considering how to apply the LP to particular school-age clients in their caseloads.

KEY COMPONENTS OF THE LIDCOMBE PROGRAM

OVERVIEW

Parents implement the LP with their school-age children during everyday conversations. For parents to know how to do this, clinicians train them during weekly, 1-hour clinic visits that continue throughout Stage 1. The clinicians' role is to train, guide, and consult with parents as they gain skill and competence in implementing the program's components. Although roles change to some extent during Stage 2, when clinic visits are less frequent, the close collaboration between clinicians and parents continues through both program stages.

In Stage 1, the parent learns to conduct the treatment, first in structured treatment conversations and later in unstructured treatment conversations. The clinician guides and consults with the parent each week while the parent and child undertake treatment conversations at home each day. During these treatment conversations, the parent listens for two essential child responses: stutter-free speech and unambiguous stuttering. These responses attract contingencies from the parent that differ according to whether the child's response was stutter-free or stuttered. In the LP, there are three contingencies for stutter-free speech and two contingencies for unambiguous stuttering. The five contingencies are presented with examples in Table 9.1.

The treatment consists of the parents' verbal contingencies used during conversations with their children. Parents selectively and carefully

Table 9.1. *Types and Examples of Parental Verbal Contingencies in the Lidcombe Program*

Parental Verbal Contingencies for the Child's Stutter-Free Speech	
Acknowledgement	"That sounded smooth."
Praise	"Hey, great talking!"
Request for self-evaluation	"Did you say that smoothly?"
Parental Verbal Contingencies for Unambiguous Stuttering	
Acknowledgment	"I heard a bump/stuttered word/stretched word/stuck word there."
Request for self-correction	"Can you try [stuttered word/phrase] again?"

use the contingencies with the aim of increasing the frequency of the child's stutter-free speech. With guidance from the clinician, the parent learns to use the contingencies correctly and in a manner that is fun for the child, typically resulting in steadily decreasing stuttering severity. Stage 1 finishes when the child achieves the Stage 2 speech criteria and maintains these criteria for 3 consecutive weeks.

In Stage 2, parents continue to provide occasional verbal contingencies for stutter-free speech and stuttering but gradually withdraw contingencies under the clinician's direction. Stage 2 is structured to help children maintain stutter-free speech. Parents detect and respond to any signs of relapse during Stage 2.

Children's progress through Stage 1 and Stage 2 is monitored by the use of a severity rating (SR) scale, a measure that parents learn to use on a daily basis. The scale has 10 points, three of which have the following definitions (Lincoln & Packman, 2003):

- 1 = no stuttering
- 2 = extremely mild stuttering
- 10 = extremely severe stuttering

An additional measure of percent syllables stuttered (%SS) is calculated during each clinic visit by the speech-language pathologist (Lincoln & Packman, 2003). Together, SR and %SS measures are used by the clinician and parent to monitor the child's progress and provide information to be used when planning changes to treatment conversations (e.g., deciding when to introduce unstructured treatment conversations).

See Video Clip 5 for this chapter on thePoint.

Expressed in terms of speech measures, the goal of Stage 1 is for children to achieve the fol-

lowing criteria and maintain them for 3 consecutive weeks:

- Less than 1% SS in clinic conversations of at least 300 syllables
- SRs for each day of the week are 1 or 2, with at least four of seven days in a week with SR of 1

The goal of Stage 2 is for children to maintain these speech criteria over subsequent months (Webber & Onslow, 2003).

SEVERITY RATINGS

The clinician introduces the SR scale to the parent and child during the first Stage 1 clinic visit. A simple verbal explanation of the scale to the parent would include the following information:

- The SR scale has 10 points.
- SR1, SR2, and SR10 are defined.
- Parents write SRs on their charts each day.
- Parents bring the charts to each clinic visit.
- SRs are used each week as the basis for discussion and making decisions about treatment.
- Blank SR charts may be downloaded from http://www3.fhs.usyd.edu.au/asrcwww/Downloads/index.htm.

The clinician adjusts the explanation as necessary for the child. This might include showing the child a graphic version of the SR scale, similar to the one in Figure 9.1

See Video Clip 2.

The main purpose of these explanations is to facilitate clear communication between parent, child, and clinician and foster the child's involvement in the treatment process. It is only of secondary importance to train the child to collect SRs and only if they are interested in doing so. It should be emphasized here that children's SRs are

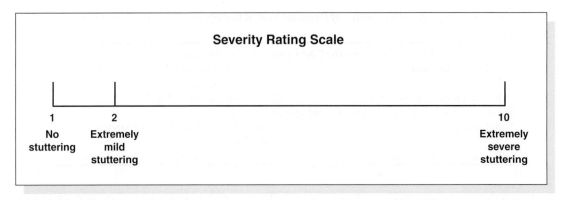

Figure 9.1. Example of a severity rating scale diagram.

not a component of the LP, so their involvement in collecting or charting them is always regarded as optional. Our experience is that school-age children generally like to hear the clinician's explanation of the scale even though they may not fully comprehend what is involved in measuring stuttering severity. However, in addition to hearing about SRs, some children will also be interested in collecting their own ratings. Although these children may enjoy writing their ratings on the standard SR chart, many prefer to use their school diary, a special notebook, or a chart of their own that they create for the purpose.

Video Clip 6 shows a clinician discussing SRs with a parent and child.

Establishing agreement between the clinician's and parent's SRs is achieved by the clinician asking the parent to assign an SR to a sample of the child's speech during a clinic visit. If the rating is within one scale value of the clinician's SR, the clinician tells the parent that they agree, shows the parent where to write the rating on the SR chart, and asks the parent to collect SRs each day. In most cases, a single SR each day is sufficient to depict the child's stuttering severity. Sometimes a parent may notice variations in severity across different times of the day, for example, less severe stuttering at breakfast and more severe stuttering in the afternoon and evening. When a parent reports such variability, the clinician asks the parent to assign two SRs each day and to either use different symbols for morning and afternoon or include short notes on the chart so that the additional information can be shared with the clinician and discussed during each clinic visit.

Occasionally, the clinician and parent SRs initially differ by more than one point. When this happens, the clinician initiates a discussion with the parent. The clinician assures the parent that there are several potential reasons why the ratings may differ at first, that there is no "right" or "wrong" SR, and that they will be able to establish agreement as time goes on. In our experience, the most common reason for lack of agreement is unfamiliarity—either by the clinician or the parent—with the extent of the child's stuttering. The parent may have missed some of the child's mild stutters. The parent's rating may be influenced by other speech-related difficulties, such as misarticulations or language symptoms. The clinician may have incorrectly identified "pauses" in the child's speech as instances of stuttering characterized by fixed postures without audible airflow (blocks). Occasionally, we review audio- or video-recorded samples of the child's speech with a parent so that specific stutters can be discussed more closely, but this is rarely needed. Most often, discussion about stutter types is sufficient to increase SR agreement to within one SR point.

Video Clip 3 shows a discussion of an SR with the clinician, child, and parent.

When children also collect their own SRs, these are regarded as supplementary to the parent SRs; they do not replace them. The reason for this is that parents have primary responsibility for delivering all LP treatment components. The primary role for children is to produce the essential responses of stutter-free speech and stuttered speech and to have fun during treatment conversations. That is, parent and child roles are essentially the same whether the program is used with preschool or school-age children.

Because child SRs are of secondary importance in the LP, it is not essential to establish close agreement between child and clinician SRs. If agreement can be achieved, using a similar process to the one described earlier with parent and clinician ratings, we regard that as a bonus. The clinician asks the child to assign a rating to a sample of the child's speech, shows the child how to record the rating, and asks the child to collect one rating each day and to bring collected ratings to each clinic visit. Older school-age children are more likely than younger children to collect their own SRs, and the ratings can give useful information about their stuttering severity when they are away from their parents, while at school or when playing with friends.

PARENTAL VERBAL CONTINGENCIES

During Stage 1, parent training is conducted in weekly 1-hour clinic visits, during which parents learn to use verbal contingencies for their child's stutter-free speech and unambiguous stuttering. Of course, not all contingencies will be used with all school-age children, and not every child utterance will be followed by a parental verbal contingency. The types and frequency of contingencies, as well as the exact wording that parents use, are all negotiated between the child, parent, and clinician during clinic visits. One important caveat on the negotiations is that contingencies for stutter-free speech will be used *at least* five times more often than contingencies for stuttering and higher ratios are routinely used.

Verbal contingencies are the foundation of this parent-implemented treatment. During the clinic visits, the speech-language pathologist guides the parent in implementing the contingencies with the child, tailoring them to the individual child's needs. The clinician observes the parent implementing the treatment program during clinic visits and collaborates with the parent and child in planning the daily treatment that they will carry out in the week ahead.

School-age children are more likely than preschool-age children to self-evaluate their speech spontaneously, so these nonessential responses can be monitored routinely. Parental verbal contingencies for these responses are praise for correct self-evaluation, regardless of whether the child evaluates stutter-free or stuttered speech.

Parents and children are encouraged to discuss the type of verbal contingencies that will be used and in what situations they will be used. It is common for school-age children to prefer their use when peers are not present. The language for verbal contingencies may be standard comments such as "Great talking" or "That sounded smooth," but some children will enjoy something that is more idiosyncratic, such as "Superhero speech!" or "Fabbo!"

STIMULUS MATERIALS

Materials used during treatment must be interesting and relevant to the particular child. Generally, age-appropriate games and books are used, particularly those that stimulate spontaneous speech when children describe the illustrations. After the first weeks of Stage 1, treatment conversations may include descriptions and ongoing discussions of movies, sports events, and hobbies and any other topics that the child chooses.

Careful consideration should be given when planning to include reading tasks in the range of therapy activities. Although reading aloud is a routine classroom task and therefore a functional goal for speech therapy, it constitutes only a small amount of children's speaking in everyday situations. Consequently, it should be only a minor therapy task, one of a range of activities that reflects the real-life talking of the child.

Some school-age children will not need tangible or token rewards to reinforce their parents' verbal contingencies. For these children, their progress is rewarding by itself, and something as simple as a tick chart or notebook with progressive scores will be sufficient to make this obvious to them. For other children, token rewards may be used when they are needed, such as when a stronger reinforcement is needed to support their motivation. In these cases, rewards can be used for gradual decreases in SRs or for participating in the therapy process. Token rewards should be structured so that the child can earn them in many speaking situations to promote generalization of fluency.

STRUCTURED AND UNSTRUCTURED TREATMENT CONVERSATIONS
Stage 1

Parents and children perform treatment each day during conversations that are carefully structured early in Stage 1 and thus are called structured treatment conversations. Later in Stage 1, treatment occurs during the everyday conversations that occur between children and parents. These conversations are naturally occurring and are no longer so carefully structured by parents; hence, the term *unstructured treatment conversations* is used. The common theme in all Stage 1 treatment conversations is that parents use verbal contingencies for children's stutter-free speech and stuttered speech and, as described earlier, that parents use those contingencies carefully and in a manner that increases the frequency of their children's stutter-free responses.

The purpose of carefully structuring treatment conversations early in Stage 1 is three-fold. First, it allows parents to learn to use the contingencies correctly. Second, children can become accustomed to treatment conversations. Third, parents can organize the conversations so that the majority of children's responses are stutter-free. These conversations usually last for 10 to 15 minutes and take place at times when children are alert and not distracted by other things. This means that structured treatment conversations for many school-age children will take place early in the day, whereas for others, the best time of day will be after school. When discussing the best time of day for treatment, parents and children will contribute their ideas. The only time of day that we routinely ask parents to avoid is just before bedtime. Because there is no single ideal time for all children, clinicians, in consultation with parents and children, often develop daily schedules for the following week to try out that schedule and see how it goes. In the subsequent clinic visit, they discuss what worked and what turned out to be impractical and use that information to devise plans for the following week. This negotiation about times of day for treatment is another aspect of the individual tailoring of the treatment that is common in LP treatment. Clinicians observe parents and children involved in structured treatment conversations during each clinic visit. They give feedback about what is working well and then discuss and demonstrate changes as necessary.

Video Clip 4 shows a clinician teaching a parent and child about structured treatment conversations.

After it becomes clear that structured treatment conversations are working well during the first weeks of Stage 1, clinicians introduce unstructured treatment conversations. They ask parents to use the same verbal contingencies in the naturally occurring interactions that they have applied with their children during their everyday lives. Clinicians typically recommend that parents begin with contingencies for stutter-free speech, although requests for children to self-correct stuttering are also used.

Video Clip 7 shows a clinician discussing treatment with a parent.

At first, unstructured treatment conversations form only a small proportion of the treatment carried out each day, and the majority of treatment still occurs in structured treatment conversations. At all clinic visits, clinicians monitor the amount and types of contingencies being used and ensure that they are being used in ways that are not constant, intensive, or invasive for children.

Video Clip 8 shows a clinician discussion treatment feedback with a child.

Although writing about preschool-age children, Onslow (2003, p. 78) elaborated on this point: "At no point must the child feel that life is permeated with parental responses to speech or that the experience is intense...if parents do so continuously during everyday childhood life, clinical disaster quickly follows. Finally, the treatment must not be invasive in the sense that the child's daily communication with family is curtailed, or that the child's relationship with the parent changes in any way."

An important feature of the LP treatment conversations with school-age children is that clinicians and parents consistently encourage children's participation in all discussions about their treatment. When they are involved routinely in treatment discussions, school-age children frequently come up with great ideas and suggestions for treatment conversations that are both unique and funny. The fact that their ideas often end up with the parent and/or clinician joining in doing silly things adds to the fun for everyone.

During Stage 1, clinicians monitor children's progress during weekly clinic visits. They accomplish this by discussing treatment in the previous week with parents and children, checking on the overall impact of treatment as indicated in SRs, and determining changes to treatment necessary for the week ahead. There is a general change from mostly structured treatment early in Stage 1 to mostly unstructured treatment conversations by the end of Stage 1; the clinician ensures that this gradual change takes place.

When it is clear that children will soon meet the Stage 2 criteria (see earlier "Overview" section for criteria), clinicians may ask parents to check with teachers and relevant other adults to confirm that they are hearing similar stutter-free speech. Children and parents may also be asked to audio- or video-record weekly 5-minute speech samples at home in natural conversations and bring them to clinic visits. Clinicians use these recordings to confirm the consistency and accuracy of parents' SRs. Children begin Stage 2 when they have achieved the criterion speech measures for 3 consecutive weeks.

Stage 2

Instead of weekly clinic visits, Stage 2 clinic visits are less frequent. The first two visits are 2 weeks apart, the next two visits are 4 weeks apart, the next two visits are 8 weeks apart, and a final visit occurs 16 weeks later. Children progress through this schedule if they maintain criterion speech measures, which consist of daily parent SRs of 1 or 2 from the week before each clinic visit and a %SS of less than 1% gathered by the clinician during each clinic visit. It is common for children not to achieve criterion speech measures in at least one Stage 2 visit. When this occurs, clinicians may decide to stall progress through the schedule of clinic visits or return the child to an earlier step of the schedule. In rare cases, clinicians may decide to return to Stage 1 treatment.

Clinicians supervise the gradual withdrawal of verbal contingencies during Stage 2, a process that seems to work best when it is done systematically. Parents may, for example, reduce the number of verbal contingencies used each day, dropping the number a little further week by week. Or, parents may decrease the number of days each week when they use verbal contingencies, increasing the number of treatment-free days by 1 day each week. Clinicians use speech measures and parents' reports to monitor child-

ren's progress; therefore, they can take an individual approach and find the ideal rate at which to withdraw treatment for each child. For some children, the rate can be sped up a little, whereas for other children, the process should be accomplished more slowly. If parents detect any signs of increased severity between clinic visits, clinicians can encourage parents to increase treatment, beginning with an increase in contingencies for stutter-free speech. They can also tell parents that, if their strategies to manage the stuttering do not result in decreased SRs within 3 or 4 days, they should contact the clinician for advice.

ASSESSMENT METHODS TO SUPPORT ONGOING DECISION MAKING

INITIAL ASSESSMENT

Initial assessment or evaluation procedures are not specified as a component of the LP. A routine stuttering evaluation would precede the diagnosis of stuttering and recommendation for intervention with the LP. For the purposes of this book, Table 9.2 is provided, which includes the topic areas and demographic information typically included in initial evaluations.

ONGOING ASSESSMENT

Ongoing assessment is performed thorough out Stages 1 and 2 of the LP. The clinician's use of measures to inform treatment decision-making and frequency of measures have been thoroughly detailed in Chapter 7. A flow chart of decisions is also delineated. The reader is referred to the Assessment Methods section on pages 133–135. The ongoing assessment process does not differ when the LP is applied with school-age children.

TAILORING TREATMENT TO THE INDIVIDUAL CHILD AND FAMILY

PARENT ROLE

In some families, it can be difficult for parents to find sufficient time to conduct LP treatment with their school-age children. This can occur even when parents are strongly motivated to

Table 9.2. *Topic Areas and Demographic Information Typically Included in Initial Evaluations*

Topic	Details

History of stuttering described by child and parent(s)	• Time of onset of child's stuttering
	• Description of stuttering at onset and more recently, including
	  • Types of stutters
	  • Variability over recent months
	• Type and frequency of feedback that parent or teacher may be giving, for example, "slow down," "take a breath first," etc., and how the child responds to this
	• Situation and/or word avoidances
	• Presence of teasing or bullying about stuttering or other issues

Previous stuttering treatment	• Formal and/or informal treatment • Types and durations of previous treatment • Child's opinions about what was helpful, successful, or enjoyable and unhelpful, unsuccessful, or not enjoyable
Current situation	• Current concerns about stuttering • Recent school progress, favorite subjects and school activities • Favorite activities, hobbies, friends outside school • Other speech and language or learning concerns

help their children but have many demands on their time due to personal circumstances. This will often become clear during discussions between parent and clinician in the first weeks of Stage 1. Sometimes, despite repeated best efforts of clinicians and parents to solve the problem, parents are able to do only a few treatment conversations, and SRs show that the minimal treatment is having very little impact on children's stuttering severity. In such cases, it may be possible for an older sibling to fill the parent role in implementing the LP, as long as there is a strong relationship between the two children and a parent is available to supervise if necessary. Regardless of who is filling the parental role—older sibling, grandparent, or other relative—training by the clinician is essential, and that person should attend all clinic visits with the client.

The other common treatment setting for school-age children is in school where an older student mentor or a teacher's aide may be able to take on the LP parent role. Again, this person would need to be trained to collect SRs and conduct treatment conversations, so it would be necessary for them to attend sessions with the client and clinician. This person would also participate in weekly clinic discussions with the client and clinician and work on joint problem solving as necessary. Leading up to school vacations, planning is required to ensure that treatment gains are maintained away from the school setting. This requires a parent, or other, to continue treatment conversations and SRs during the vacation weeks.

CLIENTS FROM CULTURALLY AND LINGUISTICALLY DIVERSE BACKGROUNDS

Adjustments for cultural and linguistic diversity (CLD) are made through consultations among the clinician, the child, and his or her family. Although discussions about individualizing treatment occur in all LP cases, there are particular issues that often arise for consideration within CLD families. One of these is the nature of parental verbal contingencies. There are some examples of non–English-language verbal contingencies in translated versions of the LP manual (http://www3.fhs.usyd.edu.au/asrcwww/downloads). In addition, parents and clinicians can determine contingencies for other languages during clinic discussions.

Another common issue for CLD families arises when parents and children do not share the same first language. For these families, it can be helpful to involve older siblings in treatment conversations at home so that LP treatment is conducted, from time to time, in the family's two languages. Individual decisions can be made about whether to conduct treatment in the first language before, or concurrent with, treatment in the second language.

CHILDREN WITH OTHER COMMUNICATION DISORDERS

For school-age children with other speech and language concerns, particularly those with concurrent cognitive impairments, progress may be slower through each of the two treatment stages. For individual clients with communication disorders, clinicians need to consider all of the child's speech and language skills and set treatment goals that are optimal for his or her needs. When working with school-age children, it may be that the child's therapy goals need to alternate over periods of time between stuttering and, for example, language. Once again, individual decisions are made about the most appropriate short-term goals at any particular time.

APPLICATION OF THE TREATMENT TO TWO INDIVIDUAL CLIENTS

CLIENT 1: MICHAEL

Assessment

Michael was age 6 years 8 months when he was assessed for the first time. His stuttering onset occurred at 2 years, and severity had remained stable prior to the assessment visit. There was no history of stuttering in his family. During the assessment, Michael said that he sometimes had bumps in his speech and that it took him "a really long time to say words." He also said that he was not bothered by his speech and was not teased at school about stuttering.

Michael's speech was evaluated during the assessment session in three different contexts: conversation, storytelling, and a "pressure" speaking task. The following measures were obtained:

Conversation – 8.6% SS
Storytelling – 10.1% SS
Pressure task – 11.7% SS

Michael was diagnosed as having moderate-severe stuttering that was characterized by syllable repetitions and audible prolongations with pitch rise. It was also noted that Michael experienced difficulty in explanation tasks and often seemed to be searching for words. The LP was recommended, along with a full language assessment.

Treatment

Michael started the LP a few weeks after completing his language assessment. His mother reported that he enjoyed the stuttering treatment process and often asked her if they could do their "smooth talking" sessions. One aspect of LP treatment that was altered for Michael was to add systematic rewards to his self-evaluation of stutter-free speech. While spontaneous self-evaluation of stutter-free speech is a routine part of the LP (Onslow, 2003, p. 72), this would usually be in a verbal exchange between child ("I'm doing lots of smooth talking!") and parent ("Yes, you are, and it sounds great."). When Michael noticed stutter-free speech, he marked checks on a wall calendar and told his mother, who praised his correct self-evaluation and gave him a sticker. His goal was to collect 10 stickers each day, and whenever he achieved this for 7 consecutive days, he received a small prize.

Five weeks after starting Stage 1, Michael's mother reported that she was having doubts about whether treatment would be effective and that she had been hoping for faster results. Consequently, she and Michael had not conducted treatment conversations for over a week. The clinician gave her information about expected Stage 1 treatment times and played her a tape of his speech recorded at the initial assessment. Michael's mom expressed surprise at the difference between his speech on the recording and his current speech; she agreed that there was an obvious reduction in severity that she had missed when observing Michael's subtle SR changes from day to day and week to week.

Another difficulty arose during Stage 2, when Michael's SRs increased concurrent with his return to school after summer holidays. At the next clinic visit, a sample of his speech was measured as 4.4% SS. The clinician recommended an increase in the number of structured and unstructured therapy conversations for a short period of time until SRs reduced to criterion levels. This strategy was successful, and he met speech criteria at subsequent Stage 2 clinic visits (see Table 9.3 and Fig. 9.2).

CLIENT 2: CURTIS

Assessment

Curtis was 8 years 11 months old when he was assessed. Stuttering onset had occurred when he

Table 9.3. *Summary of Speech Measures at Michael's Stage 1 Clinic Visits*

Clinic Visit Number	Within-Clinic %SS Measure	Average SR for Preceding Week	Clinician Comments
1	10.1	7.1	Began Stage 1; introduced structured treatment conversations
2	10.5	6.9	
3	9.2	5.7	Introduced unstructured treatment conversations
4	6.0	5.0	Mom reports he spontaneously self-corrects stutters; SR1 in structured treatment conversations; enjoys contingencies for stutter-free speech
5	5.0	5.1	Only two treatment conversations this week
6	–	5.0	Unable to attend clinic visit
7	2.6	2.4	Introduced contingencies for spontaneous self-evaluation of stutter-free speech
8	1.2	2.0	All treatment now in unstructured treatment conversations
9	1.0	1.4	
10	0.3	1.1	
11	0	1.1	Began Stage 2

was 6 years old, and severity had varied since then. His stuttering ceased for almost 6 months after onset and then returned with increased severity. It had been constant for the 2 years before assessment. Curtis had 1 year of stuttering treatment at school when he was 7 years old but had made minimal progress. According to his father, Curtis's stuttering severity decreased slightly during that year and increased again as soon as treatment finished.

Curtis indicated that his stuttering sometimes bothered him but said that he did not avoid words or situations because of stuttering. He said that he had been teased at school about his speech while playing soccer and had reacted by walking away.

During the assessment session, Curtis's father said that he was very concerned about Curtis's stuttering and that he frequently tried to help him by telling Curtis to correct his speech. He knew that his comments often caused Curtis irritation and frustration and resulted in Curtis refusing to talk, but he did not know what else to do.

At the time of assessment, Curtis's speech was evaluated during conversation, explanation, and reading tasks, with the following measures obtained:

Conversation – 7.0% SS
Explanation – 7.0% SS
Reading – 0.9% SS

Curtis was diagnosed as having moderately severe stuttering characterized by repetitions. These included part-word repetitions ("ca-ca-ca-can"), whole-word repetitions ("that-that-that-that-that one"), and fillers ("But um ah um um would you…"). The LP was recommended because the clinician recognized that the positive reinforcement, naturally built into the program, would improve the quality of feedback given by the father.

Treatment

In the first Stage 1 clinic visit, Curtis's father was asked to use only one verbal contingency, which was praise for stutter-free speech. The clinician decided to restrict contingencies in this way to facilitate positive interactions about speech between Curtis and his father. She was aware that Curtis had previously been accustomed to receiving only corrective feedback from his father.

Alongside his father's daily SRs, Curtis collected his own ratings on a separate chart. This encouraged Curtis to monitor his speech in a positive manner and compare his ratings with those of his father. As Curtis progressed through Stage 1, there were only occasional days on which his ratings differed from his father's by more than one rating point. Curtis participated in clinic discussions about the ratings with the clinician and his father and was

The Lidcombe Program of Early Stuttering Intervention

Treatment Record: Stage 1

NAME   Michael

Severity Ratings
SR1 = no stuttering
SR2 = extremely mild stuttering   O % Syllables Stuttered
SR10 = extremely severe stuttering   ● Severity Rating

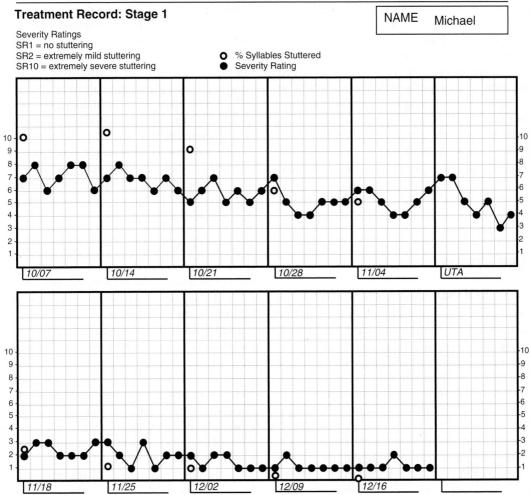

Figure 9.2. Stage 1 treatment record for Michael.

obviously pleased to see the severity ratings decrease.

Verbal contingencies for stuttering were introduced in the second Stage 1 clinic visit, after the clinician had verified with Curtis and his father that the first week of treatment had been successful. Requests for Curtis to self-correct stutters were then added, in a ratio of 1:7 (one request for self-correction to seven instances of praise for stutter-free speech).

A few weeks later, Curtis indicated that he had changed his mind and no longer liked verbal contingencies for stutter-free speech. He said that he thought that they sounded "babyish." This occurred despite the fact that his SRs were showing that he was responding well to the treatment. After discussing a few possibilities

for changes to treatment, the clinician suggested that they introduce a form of self-monitoring. To do this, Curtis would first create a wall chart and then add checkmarks whenever he evaluated his speech as stutter-free. When he added checkmarks, he also confirmed with his father that his evaluations were correct. Curtis reported that he enjoyed this and that it made him feel more "in charge" of his therapy. It also removed the need for his father to instigate verbal contingencies for stutter-free speech.

At the end of Stage 1, Curtis asked the clinician if he could finish weekly therapy sessions because his stuttering had reached a very low level. The clinician agreed with this evaluation and asked Curtis for his ideas about how he could maintain his speech gains. Curtis and the clinician agreed that he would continue daily SRs, and if his SR went above 2, he would participate in a 10-minute structured treatment conversation at home on the same day and increase the frequency of his self-monitoring in unstructured conversations. They also agreed that Curtis's progress through Stage 2 would be reinforced by small tangible rewards from his father that would be given contingent on meeting Stage 2 speech criteria at each clinic visit. Curtis's favorite reward was to get additional pocket money to spend at a local discount store. Stage 2 clinic visits were planned according to the usual schedule, and Curtis progressed through these visits without difficulty (see Table 9.4 and Fig. 9.3).

CASE STUDY

BACKGROUND AND ASSESSMENT

Darren, who was age 6 years and 1 month at assessment, started stuttering at 3 years with severity increasing gradually over the following 3 years. Darren's mother, Joan, stuttered as a child and then recovered during adolescence. Joan's brother and sister stuttered as young children, and both continue to stutter as adults.

Darren was aware of his stuttering and said he talked just like his uncle. He did not appear to be bothered by it and referred to his stuttering as "skipping." Joan described him as being very talkative and friendly and having lots of friends and a good relationship with his older sister, Kelly. Although he had had no previous formal stuttering treatment, on occasion, Joan

reminded him to "take his time" or "say the word again" when he stuttered.

Darren's school speech-language pathologist had recently conducted an evaluation of his articulation and language. Results indicated a mild-moderate delay in morphosyntactic development, a mild-moderate delay in narrative skills, and a mild delay in articulation. Assessment of his stuttering resulted in a diagnosis of severe stuttering that was characterized by prolongations (e.g., "naaaaaap") and part-word repetitions (e.g., "c-c-c-could"), along with nasal flaring and eye widening. In addition, he often spoke on residual air and took quick, audible inspirations mid-phrase.

TREATMENT

It was recommended that intervention begin with the LP to address the stuttering, with remediation of language and articulation to follow. During the first three Stage 1 clinic visits, Joan learned how to use SRs reliably and use verbal contingencies for stutter-free and stuttered speech in structured and unstructured treatment conversations. She reported using approximately 15 to 20 contingencies for stutter-free speech and five contingencies for stuttering each day during unstructured conversations. She used the same ratio of contingencies in 10-minute structured treatment conversations.

At the fourth clinic visit, Joan reported that Darren had been SR1 for part of each day in the previous week, and the SR never exceeded 2 on any day. During the baseline speech sample that day, Joan rated an SR of 2, while the clinician assigned an SR of 6.

Table 9.4. *Summary of Speech Measures at Curtis's Stage 1 and Stage 2 Clinic Visits*

Clinic Visit Number	Within-Clinic %SS Measure	Average SR for Preceding Week	Clinician Comments
1	9.3	6.3	Began Stage 1; introduced structured treatment conversations; parental verbal contingencies introduced only for stutter-free speech
2	5.4	4.0	Parental verbal contingencies introduced for unambiguous stuttering
3	2.1	2.3	Introduced unstructured treatment conversations
4	0.7	1.4	Curtis dislikes parental verbal contingencies for stutter-free speech
5	0.5	1.1	
6	0.2	1.1	
7	1.0	1.0	Began Stage 2

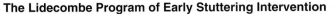

The Lidecombe Program of Early Stuttering Intervention

Treatment Record: Stage 1

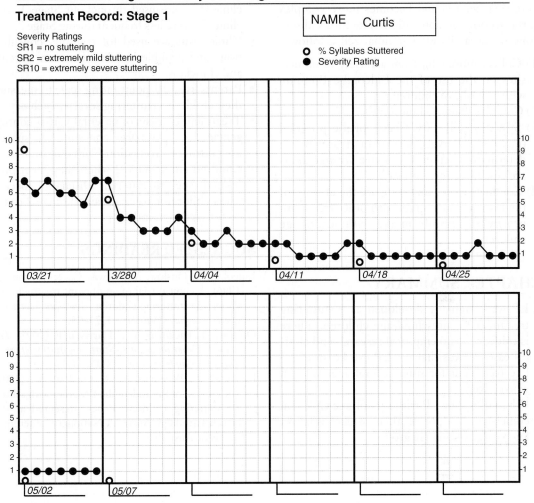

Figure 9.3. Stage 1 treatment record for Curtis.

Baseline samples of Darren's speech during the first three clinic visits were measured as having 12% SS, 8% SS, and 6% SS. At clinic visits 4 and 5, his baseline samples were 9% SS and 12% SS, respectively.

CASE STUDY QUESTIONS

1. What are three important questions to ask Joan regarding the treatment at home?
2. During a clinic visit, how can the clinician verify that the program requirements are being met?
3. There is a considerable discrepancy between Joan's and the clinician's SR on the same speech sample during clinic visit 4. What steps can the clinician take to establish interjudge reliability of their SRs within 1 rating point?
4. What are three possible reasons for the increase in Darren's %SS measures at clinic visits 4 and 5?
5. Brainstorm possible changes to Darren's LP treatment that will assist his progress toward Stage 2 speech criteria.

FUTURE DIRECTIONS

Research is needed in the way of prospective replications (i.e., clinical trials) of the Lidcombe Program with school-age children. Through carefully planned research protocols, we will advance our identification and understanding of the variables that predict treatment success as stuttering persists and becomes more complex in the school-age population. The future directions for research can be summarized as follows:

(1) Collect more data from a variety of clinical sites on the use of the Lidcombe Program with school-age children.
(2) Conduct Phase 1 clinical trials.
(3) Systematically vary aspects of the program (i.e., visit intervals, format of treatment) to determine whether alternative arrangements are equally or more effective.
(4) Conduct studies that compare the efficacy of the Lidcombe Program with other treatment programs currently in use with school-age children.

CHAPTER SUMMARY

- LP was originally developed as a stuttering treatment for preschool-age children. There is evidence from empirical research and clinical case records that the LP can be an effective treatment for some school-age children who stutter.
- When using the LP with school-age children, clinicians incorporate their wider, relevant knowledge of this age group.

- The LP consists of Stage 1 and Stage 2. Weekly clinic visits are used throughout Stage 1, and clinic visits are less frequent during Stage 2.
- Clinic visits are used for training, consultation, and troubleshooting between parents and clinicians.
- Parents use a 10-point rating scale to measure their children's stuttering severity each day.
- Treatment consists of parental verbal contingencies for stutter-free and stuttered speech used during conversations with children.
- Children enter Stage 2 when they meet prescribed speech criteria. Discharge occurs when children have maintained Stage 2 criteria for several months.

SUGGESTED READINGS

Lincoln, M., Onslow, M., Lewis, C., & Wilson, L. (1996). A clinical trial of an operant treatment for school-age stuttering children. *American Journal of Speech-Language Pathology, 5*, 73–85.

Onslow, M., Packman, A., & Harrison, E. (2003). *The Lidcombe Program of Early Stuttering Intervention: A Clinician's Guide.* Austin, TX: Pro-Ed.

Rousseau, I., Packman, A., & Onslow, M. (2005, June) A trial of the Lidcombe Program with school age stuttering children. Paper presented at the Speech Pathology Australia National Conference, Canberra, Australia.

CHAPTER 10

The Fluency Rules Program

CHARLES M. RUNYAN AND SARA ELIZABETH RUNYAN

INTRODUCTION

The Fluency Rules Program (FRP) (Runyan & Runyan, 1986; 1991; 1993; 1999; 2007) was developed in the early 1980s to provide public school speech-language pathologists (SLPs) with an effective, efficient, and easy-to-administer treatment program for preschool and early grade school-age children who stutter. Then, as now, clinicians in school settings faced a host of challenges such as large case loads, scheduling conflicts, teacher work days, and school holidays, which limited the number of treatment sessions available for children. Runyan and Bennett (1982) reported in Virginia that the average public school SLP's caseload exceeded 60 children and that these children averaged only 25 therapy sessions during the school year. In addition, the literature had established that many public school SLPs were uncomfortable conducting stuttering therapy and often excluded children who stutter from their caseload (St. Louis & Durrenberger, 1992; St. Louis & Lass, 1980; 1981). This exclusion was particularly true for children who had coexisting communication problems (Blood & Seider, 1981).

In response to these issues, the FRP—as the name implies—was created to be a rules-based stuttering treatment program. Rules were used because children as young as preschoolers are aware of the importance of following rules (e.g., "Don't talk to strangers," "Don't run at the pool") and, with the help of an SLP, a child could become fluent by "following the rules of fluency." In order for the FRP to be effective, easy to administer, and time efficient, the individual rules were designed to be simple and in language a child could comprehend regarding the concepts of fluent speech production. Since its creation, the FRP has been continually modified by eliminating unnecessary rules, strengthening effective ones, and developing new clinical techniques. Most of the program modifications have evolved during the therapeutic process with the children we have treated. The current FRP consists of three sections with different goals. The first section of the FRP contains three *Universal Rules*: (1) Speak Slowly, (2) Say a Word One Time, and (3) Say It Short. These rules are intended to reduce speech rate and eliminate the repetition of single-syllable words and/or part-words as well as prolongations. The second section, *Primary Rules*, presents three rules to help children understand the physiologic differences between stuttered and fluent speech. The final section, *Secondary Rule*, contains a single rule to eliminate secondary stuttering behaviors.

THEORETICAL BASIS FOR THE FLUENCY RULES PROGRAM

The FRP is a fluency-shaping program designed to establish fluent speech in all children who stutter. It has been our clinical experience that a particular problem for younger children who stutter is their lack of awareness of when these disfluent behaviors occur. Although children are typically globally aware that they are repeating words, the children are not aware of how frequently they are producing disfluencies or exactly when the disfluencies occur. These young children have apparently not developed the perceptual skills necessary to monitor their speech production system to an awareness level that could lead to the recognition of all instances of repetitions and then to the elimination of the repetitious speech.

For older children, stuttering presents problems of both awareness and production. That is, older children are neither aware of all instances of stuttering nor of how speech is produced. Therefore, these children must continue to improve their self-monitoring skills as well as learn the physiologic elements or fundamentals of fluent speech production. The FRP gives children specific strategies to improve their self-monitoring skills and coordinate their speech production skills.

To improve children's abilities to self-monitor and to learn the elements of speech production, the FRP uses two therapy strategies. The more basic strategy of the FRP is that children must enjoy and look forward to attending therapy (Onslow, Packman, & Harrison, 2003; Ramig & Dodge, 2005; Runyan & Runyan, 2007). Clinicians and parents are keenly aware that children who are happy in an experience (e.g., music, sports) will quickly learn new skills. This positive therapy environment can be created by conducting therapy in a play atmosphere, often seated on the floor with toys and games of the child's choice using conversational speech to implement specific Fluency Rules. Another key component to therapy being a fun and happy experience is the therapist's willingness to be uninhibited and relate to a child at his or her cognitive level during the treatment process.

Video Clip 1 for this chapter on thePoint website demonstrates this play-oriented therapeutic environment. In addition, it demonstrates the third Universal Rule—"Say It Short."

In our private practice, therapy was often gradually terminated when a child was ready for dismissal because children enjoyed the experience even though they had become fluent. This attitude allowed for a gradual decrease in scheduled sessions and may have helped prevent relapse by not ending treatment too quickly after fluency was achieved.

The second FRP treatment strategy is the liberal use of visual cues or visual reminders throughout the therapeutic program. The most important improvement to the FRP has been the development of visual or nonverbal hand signals to remind children of the Fluency Rules (Runyan & Runyan, 1999; 2007). The Fluency Rules, with corresponding hand signal cues, are displayed in Table 10.1. Prior to the development of these nonverbal cues, the clinician verbally interrupted the child to remind him or her of a "broken" fluency rule (i.e., instance of stuttering). These interruptions were time consuming and disruptive to the client's flow of speech. The substitution of nonverbal cues for verbal reminders facilitates conversational flow and maximizes clinical opportunities for the children to improve self-monitoring skills and produce fluent speech. Visual cues in the form of symbolic materials, including therapy room decorations, have also been used to remind children of previously taught rules for fluent speech (Hammett, 1994). For example, pictures and stuffed animals resembling turtles and snails have been used to encourage slow speaking rate. Finally, visual cues are important components of the carryover portion of the FRP in which SLPs, classroom teachers, and parents are encouraged to place symbolic items in the children's environment as passive reminders of the Fluency Rules while continuing to use the hand signals as active reminders of the rules when the children are talking.

EMPIRICAL BASIS FOR USE OF THE FLUENCY RULES PROGRAM

Runyan and Runyan (1991) reported treatment results based on nine children consisting of five males and four females with a mean age of 5 years

Table 10.1. *Individual Fluency Rules with Corresponding Hand Gestures*

Fluency Rule	Corresponding hand gesture
Universal Rules	
1. Speak Slowly	1. Move the hand up and down to indicate slow down
	2. Old Ears/Happy Ears
2. Say a Word One Time	1. Hold up one finger
	2. Old Ears/Happy Ears
	3. Bent finger
3. Say It Short	1. Hold thumb and forefinger close together
	2. Old Ears/Happy Ears
Primary Rules	
4. Speech Breathing	Draw a breath curve in the air
5. Start "Mr. Voice Box" Smoothly	Pull close fingers apart with the right hand with the right hand slightly elevating as if going up a gentle slope
6. Touch the "Speech Helper" Together Lightly	Touch the thumb and forefinger together lightly
Secondary Rule	
7. Use Only the "Speech Helpers" to Talk	Imitate the secondary behavior

5 months (range, 3 years 8 months to 7 years 1 month). Based on the Stuttering Severity Instrument (SSI) (Riley, 1972), three, four, and two of the children were determined to have mild, moderate, and severe fluency disorder, respectively. Five children were followed for 2 years after completion of therapy, whereas four were followed for 1 year. All had been treated with FRP in a public school and received therapy two or three times a week for 30 or 40 minutes. The data indicated that all children evidenced a significant improvement in fluency, maintained normal speaking rates, and eliminated all secondary behaviors. The improvement in fluent speech production occurred in the first year of therapy and was maintained during follow-up. However, a lingering concern remained because each child's speech still contained slight, residual signs of the stuttering consisting of infrequent part-word repetitions of two or fewer iterations. Unfortunately, these children could not be followed for longer periods of time, and no additional data were available. Also of note, these children were treated using the 1991 version of the FRP in which all seven rules were taught to every child; the Universal Rules were not always taught prior to the Primary Rules, and the development of hand signals as visual reminders had not yet been incorporated in the treatment.

Subsequently, Runyan and Runyan (1993) reported on 14 children treated in a private practice setting. This group consisted of one girl and 13 boys. Based on the Stuttering Prediction Instrument (SPI) (Riley, 1981), two, eight, and four children were classified as having severe, moderate, and mild stuttering, respectively. The mean age at the beginning of therapy was 8 years 9 months (range, 2 years 3 months to 11 years). Nine of these children demonstrated secondary behaviors. The four mild stutterers and one moderate stutterer did not exhibit secondary behavior. When dismissed from therapy, 10 children were judged by the investigators to be within the acceptable range of a score of 3 or below for speech naturalness. The four remaining children continued in treatment. The average length of therapy for the 10 children who were dismissed from treatment was 9 months (range, 3 to 20 months). One of the female preschool subjects who was dismissed as a fluency success is now in college, and her stuttering has returned. Contact with the family was lost, and the history of the relapse is unknown.

Runyan and Runyan (1999) reported on an additional six males, whose average age was 5 years 11 months, with two of the children being preschool age. Before intervention, four of the children were judged to have moderate stuttering, and two had severe stuttering. Five children were released from therapy after the elimination of stuttering behavior. Length of therapy for one preschooler was 23 months, whereas the other four children averaged 9 months of treatment. The oldest child, a second grader, continued in therapy and, although still rated as having severe stuttering, has improved markedly by reducing secondary behaviors and the number of iterations per stutter. As a fifth grader at last follow-up, he continued to stutter and attend therapy. Due to logistical factors, he attends therapy only once a month.

Results of the first group of children treated using this program (Runyan & Runyan, 1991) demonstrated that the FRP was effective with children in the public school setting. Six of the 17 children in the second group and six children in our most recent group seen at the private practice also received services in the public schools. Based on our clinical experience, we believe that the FRP can be implemented successfully in a coordinated format partnering with the public school and the private sector.

PRACTICAL REQUIREMENTS FOR THE TREATMENT

No special equipment is needed to effectively apply the FRP. Nonetheless, two clinician attributes would be beneficial to the treatment process. The first is a basic understanding of the anatomy and physiology of speech production to teach children, when necessary, the differences between fluent speech and stuttering. This knowledge is important because children are more willing to follow therapeutic directions when they understand the anatomic and physiologic differences between when they stutter and when they are fluent. The second clinical attribute is the therapist's ability to create fun, interesting, and engaging activities that maximize each client's speech output.

KEY COMPONENTS OF THE FLUENCY RULES PROGRAM

UNIVERSAL RULES

The first section of the FRP contains three Universal Rules: (1) Speak Slowly, (2) Say a Word One Time, and (3) Say It Short. These rules are used with every child from the beginning of treatment. The SLP determines which Universal Rules are appropriate for each child based on initial evaluation results. For example, if one child talks too rapidly and repeats words, then the SLP would implement Universal Rules 1 and 2. If another child presented with a normal speech rate but both repeated and prolonged words, the use of Rules 2 and 3 would be appropriate. The Universal Rules are the initial focus of therapy for all children even if the child displays more advanced aspects of stuttering such as laryngeal blocks or oral tension. Clinically, we have witnessed children who initially exhibited oral and laryngeal tension who have subsequently eliminated these behaviors after the application of the appropriate Universal Rules. That is, by working on a combination of speech rate (Rule 1: Speak Slowly), repetitions (Rule 2: Say a Word One Time), and, if needed, prolongations (Rule 3: Say It Short), laryngeal and oral tensions were eliminated without being addressed directly.

Video Clip 2 provides a description of the Universal Rules.

Rule 1: Speak Slowly

Controlling speech rate is a clinical component of many treatment programs (e.g., Cooper & Cooper, 1985; Costello, 1983; Guitar, 1998; Ingham, 1999a; 199b; Kully & Langevin, 1999; Meyers & Woodford, 1992; Neilson & Andrews, 1993; Shames & Florance, 1980) because it has been well documented that reduced speaking rate reduces stuttering (Bloodstein, 1987; Gregory & Hill, 1980; Jones & Ryan, 2001; Max & Caruso, 1998; Perkins, 1992; Ramig, 1984). Although labeled Speak Slowly, the treatment goal for this rule is actually the use of a slow normal rate. The normal speech rate for children in grades 1 through 5 is approximately 125 words per minute (wpm) for grade 1, with a somewhat systematic increase to 142 wpm in grade 5; whereas for syllables, the rate is 148 to 170 syllables per minute (spm) (Pindzola, Jenkins, & Lokken, 1989; Purcell & Runyan, 1980). A benefit of reduced rate is that it allows the child more time to detect and identify repetitions or prolongations. Use of a reduced speech rate may also simplify motor timing or allow additional time to develop the monitoring ability needed for the acquisition of physiologic skills necessary for fluent speech production (Perkins, 1992; Wall & Myers, 1995). In addition to reducing stuttering by reducing speech rate, Conture (1990), Healey and Scott (1995), and Runyan and Runyan (1993) noted a secondary benefit for this rule. These authors reported that when the speech rate of children who stutter was reduced, there appeared to be a calming effect during the treatment session. Runyan and Runyan (1999) also noted that when the clinical focus during therapy was reduced speech rate, the frequency of stuttering continued to reduce, while the slow normal rate of speech remained unchanged. This continued reduction in stuttering when using slow rate could have been in part due to the maintenance of the calm therapeutic environment due to the slow rate.

Video Clip 3 on thePoint shows the use of a hand gesture by the clinician to elicit a correction.

When introducing and implementing this rule, the clinician's modeling of speech at a slow normal rate is very important (Ramig & Dodge, 2005; Runyan & Runyan, 1991; 1993). After the clinician has modeled the age-appropriate slow, normal speech rate, the child is instructed to talk the same way the SLP is talking. Symbolic materials (e.g., turtles, rabbits, and snails versus lions, horses, and cheetahs) can be used to contrast slow and fast. To teach the concept of "speak slowly," the SLP can simulate a race between a fast and a slow animal (Meyers & Woodford, 1992). In this race, the slow animal is victorious while the fast animal has difficulties, like stumbling or falling down. These difficulties can be used to illustrate that when people talk too fast, they may stumble over words and stutter, just as when they run too fast, they may stumble and fall down. To further establish the understanding of this concept, the child and the clinician can role play by pretending to run too fast while talking too fast with the clinician producing pseudo-stuttering. Then the clinician and child can walk slowly around the therapy room talking in a slow normal fluent manner and discussing how much better they can control their balance and speech "when we walk and talk the slow way."

The visual cue for this rule is moving a hand up and down in the traditional manner that means "slow down" when the child's speech rate becomes too rapid. A second nonverbal reminder "Old Ears/Happy Ears" is implemented by having the clinician grab his ears in mock pain when the child produces rapid speech or dance around the room pointing to the "happy

ears" because slow speech rate makes the clinician's ears happy.

Rule 2: Say a Word One Time

Typically, part-word and single-syllable whole-word repetitions are the predominant speech characteristics that need therapeutic intervention in the speech of children who stutter; therefore, the "Say a Word One Time" rule is important to the success of the FRP.

To teach the concept of saying a word one time, the comparison of two contrasting series of items can be used. For example, two different series of coins can be compared. The first series contains different coins in a row (e.g., penny, dime, nickel, etc.) and represents fluent speech, and the second row of coins has some similar coins in a row (e.g., penny, penny, penny, nickel, and dime) and represents disfluent speech containing repetitive words. Other series like counting and naming the days of the week or the months of the year can illustrate the importance of each word and that none needs to be repeated for the child to understand the meaning of each word. To demonstrate, the SLP can repeat a word 10 or more times followed by asking the child if he or she needed to hear the word "that many times" to understand the meaning. Another technique for teaching this concept is the use of "different feet." To demonstrate, the SLP can talk at a slow rate as he or she walks slowly around the therapy room with the child. While walking, the SLP can explain that walking is easy and smooth when different feet are used for each step. Then, he or she can stop and hop forward several hops on one foot to demonstrate how walking becomes difficult and bumpy when the same foot is used for every step. Repeating this activity by saying a different word with each step and then by beginning to hop on the same foot while repeating a word will show that, during speech, if the same word is said "over and over," speech gets bumpy and may become difficult to understand.

The hand gesture for this rule is holding up the index finger, similar to the way sports fans demonstrate that their team is number one, to indicate when a repetition has occurred.

In Video Clip 4, the Universal Rules are reviewed. Clip 4 also demonstrates how the clinician can reinforce fluency using "Happy Ears." Video Clip 5 includes examples of the transition from child catching the clinician using one-finger gestures to identifying repetitions in the child's speech.

On a few occasions, a child has reacted negatively to the clinician identifying his repeated words. To accomplish our clinical objective of increasing the child's awareness of when a repetition occurs while not distressing the child, we have used a finger raised only halfway up or just slightly bent as the nonverbal reminder.

See Video Clip 5 for an example of using the bent finger technique.

The SLP then asks in a questioning manner, "You don't ever say your words more than once, do you?" The child may deny the production of the repetition but nonverbally indicate awareness of it. This interaction accomplishes the goal of increasing awareness without requiring the child to outwardly admit to "doing something wrong."

The Old Ears/Happy Ears nonverbal cue can be used again to increase awareness of when the child repeats a word. To ensure the child's awareness of the cue, the therapist can "fall" down on the floor holding his or her ears in mock pain.

This activity is demonstrated on thePoint in Video Clip 6.

This animated activity gains the child's attention, and fluent speech usually follows. If the fluency continues, the therapist can dance around the therapy room holding his or her ears saying, "I have happy ears because no repeated words hurt my ears." The combination of "happy ears" and "old ears" provides a constant reminder to a child to say words only one time. The happy ears cue becomes increasingly important as therapy progresses because as repetitions decrease, the need remains to maintain the therapy focus on saying each word one time, and the use of the happy ears can serve as a positive reminder of this rule.

Rule 3: Say It Short

This rule was designed to eliminate prolongations and is only taught to children whose stuttered speech exhibits prolongations. For children who demonstrate prolongations, this rule is an integral component of the treatment process and is introduced during the initial intervention session. Finger cues can also be used to guide a child to keep a repetition brief.

Video Clip 7 shows the clinician first complimenting the child for fluency and then cueing him to have only one repetition.

The concepts of long and short have been well developed in the language of children by the age most are referred for services. If needed, however, contrasting familiar long and short objects (e.g., pencils, animals) can be used to teach these concepts. A number of therapy techniques have been suggested to explain that words should not be prolonged but move quickly from syllable to syllable and word to word. Piano fingers (Runyan & Runyan, 1993) and Conture's Thumb and Opposing Finger Analogy (1982) have worked successfully to demonstrate this concept. Basically, these techniques use the thumb to touch each finger in succession or touch each object in a series quickly and lightly. The SLP explains and demonstrates that each finger represents a different sound and fluent speech moves quickly and smoothly from sound to sound. Next the SLP can demonstrate that when the thumb stays too long on a finger or an object, a prolonged sound will occur. To experience the feeling of quick and smooth flowing speech, the clinician and child repeat short phrases in unison while tapping their fingers as different sounds are produced. Conture's (1982) Lily Pad/Frog Analogy, where a frog jumps lightly and smoothly from lily pad to lilly pad without sinking, and Barrel Bridge Analogy, where a child jumps from barrel to barrel without falling into the water, have also been used to teach the smooth-flowing timing aspect of fluent speech and concept for this Fluency Rule. A final technique, which is similar to the use of excessive repetitions for the 'Say a Word One Time' rule, involves the SLP producing a word using an exaggerated prolongation (e.g., 5 seconds) and then asking the child if he or she "needed to hear the word for that long" to understand its meaning.

The hand gesture for this rule is holding the thumb and first finger close together in the traditional manner to indicate something is short.

Video Clip 8 demonstrates a child identifying prolonged words by the therapist using the hand gesture for short.

As with the previous two rules, the SLP can grab his or her ears in mock pain when the child prolongs a sound and then point to his or her "happy ears" after a period of time when no prolongations occur.

PRIMARY RULES

The Primary Rules are of primary importance (i.e., this is why these rules were label as such) for the child to understand the physiology of speech. The three Primary Rules were designed to help the child when the Universal Rules do not eliminate stuttering behavior and additional direct physiologic instruction and intervention is needed. Recall that for many children who exhibited such physiologic difficulties as laryngeal tension, airflow management, and/or oral tension, the application of the Universal Rules was sufficient to eliminate all aspects of stuttering. Therefore, the SLP must be patient and not hurry the therapy process associated with the Universal Rules and assume too quickly that more direct treatment is needed because of the presence of physiologic issues.

Ultimately, the SLP must make the determination that the Universal Rules alone cannot eliminate stuttering and that direct physiologic-based treatment is required. From our experience, when children demonstrate the understanding of the concepts of the Universal Rules by quickly and accurately identifying when repetitions and/or prolongations occur but still demonstrate a consistent pattern of stuttering, the use of the Primary Rules is warranted.

When the determination is made to use the Primary Rules, the first step is to teach the physiologic concepts needed to understand these rules by presenting an overview of the speech production process. Speech production can be explained and demonstrated to the child in simplified terms as a series of sequential physiologic events. First, speech production begins with airflow or exhalation that will "carry the words out." Second, as the air "is carried out," it goes over "Mr. Voice Box," or the vocal folds, which cause them to vibrate and make a sound. And finally, movement of the tongue and lips "forms or shapes" this

sound into words. To help explain these physiologic concepts and the Primary Rules, we have used Conture's Garden Hose Analogy (1982) in which he equates the garden hose nozzle to the lips, the garden hose to the vocal tract and tongue, and the faucet to the larynx. In this analogy, the relationship between anatomic structures and the physiology associated with air flow, voicing, and light oral contacts is explained first; this is then followed by an explanation of how correct use of each structure and movement contributes to fluent speech production. Our clinical experience suggests that the majority of children who need the Primary Rules are experiencing laryngeal tension and associated breath stream management issues. Therefore, for these children, only Primary Fluency Rules 4 and 5 are used during therapy. For children who also or only exhibit oral tension, Rule 6 is used in treatment.

Similar to the Universal Rules, patience is recommended when applying the Primary Rules because often clinicians move too quickly through the steps of teaching the physiologic components of fluent speech without realizing that these children are trying to master a very complex motor skill. Once the decision is made to use the Primary Rules, both the clinician and the child must realize that it will take a significant amount of therapy time and practice to master these rules and speak fluently.

Rule 4: Use Speech Breathing

Using methods similar to other clinicians (Conture, 2001; Healey & Scott, 1995; Ramig & Bennett, 1995), we teach speech breathing by drawing a breath curve, labeling the inhalation and exhalation phases, and explaining that for speech the focus must be on the exhalation phase. The child is then instructed that during exhalation, do not hold your breath, let the air out slowly, and let just a little bit of air out before starting to talk. When direct treatment for speech breathing is used, clinical success has been assisted using a combination of visual and tactile feedback. For example, the child can be instructed to draw the breath curve (Ramig & Dodge, 2005) on a chalkboard or piece of paper with one hand while his or her other open hand is placed on "the stomach" just below the sternum. Next, the child should visualize and feel breathing by tracing the breath curve with the index finger as he or she feels his or her "stomach" move as the air goes in and out. We explain that the inhalation phase is similar to putting gasoline into a car's gas tank, which provides the energy to run the car; whereas for speech, air intake provides energy to produce the sound for speech. Next, we place an "X" on the breath curve shortly after exhalation begins to indicate where speech should begin. Then we explain that the distance from the beginning of exhalation, "the top" of the breath curve, to the "X" is important because the vocal folds must be open so the "air can come out," which allows the vocal folds to vibrate easily and make a sound.

With older children, we have used the Computer Assisted Fluency Establishment Trainer (CAFET) (Goebel, 1984) to provide visual and tactile feedback. The CAFET integrates feedback signals from the speech and respiratory functions and visually displays these signals on a computer screen. This feedback allows the child to see and feel the breath curve and coordinate the onset of speech with the exhalation phase of speech breathing.

Video Clip 9 demonstrates the implementation of speech breathing with a grade-school child. During this segment, the child is tracing the breath curve with his finger with the clinician's hand just below the sternum. The clinician detects an unusual quick breath and comments about this movement to the child. Video Clip 10 demonstrates how a clinician can help a child feel speech breathing. Of interest is the portion when the child reverses the direction of his thoracic/abdominal wall during the production of a phrase as indicated by the book's slight "jump." This outward "pushing" behavior has been related to laryngeal tension as reported and observed in other stuttering clients.

The hand gesture for Rule Four is the clinician's drawing the breath curve in the air using his or her index finger following the rhythm of the child's breathing cycle. To signal when to start speech, the SLP makes a quick upward movement with the index finger while tracing the breath curve.

Rule 5: Start Mr. Voice Box Running Smoothly

This rule teaches children the concept of gentle onset of phonation, which is a treatment component in many fluency treatment programs (Cooper & Cooper, 1985; Costello, 1983; Culatta & Goldberg, 1995; Curlee & Perkins, 1969; Goebel, 1984; Leith, 1984; Guitar, 1998, 2006; Herring, 1986; Kully & Langevin, 1999; Leith, 1984; Nielson, 1999; Neilson & Andrews, 1993; Pindzola, 1987; Ramig & Bennett, 1995; Riley & Riley, 1984; Schwartz, 1999; Shine, 1988; Wall & Myers, 1995; Webster, 1979; 1980; Zebrowski & Kelly, 2002). The FRP defines gentle onset of phonation as a gradual increase in intensity over time that occurs at the beginning of an utterance. This rule has been effective with children who indicate during the assessment that they feel "the words get stuck in their throat" or who point to their neck when asked "Where do you feel tension when you try to talk?" (Conture, 2001).

The laryngeal lips analogy is used to teach the concept for this rule and requires an explanation that our "real" lips are similar to our vocal cords or "laryngeal" lips. The SLP then produces what is called "the raspberry sound" by blowing air between his or her "real" lips and causing them to vibrate while explaining that the sound the laryngeal lips just made is like the sound our "voice box makes in our neck" when air goes between our vocal cords and causes them to vibrate. Then the SLP explains that to make this sound, our "real lips" must be brought together lightly to allow air flow to vibrate the lips and make a sound. Then the SLP can demonstrate that if the lips come together too tightly, air flow will stop, the laryngeal lips cannot vibrate, and the noise produced by our "real lips" will stop. The SLP explains that this is what happens to the vocal cords when they touch together too tight and speech stops.

Video Clip 11 demonstrates the therapeutic use of laryngeal lips.

After the child understands the concept of gentle onset, the SLP explains that the gentle onset of the voice does not mean speech that is low in volume or intensity. To demonstrate, the SLP can slightly prolong the gentle initiation of an utterance gradually increasing volume until conversational speech intensity is reached.

There are two hand gestures for this rule; one is pointing to the laryngeal lips (i.e., real lips), and the other is to slowly elevate a finger in the air as if going up a gentle slope to indicate "to start Mr. Voice Box running smoothly" by gradually increasing intensity.

Rule 6: Touch the "Speech Helpers" Together Lightly

This rule is designed to assist children who experience tension in the area of the mouth (e.g., lips, tongue, or jaw) during stuttering. For children who display oral tension, understanding the contrast between light and hard contact is essential. Such children report that stuttering often occurs as the result of excessive tension in the oral anatomic structures (Dell, 2000; Ramig & Dodge, 2005). These children are reminded that during speech production, the "speech helpers" (i.e., lips and tongue) are responsible for taking the sound produced by air flowing over the vocal folds and shaping this sound into words. When shaping the sound into words, the best way to do this is to touch their speech helpers together lightly (Guitar, 1998; 2006; Healey & Scott, 1995; Kully & Langevin, 1999; Luper & Mulder, 1964; Neilson, 1999; Shine, 1980; Van Riper, 1982; Wall & Meyers, 1995; Williams, 1971; Zebrowski & Kelly, 2002). Often, well-meaning caregivers encourage the child to "just try harder" when he or she is trying to cope with the onset and development of stuttering. Obviously, by attempting the physiologic movements for speech with more physical effort, the child can easily develop excessive tension in speech-related anatomic structures, as well as secondary behaviors. Convince the family and the child that despite the common belief that hard work brings success, for speech, easy is better.

To demonstrate the ineffectiveness of using excessive tension to produce speech, the clinician and the child attempt a bilabial plosive (e.g., buh) by pressing the lips together as tightly as possible "until a word pops out." As the child and the clinician attempt this production, the SLP can again use humor by pressing his or her lips together with so much tension that the therapist's face becomes contorted. We have even "fallen" to the floor with exaggerated effort in an all-out attempt to produce the sound. After trying this "hard way to produce speech," we ask the child whether all this "hard work" helps to get the sound or word out. Children quickly recognize and feel the futility of trying to produce speech with excessive effort. The SLP and the child can then practice lightly touching their lips together so speech is produced with ease, not effort.

Video Clip 12 shows a child pushing his lips together too tightly and engaging in secondary behaviors. The therapist uses exaggerated effort to humorously demonstrate why his excessive effort does not help produce fluent speech.

The visual reminder used to cue this rule consists of touching the first finger and thumb together very lightly.

SECONDARY RULE
Rule 7: Use Only the Speech Helpers to Talk

The last Fluency Rule was designed to eliminate secondary behaviors that involve movement of anatomic structures (e.g., head turns, leg patting, eye blinks) not associated with fluent speech production. Our focus is to teach the concept that these nonspeech anatomic behaviors have "nothing to do with talking" and that using them will not help produce fluent speech.

To eliminate a secondary behavior, the clinician reviews how speech is produced: air flow carries the words out; this air flow vibrates the vocal folds, which produce a sound; and the movement of the lips and tongue shape the sound into words. Then the clinician tells the child that when he or she has talked about how speech is produced, he or she has only described moving the lips, tongue, jaw, and other speech structures. No extra movement is needed. The clinician explains to the child that "you do not need to move other parts of your body when you talk." Even after this explanation, the child is frequently unaware of the physical movements associated with the secondary behaviors. The use of a mirror often leads to the child's awareness and subsequent rapid elimination of the unnecessary behavior.

Another therapy technique the clinician can use with or without the mirror is to demonstrate the child's secondary behavior in an exaggerated manner to demonstrate that "this movement" does not help produce speech. For example, if the child turns his or her head when speech is initiated, the clinician explains that head turning was not one of the anatomic structures reviewed when explaining how speech is produced and, therefore, will not contribute to fluent speech production. To demonstrate this explanation, the clinician can stand in front of a mirror, if available, and says, "I am going to turn my head as often as possible until the intended word pops out." Then with considerable animation, the clinician turns his or her head a number of times. Obviously nothing happens, and it is clear that head turning to start speech is not helpful and should be eliminated. The nonverbal cue for this rule is a replication of the child's secondary movement as a reminder of the futility of its use.

IMPLEMENTING THE FLUENCY RULES PROGRAM

Universal Rules

During the evaluation, the SLP determines which Fluency Rules have been "broken" and need to be included in the treatment plan. Although the Universal Rules are always used early in therapy, the SLP should be aware of children who display oral and/or laryngeal tension with or without secondary behaviors and be prepared to implement the Primary Rules and Secondary Rule when needed. Before beginning therapy, teach any language concept(s) (e.g., say the word *once*, say the word *short*, say the word *slowly*) necessary for clear understanding of therapy instructions for the Universal Rules.

Before therapy, the SLP should review the diagnostic report and determine which of the Universal Rules need to be implemented. If more than one Universal Rule is needed for treatment, plan to begin therapy in the order presented in the text. In other words, if the child is a rapid talker and exhibits repetitions, start treatment with Rule 1—the concept of slowing the rate of speech using the appropriate hand gestures. After the speech rate has been reduced, then introduce Rule 2—Say a Word One Time. Use both Universal Rules simultaneously with more treatment emphasis on the last rule introduced. Plan to begin each therapy session by reviewing the applicable rule(s), and then use conversational speech in play situations to maximize clinical opportunities for the child to monitor his or her speech output.

In Video Clip 13, the clinicians show how each therapy session should begin with the review of the applicable Fluency Rules.

When the treatment plan includes implementing Rule 2—Say a Word One Time—for clinical

expediency, all repetitions are identified and treated as stuttering. When introducing Rule 2 during the first therapy session, the child is told that during therapy, all words are said one time. This identification strategy was adopted because early in the development of the FRP, an excessive amount of treatment time was sometimes expended discussing with children whether a disfluent event was a stutter or a normal disfluency. Therefore, our current clinical rule is that all disfluencies—both those that could be considered normal and those regarded as stuttering—are identified as behaviors to be eliminated.

When application of the Universal Rules begins, the child monitors the clinician's speech to determine when one or more of the three rules that have been targeted for therapy are "broken." Using the Say a Word One Time rule as an example, the SLP tells the child that, "Sometimes I say a word more than one time and you could help me know when this happens by raising a finger to indicate that a repeated word occurred." This clinical activity allows the child to increase his/her awareness of repeated sounds as well as to demonstrate to the SLP that the child understands the concept of saying a word one time.

In Video Clip 14, a child raises her finger to demonstrate that she understands the concept of saying a word only one time. In Video Clip 15, a child with special needs demonstrates that he also understands the concept of saying a word one time. In Video Clip 16, a clinician with two children demonstrates how one child can identify a repetition in the speech of another child. In another approach to repetitions shown in Video Clip 22, the clinician uses an exaggerated number of repetitions until both children demonstrate awareness of the repetitious behavior.

If two SLPs are involved in therapy, this awareness activity can be supplemented by having the therapists "catch" each other by raising a finger and saying "one time" when the other clinician repeats a word. After the introduction of this Universal Rule using the "catch me" (Guitar, 2006; Ramig & Dodge, 2005) or "gotcha" activity (Seltzer & Culatta, 1979), the clinician should invite the child to join in by helping "to catch" (i.e., identify) the therapist who used the repeated word. To maintain a high level of therapy interest, the therapist can turn this "catching" activity into a competitive game by keeping score to determine who will be the first person to catch the one who repeated the word.

See Video Clip 17 for an example of the "catching activity".

The clinicians continue to frequently repeat words, and "catching each other" continues until the concept of identifying repeated words is firmly established.

During this initial treatment period, the clinicians calculate the percentage of correct identifications made by the child and how rapidly these correct identifications are made. As the child's ability to correctly and rapidly identify repetitions produced by the clinician increases, the therapist introduces the idea of identifying repetitions in the speech of the child. The transition to "catching" the child when he or she repeats a word can be accomplished by the clinician excitedly saying, "I think I heard you say a word more than one time and now I can help you just like you helped me!" This transition to the identification of the repeated words in everyone's speech, including the child's, usually goes smoothly, and therapy continues using the "catch me" game format. As therapy continues, the treatment focus changes to how rapidly the child can identify repetitions in his or her own speech. The clinician encourages the child to "raise your finger as soon as you hear yourself repeat a word and before I can catch you." A positive clinical sign is when the child becomes aware of and can accurately and quickly signal when a repetition occurs in his or her speech.

Video Clip 18 shows a child identifying a repetition in his speech but then realizing that he made a social blunder.

Sometimes the transition to identifying repeated words in the child's speech meets resistance because the child feels that he or she is doing something wrong. Nevertheless, the transition can usually be accomplished by telling the child how happy the therapist is because the child has helped identify repetitions in the SLP's speech, how much better the therapist's speech sounds, and that now the SLP can help the child's speech sound better. As described in

Universal Rule 2, the bent finger therapy technique was developed because one child became concerned when "caught" repeating a word. This cue can be used when this situation arises.

As therapy with Universal Rules progresses, the child will understand the meaning and intent of each applicable rule and become skilled at monitoring his or her speech, resulting in decreased targeted behavior (for example, the frequency of repetitions gradually decreases). When the child's frequency of the targeted behavior decreases, the SLP must increase his or her disfluencies proportionately so the child can continue to recognize disfluencies in others and thus maintain the focus of therapy.

Remember to be patient and allow the children sufficient therapy time to incorporate the Universal Rules into their conversational speech. Clinical experience has indicated that for some children, the therapy process takes time, but after many sessions, stuttering may disappear abruptly. Our most dramatic clinical success was with a very uncooperative preschooler who stuttered on more than 80% of his words with some instances of stuttering containing eight iterations. After several unproductive therapy sessions and a consultation, minimal clinical progress had been achieved. Subsequently, we discovered that the child had a fascination for puzzles and incorporated this activity into the therapy program. Soon, the child began to talk more, and the Universal Rules could be applied regularly. The child quickly used the rules, and after two treatment sessions, the mother reported that the child spontaneously "caught" an inadvertent repetition in the father's speech at the dinner table. A dramatic decrease in stuttering followed this dinner table event, and by the next therapy session, the child produced no stutters. During three additional therapy sessions, no stuttering was observed, and the parents reported none at home. Twenty years later, he remains fluent.

Primary Rules

Primary Rules will be applied when a child gradually develops mastery of the Universal Rules (quickly and accurately identifying repetitions and prolongations in his or her speech) but still continues to stutter. Before introducing the Primary Rules, four treatment principles are explained and established with the child. First, the child must learn the fundamental skills of fluent speech production. This knowledge will demystify stuttering and allow the child to understand the difference between how stuttered and fluent speech is produced and what needs to be changed in how the child talks now to become a fluent talker. To assist in teaching this principle, age-appropriate physical activity analogies to which the child can relate, such as sports (Manning, 1991), playing a musical instrument, or dancing, have been beneficial. That is, if a child is playing in a basketball league concurrently with speech therapy, the SLP can compare the motor skills of speech with the motor skills of playing basketball—both require coordinated muscle movements and considerable practice to accomplish a goal. For example, shooting a free throw in basketball and fluent speech can be compared. To successfully shoot a free throw, the player must remember the fundamentals: take a deep breath, keep your eye on the basket, and follow through with your hand and arm. If one of these fundamentals is executed incorrectly, then the free throw may be missed. As previously presented, the fundamentals for fluent speech include: breath stream management (i.e., exhalation), gently vibrating the vocal folds (i.e., saying "ahhh"), and light articulation contacts to shape the sounds into words. If these fundamentals are not executed correctly, then stuttering could occur.

The second pretherapy principle involves the clinician explaining that to become a "fluent talker," the child must "feel fluency." As indicated in the first principle, when therapy begins, the child will learn the fundamental motor skills of fluent speech. This knowledge will allow the child to contrast the different feeling between fluent and stuttered speech. The example of shooting a basket can be used again, but this time to illustrate the importance of feeling the fundamental skills of a successfully completed motor event. Basketball players often know immediately as the ball leaves their hand that it will go in the basket because the shot "felt right." This instant feel or recognition of a successful motor event can only be accomplished by repeated practice of the fundamentals of a motor task. The feeling of fluency must begin with the initial "sounds" of an utterance because stuttering occurs more frequently at the initiation of speech. In addition, if

speech is begun fluently, then the remainder of the sentence is more likely to be fluent. Pushing a car illustrates this concept. An easy push gets the car moving, and once under motion, very little effort is needed to keep the car moving. Therefore, it is important for the child to feel fluency from the beginning to the end of the utterance.

The third pretherapy principle is that the child must be made aware that practice, practice, and more practice of the fundamental skills will be required to master fluent speech. Anyone who plays sports or a musical instrument or dances understands the need to practice to perfect a skill involving sequential muscle movements. After the child understands the need to practice, we point out to the child that, even though a lot of practice will be needed, every time the child begins to talk is an opportunity to practice.

The final principle of "there is no such thing as difficult sounds" is intended to dispel the child's concept of "difficult" speech sounds. To eliminate this concept, the child is asked to indicate which sounds give him or her the most trouble to say. Following this disclosure, the child is told that if he or she practices and feels the fundamentals of fluent speech that he or she is about to learn, then it will not matter which sound is attempted because all sounds will come out fluently. Two sports analogies are used to explain this concept. The first example uses basketballs that have slightly different physical characteristics. We explain that it does not matter if a new ball, an old ball, a leather ball, or a rubber ball is shot because if the fundamental skills of shooting a basketball are correct, then any ball selected will go in the basket. The second analogy relates the game of golf to speech. In golf, many different clubs are used to play the game, just like there are many different "sounds" needed to produce speech. For both skills, if the correct fundamentals are used, a person will be able to use any golf club correctly or say any word beginning with any sound fluently. However, both in speech and golf, people often believe they cannot say a word beginning with a particular "sound" or hit a certain club because, in the past, they occasionally experienced difficulty with these specific activities. Such intermittent difficulties often cause people to believe they cannot say words beginning with a particular sound or successfully hit the ball with a particular club. Again, we emphasize that if the fundamentals of speech and golf are perfected with practice, then it will not matter which word or club is selected because all can now be used successfully.

Following the explanation of these treatment principles, therapy begins by having the child model the production of groups of sounds in the initial position of phrases presented using an arbitrary hierarchical order of difficulty (i.e., vowels, semivowels, nasals, voiced fricatives, voiced stops, voiceless fricatives, and voiceless stops) (Goebel, 1984). First, the child repeats the vowel initial phrases (e.g., "Animals are your friend," "Everyone is invited," "Under the table") modeled by the SLP until three sets of 50 consecutive phrases can be produced without an instance of stuttering. The child is instructed and the SLP constantly reminds the child while repeating the material to remember the fundamental skills of speech and concentrate on how speech is being produced fluently and to feel the fluency. Once this initial therapy goal has been accomplished, the child moves to the sounds in the initial position at the next level of difficulty (i.e., semivowels). Interspersed throughout the treatment program therapy, usually after a set of 50 phrases has been successfully completed, the clinician engages the child in short periods of conversation. At first, this change in activities from repeating phrases to conversational speech may elicit stuttering. When an instance of stuttering following the successful fluent productions of 50 phrases occurs, it provides an opportunity for the clinician to remind the child to always monitor his or her speech and not lose his or her focus when producing spontaneous speech. Therapy continues until the child has successfully produced phrases at all levels of difficulty. Once these hierarchical lists have been successfully completed, the child is reminded that he or she has just produced every "sound" in our language in the initial position and has also demonstrated that there are no difficult sounds or ones that he or she cannot produce fluently if the fundamental skills of fluent speech are used to feel fluency.

The next stage of therapy involves using the newly learned fundamental skills and feeling of fluency in conversational speech. At this point in therapy, the child and clinician must be prepared for the possibility of stuttering recurring because the focus of therapy shifts from the production of

modeled phrases to more complex conversational speech. We explain that modeled speech was easier because the child did not have to think about what he or she was going to say and could focus entirely on how to produce speech. Now as conversational speech is practiced, the child must "divide" his or her attention between context and production. To reduce the impact of this shift in therapy focus to conversational speech, a question and answer format is used (Goebel, 1984) that requires the child to answer simple questions (e.g., What do policeman do? What is an ambulance?). Prior to answering the question, the child is instructed to listen to the question, think of an answer, restate the question (i.e., a similar task to the previously modeled phrases), and then answer the question. Throughout the task, the child is instructed to remember and practice the fluency rules. If stuttering occurs and continues when practicing conversational speech, therapy returns to the previous stage, which involved practicing modeled phrases containing the sounds on which stuttering occurred. The child is reminded to focus on the speech fundamentals and feel fluency while modeling the phrases to reassure the child that he or she can produce the previously stuttered words fluently. After a minimum of three sets of 50 modeled phrases are produced without one instance of stuttering, treatment returns to the question and answer format to resume practice on conversational speech.

Therapy using questions and answers continues until the child remains fluent for one therapy sessions. The treatment focus then advances to traditional conversational dialogue between the therapist and the child. If the child stutters during the practice of conversational speech, therapy again returns to fluently modeling 50 phrases containing the stuttered word. Practicing conversational speech and returning to modeled phrases when an instant of stuttering occurs continues until fluency is reached or the therapist, child, and family decide that treatment benefits have been maximized. Our experience has been that fluency is often obtained in the treatment sessions but that using fluent speech in other speaking environments has been difficult. To assist the child, we ask the child to bring a list of words on which stuttering occurred away from our office. At the beginning of the next treatment sessions and prior to practice using conversational speech, the child practices these words using the modeled phrases format. Other techniques to be used outside the treatment room will be presented in the following carryover section of this chapter.

Secondary Rule

Apply the Secondary Rule immediately after the child exhibits a secondary behavior involving nonspeech muscles. Because these secondary behaviors are counterproductive to the acquisition of fluent speech, the SLP should take immediate action when a secondary behavior occurs to eliminate its use. Application of the Secondary Rule should pre-empt application of any Fluency Rule until secondary stuttering behaviors are eliminated. When the SLP is satisfied that a child understands the concept of the Secondary Rule, therapy can return to the previous activity. If the secondary behavior recurs, the SLP should stop existing therapy and return to teaching the concept for the Secondary Rule.

Carryover and Transfer

When fluent speech is transferred or carried over from the therapy setting to the home and classroom, visual reminders are used extensively. For the FRP to be effective, the child must remember the Fluency Rules in all speaking environments. In the school environment, the SLP, the classroom teacher, subject teachers, and the child meet to select a small unobtrusive item to be placed in each room as a reminder of the Fluency Rule (e.g., stickers on notebooks or refrigerator magnets on the edge of chalkboards). Only the teacher and the child need to be aware of the item and its significance. Then, if the child forgets to use a Fluency Rule, the teacher can provide a reminder by glancing in the direction of or by touching the designated item. At home, the same procedure can be used with the same or different visual reminders. Parents can place these reminders (e.g., symbolic elephants are effective because elephants never forget) in conversation areas (e.g., the family room, kitchen, bedroom, and dining room), and family members may call attention to them as needed. Use of these subtle visual cues, as well as the individual hand signals selectively used by the parents, provides a secondary benefit for the family. These reminders elimi-

nate the need for a direct confrontation when stuttering occurs, which reduces family conflicts that may arise from frequent verbal reminders, particularly during the early stages of transfer. We recommend that the family not use the visual reminders 100% of the time, but only at select times (e.g., at the dinner table, in the car, before bed) to remind the child when to be fluent by using the Fluency Rules. Ideally, the transfer segment of therapy will result in the Fluency Rules being generalized to areas away from the therapy room and ultimately lead to fluent speech in these environments.

An effective treatment strategy combining visual reminders and games and toys can motivate the child to use the Fluency Rules in therapy and at home. During therapy, when practicing the primary rules, games or other fun activities are regularly scheduled to reward hard work and the correct application of the Fluency Rules. In other words, when the child cooperates and tries hard in therapy, then the child and the therapist will take a play break. These "play breaks" are not really breaks from therapy but serve the primary purpose of providing the child the opportunity to practice the Fluency Rules in a less structured setting. These "play breaks" also provide the opportunity to remind the child that he or she must still remember the Fluency Rules even when having fun.

To facilitate carryover at home, a lending library arrangement was created allowing the child to borrow a game or toy previously used in the office until the next therapy session if the child promises to use the Fluency Rules when playing with the borrowed item. By prearrangement, the parents agree to play with their child using the borrowed item and to implement the Fluency Rules during these activities. An additional benefit of the lending library is more parental involvement at a point in therapy when parents can make positive contributions toward their child's progress. Equally important is the motivational value of these games in the clinic with children. When our lending library started, there were two uncooperative children on the caseload who gained renewed interest and cooperation in therapy because of the inclusion of "play breaks" using video games during therapy and their ability to borrow the games when they showed progress. Both children successfully completed therapy, which we believe was due in part to the use of the library and the interest these games brought to the therapy process.

Telephone calls are also used to assist the carryover of fluency to the home environment. Typically the telephone calls occur near the end of the treatment program, when the child is using the Fluency Rules effectively in therapy sessions. To keep awareness high at home, we telephone the child and ask about his or her speech and if the Fluency Rules are being used today. At first, with the parents' permission, these calls are frequent, occurring several times a week. This frequency of calls is continued for about a week, and then calls are gradually reduced until they occur infrequently, about once a month. Periodically, however, we again call several times on randomly selected nights. The intended outcome is to have the child think that every time the phone rings, the therapist is calling again, which serves as a reminder to use the Fluency Rules. Since the creation of the lending library, calls are more effective because conversations can also be directed toward the use of the toys or games and not exclusively speech or fluency focused. These calls also provide an excellent opportunity to evaluate the child's fluency in a different setting than the clinic.

ASSESSMENT METHODS TO SUPPORT ONGOING DECISION MAKING

The two purposes of our assessment procedure are to determine if therapy intervention is needed because stuttering may persist and to educate the parents and child about the differences between stuttered and fluent speech production. To accomplish these purposes, baseline assessment information is gathered and shared during the initial family interview, the postinterview evaluation, the child's speech evaluation, and the follow-up evaluation.

When the patient and family arrive for the initial evaluation, our protocol is that one of the clinicians conducts the intake interview with the family, while a second clinician and another clinician take the child into the therapy/play room to obtain an initial clinical impression of the stuttering disorder. If the child will not separate from the family, then the child and the family are all taken to the therapy/play room to obtain the speech sample. Almost always, the child enjoys the play activities involved in collecting the speech sample, and after a short period of time, one clinician and the parents can leave the therapy/play room, and the initial interview can be conducted. The focus of this portion of the initial interview is to collect case history information and the parents' perception of the child's fluency disorder.

INITIAL INTERVIEW

Information obtained during the parent interview can be extremely important in determining what factors may be present that would increase the possibility that stuttering could persist and therapeutic intervention should be considered. These interview questions probe such factors as time since onset, family history, gender, history of stuttering, and age at onset (Yairi & Ambrose, 2005; Curlee, 2007).

Time since Onset

The length of time since the onset of stuttering is very indicative of a stuttering disorder that can continue. If the child's stuttering disorder has continued for 15 months or longer, the likelihood of stuttering continuing is greatly increased.

Family History

Another important factor supporting the need for treatment is a family history of persistent stuttering. Yairi & Ambrose (2005) reported that a history of recovered or persistent stuttering occurred in the families of children who stutter in approximately 65% of cases and is the best predictor of persisting stuttering in children.

Gender

The easiest and one of the more significant prognostic factors is the child's gender. It has been well established that the incidence of stuttering is higher among males than females and that the difference between the number of males who stutter and females who stutter increases from the childhood onset of the disorder to adulthood (Yairi & Ambrose, 2005).

History of Stuttering

If the developmental history of stuttering indicates that the frequency of stuttering-like disfluencies (SLDs) (i.e., part-word repetitions, single-syllable whole-word repetitions, and dysrhythmic phonation) is not decreasing 15 months after onset, then therapeutic intervention should be considered. Yairi and Ambrose (2005) indicated that children who naturally recover from stuttering experience a reduction in the frequency and/or severity of stuttering usually by the end of the first year after onset.

Age at Onset

A late onset of stuttering could be an important indicator of a need for services. Yairi and Ambrose (2005) reported that children whose stuttering persisted had a reported onset of stuttering 3.5 months later than those who did not continue to stutter. A late onset for males would be approximately after their third birthday, whereas for females, late onset is after 34 months of age.

POSTINTERVIEW EVALUATION

After the case history information is collected, the clinicians exchange places. The clinician originally with the child now talks with the parents and answers any questions they have about the disorder of stuttering, explains the physiologic differences between stuttered and fluent speech, and determines if today's observed behaviors are similar to those noted by the parents that prompted their seeking an evaluation. This exchange of activities allows the clinicians to compare notes after the evaluation session and before the final portion of the postevaluation interview to determine if their initial impressions are similar and if the changeover caused any increase or change in the child's disfluencies. The final component of the initial interview is a joint meeting of the two clinicians and the parents, while the child continues to interact with the third clinician. During the postevaluation interview, the authors share their initial findings with the family and, when needed, their impressions of the trial therapy conducted at the end of the evaluation session.

To determine if therapy will be recommended, the clinicians use a prognostic checklist (Table 10.2) and discuss with the parents the

importance the clinicians place on each item. The clinicians explain that this checklist is organized with the items considered by the clinicians as most important for the prognosis at the top of each category with accompanying check boxes for a yes/no response. The parents are informed that the more "yes" responses there are to the six designated questions, the greater the potential is for persistent stuttering and the need for therapy. The following are examples of how the check sheet is used. In the Initial Interview section, if the first two questions (i.e., time since onset greater than 15 months; a family history of persistent stuttering) are checked "yes," then immediate therapy is recommended. If the answers to questions 2 and 3 (i.e., a family history of persistent stuttering; gender is male) are checked "yes" but question 1 is a "no" response (i.e., time since onset less than 15 months), beginning therapy immediately is recommended after the implications of question 1 are explained. If the answers to questions 1 and 2 are "no," then the remainder of the items are explained, and the recommendation is made that the family return for a second visit so the results of the videotape analysis can be discussed and a final determination can be made regarding the possible need for therapeutic intervention.

SPEECH EVALUATION

All initial evaluations are videotape recorded and used for the speech analyses. Information obtained during the speech evaluation is focused on determining the severity of the disorder. To determine the overall severity of the stuttering disorder, the following factors are considered: number of iterations, frequency of stuttering, the presence of secondary behaviors, and the presence of coexisting communication disorders (Curlee, 2007; Yairi & Ambrose, 2005).

Number of Iterations

Number of iterations appears to be a sensitive measure of persistence of stuttering. Yairi and Ambrose (2005) reported that normally fluent children typically produced one iteration (e.g., and, and) and averaged 1.1 iterations, whereas children who stutter averaged 1.5 iterations but frequently produced more repeated units. In fact, when these authors reviewed the frequency with

Table 10.2. *Diagnostic Information Prognostic Checklist*

Evaluation			Y	N
Initial				
Interview				
	Time since onset	Is the time since onset greater than 15 months?	☐	☐
	Family history	Is there a family history of persistent stuttering?	☐	☐
	Gender	Is the child a male?	☐	☐
	History of stuttering	Has the frequency of stuttering-like disfluencies or overall severity of stuttering increased since onset?	☐	☐
	Age at onset	Did stuttering onset occur after the third birthday?	☐	☐
Postinterview		Initial diagnostic and trial therapy impressions		
Evaluation		are discussed.		
Speech				
Evaluation				
	Number of iterations	Are 2 or more iterations present?	☐	☐
	Frequency of stuttering	Record for baseline data.		
	Presence of secondary behaviors (struggle and/or tension)	Record for baseline data.		
	Coexisting articulation disorder	Determine for inclusion in treatment paradigm.		
	Coexisting language disorder	Determine for inclusion in treatment program.		
Follow-Up		Is the Yairi measure 4 or higher?	☐	☐
Evaluation				

which single and multiple iterations occurred, they found that for the stuttering children, 70% had one iteration, 18% had two iterations, 7% had three iterations, and 5% had four iterations. These percentages were strikingly different for the normally fluent children: 89% had one iteration, 10% had two iterations, and three of four iterations occurred very infrequently. The authors concluded that the repetitions produced by children who stutter often contain two or more iterations and the frequency of their occurrence per 100 syllables is greater than for nonstuttering children.

Frequency of Stuttering Behaviors

The frequency of disfluencies and/or SLDs has been cited to indicate a persistent stuttering disorder. Adams (1984), Conture and Caruso (1987), and Curlee (2007) believe there is a fluency disorder if the total of all disfluencies exceeds 10% of spoken words. When only SLDs are considered, a child who does not stutter produces less than 3% of these types of disfluencies.

Because the child who continues to stutter produces almost eight times as many SLDs as the child who does not stutter, the greater a child exceeds 3% of SLDs, the more likely it is that the child's stuttering will continue.

Secondary Behaviors

The presence of secondary behaviors close to onset does not predict a persistent stuttering disorder. However if such behaviors as muscular tension, airflow blockages, and head and neck movements continue for longer than 15 months after onset, the chances are much higher that stuttering will persist.

Coexisting Speech and/or Language Disorders

Children who also exhibit other speech and language disorders are not necessarily more likely to become persistent stutterers (Yairi & Ambrose, 2005). Although the predictive aspect of coexisting speech and language disorders is limited, determining if such communication disorders are present is extremely important to note and evaluate during the initial evaluation so that a comprehensive treatment plan can be developed for the child.

FOLLOW-UP EVALUATION

When the diagnostic information obtained during the first visit cannot establish whether a therapy intervention program is needed, a second evaluation session is scheduled so information gathered from the analysis of the videotape recorded during the initial visit can be presented to assist in the prognosis. The second visit will also allow the clinicians to determine if the child's disfluent behavior noted during this visit is consistent with that noted at the initial evaluation session.

At the second session, Yairi's weighted SLD measure, which is determined by reviewing the videotape, is presented to the parents. The weighted SLD measure uses the frequency, type, and extent of the stuttering behavior to calculate a single score that can be used to support a prognosis. This single score is calculated based on 100 syllables as follows: [(part-word repetitions + single syllable word repetitions) × average repetition units + 2 × the frequency of blocks and prolongations]. If the calculated score exceeds 4, then there is considerable evidence that the child's speech is characteristic of a persistent disorder, and treatment should commence (Yairi & Ambrose, 2005). The diagnostic checklist is again used to assist in making the final therapeutic determination. First the findings from the initial evaluation and the relevance of each previously checked item are reviewed and verified. If the results of the analysis of the videotape indicate that the child scored 4 or higher on the Yairi weighted SLD measure or exhibited two or more iterations at least three times during the speech sample, a therapy intervention program is recommended.

TAILORING THE TREATMENT TO THE INDIVIDUAL CLIENT

One of the strengths of the FRP is that it is presented the same way to every child, with the only difference being the pace at which the treatment program is implemented. The pace of presenting the FRP is determined by the child's ability to grasp the concepts of the individual Fluency Rules and the logistical availability of the family and the child to attend therapy. The simplicity of the rules has had broad appeal and has received positive comments from parents and public school clinicians because of the ease with which individuals interested in the child's environment can participate in the therapy process by reminding the child of his or her fluency rules using the designated hand signal. To date, following our directions, we have never had a parent be reluctant to selectively use the Fluency Rules and corresponding hand signals in the home environment. In fact, we strongly recommend that the best model for implementing the FRP is when the professional clinic (e.g., private practice, university, or hospital), the parents, and the public school clinician all are involved in the similar treatment program.

The most pleasant and unexpected surprise the authors have experienced using the FRP was the success experienced with cognitively challenged children. Over the years, we have successfully treated children labeled as learning disabled, autistic, or having Down syndrome.

Video Clip 6 shows a child who has Down syndrome. Video Clip 19 was taken during a consultation with a public school SLP who was having difficulty eliminating this child's repetitions. After a short period of using the FRP, the child responded to the instruction. As seen in the segment, the SLP was very excited with the response. The child no longer uses repetitions.

Although the FRP's origin was to help preschool and early grade-school children with their stuttering, this treatment program can be use with students in all grades. Of course with the older child, the focus of treatment is often the physiologic aspect of fluent speech production using the Primary Rules. With the older child, the hand signals are more than a signal to acoustically self-monitor their speech; they also serve as a reminder to use the physiologic mechanics of speech production that support fluent speech and to feel the differences between stuttered and fluent speech.

APPLICATION TO AN INDIVIDUAL CLIENT

Cody, a 4-year, 2-month-old male, was seen for six therapy sessions subsequent to his evaluation at our private practice. Based on the Stuttering Prediction Instrument (SPI) (Riley, 1981), Cody was rated a moderate stutterer. Cody stuttered on 27% of his words; the greatest number of iterations was 11, with an average of nine iterations for the three longest repetitions. No prolongations, secondary behaviors, or family history of stuttering were noted. His speech rate, language, and articulation abilities were judged to be within normal limits. The evaluation session was videotaped in our waiting room because Cody would not separate from his mother. During the evaluation session, a trial period of therapy was conducted. Based on our observations of normal rate of speech and the absence of prolongations, the application of Universal Rule 2—Say a Word One Time—was implemented. As a component of trial therapy, the two clinicians identified repeated words in their speech using the appropriate hand gestures and invited Cody to help in the identification of the repeated words. Note that, *in Video Clip 20*, Cody subtly (notice his hand near the couch) uses the raised finger hand gesture for saying a word one time. The second time he identifies the repetition he is more confident in his use of the hand gesture. The use of the gesture indicates clearly that Cody understands the concept, and therapy is recommended to be continued using the competition format of who identifies the repeated word first.

In the next session (*Video Clip 21*), Cody learned to quickly identify word repetitions produced by the clinicians with 100% accuracy. Also during that session, the concept of old ears was used, and the transition to identifying the repetitions in Cody's speech was introduced. In *Video Clip 22*, Cody continued to identify repetitions that occurred in the clinician's speech and his own speech. In *Video Clip 6 and 19*, the therapist demonstrated the use of humor by wearing large rubber ears to remind Cody that the therapist has old ears and not to hurt the therapist's ears by saying a word more than one time. On this segment, the child also indicated that he is aware of his Fluency Rule by using the hand gesture. Before the fifth session, the mother reported, and

we also observed, a marked decrease in the frequency of repetitions and an even greater reduction in the number of iterations. Because Cody produced fluent speech, the clinicians complimented Cody on using fluent speech and saying his words one time. During the sixth session, Cody produced only two repetitions, and his mother noted "virtually no repetitions at home." Therapy was discontinued, and the family was given the option of bringing Cody back to therapy if the repetitions reappeared. Eight years later, he remains a fluent speaker.

FUTURE DIRECTIONS

As was stated in previous publications (Runyan & Runyan, 1999; 2007), we continue to encourage clinicians in all therapeutic environments to use the FRP and to share their results, techniques, and experiences with us and their colleagues at professional meetings. The FRP's ultimate effectiveness and utility can only be demonstrated when larger and more diverse groups of children who stutter are treated by different therapists in different settings and followed over a longer period of time. In the years we have developed and used the FRP, there are clinical impressions we have noted and questions we have asked that hopefully will be answered as more clinicians become involved, more children are treated, and more data becomes available. Some of these questions are as follows:

- What is the best model for implementation of the Fluency Rules? Is clinical intervention more effective if the professional clinic, the public school clinician, and the parents are all involved in implementing the program? Our clinical impression is that it is more effective.
- Can the FRP be an effective treatment program for use in the public schools, considering the limited treatment schedule inherent with the public school calendar? Our clinical experience and some limited data indicate that it can be used effectively.
- After the necessary training and with professional supervision, can the FRP be administered as a parent-implemented program? Our clinical impression is that it could be administered successful by parents who have the necessary attributes. However, some of the fun activities and humor we use may be difficult for parents to use. The most effective model

may be a short intensive program with the professional speech pathologist followed by a supervised parent-driven program with intermittent visits to the professional clinic.

- Do children with coexisting articulation, language, or cognitive issues need more clinical time to eliminate stuttering behaviors? Our clinical impressions are that children with just stuttering and articulation disorders need no additional time, but language-disordered and cognitive-challenged children who also stutter need more time for treatment. However, as discussed in this chapter, children with these coexisting communication issues have been successfully treated using the FRP and have been released from therapy.
- Combining the last two bulleted items, assuming that a parent-driven treatment program is possible, can the parents implement a therapy program effectively that encompasses treatment for stuttering and coexisting communication issues? Our clinical impression is that it is doubtful parents can effectively administer a treatment program for multiple communication needs. However, parents can be used to support select aspects of the treatment program.
- Can the FRP be administered in a group as effectively as with an individual client? Our clinical impression is that it can, and in fact, a group may even make the program more efficient.
- Does the number of children who become fluent decrease if the Primary Rules are needed for therapeutic intervention? Our clinical impression is that far fewer children become fluent when direct physiologic intervention is needed. We also have the impression that when the Primary Rules are needed, the treatment process takes longer.

CHAPTER SUMMARY

The FRP was designed to provide public school SLPs with an effective and efficient stuttering treatment program for preschool and early grade-school children.

The FRP consists of three sections: Universal Rules, Primary Rules, and the Secondary Rule.

- The Universal Rules are used with every child and focus on reducing speaking rate and the elimination of repetitions and prolongations.

- The Primary Rules focus on assisting children to understand the physiologic differences between stuttered and fluent speech.
- The Secondary Rule eliminates secondary behaviors.
- Therapy should be conducted in a fun environment using the appropriate hand gestures for each rule during conversation to maximize the child's responses.
- Therapy begins with the Universal Rules increasing the child's awareness of stuttering and decreasing the frequency of occurrence.

If the Universal Rules do not eliminate stuttering, the Primary Rules are used. Before implementing the Primary Rules, the following four therapy principles are presented: learn the fundamentals of fluent speech, feel the fluency, the need for practice, and the concept that there are no difficult words to produce.

To assist in transferring fluent speech from the therapy room to other environments, clinicians should involve classroom teachers, public school therapist, private practice therapist, and parents in using the Fluency Rules' hand gestures and placement of reminders of the rules in the children's environments.

CHAPTER REVIEW QUESTIONS

1. What are the three Universal Rules?
2. What are the three Primary Rules?
3. When should the Secondary Rule be used?
4. What is the hand gesture for each Fluency Rule?
5. When should a clinician move from the Universal Rules to implementing the Primary Rules?
6. In the FRP, we explain to the children that fluent speech is composed of three sequential steps. What are these three steps?
7. How are secondary behaviors eliminated?
8. List three therapy techniques recommended to help children carry over fluent speech to the home and school environment.
9. Explain how the FRP demystifies the concept of difficult sounds for children.
10. Explain the "catch me" activity and how the clinician can transfer this activity to the child's speech.

11. Explain the criteria for determining whether a child is an incipient stutterer or a normally disfluent child.

SUGGESTED READINGS

Bennett, E. M. (2006). *Working with People Who Stutter: A Lifespan Approach*. Upper Saddle River, NJ: Pearson Merrill Prentice Hall.

Conture, E. G. (2001). *Stuttering: Its Nature, Diagnosis, and Treatment*. Needham Heights, MA: Allyn and Bacon.

Guitar, B. (2006). *Stuttering: An Integrated Approach to Its Nature and Treatment* (3rd ed.). Baltimore, MD: Lippincott, Williams & Wilkins.

Manning, W. (2001). *Clinical Decision Making in Fluency Disorders* (2nd ed.). Vancouver, British Columbia, Canada: Singular Thompson Learning.

Ramig, P. R., & Dodge, D. M. (2005). *The Child and Adolescent Stuttering Treatment and Activity Resource Guide*. New York, NY: Thompson Delmar Learning.

Yairi, E., & Ambrose, N. G. (2005). *Early Childhood Stuttering*. Austin, TX: Pro-Ed.

CHAPTER 11

Smooth Speech and Cognitive Behavior Therapy for the Treatment of Older Children and Adolescents Who Stutter

ASHLEY CRAIG

CHAPTER OUTLINE

KEY TERMS

Anti-relapse program: a psychological program designed specifically to lower risks or vulnerability to experiencing relapse after treatment for stuttering.

Cognitive behavior therapy: a psychological therapy that is based on the idea that cognitions, emotions, and behavior interact. This therapy is based on the assumption that thoughts can determine negative feelings and behavior.

Fluency shaping: a type of treatment for stuttering that completely modifies the speech of the participant rather than modifying the moment of stuttering.

Relapse: the recurrence of stuttering symptoms that are perceived as personally unacceptable after a time of improvement.

Smooth Speech: a fluency shaping technique that emphasizes continuous airflow rather than continuous vocalization in the participant's speech production.

Social anxiety disorder (social phobia): an anxiety disorder in which a person shows noticeable and persistent fear of social situations in which he or she may be embarrassed.

INTRODUCTION

Stuttering can be a chronic disorder with as yet no certain cure (Bloodstein, 1995). It is also a disorder that begins in early childhood (American Psychiatric Association, 1994). Regrettably, therefore, this means that children who continue to stutter as they grow older have to cope with and adapt to the impairment that can result from stuttering. Aspects of that impairment include involuntary speech disruption and associated problems such as embarrassment, frustration, shyness, anxiety, and social avoidance. Of grave concern is recent research indicating that many thousands of children are at risk for these problems (Craig et al., 2002). The prevalence of stuttering is approximately 1.44% in 6- to 10-year-old children (95% confidence interval, 0.66% to 2.22%), whereas the prevalence of adolescents who stutter is lower, at approximately 0.5% (95% confidence interval, 0.2% to 0.86%) (Craig et al., 2002). These data suggest that a very large number of older children and adolescents stutter in our communities. The reduction in prevalence from the older child to adolescents is probably due to a combination of factors such as spontaneous remission, avoidance of speaking, and treatment success.

A further cause for concern arises from evidence that as children who stutter grow older, the risk of decreased quality of life as a consequence of stuttering increases (Craig et al., 2003). It is reasonable to assume that appropriate speech skills are important for successful social interaction, and stuttering by its very nature can limit a child from speaking effectively (Craig et al., 2003). Additionally, longitudinal research has shown that a significant minority (approximately 15%) of children with speech disabilities (stuttering being one of these) are at increased risk for anxiety disorders in early adulthood (Beitchman et al., 2001). This means that for many children who stutter, the influence of stuttering over time will be debilitating socially and psychologically. This is supported by research findings that show that older children who stutter have increased communication fears (Blood et al., 2001; Hancock et al., 1998). Certainly, adults who stutter have been shown to have significantly higher levels of state and trait anxiety (Craig, 1990; Craig et al., 2003; Craig & Tran, 2006; Mahr & Torosian, 1999; Menzies, Onslow, & Packman, 1999). Moreover, Stein, Baird, and Walker (1996) maintain that a significant proportion of people who stutter have anxiety levels typical of those seen in people with social phobia. In fact, these authors have argued that many people who stutter should be diagnosed with **social anxiety disorder** or **social phobia**.

For these reasons, it is imperative that efficacious treatments be developed for older children and adolescents to manage their stuttering and thus reduce the impact of any possible impairment. Unfortunately, there has been a dearth of well-controlled research investigating treatment efficacy for this age group. This lack of evidence has possibly resulted in an opinion among many clinicians that treating the older child or adolescent who stutters is too difficult (Craig et al., 1996). However, a body of evidence exists that demonstrates that **Smooth Speech** (a **fluency shaping** treatment and variant of prolonged speech) within a **cognitive behavior therapy (CBT)** regimen was very successful in reducing stuttering in the majority of older child and adolescent stuttering participants (Craig et al., 1996; Craig & Hancock, 1996; Craig, Hancock, & Cobbin, 2002; Hancock et al., 1998; Hancock & Craig, 2002). Fluency shaping techniques like Smooth Speech are treatments that directly target stuttering (Craig, Feyer, & Andrews, 1987). Smooth Speech teaches participants to control their stuttering by adapting and changing their speech patterns. The combined Smooth Speech and CBT treatment teaches control of stuttering. Smooth Speech trains the participant to: (1) produce a continuous pattern of airflow just before and during spoken phrases; (2) maintain a regular phrase-pause-phrase-pause pattern of speech while ensuring that airflow is continuous during the phrase; and (3) maintain speech naturalness. CBT trains the person to (4) lower overall muscle tension activity when speaking; (5) improve conversational and social skills; (6) reduce negative thinking and fears associated with speaking; and (7) increase feelings of self-control of speech and social behavior. This chapter will describe and discuss in detail the goals, key components, practical requirements, and application of the Smooth Speech and CBT program (Craig, 1998a).

The combination of Smooth Speech fluency shaping treatment with CBT was found to be effective in reducing stuttering by more than 90% in the short term (after 1 week) and by approximately 70% to 80% in the long term (after 4 to 6 years) in a large group of older children and adolescents (Craig et al., 1996; Hancock et al., 1998). It was also found to significantly increase speech rate and lower communication fears in both the short and long term in a large group of older children (Hancock et al., 1998). The primary goal of this combination treatment is to improve the quality of life of older children and adolescents who stutter by teaching them a broad range of speech and psychological skills. These skills will assist them in controlling their stuttering symptoms, enhancing their ability to interact socially, and improving their attitudes towards communicating with others.

For the purposes of this chapter, stuttering will be defined as "interruptions to the fluency and flow of speech, where the person knows what he or she wishes to say, but is unable to because they are experiencing either: (a) involuntary repetitions of syllables, especially when starting words, (b) involuntary prolonging of sounds and (c) unintentional blocking of their speech" (Andrews et al., 1983; Craig et al., 1996, p. 811). It may also involve unnatural hesitations, interjections, restarted or incomplete phrases, and unfinished or broken words. Associated symptoms can include eye blinks, facial grimacing, jerking of the head, and arm waving (Craig et al., 1996).

THEORETICAL BASIS FOR SMOOTH SPEECH AND COGNITIVE BEHAVIOR THERAPY AS A TREATMENT FOR STUTTERING

Theorists have suggested that psychological factors such as anxiety play an independent etiologic role in stuttering (Bloodstein, 1995). However, little evidence has supported the contention that stuttering is a psychogenic disorder—that is, that psychological factors play a dominant role in its cause (Craig et al., 2003). In contrast, evidence has accumulated suggesting that stuttering is more likely to be due to a physiologic deficit (Andrews et al., 1983; Bloodstein, 1995; Hulstijn, Peters, & Van Lieshout, 1997). For example, recent research suggests that stuttering is the result of a neural deficit (Fox et al., 1996; Sommer et al., 2002) of perhaps genetic origin (Yairi, Ambrose, & Cox, 1996).

Any psychological difficulties accompanying stuttering are best viewed as secondary but nonetheless important contributing factors (Craig et al., 2003; Craig & Tran, 2006). It is accepted that secondary factors like raised levels of anxiety and social fears related to speaking can negatively influence the severity of stuttering (Craig & Tran, 2006) and consequently lower the quality of life. The assumption that stuttering is physi-

cally caused, with the possible development of secondary psychological complications with age, is the underlying rationale for the Smooth Speech and CBT combination treatment.

Given the above assumption, it was considered important that treatment primarily address the physical problem of stuttering and its associated symptoms. Therefore, Smooth Speech was initially taught to provide speech skills that allow the person to control his or her stuttering. A fluency shaping technique such as Smooth Speech was considered desirable because stuttering consists of involuntary disfluencies throughout the person's speech, often regardless of the social context. It is also complex, involving neurophysiologic, perceptual, acoustic, kinematic, neuromuscular, respiratory, and linguistic dimensions (Smith & Kelly, 1997). Consequently, it was believed that for older children who stutter, a technique was needed that reshaped all speech production rather than modifying only stuttering symptoms. Furthermore, the Smooth Speech and CBT program was also designed to reduce speech muscle tension because stuttering has been shown to involve higher levels of speech muscle tension (e.g., facial and laryngeal) before and during speaking (Bloodstein, 1995; Craig & Cleary, 1982; Freeman & Ushijima, 1975; 1978).

Theoretically, it was assumed that Smooth Speech (1) enhances the brain's capacity to process speech by improving coordination of respiratory, supralaryngeal, and laryngeal systems; (2) reduces the demands associated with speaking (e.g., via speech rate reduction therapy and increased airflow); and (3) reduces motor dysfunction (e.g., reduced muscle tension levels, increased airflow, and slowed speech rate techniques). Additionally, Smooth Speech is an intensive treatment that targets and alters speech behavior regardless of the stuttering moment (e.g. slowing down total speech rate and increasing airflow before and during phrases). Such an intensive and multifaceted treatment was believed to be necessary because the older child or adolescent has typically been stuttering since the age of 2 to 5 years. Therefore, in the opinion of the author, their stuttering symptoms have, in most cases, become entrenched or chronic and significantly more difficult to manage than stuttering in young children. However, given the remaining potential in the older child for neural plasticity changes as a consequence of an active therapy, a fluency shaping technique was desirable because of its ability to produce significant speech and fluency changes.

A fluency shaping technique alone, like Smooth Speech, may not be sufficient for treating stuttering for reasons discussed later in this chapter. Evidence (e.g., Andrews et al., 1991) indicates that stuttering is an interaction between a genetic predisposition (70%) and the influence of the environment (30%). Therefore, as suggested earlier, stuttering will be associated with factors other than the physical cause. In older children, this seems highly probable because of the increased intricacies of social interactions and maturation that begin to occur in adolescence, thereby resulting in psychological consequences. Many adolescents will become embarrassed and frustrated when speaking (and stuttering), and some may begin to learn to avoid situations in which the potential for embarrassment and frustration is high. Moreover, the chances of stuttering becoming more severe increase in more demanding social interactions, and severity also usually increases with increased fatigue or anxiety (Craig & Tran, 2006). Perceived challenging words can also be linked to more severe stuttering (Bloodstein, 1995; Craig et al., 2003). Therefore, it is important that treatment be designed to address these psychological and social aspects of the problem.

Given the increased complexity of stuttering with the appearance of secondary psychological factors, cognitive-based therapies were incorporated into the CBT component of the combined approach. These therapies included social skills and assertion training, behavioral techniques designed to overcome shyness and avoidance behavior (e.g., graded exposure techniques, reward and response cost strategies), direct anxiety management using relaxation techniques, attitude change techniques, and relapse prevention strategies.

EMPIRICAL BASIS FOR THE EFFECTIVENESS OF SMOOTH SPEECH COMBINED WITH COGNITIVE BEHAVIOR THERAPY

As stated in the Introduction, there is a scarcity of well-controlled research on fluency shaping strategies for stuttering in older children. Nonetheless, it may be beneficial to begin our exploration of the empirical basis of Smooth Speech treatments for older children by briefly describing evidence for similar treatments conducted with adults. For example, regulated breathing techniques (Azrin & Nunn, 1974) have been studied in adults using a clinical trial design. The regulated breathing program involves similar airflow techniques used in Smooth Speech treatment. It requires participants to breathe smoothly and deeply, with regular pauses, while relaxing speech and chest muscles. It has also been integrated into a CBT regimen that includes relaxation techniques, self-correction and self-control strategies, and social support and that encourages long-term maintenance by using transfer and generalization techniques. Controlled studies with adults who stutter have found significant reductions in stuttering compared to an active placebo control (Azrin, Nunn, & Frantz, 1979; Ladouceur, Boudreau, & Theberge, 1981; Saint-Laurent & Ladouceur, 1987). However, regulated breathing by itself was not found to be effective as a treatment for stuttering (Andrews & Tanner, 1982). Evesham and Fransella (1985) studied the efficacy of a fluency shaping technique similar to Smooth Speech with two types of maintenance strategies. One group received the standard fluency shaping, whereas another received additional psychological therapy called construct therapy. Although both groups were found to have significantly reduced stuttering, the group that received the construct therapy was found to have superior treatment gains after 24 months using a variety of measures such as percentage of syllables stuttered, syllables spoken per minute, and speech attitudes. Smooth Speech within a CBT regimen conducted in an intensive structured format has also been found to be very effective for adults (Craig, Feyer, & Andrews, 1987; Boberg & Kully, 1994). For instance, in what was known as the Prince Henry Hospital program (Craig, Feyer, & Andrews, 1987; Ingham & Andrews, 1973), the first week was dedicated to learning smooth speech beginning at slow speeds and increasing the speed gradually in structured rating sessions of groups of six. Regular audiovisual feedback sessions were conducted every day, and the goal was to speak at normal rates using socially acceptable conversation skills by the end of the week (for instance, not speaking in a monologue style). Transfer of the skills occurred in the second week. Participants began transfer by completing two home conversations on the weekend, and then a graded hierarchy of conversations was followed beginning with the easiest (home conversations) and progressing to the hardest (speaking in front of a group or speaking on the telephone to strangers). The third week consisted of generalization and maintenance strategies, with a meeting with family members at the end of the week to discuss ways they can help participants maintain their fluency. Small financial rewards were made contingent on success throughout the 3 weeks, and brief rating sessions were held every day of the second and third weeks to reinforce smooth speech skills. Each participant was encouraged to spend time discussing barriers to fluency with a clinician throughout the second and third weeks.

A few researchers have found fluency shaping techniques similar to Smooth Speech integrated within a cognitive behavioral regimen to be effective at reducing stuttering in the short and long term in older children and adolescents (Boberg & Kully, 1994). Boberg and Kully (1994) studied 17 adults and 25 adolescents and found that 69% maintained a "satisfactory" level of posttreatment fluency after 12 to 24 months (determined by performance on a telephone call). The Fluency Rules Program developed by Runyan and Runyan (1986) used similar skills to those used in the Smooth Speech fluency shaping program and reported that 9 (75%) of 12 school-age children significantly improved their fluency after 12 months (Runyan & Runyan, 1999). Kully and Boberg (1991) combined fluency shaping and stuttering modification (e.g., pullouts, easy vs. hard stuttering) approaches in 10 young subjects and found that 8 of the 10 children who stuttered had significantly reduced stuttering immediately after treatment. A follow-up of eight children showed improvements after 8 to 18 months.

Perhaps the most persuasive evidence to date comes from controlled trial research conducted by Craig and Hancock and colleagues (Craig et al., 1996; Hancock et al., 1998). They conducted a two-city controlled clinical trial with 97 older children and young adolescents who stuttered and investigated the efficacy of three treatments compared with a no-treatment control. The purpose of the clinical trial was to evaluate the effectiveness of an intensive Smooth Speech program integrated within a CBT regimen. A second aim was to determine the efficacy of a less intensive Smooth Speech and CBT treatment on stuttering, and a third aim, not relevant for this chapter, was to determine whether a speech muscle feedback treatment would be successful in reducing stuttering.

The mean age of the children before treatment was 10.8 years (range, 9 to 14 years), and most of the children were boys (82%). Three treatments were investigated in the clinical trial, although only results for the two Smooth Speech programs will be presented in this chapter. Both Smooth Speech groups involved participants being treated in groups of four or five by the clinicians who were trained in the therapy protocols. The clinician-to-client ratio was similar for both groups. The first treatment (n = 27) consisted of an intensive therapy format in which Smooth Speech was taught over 5 consecutive days in structured speech rating sessions beginning with slow speeds on the first day (one-quarter of the average speech rate) and gradually increasing the speed to normal rates by the fourth day. The children were required to interact in fluent conversation for at least 5 minutes in each session. Conversation styles that were not considered socially acceptable (such as a monologue) were discouraged by the clinician. Video self-assessments of performance (for fluency, speech naturalness, and conversational skills) occurred at regular intervals throughout the week, and a graded exposure approach from simple to more difficult social interactions was used for speech assignments to transfer fluency skills outside the clinic. Generalization of fluency skills and discussions with parents about maintenance occurred on the last day of the week. Success throughout each phase of the program was financially rewarded.

The second program (n = 25) involved teaching Smooth Speech in a less intensive format and was labeled "home based" in the trial (Craig et al., 1996). It was considered important to determine whether Smooth Speech could be applied in a nonintensive format because it is difficult for clinicians to arrange up to 5 or 6 straight days that are wholly dedicated to a particular therapy and group of clients. This program placed more emphasis on practice in the home environment and less emphasis on structured rating sessions in the clinic. Consequently, it required 1 day a week for 5 weeks, not including follow-up sessions. Smooth Speech was taught on the first day beginning with slow speech rates, but the goal was for the children to talk using Smooth Speech at normal speech rates by the end of the first day. Parents learned how to use and teach Smooth Speech. When the clinician believed the parents were able to use Smooth Speech, identify stuttering, reliably time speech assignments, and reliably monitor the child's use of Smooth Speech, the parents were encouraged to assume the role of clinician for their child. Smooth Speech was reinforced on the second day of the program (that is, the second week) within the context of group games involving conversations followed by suitable rewards for successful completion of speech assignments. Additional cognitive behavioral strategies were used. These consisted of discussion of related problems and fluency barriers, self-monitoring skills such as maintaining speech diaries that measured fluency/stuttering and attitudes, and transfer and maintenance procedures. Homework activities were given each week of the program over the 5 weeks. They were assessed by the clinicians and the parents.

The third treatment (n = 25), which is of minimal interest here, consisted of a speech muscle biofeedback program (Craig et al., 1996). All three programs were integrated within a CBT regimen. A no-treatment control group (n = 20) consisting of older children who stuttered was also evaluated. Subjects were conscripted over a period of 2 years and were allocated to groups when they first attended the clinic. Although they were not randomly allocated into groups, there is no compelling reason to suspect that the resulting groups were biased in a way that would have confounded outcomes. As shown in Craig et al. (1996), all four groups were similar in age, gender, makeup, and stuttering history (i.e., similar rates of stuttering and treatment history).

Most children who participated in the study had begun to stutter early (mean age of 4.7 years, with a range from 2 to 11 years) and had stuttered most of their lives (average of 6 years). Approximately two-thirds of the children had received some form of therapy prior to the study, although in most cases, the intervention had been carried out several years before. No children had received therapy in the 3 months prior to the Smooth Speech treatment. To control for language ability, only those who were progressing normally in their speech for their age were included in the program. For ethical reasons, the no-treatment control children were offered therapy after waiting 3 months. Participants were assessed immediately before treatment, immediately after treatment, and at 3 and 12 months after treatment. A long-term follow-up occurred after 2 to 6 years (mean of 5 years after treatment). However, subject attrition occurred at this long-term follow-up, with six subjects in the nonintensive and three subjects in the intensive Smooth Speech programs being lost to follow-up. It is important to note that there had been no significant fluency differences at the 12-month assessment between those who were and were not able to be reassessed (Hancock et al., 1998).

Severity of stuttering was assessed by the percentage of syllables stuttered (%SS) and rate of speech or syllables per minute (SPM). Children were assessed in three contexts: (1) having a conversation with the clinician in the clinic; (2) talking to a family member or friend on a telephone from the clinic; and (3) talking to a family member or friend in the home environment. Speech naturalness was assessed using a Likert scale (ranging from 1: poor naturalness to 5: very good naturalness) by the clinician, the parent, and the child. Anxiety was assessed using the State-Trait Inventory for Children (STAIC) (Spielberger, Grosuch, & Lushene, 1970), a measure that assesses both state anxiety (how anxious the participant feels at the time of testing) and trait anxiety (how anxious the participant feels generally). Attitudes towards speech were assessed only at the 5-year long-term follow-up; this was done using the Communication Attitude Test–Revised (CAT-R) (Brutten & Dunham, 1989; De Nil & Brutten, 1991). Children were assessed for their anxiety and attitudes towards their speech in a relaxed environment—that is, in the clinic when the child was comfortable and feeling at ease, without any pressures from the parent or clinician.

Both the intensive and the home-based Smooth Speech programs were found to be very effective for reducing stuttering in older children and adolescents (Craig et al., 1996; Hancock et al., 1998). Results over time and as a function of treatment for the two programs are found in Table 11.1 in the form of percent improvement (%Imp) scores and effect sizes. %Imp was determined by the following formula: [(pretreatment %SS – posttreatment %SS)/pretreatment %SS] × 100. Effect sizes were determined using the following formula: (pretreatment %SS – posttreatment %SS)/standard deviation [SD] of pretreatment %SS. Inspection of Table 11.1 shows that stuttering was substantially reduced in the short term (i.e., immediately after treatment) as shown by the very large effect sizes, from 1.6 to more than 2 for the clinic conversation and telephone conversation, respectively. At the 12-month and mean 5-year posttherapy sessions, the reductions in stuttering were maintained with large effect sizes ranging from 1.3 to 1.8. This is impressive considering that a large effect size is considered to be 0.8 or greater (Cohen, 1988). Although not presented here, stuttering frequency levels were similarly reduced in the home conversation measures (Craig et al., 1996; Hancock et al., 1998).

Figure 11.1 shows the short- and long-term fluency outcomes (%SS) for clinic conversation of the two Smooth Speech groups as well as for the stuttering control group (only up to 3 months). As can be seen, substantial and very significant reductions in stuttering occurred in the two Smooth Speech groups compared to the control group. Whereas the control group worsened over a period of 3 months (having slightly negative effect sizes), as shown in Figure 11.1, the Smooth Speech groups were found to have large reductions in stuttering over this period. After a mean of 5 years, both treatment groups were found to have maintained an improvement of approximately 75% or more, and this is regarded as a very desirable goal for therapy by the author. Although stuttering severity scores increased slightly at 3 months, 1 year, and a mean of 5 years after treatment, these increases were not substantial. In contrast, the stuttering severity for the age-matched control children remained elevated for the 3 months in which they participated in the study. In the absence of effective treatment, it would be unlikely that the control group would improve after the 3-month period.

The children who received the two Smooth Speech treatments within a CBT regimen significantly increased their rate of speech compared with the controls (up to 3 months). Speech rate continued to increase for the two treatment groups up to the 5-year follow-up (Hancock et al., 1998). A proportion of this increase could be due to increased maturation after 5 years (subjects ages at this point ranged from 16 to 18 years). However, there is no question that, in the long term, the participants in the Smooth Speech programs were speaking faster with less stuttering compared with their pretreatment performance and at rates typically

Table 11.1. *Mean % Improvement Scores (%Imp) and Effect Sizes (ES) for Frequency of Stuttering (%SS) for the Two Smooth Speech Treatments for the Clinic and Telephone Conversations*

Time Intervals and Contexts	Intensive Smooth Speech		Home-Based Smooth Speech Treatment	
	%Imp	ES	%Imp	ES
Pretreatment to immediate posttreatment				
Clinic conversation	95%	2.2	90%	2.1
Telephone conversation	94%	2.1	83%	1.6
Pretreatment to 1 year posttreatment				
Clinic conversation	72%	1.7	76%	1.7
Telephone conversation	72%	1.7	61%	1.3
Pretreatment to a mean 5 years posttreatment				
Clinic conversation	76%	1.8	80%	1.8
Telephone conversation	76%	1.8	71%	1.4

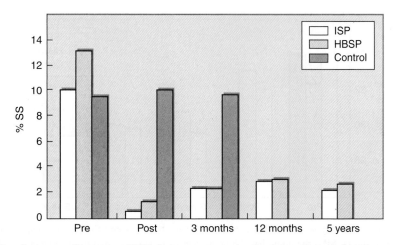

Figure 11.1. Mean frequency of stuttering (%SS) during a conversation for the two Smooth Speech groups and the control group. ISP is the Intensive Smooth Speech group, and HBSP is the home-based Smooth Speech group. (Adapted from Craig et al. [1996] and Hancock et al. [1998].)

expected in society. This decreased stuttering and increased speech rate demonstrate that a fluency shaping treatment that uses CBT techniques can be very successful in reducing stuttering severity in the long term.

The children who received Smooth Speech were speaking naturally after treatment. This was found in the perceived naturalness scores as rated by the clinician, the parents, and the children themselves (Craig et al., 1996; Hancock et al., 1998). This is an important result because of a common misconception among clinicians that people who are treated with Smooth Speech will speak in an unnatural style after treatment (Hancock et al., 1998). This may be true if the fluency shaping strategy being used emphasizes continuous vocalization (as in some forms of prolonged speech treatments) rather than continuous airflow (as taught in Smooth Speech). It also demonstrates the importance of including CBT aspects alongside the fluency shaping treatment. For example, it is imperative that participants have the opportunity to correct their speech styles using audiovisual feedback sessions in which the group provides comments on naturalness and social skills aspects of their conversation. In these sessions, negative attitudes towards speech can be challenged and adapted.

Figure 11.2 shows that trait anxiety levels of the older children receiving the Smooth Speech programs actually decreased over time to levels expected to be seen in populations with typical speech, whereas anxiety levels in the control group did not substantially change (Hancock et al., 1998). This may suggest that the treated adolescents worried less about themselves (especially their speech) than those who were not treated. These findings are similar to other research suggesting that stuttering treatments like fluency shaping are psychologically beneficial (Blood, 1995; Blood et al., 2001). The results of this clinical trial strongly suggest that older children and young adolescents who receive effective treatment will achieve lower levels of chronic anxiety than expected for their age. Additionally, negative attitudes toward communication were also found to reduce significantly for both the intensive Smooth Speech (mean = 11.8, SD = 7.7) and the less intensive Smooth Speech groups (mean = 13, SD = 8.3). These levels are lower than those that might be expected in older children who stutter (De Nil & Brutten, 1991). This suggests that the treated children were more willing to communicate verbally, providing further evidence of their enhanced psychological well-being.

A criterion of less than 1% SS represents minimal stuttering (Craig et al., 1996), and less than 2% SS has been used as a cutoff point for treatment (for example, stuttering <2% SS may suggest that the person does not need an intensive treatment program) as well as a criterion for **relapse**—that is, stuttering greater than 2% SS has been considered to indicate significant stuttering (Craig, 1998b). Therefore, it is useful to determine the proportion of subjects who were

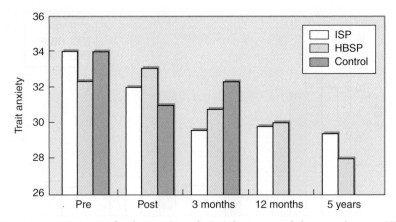

Figure 11.2. Mean trait anxiety scores for the two Smooth Speech groups and the control group. ISP is the Intensive Smooth Speech group, and HBSP is the home-based Smooth Speech group. (Adapted from Craig et al. [1996] and Hancock et al. [1998].)

stuttering at or below these levels after treatment. A large majority of children who received the intensive Smooth Speech format had less than 2% SS immediately after treatment, whereas more than 80% were stuttering negligibly (i.e., <1% SS). However, by 12 months, fewer children were stuttering at these very low levels (only 4% had <1% SS, and <50% had <2% SS). Interestingly, after 5 years, the proportion of subjects with low amounts of stuttering increased substantially (>40% had <1% SS, whereas 80% had <2% SS). A similar trend occurred in the less intensive Smooth Speech program. Just over 75% children had less than 2% SS immediately after the intervention (60% of those had <1% SS); this percentage decreased after 12 months (60% had <2% SS, and 36% had <1% SS). For unknown reasons, the participants in the less intensive program fared better after 12 months than those in the intensive program. Once again, the children and adolescents had improved at the 5-year follow-up, with 50% stuttering minimally and 64% with less than 2% SS.

If one used the 2% SS relapse criterion, one could suggest that relapse rates hover around 20% for the intensive form of Smooth Speech and around 36% for the less intensive program. Figure 11.3 shows the percentages of parents who believed their child had relapsed to pretreatment levels, had never relapsed (no significant stuttering), or still stuttered but not as high as pretreatment levels. Only 13% of the questioned parents believed their child had relapsed

back to pretreatment levels. This is a lower estimate of relapse than predicted by the use of the 2% SS criterion. However, 53% of parents believed their child had exhibited some stuttering 5 years after treatment. It is possible that some of these parents mistrusted their diagnosis of their child's stuttering as indicative of relapse. Even so, these rates of relapse are pleasing. As discussed elsewhere (Craig, 1998b), such relapse rates are not as large as seen in many other disorders such as obesity, schizophrenia, and drug addictions. Having said this, it is important to attempt to reduce these rates and lower the risk of relapse for older children once they have received Smooth Speech treatment. In fact, we have established that additional treatments that we have labeled **"anti-relapse"** or booster therapies are effective at lowering relapse risk in older children (Craig et al., 2002; Hancock & Craig, 2002).

Figure 11.4 provides evidence that additional anti-relapse treatment can benefit adolescents who have relapsed or are having problems with maintaining their fluency. This study (Hancock & Craig, 2002) investigated the effectiveness of an anti-relapse treatment for 12 adolescents who had participated in the initial treatment programs reported earlier and who were experiencing difficulties maintaining treatment gains. Groups consisted of up to four children and parents (i.e., at least eight persons per group), and the anti-relapse program was conducted 2 days a week over 2 weeks, with a fifth-day option

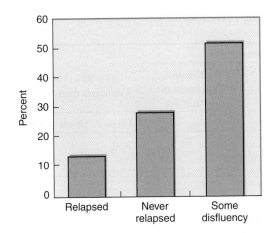

Figure 11.3. Percentage of parents who, a mean 5 years after treatment, believed that their child had relapsed to pre-treatment levels, never relapsed since treatment, or exhibited some stuttering but not serious enough to be concerning. (Adapted from Craig et al. [1996] and Hancock et al. [1998].)

in the third week if treatment skills had not been adequately transferred and generalized outside the clinic environment. An experienced clinician led the group. The anti-relapse program was successful in producing significant reductions in stuttering as well as increasing speech rate and speech naturalness 2 years after the additional booster treatment. The anti-relapse treatment program placed a stronger emphasis on CBT components (e.g., attitude change therapy, self-management therapy, relaxation therapy) com-

pared with the initial Smooth Speech programs. Hancock and Craig (2002) also provided evidence that showed that participants' speech rates increased over the period of time following the anti-relapse program compared with their speech rates following the initial program.

Table 11.2 provides further evidence that an anti-relapse program can be effective for reducing risks of relapse. Three "relapse criteria" are presented that provide an estimate of how many of the 12 adolescents had experienced relapse in a clinic conversation, a telephone call, and a conversation in their home. Two years after the initial program, all 12 adolescents had greater than 2% SS compared with only one-fourth of the 12 adolescents 2 years after the anti-relapse program. Seven of the 12 adolescents had negative communication attitudes 2 years after the initial program; 2 years after the anti-relapse program, this number was reduced slightly to five of the 12 adolescents. However, it was very pleasing to find that a fair number of adolescents achieved a stuttering rate of less than 2% SS and normal communication attitudes after the anti-relapse program. None of the 12 adolescents achieved this 2 years after the initial program, whereas seven achieved this 2 years after the anti-relapse program. This was an exciting finding and strongly suggested that a combination approach (initial and anti-relapse/booster treatments) can be very successful in the long term

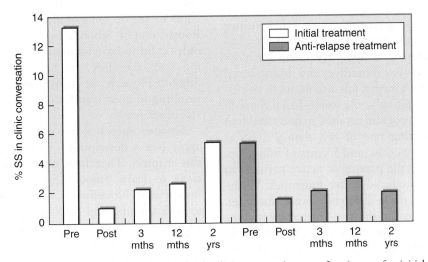

Figure 11.4. Mean percent syllables stuttered (%SS) for the clinic conversation up to 2 to 6 years after initial treatment and up to 2 years after the anti-relapse treatment. (Adapted from Hancock & Craig [2002]).

Table 11.2. *Percentage of 12 Subjects Who Relapsed Using Three Relapse Criteria for Both Initial and Anti-Relapse Programs*

| Occasion | Relapse Criteria | | | Negative Communication Attitudes | ≤2% SS and Normal Communication Attitudes | | |
| | >2% SS | | | | | | |
N = 12	Clinic	Phone	Home		Clinic	Phone	Home
Two years after initial treatment program	100	100	92	58	0	0	0
Two years after anti-relapse program	25	25	25	42	58	58	58

NOTE. The three relapse criteria were as follows: score >2% SS; negative communication attitudes; and score >2% SS and negative communication attitudes Adapted from Hancock & Craig (2002).

at reducing stuttering and removing speech-related fears.

In summary, the results of this controlled trial and anti-relapse study were very pleasing. The study's findings indicated that, for the majority of older children who participated, a Smooth Speech and CBT program resulted in a significant reduction in stuttering and anxiety levels. Furthermore, their speech production was natural. This may have been because the Smooth Speech technique was taught with an emphasis on continuous airflow rather than continuous vocalization and the participants were provided with feedback on their speech production. The children were also speaking at speeds typical of their peers (i.e., ranging from 180 to 200 SPM). Furthermore, for those at risk of relapse, anti-relapse protocols have now been established that are known to reduce risk of relapse in the long term. An unexpected positive outcome of this clinical trial was that, in addition to the fluency shaping treatment for older children, the less intensive and home-based Smooth Speech format was also found to be efficacious. Interestingly, the home-based Smooth Speech/CBT program resulted in more children with a stuttering rate of less than 2% SS at 3 months, 12 months, and 5 years of follow-up. Perhaps using the parents as active partners in the therapy produced better outcomes. Whatever the case, these differences were not large. These findings for the two related treatments provide a choice for clinicians who can confidently vary the way they use a fluency shaping program, particularly in response to individual client preferences.

PRACTICAL REQUIREMENTS FOR THE SMOOTH SPEECH AND COGNITIVE BEHAVIOR THERAPY PROGRAM

THERAPY TRAINING

Given the specialized nature of treating older children who stutter, it is imperative that the clinician planning to use Smooth Speech therapy have a reasonable level of expertise in the area of stuttering, especially child and adolescent stuttering, and have a familiarity with the requirements of the components of the Smooth Speech and CBT program. Clearly, training in Smooth Speech is essential. Smooth Speech is a skill that must be continuously used by the child, and if clinicians are unskilled in its use, it is not likely that they could teach an adolescent or older child to use it successfully and appropriately. Poorly taught Smooth Speech may lead the older child to have an unnatural style of speaking and, therefore, to be unwilling to use Smooth Speech in conversational contexts, resulting in poor transfer outcomes and a high risk of relapse.

Smooth Speech is not difficult to learn and apply (see a description of basic skills later in this chapter). Therefore, it is possible for clinicians to learn Smooth Speech from written instructions. Nonetheless, clinicians are advised to seek training and feedback from a clinician who has a track record of using a Smooth Speech style of treatment, especially Smooth Speech in which the emphasis is placed on continuous (and increased) airflow. A guide to using

Smooth Speech is provided in the relevant video clip. It is important to mention again the distinction between Smooth Speech and prolonged speech. It is possible that clinicians are still using prolonged speech in which the emphasis is placed on continuous vocalization. The author's view is that such a treatment should be regarded as an outmoded fluency shaping technique. Many people who stutter and learn prolonged speech, with its special emphasis on continuous vocalization, fail to maintain it because they are likely to be concerned about sounding abnormal and slurred (Craig & Calver, 1991). In the early days of the development of Smooth Speech (mid to late 1970s) when continuous vocalization was still emphasized, it was not unusual to hear clients voice their strong concerns about using the skills in public. Prolonged speech can seriously distort the production of voiceless sounds, creating a speech style that can sound very strange, and often a monotone and boring style of speech will be the end product. To avoid this, we recommend that clinicians seek training in Smooth Speech. Given that the best available evidence does support the use of CBT with Smooth Speech for treating older children who stutter (Craig et al., 1996), clinicians untrained in CBT methods should also seek training in cognitive behavioral techniques. CBT has a strong evidence base for its efficacy in many disorders (Hersen, 2002), and there are numerous CBT training workshops available. Alternatively, it may be prudent for a speech pathologist to seek out a working collaboration with a clinical psychologist who can assist in the application of the CBT protocol with Smooth Speech (Craig, 2003). It is also very important that clinicians interact in therapy in a supportive and professional manner. Positive relationships with older children who stutter (and their families) are vitally important for producing successful therapeutic outcomes.

TIME DEMANDS

Because stuttering is a chronic disorder, intensive therapy will be required to manage it, especially for older children, adolescents, and adults because their maladaptive learned responses will be so well inculcated. Furthermore, because of its goals, Smooth Speech will be even more time intensive than many stuttering modifica-

tion programs. Historically, the adult Smooth Speech/CBT program protocol was designed to run over 3 consecutive weeks, not including follow-up (Craig, Feyer, & Andrews, 1987). For older children and adolescents, the Smooth Speech/CBT program was designed with time demands as a major consideration. It was believed there would be little point in investigating the efficacy of a treatment that would never be used by clinicians in the community because it is too time demanding. Five straight days of intensive treatment was believed to offer a reasonable compromise. Although a period of 5 days may still be a challenge for many clinicians to arrange, designing a program with fewer days could well result in reduced effectiveness. Notwithstanding this, if 5 straight days of intensive Smooth Speech therapy is too time demanding, then evidence suggests that a less intensive structure can work if parents are trained to play a role in the therapy (Hancock et al., 1998). The home-based Smooth Speech program was designed to lessen time pressures and requires 5 days over 5 weeks. It was thought that this format would be more attractive to clinicians working in busy community clinics. Although dedicating 5 straight days or 5 days over 5 weeks does represent a challenge in terms of time, the potential significant improvements this treatment can offer undoubtedly outweigh difficulties in dedicating time to therapy.

MATERIALS NEEDED FOR SMOOTH SPEECH/COGNITIVE BEHAVIOR THERAPY PROGRAMS

Smooth Speech and CBT programs do not require high-end technology. However, a certain amount of materials and equipment will be necessary. These include all of the following:

1. Specialized equipment to conduct the structured rating sessions will be needed to rate an individual or a group of up to six participants. In the past, mechanical rating devices were used to facilitate online measurement of syllables spoken, the number of stutters, and the time spoken for each participant—the data necessary to determine %SS and SPM. There are now affordable hand-held digital devices (e.g., True-

Talk at http://www.synelec.com.au/synergy/home.html; Chopper at http://www.chop.edu/consumer/jsp/division/generic.jsp?id=79351) and computer software available to run rating sessions. Clinicians will need to participate in training themselves to count syllables and stutters accurately in order to use this equipment successfully. Normally, it is desirable to assess %SS and SPM immediately before and after treatment, as well as after a significant period of time to determine long-term outcome. This assessment can be done using conversational speech of the participants, either rating them "on line" as they speak or recording their speech and assessing afterwards "off line." Because of the use of %SS and SPM in decision making, inaccurate recording of these measures can only have a negative influence on treatment outcome.

2. Audiovisual feedback equipment. Because of the nature of feedback, clinicians will need to have a working knowledge of audiovisual technology. Feedback assessment forms will need to be developed to allow the clinician to assess each participant and each child to assess his or her own conversation as well as the conversations of other participants for normalcy and fluency. An example of such a sheet is provided in Appendix 11.1. Participants rate themselves and the other participants during the audiovisual session. The sheet has room for four participants to rate. The clinician also rates each participant, and participants compare their rating to that of the clinician. The feedback sheet should also include aspects of social skills such as whether the participant presents themselves in a socially acceptable manner (e.g., monitoring facial appearance, tension, eye contact, speed of speech, and other features that seem relevant to the individual group members).

3. Small hand-held digital or tape recorders may be needed for the participants to record their conversations in the transfer, graded-exposure phase of treatment. It is important that they are able to assess the quality of their conversation in terms of fluency (or stutters), speech rate, and naturalness. This allows them to highlight their weaknesses and discuss strategies of overcoming them. Additional recording/playback devices will be needed for the clinicians if they plan to listen

to these conversations. Assignment assessment forms are needed to allow the children to assess their conversations (Fig. 11.5).

4. Treatment manuals will be needed for distribution to the participants and the parents so that they have a thorough understanding of various phases of treatment (Craig, 1998a; email contact: feedbackent@internode.on.net). Clinicians need to be conversant with the protocol in the manual.

5. Access to psychological questionnaires will be needed to assess constructs such as anxiety and communication attitudes. I regularly use questionnaires such as Spielberger et al. (1970; 1983) Trait/State Anxiety (child and adult versions); a mood state questionnaire such as the Profile of Mood States by McNair, Lorr, and Droppleman (1971); the Communication Attitude Test by Brutten and Dunham (1989); a social anxiety questionnaire for children, such as the Revised Children's Manifest Anxiety Scale (Reynolds & Richmond, 2000) or the Social Phobia and Anxiety Inventory for Children (Beidel, Turner, & Morris, 2000); and a social anxiety scale for adults such as The Adult Manifest Anxiety Scale (Reynolds, Richmond, & Lowe, 2003) or the Social Phobia and Anxiety Inventory (Turner, Beidel, & Dancu, 1996).

KEY COMPONENTS OF THE SMOOTH SPEECH AND COGNITIVE BEHAVIOR THERAPY PROGRAMS

CHARACTERISTICS OF SMOOTH SPEECH

Given that Smooth Speech is the foundation skill for both programs, it is vital that the clinician have a methodical and comprehensive understanding of the characteristics of Smooth Speech. Smooth Speech skills allow the participant to develop regular breathing patterns, requiring the participant to expel increased airflow during spoken phrases (say 10% more), speak a little more slowly than most people (generally in the range of 160 to 200 SPM), and speak in a predictable pattern involving regular pauses between the phrases. Because Smooth Speech is different from spontaneous speech,

Date of assignment	6-09-06	6-10-06	6-11-06
Speech context	home	home	home
Person spoke to	mother	father	father (repeated)
Airflow quality Very good / good / poor airflow	good airflow	good airflow	good airflow
Speech rate Too fast / acceptable / too slow	acceptable (160 SMP)	too fast (220 SPM)	acceptable (180 SPM)
Phrasing and pausing quality Mostly present / present / most not present	present	present	present
Naturalness Very natural / natural / unnateral	natural	natural	natural
Degree of relaxation Very relaxed / relaxed / tense	relaxed	tense	relaxed
Number of stutter present	target: 3 actual: 1	target: 3 actual: 5	target: 3 actual: 2
Time spoken	5 minutes	5 minutes	5 minutes
Pass: yes / no	yes	no	yes
Things to work on in future assignments	improve phrasing / pausing quality	improve airflow, work on relaxation and lower speech rate	work on airflow and reducing stutters

Figure 11.5. A sample self-evaluation form used for rating assignment quality for three assignment assessments of a 9-year-old child who was treated for stuttering. Note that the client failed assignment 2 and repeated it successfully the next day. (Adapted from Craig [1998a].)

Table 11.3. *Typical Airflow Advice Given to the Children Who Participated in the Smooth Speech and CBT Program*

When you say a word or phrase, you must begin by first breathing out, and continue breathing out until you finish the word or phrase. If you stop breathing, your speech will become choppy and will not be smooth. Articulate your phrases so that the all the words flow together to become "one long word." Try to keep the sound natural; that is, use your natural variation in speech.

Some sounds like the vowels (a, e, i, o, and u) have very little airflow when they are being produced, so you will need to begin them with more air. We suggest that you begin them with an "h" sound (a soft airflow). Using the "h" before you begin a sound such as a vowel (especially at the start of the phrase) should not change how people hear the word if you do it gently. Here is an example: Put an "h" sound before the following phrases: "Ah-are-you," "h-I-am." Say this next one as slowly as you can, making sure your air is expelled at the beginning and throughout the phrase: "h-I want-to-go-to-the-beach."

When consonants start a phrase, make sure air is escaping between the tongue, lips, teeth, and palate. The tongue, lips, and jaw should also move smoothly, not in a jerky manner. Say the following words slowly with lots of airflow: "me," "we," "you," "no," "ray," "lie," "show," "say," "zoo," "far," "van," "thing," and "they."

Plosives sounds like "b" and "p," "d" and "t," and "k" and "g" are produced by air being trapped in your mouth and then let go in an explosive nature. Smooth Speech requires you to say these sounds with some air escaping, rather than with the air being cut off and let go. Try the difference between the two ways of saying these letters.

Adapted from Craig (1998a).

people intending to use it need to commit themselves to using the foundation skills. The challenge for older children who intend to use Smooth Speech is to monitor and control their speech in all social contexts.

The characteristics of Smooth Speech are taught in Video Clip 3 for this chapter on thePoint site.

These characteristics are as follows:

1. Airflow is increased during speech. Because stuttering is virtually eliminated when one whispers, Smooth Speech skills encourage the participant to think about increasing airflow in a continuous manner throughout his or her speech. A convenient way to learn this is to think of speech as whispering with voice on top or as speaking with whispering on top. Continuous airflow at the beginning and throughout the phrase involves having no break in airflow during the entire phrase. To achieve this, care must be taken with plosive sounds (e.g., b, p, t, d, g, k) and sounds that normally require little airflow (such as the vowels). In all words and sounds, the child who stutters must learn to produce the sound with more airflow than usual, while still achieving an articulation that is as close as possible to the

natural sound. The amount of airflow produced should be approximately 10% to 15% more than that required to speak normally. Additionally, Smooth Speech emphasizes gentle onsets—that is, continuous airflow at the beginning of phrases. Every phrase should begin with extra air, like starting with a whisper. Table 11.3 presents typical advice that could be given to the older child.

2. Speech is organized so that it is composed of a phrase-pause-phrase-pause-phrase structure. This gives a structure to speech, which allows speakers to predict and manage their speech. The phrase is accompanied by airflow all the way through and is separated by a pause, which should be 1 to 2 seconds in length. This is to provide a brief rest for the speaker as a means of enhancing speech motor capacity. Table 11.4 presents typical advice given to the child.

Video Clip 4 shows a client learning to join phrases using increased and continuous airflow.

3. Muscle tension is reduced around the lip, throat, and chest areas. This is achieved by consciously relaxing the face, chest, and throat areas or by using brief isometric exercises to reduce tension in these areas. Isometric

Table 11.4. *Typical Phrase-Pause-Phrase Advice Given to the Children Who Participated in the Smooth Speech and CBT Program*

Smooth Speech requires you to use continuous airflow throughout the phrase as you speak. It also requires that you have regular pauses between the phrases. Say the following very slowly with lots of airflow and stopping regularly for a brief pause:

I-want-to-go [pause] to-the-beach. [pause] Would-you-like-to-come-also? [pause] I-want-to-go-early. [pause] How-about-tomorrow-morning? [pause] And-we-should-bring [pause] some-food-for-lunch [pause] and-some-money [pause] so-we-can-buy-dinner.

Adapted from Craig (1998a).

exercises involve tensing up the area and holding for up to 5 seconds and then letting it all go and feeling the tension drain away (Craig, 1998a). This can be repeated if necessary. The person who stutters can also learn to control muscle tension by using speech muscle biofeedback (Craig et al., 1996; Craig, 1998a). Table 11.5 presents typical advice given to the child about achieving this characteristic.

4. Intonation is varied during speech. Natural variation in intonation should be encouraged, and monotone speech should be discouraged. The person should also be taught to stress sounds naturally. Table 11.6 presents typical advice given to the child.

When teaching Smooth Speech, it is important to emphasize that it is *not* the following:

1. Slow speech. Slowing down rate of speech is important when the child learns Smooth Speech. However, it must be pointed out that it is a different skill. It is important that the child use slower speech, using a rate of speech that is slower (160 to 200 SPM) than the normal rate in society (approximately 200 to 240 SPM). It should be emphasized that slow speech is a separate skill that must also be learned.

2. Prolonged speech. Continuously vocalizing during phrases creates a vibration type of sensation. Moreover, prolonged speech results in monotone-sounding speech, which may reduce stuttering; however, monotone speech is poorly accepted in society and should not be used. We advocate the use of Smooth Speech that requires continuous airflow rather than continuous vocalization.

3. Spontaneous speech. It is also important to distinguish between normally produced speech (spontaneous speech) and Smooth Speech. Spontaneous speech is produced without any particular pattern or control. Smooth Speech is controlled speech (airflow plus pausing) and is usually combined with slower speech (160 to 220 SPM).

WHEN SHOULD SMOOTH SPEECH BE USED?

Fluency shaping techniques require the participant to use the skills constantly. Therefore, the decision to use a fluency shaping technique will be governed by factors such as the severity of the person's stuttering, age, time available for treatment and practice, the ability of the person to use fluency skills, the priority for total fluency, and how much the person fears stuttering. Smooth Speech taught as a fluency shaping technique demands that the person who stutters use Smooth Speech as much as possible. This is the reason why initial intensive treatment is needed. The problem is that this style of treatment is very demanding because it requires consistent monitoring and regular follow-up sessions in the first year after the course. However, for a very severe stutterer, it is likely to be the most successful technique for reducing

Table 11.5. *Typical Speech Muscle Tension Advice Given to the Children Who Participated in the Smooth Speech and CBT Program*

Practice tightening up your muscles around the face and throat and hold them tight for about 5 seconds. Let the tension go slowly. Notice how much more relaxed it feels. You can do this before you speak when you are practicing using Smooth Speech. Stuttering will be greatly reduced if you do this.

Adapted from Craig (1998a).

Table 11.6. *Typical Naturalness Advice Given to the Children Who Participated in the Smooth Speech and CBT Program*

Try speaking in only one tone now. It sounds really boring doesn't it? You must learn to use your full range of tones in your speech. Now, speak as high as you can. Now speak as low as you can. Say the following phrase slowly with airflow while beginning with a high tone and finishing with a low tone. Then say it beginning with a low tone and finishing with a high tone. Make sure it sounds normal though.

"I-am-going [pause] to-the-beach-tomorrow."

Tape yourself and listen to how natural it sounds. Did you begin gently with air, and was there airflow all through the phrase?

Adapted from Craig (1998a).

stuttering. It will also require a high priority for fluency and a high level of commitment.

If a person's stutter is very mild (for example, <2% SS) or he or she does not wish to do an intensive course or commit himself or herself to consistently using Smooth Speech, a stuttering modification approach can be used. This approach requires people who stutter to use Smooth Speech skills only when they think they are at risk of stuttering. For instance, when they are speaking and think they might stutter, they can use the skills to minimize or prevent the stutter. For example, they might slow down, or stop, start with increased airflow, speak gently, and reduce their muscle tension at the moment until they feel that the risk of stuttering is reduced. This approach can be very successful. A person who does not mind occasionally stuttering and who is not prepared to change his whole speech pattern is likely to favor this approach. For older children with only mild stuttering and who do not worry excessively over their stuttering, a stuttering modification approach could be the treatment of choice. It has the added advantage of not requiring as much treatment time (e.g., this technique can be taught in weekly hour-long sessions rather than in an intensive approach). It is important to monitor the person's progress to ensure that such an approach meets his or her needs.

CORRECT BREATHING

It is important that the clinician discuss breath control when using Smooth Speech. It can facilitate the success of treatment and help the person who stutters to relax. Breathing should be full, although not too deep or too frequent (e.g., perhaps approximately 10 breaths per minute). Table 11.7 provides some suggestions made to clients about this component of treatment.

VALUE OF THE COGNITIVE BEHAVIOR THERAPY REGIMEN

The CBT regimen provides valuable strategies known to be effective in changing behavior

Table 11.7. *Advice on Breath Control*

Try some breathing exercises. For this exercise, always breathe in through your nose and out through your mouth. Don't take in too much air, just a slow, comfortable breath.

Stand up straight with the fingertips of your two hands just touching the lower rib cage.
Blow out all your air to make sure you have a full breath.
Breathe in (and count to 3 to yourself).
Blow out (and count to 3 to yourself).
Blow out all your air.
Breathe in (and count to 3 to yourself)
Blow out as you say "ah" for a count of 4.
Blow out all your air.
Breathe in (and count to 3 to yourself)
Breathe out as you say: 1, 2, 3, 4

Adapted from Craig (1998a).

(Craig, Feyer, & Andrews, 1987). CBT typically includes techniques that are designed to prioritize achievable behavioral goals and establish regular assessment of the treatment skills and cognitive behavioral goals. It is also designed to increase motivation by developing reward/response cost–based systems and implement attitude change techniques to address cognitive barriers such as anxiety and psychological upset. Schedules of rewards and behavioral assignments are used, for example, to reinforce behavioral and attitudinal change skills. Most importantly, it uses transfer, generalization, and maintenance procedures to enhance change outside the clinic and into the long term (Hersen, 2002).

SMOOTH SPEECH AND COGNITIVE BEHAVIOR THERAPY PROGRAM

Table 11.8 shows the necessary components that should be incorporated into an intensive Smooth Speech and CBT program. Details of such a pro-gram have been described elsewhere (Craig 1998a; Craig et al., 1996; Hancock et al., 1998).

Assessment

Initially, it is essential that the older child or adolescent be adequately assessed. Further details are provided in a following section in this chapter. It is necessary to assess the severity of stuttering using at least %SS, SPM, and naturalness in multiple contexts. Audio or video recordings of the child's speech should be used to determine these measures. It is also important to measure such traits as chronic and social anxiety and state anxiety measures linked to certain contexts such as the clinic, home, telephone, and so on. It is important to also measure communication attitudes. To determine how effective the treatment has been for an individual, all measures should be taken at least twice—immediately before treatment begins and immediately after treatment. Participants should also be assessed after a period

Table 11.8. *Components Used in a 1-Week Smooth Speech Intensive Fluency Shaping Program That Incorporates CBT Techniques*

Pre-, post-, and long-term treatment assessment (immediately before and after treatment, at least 3 months after)

- Behavioral assessment of the severity of stuttering (%SS, SPM, naturalness)
- Assessment of communication attitudes in different contexts (e.g., the CAT-R)
- Assessment of anxiety (trait, state and social anxiety) in different contexts (e.g., Spielberger State/Trait Anxiety Scales)

Smooth Speech training (3 consecutive days)

- Education about stuttering and Smooth Speech
- Smooth Speech rating sessions for 3 days in groups of 4 to 5
- Gradual increase in speech rate beginning from slow to normal speeds in rating sessions
- Feedback and modeling of fluency and conversational skills in rating sessions
- Audiovisual feedback sessions to ensure natural speech product
- Rewards for success in assignments
- Home practice using Smooth Speech at slower speeds each night after the daily treatment

Transfer and generalization of fluency skills (2 consecutive days)

- Graded hierarchy of difficulty of speech assignments (easy to difficult)
- Speech assignments taped for assessment purposes
- Self-evaluation of performance and clinician feedback on assignment problems
- Rewards for success in assignments
- Additional skills learned such as attitude control and relaxation skills
- Reinforcement of Smooth Speech skills via brief rating sessions in the morning and afternoon

Maintenance and long-term follow-up

- Structured maintenance procedures begun in clinic and extended to home setting
- Social support strategies provided by family and friends
- Anti-relapse therapy skills learned such as self-help and self control skills

Adapted from Craig et al. (1996) and Hancock et al. (1998).

of at least 6 to 12 months to determine whether treatment skills have been maintained.

Smooth Speech Training

In the first 3 days of an intensive program, the participants are briefly educated about stuttering and the nature of Smooth Speech. Then they begin training in Smooth Speech skills in structured conversation and fluency rating sessions conducted by the clinician over a period of up to 3 days (for example, from 9 AM to 4 PM). It is recommended that one parent or family member sit in on these sessions and that the group consist of four to five participants. The participants are taught to speak without stuttering in the rating sessions, beginning at very slow speeds (approximately 50 SPM). If they are able to speak fluently (no stuttering) while using Smooth Speech, the participants are allowed to progress up to higher speech rates in steps of 5 or 10 SPM depending on progress. If participants are having no trouble maintaining fluency at a particular rate, they may progress in steps of 10 SPM. However, if they are struggling—if they have stutters and must retry the step—then progressing by 5-SPM steps can be more effective in the long run. In addition to slowed speech, they are required to increase the amount of airflow during speaking and to prolong syllables at the slower speeds. They are trained to speak while breathing out and controlling their rate of speech, and they receive instruction on respiratory control, with easy, relaxed breathing during speech modelled by the therapist. Another fundamental characteristic of Smooth Speech is the use of gentle onsets and offsets. This involves the participant beginning their phrases with airflow and using soft articulatory contacts. In addition, a phrase-pause speech pattern is taught. Thus, gentle offsets are pauses at the ends of phrases, which serve to reduce muscle tension and may restore neural capacity, while developing a controlled breathing pattern.

Sessions involve each child speaking for a total of approximately 5 minutes, with monotone and monologue performances actively discouraged. To make these rating sessions enjoyable, it is recommended that the clinician use various group-based games (such as board or card games) to make the activity fun and thus stimulate speaking during the sessions. The older child or adolescent is also required to speak in a socially acceptable manner—that is, using a rate of speech that is not too fast or slow and not speaking with a monotone and monologue style. It is the responsibility of the clinician to guide and model acceptable speaking styles to the participants in the rating sessions.

In addition to conversational sessions, special video self-rating sessions are conducted at regular intervals throughout the 3 days (optimally twice a day), during which the rate of speaking used depends on the speed at which the group is speaking. Members of the group are recorded consecutively while speaking using Smooth Speech, and then each recording is replayed to provide feedback to the children. All group members have an opportunity to provide feedback, and all receive feedback on their performances. The clinician also provides feedback. Elements that are judged include factors like quality of fluency, amount of airflow, naturalness, acceptability of conversational style, and speech rate.

A sample of a teenager using Smooth Speech at a normal rate is shown in Video Clip 5.

To increase motivation of the participants, immediate but small financial rewards can be made contingent upon successful completion of each rating session. Success is defined as no stuttering in the 5 minutes, acceptable speaking style, and speaking at the target rate. To reinforce Smooth Speech skills, participants are asked to complete a speech assignment with a member of their family in their home environment each night after the rating sessions. They are asked to speak at the rate of speech that they complete at the end of each day. So, for example, if they reached 80 SPM on the first day, they would complete the assignment at this speed at home. Each assignment is assessed and discussed the following day with the clinician in terms of how successful the participant was in maintaining fluency at home.

In summary, participants progress through the program if they complete sessions stutter-free while using Smooth Speech with acceptable conversational skills. The therapist models and shapes appropriate speech in the participants throughout these sessions. To reinforce social acceptability, video feedback on performance is provided at regular intervals throughout the day. The desired goal of Smooth Speech consists of relaxed speech spoken at a normal rate, with continuous airflow throughout the phrases, and that sounds natural.

Segment 6 shows a sample of Smooth Speech following a model.

Transfer and Generalization of Fluency Skills

When the participants have completed the required structured rating sessions and learned to control their speech with minimal stuttering while speaking at normal speech rates in the clinic, they begin the transfer and generalization sessions in the remaining days of the program. Participants are required to complete a number of speech assignments based on a hierarchy of difficulty, beginning with easier assignments

(e.g., speaking at slower speeds with a family member) and ending with more challenging tasks (e.g., speaking for 5 minutes to a stranger on the telephone or giving a speech in front of an audience). To construct the graded hierarchy for participants, we consult with them to determine what they find easy and what they believe will be difficult.

The program requires that participants perform and audio record each assignment (performing the easiest assignment first). Then they listen to the recording and rate the quality of their performance. Self-rating sheets are provided for self-evaluation (see Fig. 11.6 for a sample self-evaluation sheet). Evaluation is based on factors such as number of stutters (ideally none, but a low target may be set, for example, 1 per minute), quality of Smooth Speech skills, and speech rate.

	Mon	Tues	Wed	Thurs	Fri	Sat	Sun
Foundation skills (slow) smooth speech (4 times a week)							
Attitude control (3 times a day)							
Real life assignment and self evaluation (3 times a week)							
Brief relaxation exercises (5 times a week)							

Figure 11.6. Practice schedule for a 1-week period, including sample goals to be achieved in that period. The number of times the activity is to be performed is shown. For example, foundation skills could be practiced 5 days a week. Attitude control could occur every day at least three times a day.

Criteria are shown in Figure 11.5. Participants only progress through assignments if they continue to satisfy assessment criteria. If problems develop at any difficulty level, the clinicians discuss this with the participants who then return to a lower level of difficulty until mastery has been achieved. Clinicians should continue to provide feedback on the participants' performance during the assignments. The participants may fail an assignment for any of several reasons—for example, too many stutters, excessively high speech rate, inappropriate conversation and communication skills, or poor intonation. In response, the clinicians should discuss difficulties associated with their failures to use fluency techniques and should suggest methods to help them, for example, by using slower speech rate or by working on attitudinal barriers. Small financial rewards are made contingent on successful completion of each assignment (usually a dollar per assignment), and the number of assignments can be set individually for each child, depending on capability and success.

Personal expectations of success should be encouraged so that the children do not become dependent on the clinician or parents for their improvements in fluency. To enhance feelings of self-control (Craig, Franklin, & Andrews, 1984), participants should be encouraged to use the self-evaluation forms included in this intervention. Using self-evaluation and self-monitoring strategies is crucial in the transfer and generalization period. As stated earlier, for each assignment, recording the number of stutters, estimated speech rate, quality of airflow, relaxation during speech, and context and to whom they spoke will assist children in developing responsible attitudes. To ensure that their goals and evaluations are realistic, the clinician should briefly review their self-evaluation in light of their recorded performance. To reinforce self-responsibility further, the children should be trained to correct any moments of stuttering that occur during the program, whether in the clinic or at home. Participants can do this by being taught to stop for 1 to 2 seconds directly after they stutter. Then they begin to speak slowly with increased airflow for 2 to 5 seconds, repeating the stuttered word and phrase fluently. It is important that the clinician and parents reinforce this practice. This has been termed "stutter and recover."

To sustain self-responsibility, short group discussions among participants are held on days 4 and 5, with topics focusing on: (1) the importance of helping themselves rather than pleasing parents or therapists, (2) the reasons that motivate them to maintain fluency, (3) strategies on how to improve motivation levels, and (4) the importance of daily practice and of varying its format to remain motivated to maintain fluency.

At home during the evenings of the program, participants can be trained to use self-reward for their own fluency and for achieving their practice goals. For instance, they can be asked to say something positive to themselves such as, "I spoke very well" and "I am in charge of my stuttering."

This is discussed and demonstrated in Video Clip 8.

Developing links between the children's thoughts, feelings, and behavior is important. These cognitive techniques can be applied to reduce any attitudinal fears or barriers. Examples of appropriate self-talk before, during, and after a difficult speaking situation can be discussed and practiced (e.g., "My stuttering is under my control. I am in charge." or "I will think about my fluency skills rather than worrying about stuttering."). Self-talk can also be used during treatment to help participants cope with the negative experience of stuttering. As stated earlier, part of the nature of control is the anticipation of all possibilities, including failure. The participants can be taught skills for dealing with failure when it occurs. For example, they can be trained to recognize high-risk situations, such as those in which they are tired or that they feel bad about, or situations they find threatening, such as speaking in front of people or speaking to someone in authority. They can then be taught methods of coping with these situations (e.g., view stuttering as a sign that they need to focus on fluency skills rather than pushing through stutters and adopting a sense of hopelessness). In addition, participants can be taught simple relaxation techniques, such as breath awareness and control, and brief isometric exercises that enable them to enhance control of their muscle tension and anxiety (Craig, 1998a). Discussions should be held regarding the value of physical relaxation to help participants think more clearly and use positive thoughts to help cope with difficult speaking situations. They should be encouraged to practice simple relaxation exercises that can be used before, during, or after an anxiety-provoking speaking situation.

A clinician discusses transfer and maintenance in Video Clip 7 of the video.

Maintenance and Long-Term Follow-Up

In the last 1 to 2 days of the program, maintenance and anti-relapse procedures are taught alongside transfer and generalization skills. If time is a problem, then an additional day or two can be arranged to teach these skills.

Anti-relapse skills and self-management techniques involve the client accepting longer-term self-responsibility, specifically adopting self-set practice goals, conducting regular evaluation, and working through any motivational barriers to maintaining the effort required to commit to a practice regimen.

Cognitive techniques should include positive and realistic self-talk aimed at enhancing levels of perceived control over stuttering (e.g., "I am the master of my speech"). Perceived control or self-mastery has been found to be related to long-term outcome for problems beyond stuttering, such as weight loss, diet change, and smoking cessation (Craig, Franklin, & Andrews, 1984). Further emphasis can also be placed on relaxation exercises, such as muscle and thematic relaxation techniques (e.g., breath awareness, isometric exercise, imaging a peaceful scene). These are designed to enhance control of muscle tension and anxiety. The value of combining relaxation with thought control techniques should be discussed and emphasized in difficult speaking situations. Figure 11.6 shows a practice schedule that can be used to encourage long-term fluency maintenance illustrating some typical goals for such a schedule.

SOCIAL SUPPORT FROM FAMILY AND FRIENDS

Given that social support is critical for the maintenance of fluency in the long term (Craig, 1998b), it is crucial that the participant's family become involved in the long-term fluency maintenance program. At the very least, the family should be educated on the use of self-control strategies that encourage and maintain fluency within home, school, and social contexts. Appointments to meet with the clinician

regarding maintenance of fluency skills should be made with the participants and their family at regular intervals for a year after the completion of the program.

There are a number of ways that the client's family can provide social support. For instance, they can reward fluent speech by praising the stutterer when he or she speaks fluently. Supports can take the form of verbal praise or nonverbal rewards, such as smiling and hugging. Praise is a very powerful motivator, although the type of praise should be negotiated with the child to avoid the frustration or embarrassment that may result if he or she is uncomfortable with the type of praise given, especially if given in the company of friends. Appropriate rewards contingent on successful achievements have the potential to make regular practice easier and more enjoyable. Rewards should be sophisticated and motivating and used in both the short and long term, and they also need to be tailored to the desires of the individual, so it will be necessary to make an individualized list of attractive rewards. It is important not to overuse a reward so that it does not lose its reinforcing power. Using natural rewards more often (such as smiles, hugs, praise, and so on) may help avoid that.

Family members must also learn not to punish the stutterer by becoming angry or frustrated or ignoring them because the effects of punishment can be detrimental. However, mild forms of punishment are unlikely to be problematic and can be used, such as bringing a moment of stuttering to the stutterer's attention and encouraging the child to repeat the sentence fluently. It is essential that such statements are said in a nonthreatening and positive manner and that this approach is negotiated with the stutterer. For example, a parent may agree to call attention to stuttering, but only if conditions are negotiated beforehand.

Family members can also assist by modeling slow and relaxed speech in the home environment. It may help the stutterer to slow his or her speech and relax facial, neck, and chest muscles. It may also help if a family member and stutterer can hold regular formal fluency sessions in which the older child practices his or her fluency skills and the family member acts in either a passive role (just listening and interacting conversationally) or an active didactic role (instructing and correcting as well as listening and conversing). Session durations of up to 10 to 15 minutes each day 3 to 4 days a week have been found to be effective.

HOME-BASED SMOOTH SPEECH/COGNITIVE BEHAVIOR THERAPY PROGRAM

The core components of the intensive form of the Smooth Speech and CBT treatment program that have been described up to this point in the chapter can be adapted to a less intensive format (Craig et al., 1996; Hancock et al., 1998). A description of such a variation in the program is also provided in this chapter under the description of the empirical basis of the treatment.

ASSESSMENT METHODS

A further requirement that must be considered before conducting the Smooth Speech/CBT program is the need for a comprehensive assessment. Purposes of an initial assessment include determining whether the individual actually does stutter, as well as determination of the nature and severity of stuttering. It is also important to determine family and personal history. This includes whether stuttering is due to genetic factors or other causes such as head injury, given that the etiology of stuttering may influence the type and course of treatment. For instance, a person who stutters as a result of receiving a traumatic injury to the head may have additional physical or psychological deficits that would need to be considered when individualizing the program. Assessment should establish the type of stuttering being exhibited and the severity of the stuttering because treatment goals may be adapted, for instance, if an individual's stuttering is dominated by severe blocking. Presently, in my view, the most effective and easy method to determine severity is to use behavioral measures such as %SS and SPM. It is important to continue to measure stuttering (at the very least with %SS and SPM) throughout treatment so that a record of fluency change exists. Naturalness should also be assessed, especially during and after treatment. Naturalness is usually assessed using a Likert scale (Craig et al., 1996; Martin, Haroldson, & Triden, 1984). As suggested in Table 11.8, it is important to assess these behavioral aspects of stuttering immediately before and after treatment, as well as in the long term (e.g., at least 3 months after the end of formal treatment).

Concomitant features of stuttering may also be assessed by video recording designed to facilitate observation of factors such as facial symptoms contingent with the stutter. Additional assessment also includes a detailed personal history, information concerning prior treatment and whether relapse has occurred, and information about any specific speaking contexts in which a higher risk of stuttering or avoidance of speaking occurs. The diagnosis should also include an assessment of trait anxiety (i.e., the person's general level of anxiety measured in a comfortable and relaxed setting) and state anxiety (i.e., anxiety linked to a specific condition or context) associated with various speech tasks (e.g., directly before and after a telephone call). Social anxiety, communication fears, and perception of control (e.g., locus of control or self-efficacy expectations) should also be assessed (Craig, Franklin, & Andrews, 1984). Although there is no evidence to suggest that children who stutter are vulnerable to depression (Craig, 2000), a comprehensive mood and personality assessment could be useful for clinical purposes (McNair, Lorr, & Droppleman, 1971). If possible, an assessment of how the stutterer interacts with family members and friends can provide valuable information about the psychosocial and interpersonal dynamics of stuttering. Furthermore, complicating factors that are likely to limit treatment efficacy should also be assessed (e.g., coexisting articulation or learning disorders).

APPLICATION TO AN INDIVIDUAL CLIENT

Mark (all names are fictitious) was 9 years old when he first presented for treatment. He had a family history of stuttering (mother and great grandfather stuttered), although neither his older brother nor younger sister had shown signs of stuttering. Mark's mother had never received or sought therapy for her mild stuttering. Mark had stuttered since the age of 2 years, and when assessed, he stuttered mildly to moderately in most contexts, with %SS values ranging from 4% SS in the home to 12% SS at school or in other demanding social contexts such as when playing sports or when interacting at a friend's house. His severity also increased when he became fatigued, stressed, or excited. His speech rate varied according to his severity, so that at home when relaxed, he spoke at approximately 160 SPM. Outside or when stressed, his speech rate decreased to 100 to 120 SPM because of his increased stuttering. Both Mark and his parents were interested in his receiving treatment.

When psychologically assessed, it was found that Mark was not particularly anxious (scoring in the normal range), although his anxiety was slightly raised on the day of assessment (state anxiety approximately one standard deviation above the norm for his age and sex). He also scored higher than normal on the CAT-R communication attitudes (Brutten & Dunham, 1989), suggesting he had increased fears about talking. Mark presented as a quiet, intelligent, and friendly boy. He had been treated before entering the Smooth Speech and CBT intensive program. For example, he had received individual therapy from two speech pathologists when young (4 and 5 years old). Therapy consisted of articulation therapy and counselling in the first instance when he was 4 years old and a behavioral program based on the Lidcombe Program in the second instance when he was 5 years old. Unfortunately, he had not improved after the first therapy, and although he had improved substantially after the behavioral parent-based program (down to low %SS values of approximately 2%), he relapsed after a period of 2 years. It was decided to place Mark in an intensive Smooth Speech program given his preadolescent age, interest in having his stuttering treated, relapse history, and moderate severity. The intensive format was also chosen rather than a home-based Smooth Speech program because his parents preferred this format after discussion of options.

Approximately 6 to 8 weeks after his initial assessment, Mark was placed in a 1-week intensive Smooth Speech and CBT program. He successfully completed the 1-week program with four other similarly aged boys. Mark's mother attended the program for 4 of the days, and his grandmother attended on 1 day. His mother and father attended on the last day for discussion of long-term maintenance. The daily schedule began at 9 AM and went to 4 PM each day except on the last day, when it finished at 5 PM. Mark enjoyed his 5 days. He mastered Smooth Speech well and completed his rating sessions on schedule on day 3, although he found the audiovisual sessions challenging, given that he was quiet and a little shy. He learned to use Smooth Speech with a natural style. He also mastered speech rate control, learning specifically to speak at slow rates (100 SPM) and at faster though slower than normal rates (160 to 180 SPM) that he could use outside the clinic.

Mark also performed well in the transfer and generalization phase of the program. He completed a number of face-to-face and telephone conversations and shopping assignments (talking to shop assistants) successfully, and he learned to tape his speech and self-evaluate his performance. He was taught how to handle failure and to accept a low level of stuttering in his speech. Figure 11.5 shows an example of his assignment assessment. When he failed assignment 2 (speaking to his father), he was encouraged to repeat the assignment immediately (the next day), concentrating on his weaknesses in using Smooth Speech that led to his failure. Therefore, he concentrated on lowering his speech rate, relaxing more before he conducted the conversation, and increasing airflow control. This resulted in a successful completion of the assignment, and he was then taught to apply his attitude control skills. This involved thought control, which involves stopping any negative thoughts going through his mind (i.e., blanking them out) and replacing them by saying realistic and positive thoughts to himself such as, "That was difficult, but I was in control," as well as relaxing before and after speaking using a quick "tense and relax" isometric approach. To maintain his motivation, a reward system was constructed for Mark in which he won $1.00 per assignment passed. His parents provided the reward monies, and the clinician administered the rewards.

After the 1-week program, Mark's stuttering had decreased by more than 90% (<1% SS) in conversations on the telephone and outside the clinic, and his speech rate was stable at around 180 SPM. His anxiety had decreased, and his communication attitudes had substantially improved. However, Mark continued to have trouble controlling his stuttering when he became excited—for example, when playing with his friends. This problem was discussed with Mark and his mother. It was decided that it would be undesirable to train Mark to control and reduce times in which he becomes excited because it is important for him to enjoy his life. Therefore, the emphasis was placed on him learning rational self-statements that would act to minimize any anxiety or guilt that might arise (e.g.,"Who cares if I stutter a little when I become excited. I know I can control my stuttering when I want to."). It was also important to work with Mark's parents on this to ensure that they were comfortable with him stuttering a little when he played and became excited.

A maintenance regimen was established on the last day of the program and developed in association with Mark and his parents. Mark continued to be fluent, with minimal stuttering 18 months after he participated in treatment. Every 3 months, he and his mother participated in a follow-up session of approximately 1 hour with the clinician to discuss his fluency maintenance and to troubleshoot. The frequency of follow-up has decreased over time as Mark continues to successfully maintain his fluency. However, if he has any difficulty, he has been encouraged to return to the clinic before a problem develops and causes relapse. Figure 11.7 shows Mark's long-term practice schedule on which he was required to log his performance each week for the first 3 months after the program. His schedule consisted of the following weekly regimen:

Foundation skills. Mark was required to perform frequent conversations at slow speeds (100 SPM) at home with a member of his family to concentrate on his Smooth Speech skills. He undertook this practice for 5 to 10 minutes 4 days a week. The time of the assignment was negotiable; for instance, he could do it in the morning before school or after school in the late afternoon depending on his homework and social timetable and also on his health status. After each foundation assignment, he was asked to evaluate his performance and note this on the sheet.

Maintaining healthy attitudes. Mark was required to write on the practice schedule each time he practiced his thought control exercises. His realistic and positive thoughts consisted of statements like, "I know I stutter but I can be fluent" or "My stuttering is under my control. I am in control." He was asked to repeat these statements to himself a minimum of three times a day for 4 days a week or more, if needed. Note that on a Friday, he had to give a speech in class; thus Mark practiced his thought control five times on this day and performed his foundation skills in the morning before his speech.

Real-life assignments. Mark completed three assignments outside his home, including shopping during which he spoke to shop assistants, talking to people on the telephone, visiting friends, and so on. He was required to tape and assess at least one of these assignments (taped assignment to be at least 5 minutes of his speech) and to assess his performance using the assessment sheet shown in Figure 11.5.

Relaxation. Mark was required to perform at least one quick relaxation isometric exercise a day 5 days a week.

FUTURE DIRECTIONS

There now exists substantial and scientifically reliable evidence from controlled clinical trial research with older children and adolescents showing conclusively that stuttering can be effectively treated and managed using a Smooth Speech and CBT regimen (Boberg & Kully, 1994; Craig et al., 1996; Craig et al., 2002; Hancock et al., 1998; Hancock & Craig, 2002; Kully & Boberg, 1991). Given the encouraging results from a variety of sources, there should now be no doubt that a fluency shaping treatment such as Smooth Speech integrated with CBT strategies is an effective treatment for older children and adolescents who stutter. Clinicians should have sufficient confidence in the Smooth Speech treatment to believe that most of the time it will result in substantially reduced stuttering, with the child speaking naturally and at normal rates. Clinicians should also be encouraged to integrate CBT components into their therapy to ensure that psychological issues are sufficiently addressed. Furthermore, they can be

	Mon	Tues	Wed	Thurs	Fri	Sat	Sun
Foundation skills (slow) smooth speech (4 times a week)	5 pm passed		5 pm passed		8 am passed	Failed first attempt, repeat, passed	
Attitude control (3 times a day)	3 times	3 times		3 times	5 times		
Real life assignment and self evaluation (3 times a week)		Telephone passed			Speech in class passed	Shopping passed	
Brief relaxation exercises (5 times a week)	Morning	Morning		Morning	Morning and afternoon	Morning	

Figure 11.7. Mark's weekly practice schedule. His daily goals are listed on the schedule with the results.

confident that Smooth Speech can be offered in variety of regimens (e.g., intensive vs. less intensive). This will enable clinicians to tailor Smooth Speech treatment to meet the particular needs of their clients, depending on factors such as the severity of the child's stuttering and psychological status, family context, and the availability of the clinician's own time. Clinicians no longer need to fear that adolescent stuttering is untreatable.

An important question remains whether the results found for older children and adolescents (both boys and girls) will extend to other age groups. We already have some evidence that suggests that Smooth Speech and CBT intensive treatment is effective for male and female adults (Andrews, Guitar, & Howie, 1980; Craig, 1998b; Craig, Feyer, & Andrews, 1987). However, all Smooth Speech treatment efficacy studies con-

ducted with adults up to this point in time have not used controlled clinical trial designs to confirm this evidence. This is a high priority for future research with adults. The question also remains as to whether Smooth Speech and CBT can be used with children younger than 8 years (the lower age limit in the Craig et al., 1996 controlled trial). It is feasible to adapt the Craig et al. (1996) treatment program and apply it in some altered form for children age 6 to 8 years. Obviously, this also needs evidence from a controlled investigation. However, given the need for significant cognitive and behavioral self-control skills (i.e., attitudinal resolve to adhere to the program and behavioral commitment) from those participating in a Smooth Speech/CBT program, it is doubtful that a Smooth Speech program could be used effectively by many children younger than 6 years old.

Future research should continue to explore issues of efficacy. For instance, we should be investigating which components of the comprehensive Smooth Speech and CBT treatment are therapeutically active and which components are not needed (i.e., redundant). We have already begun this process by examining the necessity of an intensive format (e.g., Craig et al., 1996). Furthermore, a randomized clinical trial should be mounted in the future to confirm the efficacy of Smooth Speech and CBT. Perhaps the principal challenge in the future to the use of Smooth Speech is the negative stereotype that many clinicians have of this style of treatment. Many clinicians, for example, may believe that it alters unacceptably the child's speech patterns so that they sound abnormal (slow and monotone). Based on the findings of the clinical trial reported in this chapter, this is simply not the case if it is applied correctly. It is hoped that this chapter will encourage clinicians to use Smooth Speech and CBT with their adolescent clients. Its potential to improve quality of life is considerable.

CHAPTER SUMMARY

- Many older children who stutter remain at risk of developing anxiety disorders if left untreated (Beitchman et al., 2001).
- Smooth Speech integrated within a CBT regimen has been shown to be an effective treatment for stuttering in older children and adolescents.
- Assuming that stuttering is physically caused, treatment should address primarily the physical problem.
- Additional psychologically based treatment (CBT) should address additional problems possibly linked to the stuttering, such as social fears and risks of relapse.
- Smooth Speech and CBT have been shown to reduce stuttering by at least 90% in the short term and 80% in the long term.

- Clinicians are advised to seek training in delivering Smooth Speech and CBT.
- Smooth Speech can be delivered in either a 1-week intensive or a less intensive home-based format.
- It is important to generalize fluency skills and offer anti-relapse therapy following initial treatment.

SUGGESTED READINGS

Craig, A. (1998). *Treating Stuttering in Older Children, Adolescents and Adults: A Guide for Clinicians, Parents and Those Who Stutter*. Gosford: Feedback Publications Press.

Craig, A. (2000). The developmental nature and effective treatment of stuttering in children and adolescents. *Journal of Developmental and Physical Disabilities, 12*, 173–186.

Craig, A., Hancock, K., Chang, E., McCready, C., Shepley, A., McCaul, A., Costello, D., Harding, S., Kehren, R., Masel, C., & Reilly, K. (1996). A controlled clinical trial for stuttering in persons aged 9 to 14 years. *Journal of Speech and Hearing Research, 39*, 808–826.

Hancock, K., & Craig, A. (2002). The effectiveness of re-treatment for adolescents who stutter. *Journal of Speech, Language, Hearing. Asia-Pacific, 7*, 138–156.

Hancock, K., Craig, A., Campbell, K., Costello, D., Gilmore, G., McCaul, A., & McCready, C. (1998). Two to six year controlled trial stuttering outcomes for children and adolescents. *Journal of Speech and Hearing Research, 41*, 1242–1252.

ACKNOWLEDGEMENTS

The research in this chapter was achieved with the support of the National Health and Medical Research Council in Australia, the Big Brother Movement of Australia, an Australian Rotary Health Research Grant, and the University of Technology, Sydney. I also thank Dr. Karen Hancock, my co-researchers in Sydney and in the Mater Hospital, Brisbane, and of course, the many children and adolescents who have been treated for stuttering over the years.

CHAPTER 12

Comprehensive Treatment for School-Age Children Who Stutter: Treating the Entire Disorder

J. Scott Yaruss, Kristin Pelczarski, and Robert W. Quesal

CHAPTER OUTLINE

KEY TERMS

Activity limitation: a difficulty an individual may have in performing daily activities. Relevant examples include producing verbal messages, communicating with others, and starting or maintaining conversations. One of the components of the World Health Organization's *International Classification of Functioning, Disability, and Health* (ICF) (WHO, 2001).

Cognitive restructuring: a process for helping individuals think differently about the problems they face. Involves evaluating and changing unrealistic thoughts through education, evaluation, and reconsideration of an individual's beliefs and attitudes.

Desensitization: a process for minimizing negative reactions through gradual exposure to feared situations, beginning with easier situations and moving toward increasingly difficult situations (i.e., along a hierarchy).

Impairment: a difficulty an individual may experience with body function or body structure. In the study of stuttering, the difficulty producing fluent speech represents the impairment in body function. One of the components of the World Health Organization's *International Classification of Functioning, Disability, and Health* (ICF) (WHO, 2001).

***International Classification of Functioning, Disability, and Health* (ICF)**: a framework for describing the entirety of human health experience. Includes components of body function and body structure (including *impairments*), as well as activities and participation (and either *limitations* or *restrictions*).

In addition, the ICF incorporates *personal* and *environmental* contextual factors that account for differences in individuals' health experiences.

Participation restriction: a difficulty an individual may experience in fulfilling life goals, including maintaining employment, supporting a family, interacting with others, and participating in social and civic life. One of the components of the World Health Organization's *International Classification of Functioning, Disability, and Health* (ICF) (WHO, 2001).

Pseudostuttering: intentional production of stutter-like speech behaviors; used in therapy as part of the exploration process to help individuals who stutter learn about what they do during moments of stuttering; also used to support the process of desensitization by helping people face the fear of stuttering in increasingly difficult situations.

INTRODUCTION

This chapter describes a comprehensive treatment approach that can be used with school-age children who stutter. The treatment involves the use of several related strategies, each aimed at improving a specific aspect of a child's communication abilities. The primary end point or preferred outcome for this treatment is *effective communication*, not just a given percentage of improvement in speech fluency or a specified reduction in stuttered speech. As such, this approach to treatment should not be considered "fluency" therapy per se, but rather a collection of therapy techniques aimed at ensuring that stuttering will not negatively affect a child's ability to express himself or herself and achieve his or her goals in life.

Accomplishing this broad objective requires the integration of several key principles, each of which will be explained in more detail within this chapter.

- First, the clinician must approach treatment with a solid understanding of the broad-based and multifaceted nature of the stuttering disorder, specifically, *that the experience of stuttering involves more than just the production of speech disfluencies.*
- Second, the clinician must accept the fact that *there is no guaranteed cure for stuttering in*

school-age children. As a result, it is likely that the child may continue to stutter in some fashion, even after successful treatment.

- Third, the clinician must recognize that *it is okay to stutter*, and that the goal of therapy is to ensure stuttering does not interfere with the child's ability to communicate effectively.
- Fourth, the clinician must be prepared to *work with people in the child's environment*, including parents, teachers, and peers, to help them understand the nature of stuttering and to help them come to terms with the fact that the child stutters.
- Finally, *treatment must incorporate a variety of individualized strategies* aimed at addressing each of the components of the child's experience of stuttering. The components of treatment may include: (1) changes to speech production to enhance fluency and minimize the severity of individual moments of stuttering; (2) changes to communication attitudes to reduce the child's negative reactions to stuttering, as well as the negative reactions experienced by those in the child's environment; (3) improvements in the child's communication abilities to ensure that the child can convey his or her message effectively in a variety of real-world speaking situations; and (4) reduction in the total impact of stuttering on the child's overall quality of life.

Together, these related aspects of treatment help to ensure that the child is able to *communicate effectively*, despite any stuttering that may remain in his or her speech. The purpose of this chapter is to explain each of these key principles and to provide specific strategies for accomplishing these broad goals for school-age children who stutter.

THEORETICAL BASIS FOR TREATMENT APPROACH

This treatment approach is based on a particular set of viewpoints about the nature of stuttering and the aspects of speech and communication that should be addressed in therapy. These viewpoints are not based on a specific theory about the *cause* of stuttering, but rather on a theory about how the disorder manifests itself in the lives of people who stutter.

NATURE OF STUTTERING

The most fundamental assumption of this treatment approach is that stuttering is a broad-based and multifaceted disorder. Elsewhere, we have expressed this sentiment in the statement that "stuttering is more than just stuttering" (Yaruss, 1998a; 2007; Reardon-Reeves & Yaruss, 2004; Yaruss & Quesal, 2004; 2006; see also Cooper, 1993; Manning, 1999; 2001; Murphy, 1989; Shapiro, 1999; Sheehan, 1970; Starkweather & Givens-Ackerman, 1997; Van Riper, 1982; Williams, 1957). By this, we mean that the *experience* of stuttering for school-age children (as well as for adolescents and adults) involves far more than the production of speech disfluencies. This view of stuttering begins with a consideration of the surface aspects of the child's fluency and stuttering behaviors, but it does not end there. The following sections describe each of the components of stuttering that are incorporated in this broad-based view of the disorder.

Speech Fluency and Stuttering Behaviors

The speech disfluencies exhibited by people who stutter, such as part-word repetitions, prolongations, and blocks, comprise an important component of the overall disorder. Numerous approaches have been developed over many years for helping people who stutter change their speech to enhance fluency (see reviews in Bloodstein, 1993; Bloodstein & Bernstein Ratner, 2008). Strategies aimed at improving fluency are among the most fundamental aspects of most treatment approaches, and the treatment described in this chapter includes several strategies to help children speak more fluently. Examples include strategies for changing *timing* and *tension* in the child's speech musculature, as well as strategies for reducing physical tension during stuttering. The goal of such strategies is to ensure that the child is able to both produce more fluent speech and manage instances of stuttering so that stuttering will have a minimal impact on communication.

Still, the surface characteristics represent just one component of the disorder. For some people who stutter, overt stuttering behaviors may not even be the most important component (e.g., Manning, 2001; Shapiro, 1999; Yaruss et al., 2002). Many people who stutter also experience a variety of negative *consequences* associated with

their disfluencies. These consequences can be described in terms of speakers' *reactions* to stuttering, the impact of stuttering on their *functional communication* in daily situations, and the impact of stuttering on their overall *quality of life* (Yaruss, 1998a; Yaruss & Quesal, 2004; 2006). The next sections of this chapter describe these components of stuttering in greater detail.

Affective, Behavioral, and Cognitive Reactions to Stuttering

As numerous authors have discussed (e.g., Cooper, 1993; DeNil & Brutten, 1991; Guitar, 2006; Logan & Yaruss, 1999; Manning, 2001; Murphy, 1989; Shapiro, 1999; Sheehan, 1970; Vanryckeghem & Brutten, 1996; 1997; Watson, 1998; Yaruss & Quesal, 2004; 2006), speakers of all ages can experience a wide variety of emotional or *affective* reactions to their speaking difficulties. Examples include feelings of embarrassment, anxiety and fear, shame and guilt, anger, isolation and loneliness, inadequacy, and other negative emotions accompanying both stuttered and fluent speech (e.g., Cooper, 1993; Murphy, 1989; Vanryckeghem et al., 2001; Watson, 1998; Yaruss & Quesal, 2006). These reactions may pose a particular challenge for school-age children because many youngsters do not yet possess the coping skills necessary for managing strong emotions on their own. As a result, clinicians may need to address these reactions as part of a comprehensive approach to stuttering therapy.

Many speakers also exhibit *behavioral* reactions to stuttering. Common examples include physical tension and struggle as speakers try to force their way through moments of stuttering (e.g., Johnson, 1961; Van Riper, 1982; Wingate, 1964). Other behavioral reactions include avoidance or escape behaviors, in which the child may attempt to minimize exposure to difficult speaking situations. Examples include refusing to read aloud in class, not ordering food for themselves at the school cafeteria, not talking on the phone to friends, or changing words to select only words they think they can say fluently. Although these avoidance behaviors seem to minimize stuttering, the child who avoids speaking situations is unable to participate in key activities that are important for educational or social development (Murphy, Quesal, & Gulker, 2007). Thus, these behaviors can make it more difficult for the child to communicate effectively, so they, too, should be addressed as part of a comprehensive approach to treatment.

Other negative reactions include *cognitive* reactions, such as low self-esteem, diminished self-confidence, and reduced feelings of self-efficacy (Blood & Blood, 2004; Healey & Scott, 1995; Manning, 2001; Ramig & Bennett, 1995; 1997; Ramig & Dodge, 2005; Reardon-Reeves & Yaruss, 2004; Starkweather & Givens-Ackerman, 1997; Vanryckeghem, Brutten, & Hernandez, 2005; Yaruss, 1998a; Yaruss & Quesal, 2004; 2006). Children who stutter may spend a considerable amount of time worrying about stuttering and wondering what other people might be thinking about them. Low self-esteem and self-confidence can also have a broader impact on the child's life in areas not related to stuttering (e.g., social interaction), so addressing these reactions is a particularly important component of treatment.

Functional Communication Abilities

As noted at the outset of this chapter, a central goal of this approach to treatment is to ensure that the child is able to communicate effectively in a variety of "real-world" speaking situations. This ability to communicate is determined not by the amount of stuttering a child exhibits in a given situation, but by how easily and completely the child is able to convey his or her message in that situation. Certainly, improved fluency can help a child convey his or her message effectively. Still, communication effectiveness can be diminished if gains in fluency are achieved through avoidance of feared words or through the use of speaking techniques that are so burdensome that the child has difficulty using them on a consistent basis. Maintaining an emphasis on effective communication ensures that treatment will not focus exclusively on the acquisition of speaking techniques or the reduction of negative reactions.

Focusing on effective communication also helps clinicians address the variability that children who stutter may exhibit in their stuttering behaviors. Many authors have commented on the differences in stuttering frequency that can be observed over time and across speaking situations (see Costello & Ingham, 1984; Yaruss, 1997a). This variability can complicate treat-

ment significantly because a child's ability to use a given strategy within the therapy room may not be indicative of his or her ability to use that same technique in another setting, such as the classroom or the cafeteria. Variability is often addressed in treatment through the use of hierarchies and generalization plans to ensure that speakers can use techniques across a variety of situations (e.g., Brutten & Shoemaker, 1967; 1974; Darley & Spriestersbach, 1978; Shumak, 1955; see also Hillis & McHugh, 1998; Ingham & Onslow, 1987). The same is true for the treatment approach described in this chapter. Here, however, situational differences are viewed less in terms of the effect they have on the child's *fluency* and more in terms of the effect they have on the child's ability to convey his or her message and speak freely, regardless of the amount of stuttering the child exhibits. Thus, these components of treatment are framed in terms of *functional* communication (Frattali, 1998) rather than in terms of stuttering frequency, and addressing functional communication represents a significant part of the effort in ongoing therapy sessions.

Quality of Life

Stuttering can have a far-reaching and sometimes devastating effect on people's lives. In addition to causing negative emotional and cognitive reactions and difficulties communicating in daily situations, stuttering can also affect a speaker's overall quality of life (Frattali, 1998). Many people have described how stuttering kept them from doing the things they wanted to do in their lives, such as pursuing careers, participating in social events, developing friendships, and succeeding in school (Hayhow, Cray, & Enderby, 2002; Hugh-Jones & Smith, 1999; Yaruss et al., 2002). Children, in particular, may experience negative reactions on the part of those in their environment (e.g., bullying and teasing) (see Blood & Blood, 2004; Davis, Howell, & Cook, 2002; Langevin, 1997; 2000; Langevin et al., 1998; Murphy & Quesal, 2002; Murphy, Yaruss, & Quesal, 2007a; 2007b; Yaruss et al., 2004). This, in turn, can negatively affect their participation in life and their acceptance of themselves and their speaking difficulties.

In this treatment approach, the ultimate goal, and the ultimate measure of success, is ensuring that stuttering does not have a negative consequence on the child's life. Improvements in quality of life can be achieved even if the child continues to stutter to some degree following treatment. If the child knows how to manage tension during fluent and disfluent speech, if he or she experiences minimal negative reactions, and if he or she can communicate effectively in a broad range of situations, then the resulting impact on the child's overall quality of life will be greatly reduced. The result will be a child who may still exhibit the stuttering *behavior* but who does not experience a stuttering *disorder*. This outcome will be taken as the overall definition of success in this chapter.

THEORETICAL FRAMEWORK

To formalize our views about the broad-based nature of stuttering and our multifaceted treatment for school-age children (as well as for adolescents and adults) who stutter, we have grounded our research and clinical practice in a theoretical framework that was specifically designed to account for complicated disorders such as stuttering. This framework, developed by the World Health Organization (WHO), is called the *International Classification of Functioning, Disability, and Health* (ICF) (WHO, 2001). The ICF describes human health experience, including both normal and disordered functioning, in terms of three primary components: (1) body function and structure, (2) activities and participation, and (3) personal and environmental contextual factors. The ICF is particularly relevant for speech-language pathologists because the American Speech-Language-Hearing Association (ASHA) has specified that the scope of practice "encompasses all components and factors identified in the WHO framework" (ASHA, 2001). Stuttering can be described in this framework as follows.

Body Structure and Function

The first component of ICF describes all of the major structures of the human body (e.g., nervous system, skeletal and muscular systems, systems involved in producing speech), as well as all of the functions those structures can perform (e.g., thinking and cognition, movement, speaking). If a person experiences difficulty with body structure or function, this is referred to as an *impairment*. Examples of communication disorders that involve impairments in body structure include cleft palate, aphasia, closed head injury, and certain voice disorders.

People who stutter are not known to have a clearly defined impairment in body structure, although research has highlighted neuroanatomic differences in adults who stutter (Foundas et al., 2001; 2003; Giraud et al., 2008; Jäncke, Hänggi, & Steinmetz, 2004; Sommer et al., 2002). People who stutter do exhibit an impairment in body *function*, however. This functional impairment is seen in the surface behaviors of stuttering (i.e., the repetitions, prolongations, and blocks). All people who stutter exhibit this impairment in body function to some degree.

Activities and Participation

The second component of the ICF describes the daily activities in which people engage as they participate in their lives. These categories relate directly to the "functional communication" and "quality of life" aspects of treatment described earlier. Examples of daily activities associated with communication include initiating or maintaining conversations, talking on the phone, and participating in social events or community life. Difficulties with daily activities are referred to as **activity limitations** (e.g., limitations in the ability to initiate conversations); difficulties with participation are referred to as **participation restrictions** (e.g., restrictions in the ability to participate in social activities).

Examples of activity limitations experienced by school-age children who stutter may include difficulties reading out loud in class, solving problems at the board, socializing with friends, and talking on the phone. If children experience these limitations in their communication abilities, they may experience a broader restriction in their ability to participate in life in the ways they are supposed to. For school-age children, this participation includes the ability to achieve educational and social objectives. Recognizing activity limitations and participation restrictions in school-age children who stutter is particularly relevant for clinicians who work in the public schools because federal legislation (i.e., the Individuals with Disabilities Education Act [IDEA]) (United States Congress, 1997; United States Department of Education, 2001; 2002) mandates that children be qualified for therapy when they experience adverse impact on their ability to achieve educational objectives.

Personal and Environmental Contextual Factors

The final component of the ICF describes the personal and environmental factors that affect people's experience of their daily lives. These contextual factors help to explain why people with the same disorder can have different experiences (e.g., why some people who stutter are not limited by their speaking difficulties, whereas others are), as well as why a given individual's experience with stuttering can differ so greatly from one situation to another.

Personal factors, including the affective, behavioral, and cognitive reactions described earlier, are particularly relevant because they mediate, to a large extent, the speaker's experience of activity limitation or participation restriction (Yaruss, 1998a; Yaruss & Quesal, 2004). If a speaker reacts negatively to his or her stuttering, he or she is more likely to avoid speaking situations and engage in other behaviors that limit his or her ability to perform daily activities and participate in life. Environmental factors include the speaker's support systems (including therapists and family members), the reactions of others (including negative experiences such as bullying and teasing by peers), and the influences of different speaking situations. If the environmental reactions are negative, this, too, will affect the speaker's ability to achieve his or her goals in life. Because the speaker's experience of stuttering is largely determined by these personal and environmental reactions, it is important for them to be addressed within a comprehensive approach to treatment. (In fact, to recognize the important role that these contextual factors play in mediating the occurrence of negative impact, they will be discussed *before* the activities and participation components of treatment in the sections that follow.)

RATIONALE FOR TREATMENT

The ICF framework is useful for describing stuttering because it outlines the key components of the speaker's experience of the disorder and captures the meaning of the phrase "stuttering is more than just stuttering." Thus, the ICF provides a justification for each of the various components that should be included in a comprehensive treatment program for children who stutter. To "treat the entire disorder," clinicians can follow the ICF to ensure that all relevant aspects of the disorder are addressed.

NATURE OF TREATMENT GOALS

One of the most important steps a clinician can take to enhance treatment success is to state treatment goals in a manner that can be clearly described, understood by others, and evaluated through research—both to ensure the efficacy of the treatment and to facilitate follow-up by other clinicians. School-based clinicians, in particular, must write treatment goals that address adverse educational impact, in keeping with the requirements of IDEA and state learning standards. (Note that the phrase "adverse educational impact" refers to the same activity limitations and participation restrictions described within the ICF. Therefore, minimizing activity limitation and participation restriction should be the primary focus of treatment.)

When considering a multifaceted treatment program, however, it can be confusing for both clients and clinicians to have long lists of seemingly unrelated goals. The ICF can help clinicians organize their goals in a more consistent, comprehensive manner. Specifically, clinicians can write goals in each of the three primary components of the ICF, as follows:

- Body Function: Goals aimed at minimizing the impairment in body function include teaching the child to use speech modification strategies designed to increase fluency and stuttering modification strategies designed to reduce tension during stuttering.
- Personal and Environmental Contextual Factors: Goals aimed at minimizing personal and environmental reactions include desensitization and education to help the child and those in his or her environment become more accepting of stuttering.
- Activities and Participation: Goals aimed at minimizing activity limitation and participation restriction include ensuring that the child can participate in all daily activities necessary for achieving success in educational and social endeavors.

The goals that are included in a given child's treatment plan will vary according to the specific needs of that child. For some children, goals will be written in each of the three categories of the ICF; for others (or for the same child at different points in therapy), goals may be written in just one or two categories. Taken together, these goals provide a comprehensive treatment approach that is consistent with both IDEA and the ASHA scope of practice.

EMPIRICAL BASIS FOR THE TREATMENT APPROACH

When selecting treatment goals, clinicians must be mindful of the differing needs of the children with whom they work. For this reason, we believe that clinicians should not apply treatment in a "one size fits all" fashion, using the same procedures for all clients they treat (Quesal, Yaruss, & Molt, 2004). Because treatment goals are defined individually for each child, the techniques and strategies used to achieve those goals must also be selected individually. One consequence of using an individualized treatment approach is that it makes it more difficult to document outcomes via standard treatment efficacy research. Because each client is working toward his or her own unique goals, the client is essentially receiving his or her own unique treatment. Thus, the same outcomes measures are not necessarily relevant for everybody participating in treatment.

Although many studies on the efficacy of treatment use measures of speech fluency as a primary metric for determining success (Bothe et al., 2006; Davidow, Bothe, & Bramlett, 2006), clinicians using an individualized treatment program might find that, for some speakers, improved fluency is *not* the most important measure of success (Manning, 2001; Murphy, 1989). For those individuals, it may be more important, at least in some stages of therapy, to help them become less concerned about their stuttering so they can participate in educational activities, regardless of the amount of stuttering they exhibit. At that point, changes in the reactions or activity and participation components of the disorder would be more important than changes in the impairment. Thus, comparisons of *fluency* before and after treatment would not be sufficient to capture the true outcomes of individualized treatment and should therefore

only be used as a part of the overall treatment evaluation plan.

For these reasons, there are, as yet, no published reports of the efficacy of the *entire*, broad-based treatment approach for school-age children who stutter described in this chapter. One might question whether the treatment can be used as an example of evidence-based practice, although we would argue that it is possible to assess whether the individual *components* of the treatment are effective for the specific children for whom they are recommended. In our clinical research (Murphy, Yaruss, & Quesal, 2007a; 2007b; Quesal, Yaruss, & Molt, 2004; Yaruss & Quesal, 2004; 2006), we have sought to do just that by ensuring that the treatment that is used for each individual child is appropriate and efficacious for that child.

EXISTING EMPIRICAL DATA

In this section, empirical data supporting the various components of treatment are presented in terms of the ICF.

Impairment in Body Function

Numerous authors have described strategies for helping individuals who stutter improve their speech fluency and change their stuttering (see reviews in Bloodstein & Bernstein Ratner, 2008; Conture, 2001; Guitar, 2006; Manning, 2001; Shapiro, 1999). Traditionally, these approaches have been divided into "speech modification" and "stuttering modification" strategies. Put simply, speech modification involves helping clients learn to change the way they speak to enhance fluency, whereas "stuttering modification" involves helping clients change the way they stutter so that stuttering is less disruptive to their communication. Regardless of the approach that is used, many of these changes involve adjustments to the *timing* of speech, such as speaking more slowly, as well as changes to the *tension* of speech muscles, such as reducing physical tension in the oral articulators during speech production (Conture, 2001).

Speech modification approaches are supported by a large empirical research literature that demonstrates that when individuals speak more slowly or reduce the physical tension involved in speech production, they are able to speak more fluently while they are using those techniques (Andrews, Guitar, & Howie, 1980;

Boberg & Kully, 1994; Bothe, 2002; Bothe et al., 2006). Stuttering modification techniques are supported by a smaller number of studies showing that when speakers adjust the tension in their speech mechanisms, they are able to stutter in a less disruptive manner (Laiho & Klippi, 2007; Prins & Miller, 1973; Starke, 1994; see also Van Riper, 1958; Williams & Dugan, 2002). Many papers have highlighted the value of incorporating elements of both approaches, as needed, in order to ensure that the individual is able to speak freely, with both increases in speech fluency and decreases in tension associated with stuttering (Healey & Scott, 1995; Ramig & Bennett, 1995; 1997; Ramig & Dodge, 2005; Reardon-Reeves & Yaruss, 2004; Williams & Dugan, 2002).

Personal and Environmental Contextual Factors

Many authors have discussed the importance of addressing personal contextual factors (often termed, simply, "communication attitudes") in a comprehensive approach to treatment (see reviews in Manning, 2001; Reardon-Reeves & Yaruss, 2004). Still, there are relatively few studies that specifically describe the efficacy of treatment strategies that are designed to minimize negative communication attitudes. To address this concern, the authors and colleagues have drawn upon a larger literature from counseling psychology and other forms of cognitive and behavioral therapy to highlight the efficacy of various methods for helping people achieve changes in attitudinal reactions (Murphy, Yaruss, & Quesal, 2007a; 2007b). Most notable among these are strategies for cognitive restructuring and desensitization (Barret, Dadds, & Rapee, 1996; A. Beck, 1976; J. S. Beck, 1995; Murphy, Yaruss, & Quesal, 2007a; Rapee et al., 2000), which are well documented in the counseling psychology literature.

There is also a significant literature examining environmental contextual factors, such as society's views about stuttering, discrimination, and the difficulties that children face associated with experiences such as bullying and teasing (Blood & Blood, 2004; Davis, Howell, & Cook, 2002; Langevin, 1997; 2000; Murphy, Yaruss, & Quesal, 2007a; 2007b). At the same time, there is relatively little research examining whether or how

clinicians can specifically help children who stutter to make changes in the responses of those in their environment. As with the personal contextual factors, the present authors have attempted to address this shortcoming in the stuttering research by drawing upon other bodies of literature (see review in Murphy, Yaruss, & Quesal, 2007b). Again, it is clear that there is strong empirical support for treatment strategies designed to minimize the impact of negative reactions by those in a child's environment.

Activities and Participation

In recent years, some treatment programs for adults who stutter have begun to document changes in the negative impact of stuttering in real-world situations (Montgomery, 2006; Yaruss 1997b). For children who stutter, however, studies examining changes in quality of life or functional communication in classroom and social situations have not yet been undertaken. Researchers may have assumed that treatment aimed at improving fluency will necessarily result in improvements in activities or participation. Still, empirical data are needed to demonstrate that children who stutter experience changes in their ability to perform daily activities and participate fully in life following treatment.

COLLECTING COMPREHENSIVE EMPIRICAL DATA IN TREATMENT OUTCOMES RESEARCH

To aid in the collection of needed empirical data, the present authors and colleagues have created a series of measurement instruments that can be used to: (1) help clinicians determine children's eligibility for treatment based on an assessment of the adverse impact of stuttering on their lives; (2) support the empirical evaluation of a variety of treatment approaches based on an understanding of the entirety of the stuttering disorder; and (3) facilitate clinicians' assessment of the changes a child experiences during the course of therapy. These instruments, called the *Overall Assessment of the Speaker's Experience of Stuttering (OASES)* (Yaruss & Quesal, 2006; Yaruss, Coleman, & Quesal, 2007a; 2007b), were specifically designed as a means of measuring the key constructs of stuttering that were proposed by the WHO in the creation of the ICF.

Of course, these are not the only measurement instruments that have been developed in an attempt to address aspects of the stuttering disorder beyond observable stuttering behaviors. Many such tools have been presented (see review in Yaruss & Quesal, 2006), although relatively few have addressed the needs of school-age children (see Brutten & Vanryckeghem, 2006; DeNil & Brutten, 1991; Manning, 2001). We hope that future research will see an increase in the use of such measures to document changes school-age children experience during the course of treatment so that clinicians will have access to a more robust literature to support them in making treatment decisions.

DATA TO BE COLLECTED BY CLINICIANS IN INDIVIDUALIZED TREATMENT

Even after comprehensive research data are available to support various treatment approaches, clinicians will still need to demonstrate whether their treatment is effective for each child with whom they work. Thus, clinicians will need to collect data before, during, and after treatment for all of the various aspects of the disorder they are addressing for a particular child in order to document the effectiveness of their intervention. Specific examples of the types of data to be considered are provided in the section on assessment methods later in this chapter. At this point, it should simply be noted that the data collected and evaluated by the clinician during the intervention process form an indispensable aspect of the application of evidence-based practice.

PRACTICAL REQUIREMENTS FOR TREATMENT

TIME DEMANDS AND MATERIALS

One of the many challenges associated with an individualized treatment approach is that it is not possible to determine a priori how long a child will need to be in therapy. Because the goals will differ from one child to the next and because each child's ability to achieve those goals will differ, then it must also be true that the length of time the child is in therapy and the number of sessions needed per week will also

differ. Thus, some children will benefit from (or be able to participate in) treatment scheduled one time per week, whereas another child may be scheduled twice a week. Many children benefit from the focused attention that goes with individual treatment sessions; others benefit from working in groups. The scheduling and format of treatment sessions will also differ depending on where the child is in the therapy process and what specific goals are being addressed at that time. For example, it may be beneficial for a child to be scheduled for treatment more frequently when doing drill work for practicing speaking techniques and then be scheduled less frequently when working on generalization or addressing personal reactions.

The scheduling of the treatment sessions is not as important as the work the child performs *in between* sessions. For the type of treatment described in this chapter, the real work comes when the child attempts to use speaking techniques, make changes in personal reactions, and expand functional communication abilities in real-world settings. The purpose of the treatment sessions, then, is to teach the child what he needs to practice in between sessions. (In this way, treatment sessions can be viewed like piano lessons. The piano teacher's goal during a lesson is not to teach a child to "play the piano," but rather to teach the child what he or she will need to practice *in between* lessons in order to learn to play the piano.) A consequence of this approach is the fact that the child's participation in therapy is a particularly important determiner of ultimate success. Of course, this is likely to be true for all treatments that involve helping a child make changes in speaking or communication patterns.

CLINICIAN EXPERTISE

Numerous authors have highlighted the fact that many practicing speech-language pathologists feel uncomfortable working with children who stutter (Brisk, Healey, & Hux, 1997; Cooper & Cooper, 1985; 1996; Kelly et al., 1997; Mallard, Gardner, & Downey, 1988; St. Louis & Durrenberger, 1993; St. Louis & Lass, 1980; Sommers & Caruso, 1995; Van Riper, 1977; Wingate, 1971). Therefore, the practical requirements of treatment are of critical importance. Even a therapy that has been proven to be effective through empirical research cannot be successfully applied if practitioners are not comfortable with the strategies. For example, if a clinician feels that it is not acceptable for a child to exhibit stuttering in his or her speech, then that clinician might have particular difficulty with the desensitization components of therapy. Therefore, an important requirement for this approach to treatment is that the *clinician* learn about, come to terms with, and ultimately, accept stuttering and the fact that it is okay for children to stutter. Fortunately, the experiences that clinicians must undergo to come to terms with stuttering are exactly the same experiences that children who stutter must undergo. Children who stutter need to learn about stuttering, become desensitized to stuttering, reduce their fear of stuttering, and learn strategies for managing tension in the speech muscles. Clinicians need to do these things too. It is our belief that clinicians can acquire this knowledge and develop these skills right alongside their clients, by simply participating in the therapy and doing what they ask the child to do. By engaging in therapy, clinicians will develop a better understanding of stuttering, while enhancing their ability to help children who stutter.

KEY COMPONENTS OF THE TREATMENT APPROACH

Throughout this chapter, we have used the ICF to ensure that we considered the entire stuttering disorder in treatment. Keeping with this theme, we will present the key components of the treatment approach in terms of the ICF. Although we describe each component (impairment, personal and environmental reactions, and activity limitation/participation restriction) in turn, the treatment itself is not provided in a sequential fashion. In other words, treatment does not address the impairment first, followed by personal reactions, followed by environmental reactions, etc. Instead, the components of treatment overlap and interact with one another (e.g., tension reduction activities address both the impairment and the negative personal reactions), and some components are addressed repeatedly at different times throughout treatment. Also, each child receives treatment based on his or her specific needs. In other words,

although all of the components of the ICF are *considered* for every child, that does not necessarily mean each of those components are *addressed* in treatment for every child. (For example, a child who experiences minimal negative reactions to stuttering may not spend much time addressing the reactions component of the disorder.) Clinicians should draw upon the various components of treatment *as needed* to address the unique challenges faced by each child who enters treatment.

MINIMIZING IMPAIRMENT

Minimizing the stuttering impairment involves helping children learn to speak more fluently. As noted earlier, most techniques used to accomplish this involve changes to *timing* and *tension* of speech production. Importantly, minimizing the impairment also involves helping children change their stuttering behaviors so they are less disruptive to communication. Therefore, after strategies for enhancing fluency are described, strategies for minimizing tension and struggle during stuttering are also reviewed.

Changing Timing to Enhance Fluency (Slower Speech and Pausing)

Perhaps the most common strategies for helping children (and adults) modify the timing of their speech to enhance fluency involve: (1) reductions in *speaking rate* (Andrews & Ingham, 1972; Boberg & Kully, 1985; O'Brian et al., 2003; Webster, 1980) or (2) increases in *pausing* (Conture, 2001; Gregory, 2003). Some approaches use significant slowing (as in prolonged speech) and relatively longer pauses (e.g., "delaying response"), whereas others incorporate less noticeable changes to timing. Like many others, we use reduced speaking rate and increased pausing to minimize stuttering; however, we feel that these changes in timing must not be so drastic that they result in a reduction in speech *naturalness*.

Speakers who use a reduced rate of speech face a difficult trade-off: the more slowly they speak, the more fluent they are likely to be, but the less natural they are likely to sound and the less natural they are likely to feel. Speaking slowly and pausing also requires more effort. This trade-off puts school-age children in an awkward position. They do not want to sound different from their peers by stuttering. At the same time, they do not want to sound different from their peers by talking too slowly. As a result, they may choose to do nothing and thus gain no benefit from the techniques. This is one of the primary reasons that many children experience difficulty with *generalization* of therapy gains. To minimize these challenges, children can be taught to use *minimal* reductions in speaking rate and relatively *short* pauses. Fortunately, only a small change in timing is necessary to enhance fluency (as seen in the later stages of prolonged speech therapy) (O'Brian et al., 2003; Onslow et al., 1996). Thus, children can learn to slow their rate and increase their pausing *slightly* and to use these modifications only when they want to enhance their fluency.

Of course, children will be more fluent if they slow their rate more dramatically or use the slower rate more frequently. Still, it should be up to the child to determine when, or how much, to slow their speech. The goal is for children to achieve a *balance* between modifying speech timing to enhance fluency, without requiring that modifications be so dramatic that the child finds it impossible to maintain them in conversational speech. Inherent in this balance is the recognition that treatment does not require children to achieve "perfect" or "normal" fluency but, instead, to achieve "improved" fluency.

Modifying speaking rate and increasing pausing in this way is actually a common strategy for nonstuttering speakers (Goldman-Eisler, 1954; 1956). For example, when a speaker comes to a new or unfamiliar word, he or she has the option of slowing down to say the word correctly. Nonstutterers do this effortlessly; children who stutter may require practice to be able to reduce their rate to help them get through a difficult word and then to increase their rate to their normal level after the difficulty has passed. It is worth noting that children can modulate their rate when they are performing other motor tasks, such as walking or riding a bicycle (Coleman, Yaruss, & Hammer, 2007). When a child rides a bicycle, the child knows that there are certain times when he or she can ride relatively fast, like on a straight road. At other times, such as when approaching a curve or riding on a bumpy road, the child may need to slow down to ensure that he or she does not crash. With

practice, children learn to make these adjustments so they can continue riding as smoothly as possible. In the same way, with practice, children can learn to make adjustments in their speaking rate so they can continue speaking as smoothly as possible.

Furthermore, when a child rides a bicycle, there is no set rate (in miles per hour) that the child must use. Riding rate is based on factors such as inherent ability, riding experience, road conditions, etc. The child learns to evaluate these parameters so he or she can ride as smoothly as possible given conditions. In the same way, changes in speech timing should not be based on a specified speaking rate. That is, the child is not required to speak at a rate of "X" syllables per second or to use a pause of "Y" milliseconds. Every child has different inherent abilities, and every speaking situation is different. Therefore, the child who stutters must learn to manipulate timing as needed to achieve optimal smoothness (fluency) in different situations.

Although minimal changes in timing are easier for children to learn and maintain than more dramatic changes, these modifications still require practice. Thus, clinicians should be prepared to spend adequate time in therapy helping children learn to master new speaking skills. This can be accomplished by working through a hierarchy of easier to harder situations (Yaruss & Reardon, 2003). For example, a child may learn to use slower rates in an easy task, such as imitation or reading, and then move toward more difficult tasks, such as structured or spontaneous speech. After a hierarchy of speaking tasks is completed, the child can work through a hierarchy of easier to harder speaking *situations*. Examples of easier situations include the therapy room or home environment; examples of harder situations include the school cafeteria, the playground, or the classroom. Different children find different tasks or settings to be easier or harder. As a result, clinicians will need to work with the child outside of the therapy room and follow the child's lead in developing a hierarchy. Additional details about the use of hierarchies to facilitate generalization are discussed in the section "Activities and Participation."

In sum, there are four fundamental considerations for using timing changes to enhance children's speech fluency: (1) timing changes should not be too drastic; (2) the changes do not need to be used all of the time; (3) there is no arbitrary standard of timing that must be achieved; and (4) timing changes should be practiced along a hierarchy of easier to harder situations so the child can learn to use them successfully.

Changing Tension to Enhance Fluency (Light Contact)

The less physical tension a child uses when speaking, the less likely he or she is to experience increased tension associated with stuttering. Therefore, another change that can enhance fluency is reducing physical tension in the articulators, as seen in "light contact" or "gentle onset" (Reardon-Reeves & Yaruss, 2004; Runyan & Runyan, 1986; 1993). With these techniques, the child learns to touch the articulators together with less physical tension. The problem with light contact is that it is difficult for children to do, particularly in conversational speech. This is especially true when children are rushed or excited, and they may simply abandon the technique in difficult situations even though they may find it helpful for minimizing stuttering.

As with the changes to speaking rate described earlier, children should not try to use light contact all of the time. Instead, they can use light contact just at those moments when they feel their tension increasing. To accomplish this, they must learn about the tension in their speech musculature. Thus, teaching light contact also involves teaching the child about the muscles involved in speaking (including muscles for respiration, phonation, and articulation) and helping the child learn that during speech production his or her muscles tense in different ways. The more the child understands about his or her speech mechanism, the more the child will be able to make changes that facilitate fluency. The more skilled the child becomes at sensing tension in his or her muscles, the more the child will be able to determine when to use light contact. As with the timing changes, this technique requires a considerable amount of practice. Over time, though, the child will find it easier to reduce tension in his or her speech muscles in order to enhance fluency.

Changing Timing and Tension to Enhance Fluency (Easy Starts)

Children can minimize the difficulties they face when trying to enhance fluency through changes

to timing and tension by not trying to make changes all of the time. Instead, they can use modifications judiciously, slowing their speech enough to increase fluency, but not so much that it becomes too difficult, interferes with speech naturalness, or limits their ability to communicate freely. Finding that balance takes practice, although as children work toward this goal, they develop the ability to manage their speech in a flexible and sustainable manner.

One way clinicians can help children achieve this balance is to recognize that children do not stutter on every word they produce, and the distribution of stuttered words is not random. Most of the time (although not always), stuttering occurs at the *beginnings* of utterances (Brown, 1938; 1945; Taylor, 1966). Once a speaker produces the first word (or even just the first sounds) of an utterance, the rest of the utterance is often produced fluently. Thus, the task of modifying speech to enhance fluency can be simplified if children focus their timing and tension modifications not on the entire utterance, but only on the first *sounds* of the utterance.

The result is a technique that has been called "easy starts" or "easy beginnings" (see Gregory, 2003; Reardon-Reeves & Yaruss, 2004), in which the speaker begins an utterance with a slightly slowed rate of speech (reduced timing) and a light contact (reduced physical tension) and transitions to a normal rate for the remainder of the phrase. The use of a normal rate and normal tension throughout the rest of the phrase makes the technique easier to use than more pervasive slowing and light contact, while allowing the speaker to maintain speech naturalness. The child can then incorporate pausing and phrasing to provide many opportunities to use easy starts, although it is not necessary for the child to use an easy start on *every* phrase. Much as a child occasionally adds movement when spinning a basketball on his finger, he can occasionally add "movement" to his speech by using easy starts. This allows the child to enhance his or her fluency through changes to timing and tension while maintaining the forward flow of speech.

Video Clip 1 on thePoint shows an example of how to introduce easy starts, including an explanation of the technique and several examples of the child's productions.

As with all of the techniques presented in this chapter, learning how often and when to use easy starts requires practice. Younger children and children with language or cognitive impairments may find this too difficult, so they may need to use a more pervasive modification to achieve increased fluency. Children should use as much modification in timing and tension as they need in order to improve their fluency, but not so much modification that the task becomes too difficult or communication is compromised. (Again, this requires that clinicians accept the notion that the goal of treatment is improved *communication* and that improved fluency is just part of the overall improvements in communication that this treatment aims to achieve.)

Changing Tension to Reduce the Severity of Stuttering (Exploration and Pseudostuttering)

Changing timing and tension can help children speak more fluently, although the techniques are not perfect. As noted earlier, the techniques are difficult to use, so children cannot use them all the time. Furthermore, even when children do use techniques, they will still stutter sometimes, so it is important for clinicians to help children learn that it is okay to stutter, even when they are trying to use techniques.

Video Clip 2 shows the clinician discussing the flexible use of techniques with the child, with a reminder that it is okay to stutter.

When children stutter, they can do so in different ways. They can exhibit a high degree of physical tension, or they can stutter with less tension. The more tension they exhibit during stuttering, the more disruption they experience in communication. "Easier" stuttering affects communication less. Thus, in addition to helping children learn to *speak* more easily, clinicians can also help children improve communication by helping them *stutter* more easily.

Changing physical tension can be difficult. Although children may be aware that they are physically tense during stuttering (especially during prolongations or blocks), they may not understand how tension arises (e.g., which muscles are involved) and how they can reduce that tension while speaking (Williams, 1971;

1983). Parents and clinicians may have told them to "relax" their muscles, but the children may not have understood how to do so, and they may find it difficult to reduce tension while speaking. Therefore, an important first step in helping children learn to change tension during stuttering is to help them learn what they *do* during the moment of stuttering. Some children tense the muscles of the jaw, whereas others tense the muscles of the larynx, and still others restrict their breathing. Children may exhibit other behaviors like eye blinking, curling of the lip, and other physically tense movements (Conture & Kelly, 1991; see also Bloodstein & Bernstein Ratner, 2008; Van Riper, 1982; Wingate, 1964). The more they understand how they are tensing their muscles, the more likely they will be to be able to *change* that tension.

One way children can learn about how they stutter is by "exploring" the moment of stuttering and describing what they do with their mouths or throats or breathing mechanism when they stutter. To help them do this, children can watch themselves stuttering using a mirror or videotape, or they can imitate their stuttering using "pseudostuttering" (discussed more later in this section). After learning about the "speech machine" (the parts of their body that are involved in speaking) (Reardon-Reeves & Yaruss, 2004), children can discuss how the parts of the speech machine work together during fluent speech and how they tense in opposition to one another during stuttered speech.

In Video Clip 3, in the middle of the discussion about the parts of the body used in producing speech, the clinician uses the analogy of a fist to indicate physical tension. There is also an example of easing out of (pseudo)stutters.

One way children can learn about stuttering is to "freeze" during the moment of stuttering. By "staying in the block" (or repetition), children gain time to think about what they are doing with their speech mechanism. The clinician can facilitate guiding the child to think about physical tension in the breathing mechanism or in the muscles involved in producing voice or speech sounds while he or she is "holding on" to the moment of stuttering. After the child understands how physical tension builds, the child can begin to experiment with ways to *reduce* that tension. This can be introduced by means of a nonspeech analogy, in which the child is directed to make a fist and then modify the tension in the fist. The clinician can explain to the child that when he makes a fist, he is in control of the amount of tension present in the muscles of his hand. If the child chooses to increase the tension in the muscles of his hand, he can do that because he is in charge of the tension in his hand. Similarly, if the child chooses to *decrease* the tension in the muscles of his hand, he can do that because he is in charge of the muscles in his hand. Through such analogies, the clinician can help the child learn that even though he may not be able to control *when* he stutters, he can, with practice, learn to change *how* he stutters by decreasing the physical tension in the muscles used for speaking.

Video Clip 4 shows a discussion of relaxing muscles following a moment of stuttering. In addition, following the discussion of the parts of the body used in producing speech, there is an example of using pseudostuttering as a way of learning about where tension is held in the body during stuttering.

Staying in a moment of stuttering can be quite difficult for children in the early stages of therapy. In part, this is due to the fact that it can be uncomfortable for children to face their stuttering in this way. Still, they need to face their stuttering, and doing this through exploration may be less frightening than other means of confronting their fears. (This will be discussed in more detail in the following sections addressing desensitization.) Children may also find this exercise difficult because when they first begin treatment, they may not yet possess sufficient self-monitoring to be able to keep track of their speech. Learning to "catch" a moment of stuttering can help children develop these self-monitoring skills, and this provides a foundation for the successful use of a wide variety of techniques used in treatment.

Another way to help children learn about what they do when they stutter is through the use of **pseudostuttering**. Pseudostuttering, or "voluntary stuttering" (Sheehan, 1970; Van Riper, 1973), means stuttering on purpose. It can be done on its own as part of an exploration

exercise, or it can be done in the context of conversational speech as part of a desensitization exercise. Pseudostuttering can help children learn about their stuttering and about how to change the tension they exhibit during stuttering. As with the exploration exercise described earlier, the clinician can ask the child what he or she is doing with his or her respiratory, phonatory, and articulatory systems during the moment of stuttering, and then guide the child toward *reducing* tension. As the child gains experience with type of negative practice exercise, he or she prepares a solid foundation for being able to use classic stuttering modification techniques, such as cancellations or pull-outs (Van Riper, 1973). Techniques for reducing the amount of physical tension during stuttering can help children communicate more easily, although they do not necessarily help children speak more fluently. For this reason, tension reduction techniques must be combined with other techniques for modifying timing and tension, as described earlier, to help the child speak more fluently (Healey & Scott, 1995; Ramig & Bennett, 1997). Every child will need a different combination of timing and tension modification strategies to minimize the effects of the child's stuttering impairment on communication. Many children will also need help to address the negative affective, behavioral, and cognitive reactions that accompany their stuttering. The next section addresses those aspects of the child's overall experience of the stuttering disorder.

MINIMIZING NEGATIVE PERSONAL REACTIONS

Stuttering can be embarrassing. It can lead to feelings of shame and reduced self-worth, and it can have significant negative social consequences. It can cause children to substitute words to try to minimize overt stuttering or to avoid entire speaking situations so they do not have to experience these negative emotional and cognitive reactions. Helping children minimize their impairment (through changes to timing and tension) can help them minimize these negative reactions. Unfortunately, however, for many children, this is not enough. As long as some stuttering still remains in their speech, the potential for experiencing negative reactions also remains. Many school-age children do not possess the skills they need to cope with these affective, behavioral, and cognitive reactions, so speech-language pathologists may need to help. Fortunately, there is much that can be done.

Desensitization

One way clinicians can help children overcome their fears about stuttering is to use **desensitization** strategies in treatment (Beck, 1995; Kaufman, 1985; Rapee et al., 2000; for applications in stuttering treatment, see Dell, 1993; Murphy, 1989; 1999; Murphy, Yaruss, & Quesal, 2007a; Sheehan, 1958; Van Riper, 1958). Desensitization is the process of helping individuals become less reactive to and more accepting of the behaviors or events that bother them. For example, when people experience fears of heights or spiders, they can engage in desensitization to help them overcome those fears. Desensitization involves exposing people to the things they fear (e.g., heights, spiders, or, in this case, stuttering). Desensitization is not accomplished all at once. Putting an individual who fears spiders into a room full of spiders could actually increase the individual's fear. Instead, desensitization must be accomplished *gradually*, beginning with easier situations and moving toward more difficult situations (i.e., along a hierarchy) as the fear diminishes. Thus, a person with a fear of heights may begin on the first floor of a building, and then gradually *desensitize* herself to her fears on the second floor, the third floor, and so on.

For children who stutter, it may be necessary to begin desensitization with very easy examples of stuttering behaviors (e.g., easy repetitions) in safe settings, such as in the therapy room. Although the child may have stuttered numerous times in the therapy room and in other settings, that, by itself, has not been desensitizing. The key to desensitization is the *intentionality* that goes with actively facing the anxiety and performing the feared behavior on purpose. Earlier in this chapter, the concept of stuttering on purpose, or pseudostuttering, was introduced as a way of helping the child *explore* the moment of stuttering. At this point in therapy, the clinician can again use pseudostuttering as a way of helping the child become desensitized to stuttering by intentionally facing the fear and asso-

ciating stuttering with a positive, empowering experience, rather than a negative experience.

Initially, when a child is asked to stutter on purpose, he or she may find it very uncomfortable. This is not surprising because the clinician is asking the child to face the thing he or she fears (and dislikes) the most. Nevertheless, if the child is going to be able to overcome that fear, there is no other way to do it other than to perform the feared behavior repeatedly until the fear diminishes. This is why the use of hierarchies is so important. Using a hierarchy, the clinician can identify a situation that is so easy that the child can approach it. Examples include pseudostuttering in unison with the clinician, in a room by himself or herself with the door closed, or as part of an exploration activity as described earlier. Once the child can produce even a small pseudostutter in a carefully controlled situation, the child is ready to begin the process of "climbing the ladder" of his or her hierarchy so he or she can stutter more openly in increasingly harder situations. Ultimately, the goal is for the child to be able to speak (and stutter) freely in any situation, without fear, so that stuttering will be less likely to interfere with the child's ability to say what he or she wants to say. This will take time, but with the clinician's help, the child will be able to diminish his or her fear, and this, in turn, will help the child to reduce the tension, struggle, and avoidance that results from his or her fear of stuttering.

Cognitive Restructuring

Another way clinicians can help children minimize their negative reactions to stuttering is through the process of **cognitive restructuring** (Barrett, Dadds, & Rapee, 1996; A. Beck, 1976; J. S. Beck, 1995; Cooper, 2000; Kaufman, 1985; Kaufman, Raphael, & Espeland, 1999; Rapee et al., 2000; Starkweather & Givens-Ackerman, 1997; see also Murphy, Yaruss, & Quesal, 2007a). Cognitive restructuring helps people think differently about the problems they face in their lives. In essence, the goal is to change unrealistic thoughts and beliefs into more realistic ones by examining those beliefs and comparing them to available evidence. The process involves helping individuals identify their current thoughts about a problem and then gradually modifying those thoughts to minimize the difficulty the problem causes. These steps might include learning about fluent and stuttered speech, identifying the source of the fear associated with stutters (e.g., listeners' reactions), determining whether those fears are realistic by testing out situations that create anxiety, and creating a different set of thoughts and beliefs based on new evidence.

Thus, after a child learns about what he or she does during a moment of stuttering (as in the "exploring stuttering" exercise), the child can create a list of what causes him or her anxiety in a particular speaking situation. For example, if the feared situation is reading out loud in class, the clinician and child can use a brainstorming activity (Murphy, Yaruss, & Quesal, 2007b) to help the child think of all of the reasons that he is afraid of that situation. To make this easier, the clinician can help the child relate his fears to a list of all of the things that might go wrong when the child reads out loud. Perhaps the list includes producing a long block, having other children laugh at him, losing his place, mispronouncing a word, etc. The clinician should validate these fears and help the child see that it is understandable that he might feel that way. At the same time, the clinician can help the child consider what would really happen if one of the feared events were to occur. If the child views these possibilities as catastrophic, then the clinician can use a desensitization hierarchy to help the child *experience* those feared events in a relatively safe and supportive situation. The clinician and child can engage in role-playing activities to see what actually *would* happen if the child were to exhibit a long block when reading. (Here again, the child can use pseudostuttering as a way of exploring different ways of stuttering while simultaneously becoming desensitized to the moment of stuttering itself.)

Initially, these activities would be performed in the therapy room, although the child ultimately must work his way up a hierarchy of situations (e.g., reading in the therapy room when a friend is there, reading in the classroom when only the speech therapist is there, reading in the classroom when the therapist and teacher are there, etc.) to the point where he is able face the feared situation in the "real world" and re-evaluate his fears. Because the child has engaged in desensitization along the way, he will find that the feared situation is not as frightening as he had anticipated, and he will find that he can

now begin to think differently about that situation. Through these types of cognitive restructuring and desensitization tasks, the clinician can help the child change his thoughts and feelings about stuttering so he will be able to communicate more freely and react less negatively to stuttering.

Self-Help and Support Groups

Another way children can learn to overcome their negative reactions to stuttering is through self-help and support groups (Bradberry, 1997; Ramig, 1993; Reardon & Reeves, 2002; Reeves, 2006; Starkweather & Givens-Ackerman, 1997; Yaruss, Quesal, & Reeves, 2007). Many self-help groups for people who stutter have been started around the world (Krall, 2001). In the United States, the National Stuttering Association (NSA) and Friends: The National Association for Young People Who Stutter both have active programs designed to help children learn that they are not alone in facing their stuttering. Self-help groups not only help the child meet other children who stutter, but they also provide a safe environment for talking about stuttering, for exploring different ways of reacting to stuttering, and for learning that it is okay to stutter.

Self-help groups also help children meet with adults who have overcome the *burden* of stuttering. This helps children learn that they can do the things they want to do in life even if they continue to stutter. This, too, helps diminish children's fear and anxiety. Self-help groups can even help the parents of children who stutter by giving them the chance to see how other families cope with the challenges associated with stuttering. Thus, the authors encourage all the families they treat to become involved in stuttering self-help groups in some fashion (Yaruss, Quesal, & Reeves, 2007).

The Link between Reactions and Impairment

Readers may note that many of the strategies for helping children minimize negative reactions to stuttering were actually introduced earlier, in the section on the stuttering impairment. Although the techniques of reducing timing and tension in both fluent and disfluent speech can be introduced in a variety of ways, we prefer to do so *through* the process of learning about and exploring stuttering, which incorporates aspects of cognitive restructuring and desensitization. In this way, much of what is done to address the impairment *also* addresses the negative reactions, and the child gains fluency while simultaneously gaining improvements in his or her reactions to stuttering. The same process will also be seen when examining the negative impact of stuttering on the child's activities and participation. Before those components of the disorder are addressed, however, the role of the environment must be considered.

MINIMIZING NEGATIVE ENVIRONMENTAL REACTIONS

Children who stutter are not the only ones affected by stuttering. Parents, teachers, peers, and others also experience the effects of the disorder. Some of these people may feel confused about the nature of stuttering. Others may experience anxiety about what stuttering means for the child's future. Parents, in particular, may harbor feelings of guilt about the role they may have played in the onset or development of the disorder, even though current research suggests that stuttering is *not* caused by parents. Still others may feel embarrassment, shame, or even pity for the child because of the obvious struggle and unusual overt characteristics of stuttering.

The child's environment can also affect the child himself. Peers may bully and tease the child about his or her speaking difficulties (Murphy, Yaruss, & Quesal, 2007b). Teachers may be uncertain about how to help the child, not knowing whether to call on the child first, or last, or not at all (Crowe & Walton, 1981; Lass et al., 1992). Parents, understandably, want the child to overcome the stuttering, and in their desire to see the child recover, they may place additional pressures on the child to maintain fluent speech (Crowe & Cooper, 1977). In addition, as noted earlier, even many speech-language pathologists are uncomfortable with their skills for helping children who stutter, and this, too, can affect the child's willingness and ability to communicate.

Put simply, children who stutter live in an environment that does not understand their disorder, although what the child needs most is acceptance and understanding of his or her speaking difficulties. The best way clinicians can help to bring this about is through *education*—about the nature of stuttering, about the goals and procedures of treatment, about bullying and teasing, and about the potential impact of stuttering on the child's life. Unfortunately, providing this education can be challenging because it can be difficult for clinicians to have access to individuals in the child's environment (Gottwald & Hall, 2003). In the end, the child must help to educate the people in his or her environment. The clinician plays an important supportive role in this process, but it is the child who must become empowered to educate peers, teachers, and parents.

Peers: Bullying and Teasing

One of the primary problems that children who stutter face with respect to their peers is bullying (Blood & Blood, 2004; Davis, Howell, & Cook, 2002; Langevin et al., 1998; Murphy, Yaruss, & Quesal, 2007b). Peers may bully children who stutter for many reasons, including the fact that stuttering behaviors draw attention to themselves and vary in a seemingly unpredictable fashion. Bullying can be particularly difficult for children who stutter because it is hard for them to respond verbally (due in part to the heightened emotions that bullying evokes). Often, children who are being bullied are told to "just ignore it" or to "walk away," although it is very difficult for children to ignore hurtful comments that are made about something so personal. Speech-language pathologists can help with this in three key ways.

First, much of the treatment described throughout this chapter is aimed at helping minimize children's negative emotional and cognitive reactions. Education, desensitization, and acceptance exercises help to reduce the fear, embarrassment, and shame children experience due to their stuttering. These exercises do not completely eliminate the fear, but they do reduce it. As children become less concerned about and more accepting of stuttering, this lays the foundation for them to be able to respond in less emotionally charged ways when they are being bullied.

Second, clinicians can help children learn to respond to hurtful comments made by others in a way that will minimize the likelihood of further bullying (Langevin, 2000; Murphy, Yaruss,

& Quesal, 2007b; Yaruss et al., 2004). Typically, when bullies make comments about a child's speech (or other characteristic), they are seeking to evoke a negative reaction. Because many children who stutter harbor strong negative feelings about their speech, they provide an easy target. If they respond with less negative emotion, the bully will not find the same satisfaction, and ultimately, will move on to another target (Kaufman, Raphael, & Espeland, 1999). To minimize comments by bullies, therefore, children who stutter can learn to respond with simple, matter-of-fact comments that indicate to bullies that they will not receive the negative reactions they are seeking. Examples include acknowledgement of the stuttering ("Yes, you're right, I stutter") or indications that the comments are obvious or boring ("Yeah, I know" or "You said that before," or simply, "So?"). Note that it will likely take many such responses in order to redirect the bully because the bully is accustomed to receiving negative reactions from the child who stutters (Murphy, Yaruss, & Quesal, 2007b). Also, it may be difficult for the child who stutters to provide such responses, given his speech production difficulties. (It is not necessary that the child be able to provide these responses *fluently*—fluency is irrelevant to the success of this approach. It is necessary that the child be able to produce the responses in an open and straightforward manner that communicates to the bully the acceptance of stuttering.) Clinicians can help children practice these responses in therapy. Through the use of brainstorming and problem-solving strategies, role playing, and repeated practice, children who stutter can determine how they want to respond to bullies and they can gain experience preparing themselves to use those responses in real-world situations.

Video Clip 5 contains a discussion about how other children respond to the child's stuttering and how he responds to them.

Third, clinicians can minimize the likelihood that other children will participate in the hurtful comments made by the bully. In fact, other children (or "bystanders") (Coloroso, 2003) can actually play a helpful role in minimizing the negative impact of bullying (Craig & Pepler,

1995; Smith & Sharp, 1994). The problem is that they, too, may be confused about stuttering, and they may not understand the hurtful effects of their comments. Clinicians can help to minimize this by educating other children in the class about the disorder. Ideally, however, the best person to educate other children about stuttering is the child who stutters.

This process can be started as the child learns to provide simple, matter-of-fact comments that acknowledge stuttering, as described earlier. These comments help to bring stuttering out into the open and show other children that stuttering is not something to fear or ridicule. The process can continue as the child moves toward being able to acknowledge stuttering and to educate other children in the class in a more formal way. This can be done as part of a book report (e.g., "I chose this book because it has a character in it who stutters, just like me.") or even part of a more formal presentation (e.g., as part of Better Hearing and Speech Month, National Stuttering Awareness Week, or International Stuttering Awareness Day).

Class presentations (Murphy, Reardon, & Yaruss, 2004; Murphy, Yaruss, & Quesal, 2007b; Yaruss et al., 2004) give children who stutter the chance to tell others "the facts" about stuttering, including the following: stuttering is not the child's fault, speech techniques do not always work and are hard to use, it is not fair to tease children about stuttering, and there are many people who stutter yet still achieve great things in their lives. The more children who stutter can teach other children about stuttering, the less likely those other children are to participate in bullying and teasing (Atlas & Pepler, 1997), and this helps to create a safer environment in which children who stutter can communicate freely, without fear of being ridiculed because of their speaking difficulties.

Note that the goal of these activities is not to *fix* the bully through any actions of the child who stutters; research suggests that many bullies do the things they do because of their own low self-esteem or difficulty accepting differences in others (Coloroso, 2003). In other words, bullies bully because of the problems they themselves are facing, not because of any characteristic exhibited by the child they are bullying. Instead, the goal of helping the child learn to respond appropriately to bullying is simply to *redirect* the bully away from the child's stuttering and to minimize the likelihood that other children in the class will support the bully. Fortunately, there is a large and growing literature on how to minimize the effects of bullying on children who stutter, as well as children experiencing other difficulties (Gertner, Rice, & Hadley, 1994; Guralnick et al., 1996). One of the key ways that clinicians can ensure that such plans are successful is to enlist the participation and support of classroom teachers.

Educating Teachers

It has been our experience that many teachers want to help children who stutter; however, they are unsure about what to do. Just as many speech-language pathologists hold outdated or inaccurate views about stuttering (Cooper & Cooper, 1985; 1996), many teachers are also misinformed about the disorder (Crowe & Walton, 1981; Lass et al., 1992). Because of long-standing taboos about talking openly about stuttering (for fear of drawing attention to the disorder or making the child self-conscious), teachers have, in essence, participated in the "conspiracy of silence" (Starkweather & Givens-Ackerman, 1997) that affects many people who stutter. To break through this barrier, teachers and children must talk about stuttering.

By initiating a dialogue between teachers and children who stutter, clinicians can empower children to educate teachers about stuttering in the same way that they educate their peers. The child's use of simple, matter-of-fact comments that acknowledge stuttering can help teachers see that stuttering is not something to be feared. Clinicians can help children identify specific facts that they want to share with their teacher, and these can be provided in the form of a brochure ("My Facts about Stuttering") or a letter to the teacher that openly acknowledges stuttering and provides suggestions about how the teacher can help the child minimize the educational impact of stuttering. Some of the suggestions that children have provided in such brochures and letters include: "Please call on me first so I don't get too scared while I'm waiting my turn," "Please don't call on me at all unless I raise my hand," and "Please let me do my book report one-on-one instead of in front of the entire class." Doing this

puts the child in the position of being the "expert" about his or her speech (Murphy, 1989; Murphy, Yaruss, & Quesal, 2007a) and empowers the child to learn that he or she can make changes in his or her environment.

Video Clip 6 contains a section about the child being the expert about his speech and teaching others about speech.

The specific solutions that a child seeks will depend on several factors, such as the child's goals in therapy, where the child is in the therapy process, and the level of support the teacher is able to provide. Classroom accommodations can be used to help ease the burden the child faces while he or she is working up the desensitization hierarchy. The goal is to help the child work directly with the teacher to find ways of supporting the child's communication. More will be said about helping the child extend his or her skills into the real world in the section on activity limitation and participation restriction. To prepare for that critical transition and to further enhance the child's success in the classroom, clinicians must help parents participate actively in supporting the child.

Helping Parents Be Supportive

Ideally, parents will be active participants in the therapy process, offering the child support and understanding, helping the child work through the challenges he or she faces due to stuttering, and giving the child opportunities to practice speaking strategies while providing a safe environment where the child knows it is okay to stutter. Achieving this situation can pose a unique challenge for many speech-language pathologists, however, because they may have relatively little contact with parents (Gottwald & Hall, 2003). They may only get to see them at Individualized Education Program (IEP) meetings, and the only source of regular contact may be through forms and worksheets that the child may (or may not) bring home after treatment sessions. In private or clinical settings, parents may be present; however, they may still expect the session to be conducted mainly or exclusively with the child. They may view their role in the child's therapy as being limited, and they may expect that the therapist will do most of the work. To optimize success in treatment, parents must be supportive of the child, and to do this, they must have a thorough understanding of the nature of stuttering and of the goals of therapy.

One of the key tasks that clinicians must perform when working with parents of children who stutter is educating them about the disorder and about therapy in general. We have found it helpful to begin this task by presenting to the parents the basic structure of the WHO's ICF model. The multifaceted ICF framework captures the broad-based essence of the stuttering disorder and helps parents recognize that "stuttering is more than just stuttering" and "therapy for stuttering addresses more than just stuttering." Parents need to understand that goals addressing the child's negative reactions to stuttering, the reactions of people in the child's environment, and the child's participation in daily activities are all part of successful treatment. This stands in contrast to what parents might expect because they might think that they are sending the child to therapy so he or she will "stop stuttering." Of course, minimizing stuttering is a significant part of the therapy program; however, it is only *one part* of that overall approach. The ICF model helps parents understand the broader goals of therapy and helps them see the justification for why the clinician is doing what he or she is doing in therapy.

Just as was seen with educating peers and teachers, however, the best person to educate parents about the nature of stuttering is actually the child who stutters. Helping the child educate his parents teaches him valuable lessons about how to talk openly about stuttering, empowers him to make changes in his own personal environment, and helps parents learn that stuttering does not have to hold the child back in his life. Initiating this dialogue between the child and parents can be done in much the same way as was suggested earlier for the dialogue between the child and teachers. Often, it will be the clinician who initiates the process, but then, the child must be supported in telling his parents what he wants them to know. Examples of the types of messages children might provide include suggestions about what helps him communicate more easily (and what does not), descriptions about what it feels like to stutter, explanations about treatment strategies and why

they are difficult to use all of the time, and so on. The purpose of this dialogue is not for the parents to tell the child about stuttering. Rather, the reverse is true. The child is the expert about his speech, so it is the child who must tell the parents about stuttering.

Unfortunately, not all parents will be open to such a dialogue, so it may be necessary for the clinician to be more directly involved in educating the parents about stuttering. Some parents may cling to the idea that the child should be able to overcome stuttering if he or she only tries hard enough. Although it is understandable that parents might have a hard time accepting stuttering, such unrealistic pressures can be detrimental to the child's attempts to come to terms with his or her speaking difficulties. We have found that at such times, participation in self-help and support groups (e.g., the NSA and Friends) can help. Just as self-help groups can help children come to terms with their stuttering, self-help groups can also help parents learn that stuttering does not have to prevent their children from doing the things they want to do in their life (Yaruss, Quesal, & Reeves, 2007). This is where the primary concern often lies: the parent is worried that stuttering may "ruin" the child's life, and so the parent clings to the hope that the child will somehow just stop stuttering. Seeing that the child can be okay even if he or she does continue to stutter can help the parents reduce their anxiety. Ultimately, this will help them become more active and more supportive participants in the therapy process.

Video Clip 7 includes a review of using the tense fist as an analogy for speech tension and easing out of tension. In this example, the child teaches his mother about the tense fist and then moves to modeling pullout, using pseudostutters, and reviewing where the physical tension is.

Another factor that helps parents reduce their concerns is seeing their children succeed in the things they want to do, such as talking to friends and participating at school. As children become more skilled at using techniques and more accepting of their stuttering, the parents will see that the children will indeed be okay. Clinicians must help children move their therapy strategies out of the clinic and into everyday, real-world experiences so the parents can see the changes that the children are making. Ultimately, this is what helps to minimize the negative impact of stuttering on the child's life, in terms of limitations in daily activities and restriction in participation, and this is the final component of therapy that we will discuss in this chapter.

MINIMIZING ACTIVITY LIMITATION AND PARTICIPATION RESTRICTION

The overall goal of treatment is to help the child minimize the negative impact associated with stuttering, and many of the treatment strategies described earlier have already helped to accomplish this. The child has learned ways of minimizing the stuttering impairment by enhancing fluency and changing stuttering through modifications to timing and tension. The child has reduced anxiety and fear; tension, struggle, and avoidance; negative attitudes; and other affective, behavioral, and cognitive reactions through desensitization and cognitive restructuring. The child has learned to minimize the negative influences of the environment by educating parents, teachers, and peers about stuttering. And, finally, the child has learned that stuttering does not have to hold him or her back in life. All of these changes make it more likely that the child will take part in daily activities and participate in life events, regardless of the fact that he or she stutters.

The clinician can do even more to help the child minimize the negative impact of stuttering by working to ensure that the child is able to *use* the techniques that he or she has learned in therapy in a variety of real-life situations. In other words, the key to minimizing negative impact is increasing *generalization*. Unfortunately, generalization can be challenging. Many authors have written about the difficulties people face in generalizing their skills out of the therapy room, and many programmatic therapy approaches incorporate detailed generalization strategies to assist with this (Hillis & McHugh, 1998; Ingham, 1999; Ryan, 1974). Unless generalization is achieved, the outcomes of therapy are in doubt. Fluency within the confines of the therapy room is nice, but fluency *only* within the confines of the therapy room is useless. Likewise, acceptance, the ability to speak freely, the ability to manage tension, and other treatment gains are useless if they are limited to the safety of a single (admittedly artificial) location. Therefore, the clinician has to help the child move these skills out of the therapy room.

The classroom and school are among the most important settings in a child's life, so school-based clinicians would seem to have an advantage in helping the child with generalization. Due to the size of their caseloads and the need to work with children in groups, however, many school-based clinicians find it difficult to work outside of the therapy room. Clinicians in private or clinical settings may be better able to work with children individually, although they may also find themselves in more isolated settings, where the "real world" is far away. The clinician can arrange "field trips" (Reardon-Reeves & Yaruss, 2004; Yaruss & Reeves, 2003), such as meetings at a mall or other locations, but even so, the situations are contrived and different from the child's everyday experience. Ultimately, the child will have to work on his own to bring therapy gains into the real world. The clinician can support the child in doing this, but in the end, the child must bridge that gap.

Clinicians can foster generalization by relying on the principles of the hierarchy and desensitization described earlier. One reason children have difficulty using therapy techniques outside of the therapy room is that the techniques are uncomfortable to use. Although the techniques help the child speak more fluently, they also stand out and sound different from the child's normal speech (and from the speech of other children). Through a process of gradual desensitization, children can become more comfortable with their new speaking methods in situations outside of the therapy room.

One way we have helped our students improve generalization is through an activity we call the "generalization scavenger hunt." In this activity, the clinician works with the child to create a list of all of the key situations he or she faces in a typical day. Examples include talking to parents and siblings at home in the morning before going to school, talking with friends while waiting for the bus and riding it to school, talking with teachers in various classes throughout the day, talking with friends in classroom and social settings at school, talking with coaches or other teachers in extracurricular activities, talking with friends in social settings outside of school, and more. Each child's list of speaking situations will differ, so the clinician will have to work with each child to create an individualized list of situations. Next, the child ranks the situations from easier to harder to create a hierarchy. Only the child knows which situations are easier and which situations are harder for him, so the clinician will need to work with the child to set up this activity. Finally, the clinician can help the child turn this list of situations into a grid, listing the situations in the rows and the primary speech therapy techniques the child is practicing in the columns. (We create this grid in a spreadsheet or word processing program so the list can be sorted in the order the situations occur during the day or in order of the child's hierarchy.)

To complete the generalization scavenger hunt, the child goes through his day with the scavenger hunt print-out. When the child enters a situation that appears on the list, he chooses to use one of the techniques he needs to practice. Because the situations on his list are sorted in order of difficulty, he can start in easy situations where he is most likely to be successful. Then, as he works toward more difficult situations, he will find that he is able to use techniques and strategies in situations he previously thought were too hard. Note that the child is not required to *always* use the techniques in those situations; he is simply required to demonstrate that he *is able to* do so. This enhances his sense of self-efficacy (Manning, 2001; Ornstein & Manning, 1985) about the techniques and helps desensitize him to using the techniques. As a result, the generalization scavenger hunt increases the likelihood that he will use the techniques in real-world situations. As the child uses his techniques more often, he decreases the negative impact of stuttering on his life, thereby minimizing activity limitation and participation restriction.

Video Clip 8 shows the introduction of the generalization scavenger hunt.

SUMMARY OF TREATMENT COMPONENTS

Together, the components of treatment help the child communicate effectively in all of the situations he or she faces in life. Timing and tension

modifications minimize the impairment, desensitization and cognitive restructuring activities minimize the child's negative reactions, education and empowerment strategies minimize the negative reactions of people in the child's environment, and generalization procedures minimize the negative impact of stuttering. The next two sections of the chapter describe methods the clinicians can use to ensure that the treatment is successful for each individual child who receives the treatment.

ASSESSMENT METHODS

A comprehensive approach to treatment requires a comprehensive approach to assessment. Because stuttering includes features that are more easily measured (e.g., surface disfluency) as well as features that are less easily measured (e.g., reactions to stuttering), we use a variety of assessment techniques. Furthermore, because we base treatment on the ICF, we believe that assessment should also be based on the ICF. It is for this reason that we developed the OASES described earlier; the OASES provides information on the child's perspective of the impairment, reactions, functional communication abilities (which incorporates both activity limitations and environmental influences), and quality of life (which incorporates participation restriction and environmental influences). Numerous other measures can be made as well.

For measures of surface disfluency ("impairment"), various techniques for fluency counts can be used (see reviews in Conture, 2001; Yaruss, 1997b; 1998b), as well as surface severity measures such as the Stuttering Severity Instrument (SSI-4) (Riley, 2009). For assessing reactions, clinicians can use components of the Behavior Assessment Battery for School-Age Children Who Stutter (BAB) (Brutten & Vanryckeghem, 2006). Clinicians can also document reactions through "portfolio-based assessment" procedures (Reardon-Reeves & Yaruss, 2004), including reports from the child, parents, teachers, and others. Paper-and-pencil assessments, such as "Hands Down" (in which the child lists positive and negative attributes) and "Worry Ladder" (in which the child lists "worries" in rank order), can also be used (Chmela & Reardon, 2001), as well as various "Checking

In" questionnaires for children, parents, and teachers (Reardon-Reeves & Yaruss, 2004). Finally, clinicians can use various other measures that are designed specifically for an individual client (see Murphy, Yaruss, & Quesal 2007a; 2007b for a case study example of using a variety of assessments to determine treatment outcomes).

Assessment should be performed throughout the diagnostic and treatment process. Repeated measures not only provide information about the presence and severity of the disorder, but they also provide information that can be used to direct goal writing and treatment planning, to document changes over time, to determine when the child's communication skills are sufficiently improved to warrant dismissal from treatment, and to follow-up with the child after dismissal to ensure that the communication improvements have been maintained. By evaluating the entirety of the child's stuttering disorder, clinicians will be able to ensure that their treatment accomplishes the goal of reducing the negative impact of stuttering on the child's life.

TAILORING THE TREATMENT TO THE INDIVIDUAL CLIENT

The stuttering disorder evolves differently for different children based on a wide variety of factors, including the severity of stuttering, the child's temperament, the child's reactions and the reactions of others in the child's environment, the social penalties that result from stuttering, and numerous other factors. Thus, a "one size fits all" approach cannot address every child's individual experiences. Because the ICF was designed to account for differences between individuals, the resulting treatment can also account for these differences. Clinicians can take advantage of this flexibility to examine the entirety of the disorder, to consider the disorder from the child's perspective, and to adjust treatment to meet each individual child's needs.

To do this effectively, the clinician must be empathetic to the child's experiences. Managing stuttering is not easy, and the more the clinician can understand the child, the more effectively the clinician can help. It takes time to learn about the child's experiences, but that is the foundation of this therapy—the clinician must

become familiar with the child's speech, the child's reactions to stuttering, the ways the child copes with the loss of control that is the essence of stuttering (Perkins, 1990), and the feelings associated with that loss of control.

For example, children who have strongly negative reactions to stuttering need to work on desensitization. For these children, techniques to reduce the tension during stuttering would precede techniques to enhance fluency because it can be difficult to modify timing when the child is already physically tense. Techniques for reducing tension include helping the child explore moments of stuttering, and this has a desensitizing effect. As the child becomes desensitized, he or she will be better able to make changes in timing and tension and speak with less effort. The child may also become more open about stuttering, and this can help the child use techniques such as voluntary stuttering and talking with others about stuttering. Thus, as the child learns to manage the feelings of loss of control associated with stuttering, he or she becomes better able to use fluency skills, such as slowed rate and pausing. Children with less negative reaction to stuttering, on the other hand, are less likely to need desensitization or techniques for reducing tension during stuttering. These children are likely to show more rapid progress in fluency and treatment may only need to focus on fluency skills.

It is also important to consider the reactions of others in the child's environment. For that reason, parents, teachers, siblings, peers, and others may also be included in the treatment process. Parents always play an important role in treatment, but this role will be different for different families. In some families, parents may learn how to make the home a more fluency-facilitating environment. In other families, parents may need to change their attitudes about stuttering to show their child that they are accepting of the child's stuttering. In school, teachers can help the child to use newly learned skills in the classroom (e.g., while reading aloud). Teachers may also assist the child and speech-language pathologist in developing and conducting a classroom presentation about stuttering. Peers can be taught about bullying and teasing and can help to support the child who stutters if he or she is being teased about stuttering.

In sum, the adaptations to treatment are based on the degree to which reactions, tension and struggle, and other affective and cognitive factors interfere with a child's communication. The goal is for children who stutter to feel more confident about their speech so they can say what they want, when they want, without worrying about stuttering, and to improve their overall communication skills so they can achieve success in educational and social endeavors.

APPLICATION TO AN INDIVIDUAL CLIENT

Dean began stuttering when he was approximately 4 years of age and received treatment in a clinical setting between the ages of 6 and 9 years. Following the ICF model, treatment goals were developed to address Dean's (1) stuttering impairment, (2) personal and environmental contextual factors, and (3) activity limitation and participation restriction.

IMPAIRMENT IN BODY FUNCTION

At the onset of treatment, Dean exhibited moderate-to-severe stuttering behaviors (scoring 25 on the SSI-3; Riley, 1994), consisting of part-word repetitions, occasional prolongations, and blocks with moderate physical tension. The impairment level goal was to teach Dean stuttering modification and speech modification strategies to enable him to communicate more easily.

Learning about the Speech System

First, Dean learned about the parts of the body involved in speaking, using diagrams and models to represent the respiratory, phonatory, and articulatory systems. (This can also be done with clay models or using the child's own body as a reference.) These discussions were continued until Dean could demonstrate his own knowledge of the speech mechanism. (*See Video Clip 3*) He then reviewed the relevant systems with his mother to reinforce lessons learned in therapy and to allow the clinician to assess Dean's understanding. Knowledge of the speech mechanism provides the foundation for later discussions about physical tension.

Increasing Awareness of Physical Tension

Next, Dean learned how physical tension builds in the speech mechanism. Initially, large muscle groups, such as legs and arms, were used as examples so Dean could visualize increased and decreased tension. Dean identified higher and lower levels of tension in a discrimination task and then practiced changing his own tension level. Later exercises incorporated finer muscle groups, such as fingers and lips. (*See Video Clip 4*)

To help Dean learn to manage tension, the clinician modeled single words and short phrases, first in a physically tense way, then in a more relaxed way, and finally, in an "in between" way. The clinician then guided Dean to identify the tension in his own body (e.g., by asking, "Did you tense your tongue? What about your cheeks?") until all of the relevant parts of the speech mechanism had been considered. Again, Dean's mother was involved in therapy to reinforce the lessons Dean was learning. At the conclusion of these activities, Dean was able to increase and decrease physical tension at will, both in isolated speech and non-speech activities as well as in structured speaking tasks.

Pseudostuttering

Next, Dean was introduced to pseudostuttering to enhance his understanding of the tension in his speech muscles. In the early stages of therapy, pseudostuttering was used to help Dean learn how he produced different types of disfluencies (e.g., part-word repetitions, prolongations, blocks). This activity also reinforced his ability to manage physical tension and laid the foundation for later desensitization exercises. (*See Video Clip 3*)

Once Dean was able to pseudostutter, the clinician introduced a game in which different disfluency types were printed on strips of paper, folded up, and put in a hat. Then Dean was invited to select one from the hat to determine which type of pseudostutter he would produce. The clinician and Dean took turns choosing whether the pseudostutter would be produced in a tense way, a relaxed way, or an "in between" way. This activity provided another opportunity for Dean to practice modifying tension and to actively participate in decision making about his speech.

Stuttering Modification Strategies

Once Dean mastered techniques for creating and modifying physical tension in nonspeech activities and pseudostuttering, he progressed to "staying in the block." In this activity, Dean was helped to "stay" in a moment of pseudostuttering for longer than normal, so he could think about where he was increasing physical tension. He had already learned how to evaluate physical tension in his speech mechanism, so he was able to quickly sense where he was tensing. Dean drew a picture of his body and colored in darker areas where he felt more tension and lighter areas where he felt less tension. This activity helped him consolidate all he learned about the parts of his body used for speech and how tension varies during stuttered and fluent speech.

Dean then progressed to learning "pull-outs" (Van Riper, 1973) by gradually reducing tension and "sliding out" of a moment of stuttering. With Dean, the term "slide-out" was used instead of the more traditional "pull-out" so that the analogy of "sliding down a slide" could be introduced. This analogy helped him visualize the change in tension as he moved through the stuttered word (see Reardon-Reeves & Yaruss, 1994). Dean first practiced the technique using pseudostuttering in single words. He then moved up a hierarchy, working on two-word phrases provided by the clinician, then two-word phrases that he generated himself, then shorter and longer sentences provided by the clinician, and ultimately, spontaneously generated sentences. Dean found this strategy to be most useful when he was unable to predict a moment of stuttering in advance. When he found himself in the midst of a stutter, he would "catch" himself and then use this stuttering modification technique to minimize tension and continue speaking more easily. (*See Video Clip 3 and 4*)

Speech Modification Strategies

To reinforce the message that the primary goal of treatment is effective communication, stuttering modification techniques were taught *before* speech modifications were introduced.

Improving speech fluency is still an essential component of addressing the stuttering impairment, however, so the following activities were used to help Dean improve his speech fluency by changing timing and tension during both fluent and stuttered speech.

Dean's speech modifications included reducing his speaking rate and increasing pausing at phrase boundaries and between conversation turns, and the clinician used a variety of drill and play activities to give Dean opportunities to practice these changes. These activities were organized along a hierarchy, starting with structured imitation and modeling activities and then moving to reading, clinician-generated sentences, self-generated sentences, and, ultimately, conversational speech. The clinician helped Dean learn that these speech techniques did not need to be used all the time and that he could use them whenever he wanted to enhance his fluency.

Next, the clinician helped Dean combine what he had learned about tension modification with what he had learned about slowing his rate of speech through the use of "easy starts." As noted previously, easy starts involve slightly slowing the speaking rate and reducing tension at the beginning of phrases, where stuttering is most likely to occur. After initiation, the rest of the phrase is produced at a normal rate. To help Dean practice easy starts, he began by reading from a list of short phrases in which the first sound was a nasal, glide, or liquid (because these are among the easiest sounds to produce with this technique). Dean then progressed through increasingly more difficult sounds (fricatives and plosives). As he continued to practice along a hierarchy of increasingly difficult situations, Dean found the easy start technique to be a useful strategy for minimizing the likelihood of stuttering.

When these speech modification strategies were combined with the stuttering modification techniques learned earlier in therapy, Dean was equipped to deal with the stuttering impairment. Nevertheless, there were several additional goals that still needed to be considered, including minimizing negative reactions and ensuring that he was not limited in his daily activities or restricted in his ability to participate in life. (*See Video Clip 1*)

PERSONAL AND ENVIRONMENTAL CONTEXTUAL FACTORS

To minimize negative personal and environmental reactions associated with stuttering, the clinician used activities designed to increase acceptance of stuttering, both by Dean and by people in his environment. This enabled him to feel more comfortable with his speaking abilities so he could communicate effectively, regardless of whether or not he stuttered. This goal was addressed through several related activities.

Personal Contextual Factors

Diagnostic testing, based on a detailed interview and results of an early version of the OASES, revealed that Dean harbored a number of negative affective, behavioral, and cognitive reactions to his stuttering. For example, he indicated that he was helpless to change his speech and that he could not say what he wanted to say because of his stuttering. He stated that he used escape and avoidance behaviors that affected his communication, and he reported that he sometimes used filler words like "uh" or "um" in an effort to try not to stutter. These aspects of stuttering were primarily managed through desensitization activities.

Because Dean exhibited strong fears of stuttering, the clinician helped him engage in desensitization exercises. Earlier in therapy, he had used pseudostuttering as part of his exploration of stuttering. Now, he used pseudostuttering to help him experience speech disruptions without feeling a "loss of control," which, in turn, helped to reduce his fear. One pseudostuttering activity involved playing a board game in which both Dean and the clinician were required to pseudostutter before they could take their turns. In other activities, Dean and the clinician described pictures or told stories using pseudostuttering. To enhance desensitization, Dean and the clinician also took turns to see who could produce the "longest," "highest," "silliest," or "loudest" pseudostutters. As before, Dean approached feared situations gradually, following a hierarchy. Dean's initial goal was to pseudostutter in the therapy room with just the clinician present. After Dean became more comfortable with this, he gradually progressed along his hierarchy until he was able to pseudostutter outside of the therapy room, with other children, with the clinic receptionist, and others.

Together, these activities helped Dean reduce his discomfort with stuttering so he would be less likely to engage in avoidance behaviors.

The clinician also helped Dean engage in cognitive restructuring so he could evaluate his beliefs about stuttering. First, the clinician talked with Dean about his negative thoughts (e.g., that he could not say what he wanted) and helped Dean identify the reasons for those thoughts (e.g., that other people would not listen to him if he stuttered). Next, Dean tested these thoughts (in this case, using pseudostuttering with other people) to see if they were true. Dean found that most people were not concerned about his stuttering, and this helped him develop a new set of beliefs that allowed him to worry less about stuttering so he could speak more freely.

Environmental Contextual Factors

A key contributor to Dean's concerns about stuttering was his perception of how other people viewed his stuttering. Therefore, in addition to helping Dean (re)evaluate his own thoughts about stuttering, therapy involved educating the people in Dean's environment, such as his family and his peers, about the disorder. For example, Dean's mother was frequently invited to treatment so Dean could review with her what he had learned. This reinforced Dean's status as the "expert" about his speech (another strategy that minimizes negative reactions) and ensured that Dean and his mother maintained an open interaction about stuttering. In this way, Dean was able to share his thoughts and feelings about stuttering, and his mother was able to become accepting of Dean's stuttering.

In addition, Dean learned how to respond when others, such as peers, made comments about stuttering. Even though Dean was not experiencing bullying or other inappropriate reactions to his stuttering, he was still fearful that his friends might comment about his speech. Dean was taught that even though he had learned about his speech, his peers still did not know much about stuttering. As a result, it would not be surprising if they asked him questions, such as why he talked differently or why he sometimes couldn't say what he wanted to say. At the start of treatment, Dean thought that these comments would be hurtful, although he quickly learned that there is a difference between inquisitive comments (e.g., "Why do you talk differently?") and comments that are intended to be hurtful (i.e., instances of bullying). Dean learned that he could respond to inquisitive comments by providing information about stuttering. In instances where the comments were hurtful, Dean found that he could still respond in a matter-of-fact manner, with statements such as, "Yes, I stutter. This is just the way I talk." Dean found that it was not just *what* he said, but *how* he said it that made the difference. Using such responses took practice, so he engaged in brainstorming and role-playing activities in therapy so he could successfully respond when other people commented about his speech. (*See Video Clip 8*)

ACTIVITY LIMITATIONS AND PARTICIPATION RESTRICTIONS

Dean's responses on the OASES indicated that he was having difficulty communicating in certain situations at school. For example, he indicated that he was reluctant to read out loud and that he did not always raise his hand to ask or answer questions. Although the desensitization and cognitive restructuring activities described earlier had reduced Dean's avoidance, he still reported having trouble with more difficult situations. To help Dean communicate effectively even in difficult situations, the "generalization scavenger hunt" activity was introduced. Dean and the clinician worked together to create a rank-ordered list of all of the situations he faced on a typical day. These included relatively easy situations such as saying good morning to his mother and talking to his brother at breakfast, as well as harder situations such as reading out loud in class, asking his teacher a question, and introducing himself. He then used this list as a guide while he practiced in different situations. Dean began by using easy starts and pseudostuttering in easier situations, and he used the checklist to keep track of how many times he used each technique. As he continued along the hierarchy, he used strategies in increasingly difficult situations, until he could use all of his techniques in all of his daily situations. In doing so, he found that his fears about "hard" situations had diminished. As a result, the negative impact of stuttering on his communication was greatly diminished, and he found

that he could speak freely in any situation. (*See Video Clip 7*)

SUMMARY

By the end of treatment, Dean had reduced the amount of stuttering in his speech, minimized negative personal and environmental reactions, and reduced activity limitations and participation restrictions. Although he continued to stutter, he had acquired tools that helped him communicate effectively across a variety of situations. He indicated that stuttering no longer kept him from saying what he wanted to say, from participating in school activities, and from interacting with friends. These positive results were confirmed by SSI-3 scores, which indicated that overt stuttering had diminished to "mild-to-moderate," and by responses on the OASES, which confirmed that the overall negative impact of stuttering was significantly reduced.

FUTURE DIRECTIONS

The most pressing need related to this treatment approach is empirical documentation that it is effective in helping children who stutter improve their fluency, minimize negative reactions, and reduce the negative impact of their disorder on communication in daily activities and participation in life. The authors and colleagues have worked toward providing such documentation through the development of a comprehensive measurement instrument for evaluating the entirety of the stuttering disorder, from the perspective of the child who stutters. Empirical research will be needed to address questions about the efficacy of this approach to treatment. Meanwhile, clinicians can draw on the techniques presented here while evaluating the outcomes of their treatment to ensure that they reduce the negative impact of stuttering on the lives of school-age children who stutter.

CHAPTER SUMMARY

- Stuttering is a multifaceted disorder that can affect many aspects of children's lives, including their ability to communicate in key situations and their quality of life.

- Clinicians should treat the entire disorder, as required by the ASHA scope of practice, embodied in the principles of IDEA, and described in the WHO's ICF.
- Treatment can draw on a variety of strategies to address the *impairment* (i.e., the observable stuttering behaviors), the personal and environmental *contextual factors* (including affective, behavioral, and cognitive reactions on the part of the child and people in the child's environment), and *activity limitation and participation restrictions*.
- Minimizing the *impairment* involves changes to timing and tension in speech production. These techniques are straightforward to teach but difficult to use and maintain over time, particularly in more challenging speaking situations.
- Reducing the child's negative *reactions* involves desensitization and cognitive restructuring tasks for helping the child think differently about the problems he or she faces.
- Reducing negative reactions among people in the child's *environment*, including parents, teachers, and peers, involves desensitization and education about the nature of stuttering and stuttering treatment.
- Minimizing *activity limitations and participation restrictions* involves strategies for supporting generalization of treatment gains to real-world situations and ensuring that the child is able to communicate effectively in all of the situations he or she faces.
- Clinicians must document the efficacy of their treatment by collecting data about the entirety of the child's experience of stuttering, before, during, and after treatment. Measures that focus only on the impairment may not adequately reflect the overall changes the child experiences as part of a comprehensive treatment approach.

CHAPTER REVIEW QUESTIONS

1. The *primary* goal of the treatment described in this chapter is:
   (A) stutter-free speech
   (B) speech that contains less than 2% stuttered syllables
   (C) effective communication
   (D) stuttering with less effort
   (E) all of the above

2. The framework on which the treatment is based is the:
   (A) *International Classification of Impairment, Disability, and Handicap*
   (B) *International Classification of Functioning, Disability, and Health*
   (C) *International Classification of Diseases*
   (D) *Diagnostic and Statistical Manual of Mental Disorders*
   (E) none of the above

3. In the treatment described in this chapter, the two primary parameters that are manipulated to help children speak more fluently are:
   (A) timing and tension
   (B) effort and struggle
   (C) rate and timing
   (D) avoidance and postponement
   (E) all of the above

4. The authors of this chapter believe that:
   (A) all children who stutter can achieve normal fluency if given the proper treatment
   (B) some children may continue to stutter in some fashion, even after successful treatment
   (C) if children continue to stutter after treatment, the clinician has not applied the treatment correctly
   (D) A and C
   (E) none of the above

5. The therapy described in this chapter includes strategies to:
   (A) change speech production to enhance fluency and minimize the severity of stuttering
   (B) change communication attitudes to reduce the child's negative reactions to stuttering
   (C) improve communication abilities to ensure that the child can convey his or her message effectively
   (D) reduce the impact of stuttering on the child's overall quality of life
   (E) all of the above

6. Which of the following is *not* an example of an affective reaction to stuttering?
   (A) Embarrassment
   (B) Anxiety and fear
   (C) Shame and guilt
   (D) Struggle
   (E) Anger

7. When a child refuses to read aloud in class, he or she is demonstrating:
   (A) avoidance
   (B) a behavioral reaction to stuttering
   (C) normal disfluency
   (D) A and B
   (E) all of the above

8. The *variability* of stuttering manifests itself primarily:
   (A) between different individuals who stutter
   (B) within a given individual
   (C) from one moment to another
   (D) from one situation to another
   (E) all of the above

9. "Portfolio-based assessment":
   (A) is a means to document change over time
   (B) may include reports from the child who stutters, parents, teacher, and others
   (C) is a standardized assessment procedure
   (D) A and B
   (E) should not be used with children who stutter

10. Which of the following would be used to assess the *impairment* level of the stuttering disorder?
    (A) Fluency counts
    (B) Stuttering Severity Instrument (SSI-4)
    (C) Communication Attitude Test (CAT)
    (D) Overall Assessment of the Speaker's Experience of Stuttering — School-Age (OASES-S)
    (E) A and B

11. Which of the following would ***not*** be a goal to address the *personal and environmental contextual level* of the stuttering disorder?
    (A) Reduce stuttering to less than 2% stuttered syllables
    (B) Desensitize the child to stuttering
    (C) Educate the child so that he or she becomes more accepting of stuttering
    (D) Educate the parents so that they become more accepting of stuttering
    (E) Educate teachers so that they become more accepting of stuttering

12. Within the treatment framework described in this chapter, treatment goals:
    (A) will always be written in all three categories (impairment, activity limitation and participation restriction, and personal and environmental contextual factors) for all children
    (B) may be written in just one or two categories for some children
    (C) may be written in just one or two categories for the same child at different points in therapy
    (D) B and C
    (E) All of the above

13. The most important outcome measure for children who receive this treatment is:
    (A) a reduction in the amount of stuttering
    (B) reduced struggle while stuttering
    (C) reduced postponement and avoidance
    (D) desensitization to stuttering
    (E) There is no single measure—different outcome measures will have differing degrees of relevance for different children.

14. The best method for delivering this treatment is:
    (A) one session per week, in individual sessions
    (B) at least two sessions per week, in individual sessions
    (C) one session per week, in group sessions
    (D) at least two sessions per week, in group sessions
    (E) it is not possible to determine, a priori, the best way to deliver individualized treatment

15. Clinicians who work with children who stutter should:
    (A) learn about stuttering
    (B) become desensitized to stuttering
    (C) learn not to fear stuttering
    (D) learn strategies for managing tension associated with stuttering
    (E) all of the above

SUGGESTED READINGS

Murphy, W., Yaruss, J. S., & Quesal, R. W. (2007). Enhancing treatment for school-age children who stutter. I: Reducing negative reactions through desensitization and cognitive restructuring. *Journal of Fluency Disorders, 32*, 121–138.

Murphy, W., Yaruss, J. S., & Quesal, R. W. (2007). Enhancing treatment for school-age children who stutter. II: Reducing bullying through role-playing and self-disclosure. *Journal of Fluency Disorders, 32,* 139–162.

Reardon-Reeves, N. A., & Yaruss, J. S. (2004). *The Source for Stuttering: Ages 7–18.* East Moline, IL: LinguiSystems.

Yaruss, J. S., & Quesal, R. W. (2004). Stuttering and the International Classification of Functioning, Disability, and Health (ICF): An update. *Journal of Communication Disorders, 37,* 35–52.

Yaruss, J. S. (Ed.) (2002, 2003). Facing the challenge of treating stuttering in the schools (Part I: Selecting goals and strategies for success; Part II: One size does not fit all). *Seminars in Speech and Language, Vol. 23 (3), 24 (1).*

CHAPTER 13

Overview of Treatments for Adults and Adolescents Who Stutter

REBECCA J. McCAULEY AND BARRY E. GUITAR

CHAPTER OUTLINE

INTRODUCTION

The four interventions included in this section are the most varied of those we present. Among the four, there are two behavioral approaches and two controversial interventions that entail the use of a mechanical device and pharmaceutical agents. Interventions for this population are perhaps so varied because stuttering in adults is notoriously resistant to change. This resistance motivates stutterers, and those who would help them, to contemplate a wide range of different interventions, even ones that invite suspicion and skepticism among many clinicians.

Some adults seeking treatment will have never had intervention for their speech problems. Thus, they may know little about how researchers and clinicians view the nature of stuttering and may have had little contact with others who stutter. For them, logical grounds on which to evaluate the quality of an intervention may not be obvious. Moreover, for adults who have not had any treatment, psychological barriers associated with embarrassment or shame can be particularly entrenched.

On the other hand, many adults seeking intervention will have had at least some previous exposure to treatment. For those whose past treatment did not help them or helped only briefly, with subsequent relapse, the act of seeking treatment entails the risk of disappointment and frustration. Consequently, both new and experienced treatment seekers, as well as those

interacting with them as therapists or significant others, may be particularly assisted by this chapter's structured comparisons and by the shared organization of the chapters that follow.

In this overview, we will describe each of the four interventions in turn, using terminology related to the model of treatment described in Chapter 2. Thus we will describe treatment goals, procedures, and activities. We will also summarize the theory or theories on which these treatments are based and the empirical evidence supporting their claims of effectiveness. Finally, we will compare and contrast the interventions.

THE CAMPERDOWN PROGRAM (CHAPTER 14 BY O'BRIAN, PACKMAN, AND ONSLOW)

This approach is intended for adults and, more recently, adolescents who stutter. As authorship of the chapter on the Camperdown Program implies, it has been developed by many of the same researchers and clinicians involved in the Lidcombe Programs for preschoolers (Chapter 7) and for school-age children (Chapter 9). Its basic goal is improvement or elimination of stuttering in typical speaking situations. Intermediate goals consist of clients' learning to (1) control their stuttering using prolonged speech, (2) use rating scales for stuttering severity and speech naturalness, and (3) use problem-solving strategies to help them work toward the generalization of their control of stuttering from clinical to everyday speaking situations. The final intermediate goal consists of clients' accepting responsibility for independent work designed to maintain their control.

The Camperdown Program is implemented in four stages. In the first stage, participants gain experience in using exaggerated prolonged speech and reliably applying rating scales for stuttering severity and naturalness. In the second stage, they explore and adopt aspects of that mode of speaking within the clinic to control stuttering, while maintaining speech naturalness. In the third stage, group sessions provide participants with experience in problem-solving tasks to help them gain skills required for further generalization and maintenance. These stages are followed by the fourth and final one, which entails activities that individual clients plan and execute themselves as a means of maintaining their fluency gains in everyday situations. A manual describing procedures and activities comprising the program is available on the internet.

Although O'Brian and her colleagues characterize the Camperdown Program as atheoretical, they briefly describe their emerging understanding of the causes of stuttering and allude to behavioral methods that form the foundation for the program. They explain that the program has been developed eclectically through the incorporation of elements and procedures taken from treatments previously found to promote fluency in adults who stutter. Therefore, it is not surprising that, in addition to evidence supporting the Camperdown Program itself, they describe evidence for several specific procedural components (e.g., teaching prolonged speech solely by having clients listen to examples from a single speaker).

Evidence provided by the authors of this chapter regarding the Camperdown Program as a whole focuses primarily on a version intended for adults who are seen in individual weekly sessions and day-long group practice sessions (O'Brian et al., 2001). Additional evidence associated with the program's ongoing development is also summarized, including preliminary evidence concerning the use of the program with a small number of adolescents (Hearne, 2006).

Most recently, the Camperdown Program has also been shown to be effective when provided within a telehealth format, in which the individual's use of written, audio, and audiovisual materials is supplemented by weekly or biweekly telephone sessions with the treating speech-language pathologist (O'Brian, Packman, & Onslow, 2008). This type of format is of particular interest in Australia because of the treatment challenges presented by extremely isolated, rural communities.

THE FLUENCY PLUS PROGRAM (CHAPTER 15 BY KROLL AND SCOTT-SULSKI)

The Fluency Plus Program is an intensive treatment intended for adolescents and adults who stutter. It has been developed over a 25-year period by Kroll and his colleagues at the Stuttering Centre of Toronto. Program features that the developers consider unique are the guiding role of research in its development, the emphasis placed on creating a highly structured maintenance component, and the importance attached to initial assessments designed to identify highly motivated potential clients who are most likely to benefit from the program. In fact, the first two of these elements are ones that might also be claimed for the Camperdown Program.

The Fluency Plus Program follows an integrative treatment model that strives for simultaneous effects on communication as well as speech. The program's basic goal is the achievement of the "communication mentality," which is described as "the ability to speak to anyone at any time, in any place, effectively and efficiently, and with little more than a normal amount of negative emotion" (Chapter 15, p. 286). To achieve that goal, clients focus on three intermediate goals: (1) learning to use a style of speech that facilitates fluency, (2) developing skills and attitudes that help them use this controlled speaking style in all social situations, and (3) developing self-directed problem-solving skills and practice routines to support maintenance.

The Fluency Plus Program requires a year-long commitment by its participants. It begins with a 3-week intensive phase comprised of five 4.5-hour sessions per week and 2 to 4 hours of almost daily homework. After the intensive phase, participants undertake 11 months of less frequent clinic sessions, each an hour in length. Once formal participation in the program is ended, clients are encouraged to participate in an ongoing support group made up of program alumni and to return for brief, but intensive refresher courses, which are offered two times a year.

Activities associated with the Fluency Plus Program include highly structured practice of eight fluency-enhancing behaviors (also called "targets"), such as the use of "stretched" syllables. Other activities are designed to promote "cognitive restructuring," in which clients work to change the way they think and feel about stuttering and communication. Speech production and cognitive restructuring activities fall within three overlapping stages described by the authors as: (1) establishment of fluency-facilitating targets, (2) transfer and cognitive restructuring, and (3) maintenance and staying connected.

The theoretical origins of the Fluency Plus Program lie in a conception of stuttering as a condition that is multidimensional in etiology and consists of learned behavioral and emotional responses to maladaptive speech behaviors. As learned behaviors, these maladaptive behaviors and emotions are viewed as open to modification through additional learning. The program's integrated framework draws on fluency shaping and what the authors consider to be stuttering modification procedures to address the core speech behaviors, accessory nonspeech behaviors (e.g., eye blinks), and attitudes and emotions associated with stuttering.

To support the Fluency Plus Program, Kroll and his co-author, Scott-Sulsky, review several kinds of evidence that have been accumulated over the course of the program's 30-year evolution. First, they begin by discussing evidence obtained for a highly structured and intensive (3-week long) behavioral therapy developed by Webster (1974). A retrospective study by Leibovitz and Kroll (1980), as well as an earlier pre- and posttreatment design (Woolf, 1967), suggested good effects of behavioral treatments on outcomes related to fluency and attitudes toward speaking, respectively; however, concerns that relapses were frequent and significant led to further studies. These studies (Kroll, Gaulin, & Tammsalu, 1981) showed that, despite some reduction over time, gains in fluency and attitudes remained well above pretreatment levels 1 to 2 years after participation.

Based on research and their clinical experience with clients, Kroll and his colleagues modified

the intensive part of the program to incorporate cognitive restructuring activities. These were designed to keep clients from returning to negative attitudes while they continue to develop behavioral strategies for avoiding relapse. In addition, Kroll and his colleagues incorporated maintenance activities over a 1-year period during which clients met less and less frequently, thus allowing them to gradually accustom themselves to independent work on their fluency and attitudes. Recent research conducted by this group (De Nil & Kroll, 1995; De Nil et al., 2003) have suggested that dramatic improvements in fluency during intensive treatment can be continued, with regression limited to 5% to 20% of participants when examined 1 to 2 years later.

A series of longitudinal neuroimaging studies (De Nil et al., 2003; Kroll & De Nil, 2000; Kroll, De Nil, & Houle, 1999) provided a novel form of evidence suggesting how brain activity changes during effective intervention and maintenance, thus providing clues that may highlight the key elements and biologic mechanisms of effective treatment. These researchers used positron emission tomography (PET) to examine brain activity during three verbal tasks (i.e., silent and oral reading, and verb generation) performed by a group of 13 stutterers at the following three points in time: before, immediately after, and 1 year after the 3-week intensive portion of the program (i.e., at the end of formal maintenance activities). In addition, the researchers compared these results to those obtained by a group of 10 individuals with normal fluency.

In these studies (De Nil et al., 2003; Kroll & De Nil, 2000; Kroll, De Nil, & Houle, 1999), stutterers showed high levels of brain activity (compared to nonstutterers) for the oral tasks before intensive treatment, relative to the nonstuttering individuals. These increased activity levels were thought to reflect relatively increased effort during speech. At the end of the intensive treatment, although the stutterers continued to show increased levels of activation, they showed greater activation in the left hemisphere. The researchers interpreted this greater activation as consistent with effortful use of the fluency-monitoring behaviors targeted in treatment. Approximately 1 year later, at the end of the 1-year period of maintenance activities, the activation patterns of the treated stutterers more closely approximated those of the nonstutterers. These findings were preliminarily interpreted as suggesting that decreasing cognitive resources were required for fluent speech because of ongoing independent fluency maintenance activities by the treated stutterers. Although only individuals who had been successfully treated (as defined in terms of measures of stuttering and attitudes) were studied, the authors noted the potential value of examining brain activity in individuals who fail to maintain their fluency.

Adding measures obtained through neuroimaging as supplementary outcome measures represents an exciting direction for treatment research because it allows researchers to go beyond providing simple support for the use of the treatment with individuals similar to study participants. Such outcome measures may shed light on the importance of specific treatment components and on the brain mechanisms underlying success in individuals who are able to maintain fluency, despite their continuing potential for stuttering. Further research that includes *unsuccessfully* treated individuals and *successfully* treated individuals who subsequently relapse after varying lengths of time may provide additional insights that can help clinicians tailor treatment selection to individual needs. Increasing the number of points in time at which the neurophysiologic correlates of treatment are examined also seems likely to prove beneficial, for example, by providing data that could constrain and therefore clarify interpretations of group differences. Such rich information would be particularly welcome given the rarity of complete and long-lasting recovery from stuttering in adults.

THE SPEECHEASY DIGITAL FLUENCY AID (CHAPTER 16 BY RAMIG, ELLIS, AND RYAN)

The SpeechEasy represents one of two stuttering interventions described in this book that incorporates nonbehavioral methods. The SpeechEasy is a hearing aid–like device that is available in three versions (in-the-ear-canal, behind-the-ear, and completely-in-the-canal). Each alters the frequency characteristics of the user's speech online and then plays it back to the user at a slight delay through the device. Thus, the device uses both delayed auditory feedback and frequency altered

feedback as its principal therapeutic manipulation. The SpeechEasy is often, but not always, used in combination with behavioral methods. This chapter is particularly valuable because the authors articulately discuss behavioral methods that should be combined with its use and do so from the independent perspective that may come more easily to authors who were not directly involved in its development.

The SpeechEasy is primarily intended to be used by adults but has sometimes been used with children. The manufacturer, the Janus Development Group, recommends use with children 10 years and older, under the assumption that at about that age, children can understand the nature of stuttering and therefore be able to understand how the device may be useful. Ramig and his coauthors stress that both they and the device's manufacturer recommend that it be considered only after the child has had an opportunity to participate in more traditional approaches. At least in part, this is because regardless of age, candidates with a previous history of behavioral treatment are considered more likely to be successful users. This may be because they are more likely to have had experience in altering their speech patterns in ways that may not only increase fluency, but also render the device more effective, such as using more sustained voicing as they speak.

Ramig and his coauthors advance two related rationales for the SpeechEasy. In the first, they tie the etiology of stuttering to abnormalities in auditory processing for speech production, thus providing a reason to view the modification of stutterers' auditory input during speech as a way of bypassing ingrained but disadvantageous processing patterns. As a second rationale, they point out results showing positive effects of altered auditory feedback on stuttering from studies predating the development of the SpeechEasy. Because several kinds of altered auditory feedback (delayed, frequency-altered, etc.) have been shown to provide fluency benefits in some stutterers (Armson & Stuart, 1998; Curlee & Perkins, 1973), the developers of the SpeechEasy decided to design their device so that it incorporates both a time delay and frequency alterations.

Unfortunately, much of the empirical support for the SpeechEasy has been obtained by the research group that created it, in association with the device's manufacturer. This research support came from studies showing benefits of Speech-Easy use for groups of stutterers across different situations, such as different audience sizes and speech tasks (e.g., scripted telephone calls). The "in-house" nature of this research, however, has led to severe criticism of the investigators and of the device (Finn, Bothe, & Bramlett, 2005). Finn and his colleagues went so far as to accuse the researchers of practicing "pseudoscience," an accusation at least in part associated with the difficulties all researchers have in controlling even unconscious bias (Dollaghan, 2007).

Ramig and his colleagues (Pollard et al., 2007) have been responsible for an independent report showing variable outcomes for participants using the SpeechEasy over a 4-month period. In their chapter in this book, Ramig and his colleagues argue that, in studies using altered auditory feedback during speech, individual variability in response to intervention has been the rule rather than the exception, thus making it quite understandable that the device would be less effective for some potential users than others. Furthermore, they cite reports that users incongruously express satisfaction with the device even as its effects on their stuttering wane (Molt, 2006; Runyan, Runyan, & Hibbard, 2006). Because of these equivocal findings, Ramig and his colleagues call for further research designed to identify *which* potential users would be most likely to experience benefits that include generalization to natural speaking situations as well as to examine the effects of continued use for periods longer than those studied thus far. Questions to be asked include the following: Do long-term users experience adaptation and loss of the benefits? Do they experience carryover of benefits when not wearing the device?

As was the case with the Fluency Plus Program, researchers interested in SpeechEasy have begun to explore hypotheses about the neurophysiology that may underlie fluency gains resulting from this treatment using contemporary neuroimaging techniques. In contrast to expectations held for the Fluency Plus Program, however, changes in brain function with the SpeechEasy are hypothesized to be limited to instances when the device is actually being used, rather than to enduring changes caused by the intervention.

Ramig and his colleagues describe research that makes use of neuroimaging (e.g., Foundas et al.,

2004) to suggest how the SpeechEasy may work. During comparisons of neurophysiology under normal listening conditions versus listening conditions that are somewhat similar to those produced by the device, areas of the brain involved in auditory processing seem to be among those most affected. This finding provides indirect support for the developers' hypotheses about how the device would produce beneficial effects. Examination of brain behavior during use of the device itself is precluded because metal devices may not be worn during any kind of magnetic resonance imaging.

PHARMACOLOGIC TREATMENT OF STUTTERING (CHAPTER 17 BY MAGUIRE, RILEY, FRANKLIN, AND GUMUSANELI)

How many stutterers have wished for a magic pill that would free them from their speaking difficulties? In Chapter 17, Maguire, Riley, Franklin, and Gumusaneli describe several drugs—none of them a magic pill—that have been used experimentally to ameliorate stuttering and its effects in relatively small groups of stutterers. In their introduction, the authors anticipate that drugs are likely to prove most useful when accompanied by behavioral interventions, as has been observed in drug therapies for the treatment of psychiatric disorders (Simon et al., 2006; Kim, 1996). In addition, they suggest that social phobia, which can be a particularly challenging concomitant to stuttering (Stein, Baird, & Walker, 1996), may be another appropriate target of drug therapy for individuals who stutter.

As would be expected, the use of drugs in the treatment of any disorder is a medical issue. Therefore, decision making about such treatment for stuttering necessitates that the stutterer work with a neurologist or psychiatrist, the physicians likely to be most familiar with the classes of drugs currently considered for stuttering. Ideally, a speech-language pathologist would also be part of the clinical team. In fact, the first two authors of this chapter comprise such a psychiatrist–speech-language pathologist team.

Medical recommendations, such as those related to dosage and continued use, are the responsibility of the physician, with advisory input provided by other professionals, such as the speech-language pathologist. Even for clients not interested in the use of drugs to address their stuttering, a physician who is knowledgeable about drugs and stuttering may be a valuable resource to warn about drugs that exacerbate stuttering. Within the team approach, the speech-language pathologist is responsible for the measurement of behavioral outcomes and pursuit of additional, behavioral treatment strategies and activities designed to address continuing negative attitudes. Maguire and his colleagues suggest a range of outcome measures, including observations by family members about stuttering severity. The authors further propose that a 30% reduction in any of the measures should be viewed as clinically significant.

Despite the expectation that drug therapies would rarely, if ever, be used alone as a treatment for stuttering, the authors focus their attention on the rationales, procedures, and evidence for interventions in which a pharmacologic agent *is* the sole treatment. This narrow focus is appropriate as an initial step in determining whether an intervention should be used at all, particularly in the case of an intervention that might be expected to have serious drawbacks as well as benefits.

In principle, pharmacologic interventions may seem especially desirable because they apparently require lower amounts of effort and commitment from the client than behavioral interventions alone. Nonetheless, the possibility of side effects associated with any drug, especially those designed to affect the function of the brain, necessitate an even more careful consideration of risks and benefits before selection than the other interventions discussed in this volume.

Hypotheses about which drugs to consider for use in stuttering have largely been based on emerging information about differences in the brain structure and function of stutterers. In particular, hypotheses are based on inferences about the role of neurotransmitters in stuttering and on a model of the neurologic bases of stuttering. This model postulates that two sets of structures are primarily responsible for planning and executing movement: the medial and lateral premotor systems (Alm, 2004; Goldberg, 1985; Nudelman et al., 1992).

Dopamine, a neurotransmitter known to act on the *medial* premotor system, has been shown in some studies to play a role in exacerbating

stuttering (Maguire et al., 2000b). The medial premotor system is thought to encompass the basal ganglia (particularly an area called the striatum) as well as the supplementary motor cortex and to affect movement planning and initiation during more automatic speech production. In contrast, the *lateral* premotor system is thought to affect movement planning and initiation during deliberate and attention-intensive speech production—conditions for speaking that involve greater use of sensory feedback (both auditory and somatosensory). Importantly, these conditions are central to stuttering interventions such as choral reading, role playing, and speaking in time to a metronome feedback (Alm, 2005). The lateral premotor system is comprised of the lateral premotor cortex and the cerebellum.

According to the authors, because the neurotransmitter dopamine plays an influential role in the function of the medial premotor system, drugs that reduce its activity have received the most research attention for use in stuttering. Another support for use of such drugs is their effectiveness in reducing the symptoms of Tourette's syndrome—a disorder that, the authors note, shares certain developmental, environmental, and genetic factors with stuttering.

In their review of the evidence, Maguire and colleagues focus on research for two drugs whose effects include the direct reduction of dopamine activity—risperidone and olanzapine. These two drugs are related to other drugs that had previously been used to treat schizophrenia and had been shown to reduce stuttering (e.g., haloperidol); hence, they are termed second-generation antipsychotics. This newer class of antipsychotic drugs was designed in the hopes of avoiding serious side effects that had often made the use of the older drugs untenable.

Maguire and his colleagues reviewed a randomized controlled trial from their own laboratory (Maguire et al., 2000a) that they considered as providing the best evidence at the time of publication examining the effects of drug treatment on stuttering. The study lasted 6 weeks and tracked the stuttering severity of 12 men and 4 women who stuttered while they were taking risperidone or a placebo. Neither the participants nor the evaluators knew whether risperidone or the placebo was being taken; thus, the study incorporated the elements of double blinding and random assignment to groups, which are both design features that are seen as hallmarks of quality in treatment studies (Dollaghan, 2007). Four measures of stuttering severity were used (i.e. percent syllables stuttered [%SS], duration of longest stutter, percentage of total speaking time that was stuttered [TS%], and performance on the Stuttering Severity Instrument–Third Edition [SSI-3]) (Riley, 1994). In addition, data were also obtained for measures of compliance and measures of extraneous movement abnormalities and other potential side effects.

After 6 weeks of treatment, results of Maguire et al. (2000a) showed levels of stuttering severity for the participants receiving risperidone that were significantly lower than those for the placebo group at the same point in time. In addition, the posttreatment stuttering severity for the treated participants was significantly lower than their own baseline levels. These positive findings were made for three of the four measures of stuttering severity (i.e., %SS, %TS, and overall results on the SSI-3). Side effects of risperidone consisted of sleepiness in several participants and hormonal effects in one of the female participants. The hormonal effects experienced by this participant included a disruption in her menstrual cycle and secretion of breast milk—an unpleasant side effect that ended after the medication was stopped. The absence of movement abnormalities that had been reported in earlier antipsychotics used in stuttering was seen as particularly advantageous.

In their chapter, Maguire and his colleagues also report on a study of a second drug in the same class as risperidone, namely, olanzapine (Maguire et al., 2004). Olanzapine, which affects a broader range of neurotransmitters than risperidone, was selected for study in part as a means of avoiding the unwanted hormonal effects of risperidone. In their 2004 report, Maguire et al. looked at olanzapine's effects on 23 stutterers over 12 weeks. Double blinding and most of the other methods used in the study of risperidone (Maguire et al., 2000a) were followed in the study of olanzapine. Stuttering severity was examined using the SSI-3 and two additional measures—one completed by the clinician and the other examining participants' perceptions of their own stuttering severity, locus of control, and avoidance behaviors. Potential movement side effects

and side effects related to blood glucose levels were also tracked.

Improvements in stuttering severity in Maguire et al. (2004) were significantly greater in the treated versus the placebo groups on all three stuttering measures, although effect sizes were not reported. Movement, hormonal, and potential metabolic side effects appeared to have been avoided, but sleepiness and an average weight gain of approximately 8 pounds were reported. Perhaps the most naturalistic demonstration of participant satisfaction reported in this chapter was the authors' report that all 23 participants decided to continue taking olanzapine after the study ended. Despite its positive results and low level of side effects reported, the authors of the chapter acknowledged the study's small sample size and warned about the need for continued studies of the risks and benefits associated with use of this drug for stuttering.

In the section of this chapter that may pose the most difficult reading challenge for those of us who are less familiar with pharmacologic terminology, Maguire and colleagues discuss the potential for drugs (e.g., pagoclone) that provide an indirect attack on the excessive dopamine levels associated with stuttering. Specifically, these drugs should work as follows. Rather than addressing dopamine levels directly, drugs such as pagoclone seem to work as an *agonist* (or, you might say, ally) to gamma-aminobutyric acid (GABA), a neurotransmitter thought to reduce the activity of dopaminergic cells (i.e., dopamine-producing cells). Thus, pagoclone does not work *directly* against dopamine *after* it is produced; instead, it works *indirectly* by keeping dopamine from *being* produced, thereby potentially having a beneficial effect while at the same time avoiding some of the side effects associated with drugs that work as *antagonists* to dopamine (or, you might say, blocking agents to dopamine).

In their chapter, the authors describe a particularly large study of pagoclone (Maguire et al., in submission). In this study, 132 participants from several centers were studied in an 8-week research project that incorporated placebo, double blinding, and random assignment to groups. The authors reported on five outcome measures addressing stuttering behavior, speech naturalness, social anxiety, and perceptions of stuttering by the client and clinician. The preliminary outcomes on all five measures suggested improvements for the participants taking pagoclone. Especially notable were the findings related to reduced social anxiety and improved speech naturalness. Initial data also suggested that side effects were infrequent and relatively minor (primarily headache and fatigue).

Like the studies of SpeechEasy, studies of drug therapies have been roundly criticized for a lack of rigor (Bothe et al., 2006). In addition, the review detailed in this chapter might also be criticized for its exclusive focus on studies from the authors' laboratory. To their credit, however, the authors acknowledge the seriousness of the risks associated with pharmacologic interventions for stuttering while at the same time attempting to point the way forward for newer drug interventions based on relatively rigorous studies.

In their discussion of future directions for research, the authors note the need for longer randomized controlled trials using larger groups of participants to provide clearer estimates of risks and benefits. More controversially, they suggest that drug interventions might eventually be used with adolescents and children, while also admitting that U.S. Food and Drug Administration approval has not yet been given for its use in treating stuttering in adults. They express optimism that pagoclone may receive such approval based on the study they described in this chapter.

COMPARISON

As we indicated at the outset of this chapter, the four stuttering interventions for adults that we have included in this volume incorporate both more traditional and highly unconventional tools for battling persistent stuttering. Table 13.1 is intended to help readers appreciate the variety of these tools.

Use of SpeechEasy and drug interventions may strike some readers as a desperate, even fool hardy, undertaking. For most of the adults who might choose them, however, they can be seen as complementary to behavioral interventions. For some adults who choose them, they may be preferred as alternative and sole avenues of intervention simply because they are not behavioral in nature and are therefore simpler to implement.

Both SpeechEasy and drug intervention for stuttering have engendered heated criticism and even condemnation by thoughtful researchers and clinicians who fear their negative impact. Nevertheless, such interventions may provide a few different benefits. The most obvious and, of course, most immediately exciting benefit would when a stutterer believes his or her fluency is enhanced through their use—either when used alone or in combination with behavioral interventions. Another potential benefit of such controversial interventions, however, might derive from studies designed to prove their efficacy and elucidate the mechanisms by which they work. Specifically, such studies may contribute to our understanding of the lower level physiologic mechanisms that maintain stuttering in adults and that, therefore, might be used to undermine its chronicity.

Examination of the two traditional interventions included in this section, the Camperdown Program and Fluency Plus Program, highlights at least one treatment element that may be particularly valuable or even crucial for this population. That element consists of a focus on having clients become active agents in the maintenance of fluency gains. Although it has always been implied that adults who stutter will need to remember to use the speech techniques they have been taught in treatment, it is the idea that that is very unlikely to happen without concerted lifelong and intermittently supported effort on the part of the individual that is emphasized. In fact, in all four of the interventions in this section, at least periodic contact with knowledgeable professionals is assumed as necessary.

Both of the behavioral interventions incorporate fluency shaping techniques built on principles of behavior modification. In addition, the Fluency Plus Program indicates that it incorporates cognitive restructuring designed to help clients deal with fear and anxiety as well as cope with avoidance behavior. However, the foundation of each program appears to be learning fluency skills derived from "prolonged speech," which was used as a treatment for stuttering more than 40 years ago (Goldiamond, 1965; Webster & Lubker, 1968). Fluency skills focus on preventing stuttering rather than unlearning the maladaptive conditioned tension, escape, and avoidance responses that characterize chronic stuttering in adults (Guitar, 2006). Research suggests that although some adults can

Table 13.1. *Characteristics of Interventions for Adults and Adolescents Who Stutter*

Characteristics		Treatment		
	Chapter 14: The Camperdown Program	Chapter 15: The Fluency Plus Program	Chapter 16: The SpeechEasy Device	Chapter 17: Pharmacologic Interventions
Nature of Goal	To eliminate or significantly reduce stuttering in everyday speech situations	To be able to communicate effectively and efficiently in all situations and with minimally affected emotions and attitudes	To support fluency in everyday speaking situations through alteration of auditory feedback	To alter brain chemistry in a way that enhances fluency
Client Population	Primarily adults who stutter, but also, more recently, adolescents who stutter	Primarily adults who stutter and are willing to accept responsibility for their progress in the program and later maintenance of fluency	Adults and teenagers, ideally those with previous treatment for their stuttering	Adults
Intervention Agents	Initially speech-language pathologists lead individual and group activities, with clients assuming greater responsibilities in later stages of the intervention	Speech-language pathologists who gradually relinquish responsibility to clients, with clients playing a significant role in their own treatment	Speech-language pathologists fit the device and work with the user; audiologists provide hearing testing and ear mold preparations, as well as consultation with the speech-language pathologist	Neurologists and/or psychiatrists with knowledge of drugs that might be considered for use; psychiatrists may also contribute special expertise in cognitive behavioral therapy; speech-language pathologists who monitor behavioral outcomes and provide behavioral intervention
Nature of Session	Early sessions involve modeling and instruction in prolonged speech and ratings of fluency and naturalness; later sessions involve problem solving and client's taking responsibility for maintenance	Early intensive sessions involve highly structured practice of fluency-enhancing behaviors as well as group counseling related to cognitive restructuring goals; later sessions involve transfer of fluency goals into everyday situations	Individual informational and counseling sessions	Individual meetings to discuss decisions about pharmaceutical intervention and provide subsequent monitoring of physical and behavioral effects
Demands for Technology	Copy of prolonged speech recording and means of playing it (either audio or audiovisual) and an individual	Video and audio recording and playback equipment; voice onset biofeedback device;	In addition to the device itself, audiologic equipment is used for hearing evaluation and ear mold preparation	Laboratory equipment used in medical monitoring of potential side effects by the

Table 13.1. *Characteristics of Interventions for Adults and Adolescents Who Stutter* (Continued)

Characteristics	Chapter 14: The Camperdown Program	Chapter 15: The Fluency Plus Program	Chapter 16: The SpeechEasy Device	Chapter 17: Pharmacologic Interventions
	recording device for self-evaluations	Dr. Fluency computer software		physician member of the intervention team
Frequency of Sessions	Initially developed using a combination of individual weekly sessions and one intensive group session	Three weeks of intensive sessions for 5 hours a day/5 days a week followed by an 11-month series of maintenance sessions planned to shift from biweekly to monthly to bimonthly in frequency (from once every other week, to once a month, to once every other month)	A minimum of two sessions—one for evaluation and the other when the custom-made device arrives from the manufacturer; in addition, ongoing behavioral treatment is recommended in conjunction with use of the device	Initial weekly assessment visits during baseline and placebo/medication periods (8 to 24 weeks); subsequent follow-up visits to monitor treatment and side effects
Overall Duration of Treatment	Variable; one example in the chapter shows approximately 13 weeks plus 6 months of decreasing frequency of sessions during maintenance	One year, including 3 weeks of intensive treatment and 11 months nonintensive maintenance	Variable, depending on the client's needs; however, the authors suggest that the benefits of the device are likely to be limited to when it is worn, so in some sense, the overall duration is underdetermined	Variable, depending on the client's needs and risks for potential side effects
General Characterization of Methods	Behavioral methods with individual clients imitating a single exemplar of prolonged speech to establish fluency; once fluency is achieved, clients modify their speech to achieve fluency and naturalness goals	Behavioral methods are used to foster fluency, whereas cognitive methods are used to help improve communication attitudes	Instructional sessions inform clients about use and limitations of the device; ongoing behavioral treatment fosters maintenance of phonation during stuttering so the device can alter feedback from the voice signal	Medical testing and history taking associated with drug prescription performed by the physician associated with the team; monitoring of outcomes and implementation of behavioral intervention, as considered appropriate, by the speech-language pathologist

maintain fluency after learning and generalizing fluency skills, most do not (Guitar, 1976; Guitar & Bass, 1978). Although the reasons for relapse after fluency skills training are not precisely known, it might be hypothesized that unlearning the maladaptive responses to the experience of stuttering (rather than only trying to prevent stuttering) could be an important component of treatment. Voluntary stuttering and other methods of desensitizing the client to the experience of stuttering may be testable, valuable adjuncts to the fluency skills and cognitive restructuring in the two behavioral interventions described.

Unique features of each of these two interventions may also suggest differences deserving wider investigation. For example, researchers associated with the Camperdown Program have explored modifications in program delivery making use of features associated with telehealth. This type of service delivery may increase the attractiveness and accessibility of treatment among adults who live in geographically isolated areas or are otherwise unable to take advantage of center-based interventions. Although its efficiency does not yet support this notion, it would also appear to address the problem of shortages of speech-language pathologists who feel competent to practice in the area of fluency disorders (O'Brian, Packman, & Onslow, 2008).

Two sets of authors—those associated with the Fluency Plus Program and those with pharmacologic intervention for stuttering—point to the potential value of cognitive therapy techniques in treatment as important aspects of the stuttering problem. Given the preeminence of cognitive behavioral therapy (Beck, 1995) in current psychological and psychiatric interventions, more explicit incorporation of these methods in stuttering treatments seems timely and worth more explicit investigation. Such methods seem especially well suited for addressing the social limitations that are experienced by stutterers and may also constitute critical barriers to lasting changes in fluency (Guitar, 1976; Guitar & Bass, 1978).

The range of measures used to describe the problem of stuttering and treatment outcomes is yet another aspect of the chapters included in this section warranting the readers' rapt attention. These measures include conventional behavioral measures of stuttering (e.g., %SS), more recently developed tools for examining the social and attitudinal effects of stuttering, and the use of brain imaging tools in the study of treatment efficacy, the underlying mechanisms of treatment, and the disorder itself. Including the entire range of measures offers immense promise for future clients and clinicians, not only by providing a comprehensive picture of what is helped by effective treatments, but also by providing critical insights into how effective interventions (regardless of their surface characteristics) work. Such insights could lead to further refinements in traditional approaches that will produce more rapid and enduring changes in the speech and social lives of stutterers. In addition, they may contribute to rendering controversial interventions more rigorously tested, better understood, and available for thoughtful adoption in appropriate circumstances.

CHAPTER 14

The Camperdown Program

Sᴜᴇ O'Bʀɪᴀɴ, Aɴɴ Pᴀᴄᴋᴍᴀɴ, ᴀɴᴅ Mᴀʀᴋ Oɴsʟᴏᴡ

KEY TERMS

Exemplar recording: an audio or audiovisual recording of the first three sentences of the Rainbow Passage (Fairbanks, 1960) spoken with exaggerated prolonged speech by author Mark Onslow.

Fluency cycle: a three-stage procedure where the client (1) practices the technique of prolonged speech in an exaggerated manner, then (2) practices speaking using whatever features of this pattern he or she needs to eliminate stuttering while sounding as natural as possible, and finally (3) listens to a recording of this speech to assess the presence and severity of any stuttering and how natural the speech sounded (see Fig. 14.2).

Self-evaluation: a process in which clients routinely evaluate their speech, within and outside the clinic environment, for how much stuttering is present and how normal the stutter-free speech sounds.

Severity rating (SR) scale: a 9-point equal-interval perceptual rating scale that quantifies the severity of stuttering. In this scale, 1 = no

stuttering; 2 = very mild stuttering, and 9 = extremely severe stuttering.

Speech naturalness (NAT) rating scale: a 9-point equal-interval perceptual rating scale that quantifies how natural stutter-free speech sounds. In this scale, 1 = natural-sounding speech and 9 = extremely unnatural-sounding speech.

Speech restructuring: any treatment technique that requires the client to change the way he or she speaks in order to eliminate stuttering. Examples would include prolonged speech, smooth speech, and rhythmic speech.

INTRODUCTION

The Camperdown Program is a speech restructuring treatment for adults who stutter. The term **"speech restructuring"** is intended to refer to any treatment that requires the client to learn a novel speech pattern that is incompatible with stuttering. Examples include prolonged speech, smooth speech, and rhythmic speech. In the Camperdown Program, the treatment technique used to control stuttering is prolonged speech. The origins of this technique relate back to the prolonged speech treatment pioneered by Goldiamond (1965) and developed into various treatment regimens by Webster and Lubker (1968), Curlee and Perkins (1969), Ryan (1971), and Ingham and Andrews (1973).

In the Ingham and Andrews (1973) program, the features of prolonged speech—soft contacts, gentle onsets, and continuous vocalization—were taught using a combination of clinician instruction and model tapes. However, in the Camperdown Program, prolonged speech is taught without reference to explicit instruction regarding its features. Instead, clients are instructed to imitate a standard video or audio **exemplar** of a man (author Mark Onslow) using a slow and exaggerated presentation of the speech pattern while reciting the initial sentences of the "Rainbow Passage" (Fairbanks, 1960).

See Video Clip 1 for this chapter on thePoint for an example of the prolonged speech exemplar.

There is no programmed instruction to instate stutter-free speech in the clinic. Instead, clients practice the skill of controlling their stuttering using exaggerated prolonged speech. Then they use whatever individual features of this pattern they need to control their stuttering while experimenting with more natural-sounding speech.

The use of a 9-point stuttering **severity rating (SR) scale** by the client and speech-language pathologist (SLP) replaces more traditional measures of stuttering frequency during the course of the treatment. Clients are taught and encouraged to **self-evaluate** their stuttering severity and **speech naturalness (NAT)** from the first session. These skills are used in later problem-solving strategies when assisting clients to generalize their control of stuttering from the clinic environment to everyday speech situations. This problem-solving replaces formal transfer tasks.

The goal of the program is to eliminate or significantly reduce stuttering in everyday speech situations. Although the initial trial was conducted with adults (O'Brian et al., 2001; 2003a), the program has also recently been used with a small number of adolescents (Hearne, 2006). The program was initially conducted using a combination of one-on-one weekly treatment sessions and one intensive group practice day. However, subsequent trials have suggested it to be efficacious when presented entirely in weekly or fortnightly sessions using a telehealth service delivery model (O'Brian, Packman, & Onslow, 2008).

The program consists of the following four stages (Fig. 14.1): (1) *teaching sessions*, where clients learn how to produce prolonged speech in an exaggerated manner to control their stuttering and also to use 9-point stuttering SR and NAT scales; (2) *within-clinic instatement of stutter-free speech*, where clients practice prolonged speech and learn to vary features of speech production until they can consistently produce acceptable-sounding (3 or lower on the 9-point NAT scale) stutter-free speech in the clinic; (3) *problem-solving sessions*, where clients experiment with strategies to help generalize their stutter-free speech to everyday speaking situations, and (4) *maintenance*, where clients assume responsibility for maintaining treatment gains. The manual can be downloaded from the Australian Stuttering Research Centre, The University of Sydney website (http://www.fhs.usyd.edu.au/asrc).

THEORETICAL BASIS FOR THE CAMPERDOWN PROGRAM

Stuttering can be described in terms of its observable behaviors: *repeated movements, fixed postures,* and *superfluous behaviors* (see Teeson, Packman, & Onslow, 2003, for a description of these terms). Such speech disruptions may interfere with normal communication and can seriously affect quality of life. Stuttering can lead to distress in everyday speaking situations and may also lead to difficulties in attaining and maintaining occupational potential (Craig & Calver, 1991; Hayhow, Cray, & Enderby, 2002). Stuttering is known to be associated with social anxiety, with half of adults seeking clinical help warranting a comorbid psychiatric diagnosis of social phobia (Kraaimaat, Vanryckeghem, & Van Dam-Baggen, 2002; Menzies, O'Brian, Onslow, Packman, St Clare & Block, 2008).

Evidence suggests that stuttering is caused by a deficit in neural processing for speech (Buchel & Sommer, 2004). We have proposed that this deficit involves the initiation of syllables (see Packman, Code, & Onslow, 2007). Our syllable initiation (SI) theory was developed

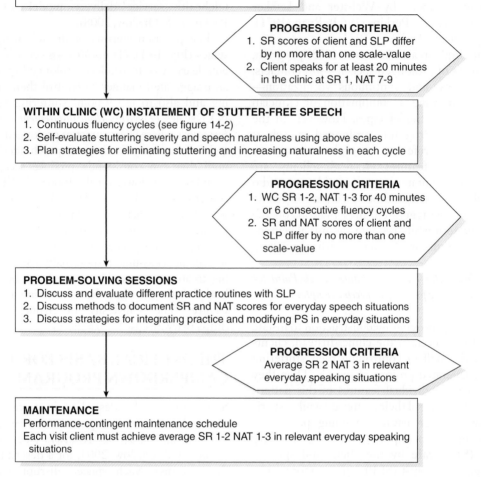

Figure 14.1. Summary of Camperdown Program stages.

from our working model of stuttering, the variability model (Vmodel) (Packman et al., 1996). According to SI theory, stuttering is triggered by the variability in motoric effort from syllable to syllable that is required to realize variable linguistic (syllabic) stress. The task demands of linguistic stress trigger the syllable initiation problem when variation in effort between syllables is greatest. The threshold for this triggering is different across individuals and varies within individuals according to their level of arousal in different speaking contexts.

Although we have outlined our theoretical position about the cause of stuttering, we emphasize that the Camperdown Program has not developed from causal theory; that is, the program is not theory driven and operates independently of a

specific understanding of causal factors of stuttering. In fact, the development of the Camperdown Program was pragmatically driven; the use of almost all its components is supported by sound laboratory and/or clinical research. This is discussed in detail in the next section.

Although many of the components of traditional speech restructuring programs were dispensed with (see below), the program is a package of procedures, and at the time of writing, we do not know which components are necessary for its efficacy. Treatment effects are most likely due to a combination of components, the identification of which will require careful, controlled research.

The goals of the Camperdown Program are to assist clients in attaining natural-sounding stutter-free speech and maintaining this in everyday speaking situations for as long as possible. To achieve these goals, clients learn to restructure their speech with prolonged speech, shape it toward natural-sounding speech, and then generalize this speech using self-monitoring of stuttering severity and speech naturalness. The use of these self-managed procedures is consistent with the idea of clients ultimately assuming responsibility for their own progress.

It has long been argued that simply attaining stutter-free speech, as occurs with speech restructuring, does not address the negative attitudes toward speaking and avoidances experienced by many people who stutter. Recent research conducted by our group (Cream et al., 2003) found that although adults may be able to control their stuttering with prolonged speech, maintaining this control in their everyday lives is challenging. Not only is it difficult to do, but individuals may feel they are not truly themselves when using it. They may still feel different from normally fluent speakers, even when they are controlling their stuttering effectively. Also, because many people who stutter suffer from social anxiety, negative attitudes toward speaking may be an important issue for treatment participants.

The Camperdown Program does not directly aim to reduce negative attitudes and feelings; however, it does take these into account in the problem-solving stage of the program. In this stage, the client and the SLP explore together the different ways for the client to maximize the effective use of prolonged speech in everyday situations. Where social anxiety is a serious problem, we advise clients to consider seeking cognitive behavior therapy (see McColl et al., 2001).

EMPIRICAL BASIS FOR USE

There are two types of evidence presented in this section: (1) evidence underpinning the treatment processes, and (2) evidence for the efficacy of the program itself.

EVIDENCE FOR THE TREATMENT PROCESSES

The Camperdown Program was developed in response to experimental research findings that challenged some of the basic assumptions on which traditional prolonged speech programs had been designed. The first step in this research was a study by Harrison et al. (1998), which reported successful outcomes from a clinical trial of prolonged speech in which the intensity of the Instatement Phase was reduced to one 12-hour day and the Transfer Phase was omitted altogether. Previously researched prolonged speech programs (Boberg & Kully, 1985; 1994; Ingham, 1987; Neilson & Andrews, 1993; Onslow et al., 1996) had been conducted over much longer periods, typically 2 to 3 weeks of intensive clinic attendance, with many programs involving a residential component. Most programs had also incorporated formal transfer tasks—for example, performance-contingent progression through a number of rating trials of a predetermined standard series of hierarchical tasks. A comparison between the outcomes for the more abbreviated program (Harrison et al., 1998) versus a more elaborate program (Onslow et al., 1996) is shown in Table 14.1.

The results of the study by Harrison et al. (1998) presented grounds on which to question the need to retain either a formal Transfer Phase or a longer instatement period, especially given the time and resources consumed for the latter by both clients and SLPs. It also seemed counterintuitive to isolate clients from the real world for long periods, given that the ultimate goal of any prolonged speech treatment is for clients to be stutter-free in everyday speaking situations beyond the clinic. This decision was supported in a study by James et al. (1989). They demonstrated

Table 14.1. *Comparison of Outcomes for Onslow et al. (1996) and Harrison et al. (1998)*

	Posttreatment Mean %SS	Posttreatment Mean %SS Reduction	Treatment Hours
Onslow et al. (1996)	0.57	96.5	130
Harrison et al. (1998)	0.38	93.7	24

that 2-hour sessions held twice weekly produced equally efficacious results compared with intensive 8-hour daily treatment.

A second concern regarding traditional prolonged speech treatment processes is the problem of operationalization (Ingham, 1984). None of the features of prolonged speech—soft contacts, gentle onsets, and so on—have been operationally defined. In addition, there was evidence that SLPs were unable to reliably identify prolonged speech target behaviors (Onslow & O'Brian, 1998). The latter study investigated the reliability with which experienced SLPs identified the presence and accuracy of target prolonged speech behaviors—specifically, soft contacts, gentle onsets, and continuous vocalization—as they would in a routine clinical program. These SLPs were asked to watch video samples of participants using prolonged speech and to decide (1) whether these participants were using any soft contacts, gentle onsets, or continuous vocalization and (2) if used at all, whether the participants were using these target behaviors correctly. Onslow and O'Brian (1998) reported that SLPs did not agree when attempting to identify correct use of prolonged speech target behaviors in these participants and could not even reliably judge whether or not the target speech behaviors were present in the participants' speech. This result suggested that, during treatment, the program SLPs would probably have given inconsistent feedback to clients about their prolonged speech target behaviors. Therefore, the teaching of the target behaviors in this study did not seem to be essential to the effects of the treatment.

Another assumption of the prolonged speech therapies has been that all components of this speech pattern are essential for effective control of stuttering. In previous programs, there had been little opportunity for clients to experiment with prolonged speech and use only the features of the speech pattern they needed to control their stuttered speech. A laboratory study by Packman, Onslow, and van Doorn (1994) investigated changes in the speech patterns of participants when they used prolonged speech to control their stuttering but were not instructed in how this should be done. Three participants, who had never received therapy for their stuttering, were taught prolonged speech at approximately 40 syllables per minute (SPM) and then instructed to use whatever features of the speech pattern they required to control their stuttering. All subjects achieved near-zero stuttering rates in the laboratory, and subsequent acoustic analysis of their speech demonstrated speech pattern changes that were different across all three subjects. These data suggested that people who stutter may benefit from being able to use only selected features of the prolonged speech pattern.

The study by Packman, et al. (1994) also caused us to question the need for programmed instruction for instating stutter-free speech in the clinic. In traditional programs, clients learned prolonged speech at a slow and unnatural level and then progressed systematically through a number of steps, meeting either speech rate or speech naturalness criteria, until a target rate or naturalness level was achieved. The subjects in the Packman, et al. (1994) study, however, achieved their natural-sounding stutter-free speech despite bypassing these steps. These participants achieved a reduction in stuttering just from exposure to, and practice of, very slow prolonged speech.

Finally, traditional prolonged speech programs have relied on clinician identification of individual moments of stuttering for clients to pass through the various stages of the program. However, research has also shown that SLPs typically do not agree to an acceptable level about either the number or location of stutters in a sample, although they are able to reliably track trends in data (Curlee, 1981; Ingham & Cordes, 1992; 1997; Kully & Boberg, 1988; Packman & Onslow, 1995). Fortunately, there is abundant evidence that stuttering severity can be measured reliably by individuals with limited or no training when scaling procedures are used (Cullinan & Prather, 1968; Eve et al., 1995; Martin & Haroldson, 1992; Onslow, Andrews, & Costa, 1990; Yairi & Ambrose, 1999). Evidence also suggested that adults who stutter can reliably self-evaluate their stuttering severity using the same rating scales (Aron, 1967; Naylor, 1953).

In summary, the procedures used in the Camperdown Program were developed with reference to preclinical laboratory evidence combined with evidence from phase I and phase II clinical trials (Harrison et al., 1998; James et al., 1989; Onslow & O'Brian, 1998; Packman, et al. 1994). Phase I clinical trials are preliminary investigations into the possibility of a new treatment conducted on only a few participants. The primary considerations in such trials are fundamental safety issues with the treatment and whether the treatment is viable from the perspective of the client and the service provider. Phase II trials are usually conducted with larger subject numbers and primarily establish estimates of how many participants will respond to a treatment. The research from the previously mentioned trials suggested that the following elements might not be necessary for the successful instatement of stutter-free speech in prolonged speech treatment programs:

1. Multiday, intensive treatment format
2. A standardized, prescriptive prolonged speech pattern
3. Programmed instruction
4. Formal transfer procedures
5. Counting instances of stuttering online

Therefore, the first clinical trials of the Camperdown Program did not incorporate any of these processes.

EVIDENCE OF EFFICACY

There are six clinical trial sources of efficacy for the Camperdown Program (Carey, et al., in press; O'Brian et al., 2001; 2003a; Hearne, 2008; O'Brian, Packman, & Onslow, 2008; and Cocomazzo, 2009 publication). The strongest evidence for the efficacy of this program comes from four phase II, clinical trials (Carey et al. in press; O'Brian et al., 2003a; Packman, & Onslow, 2008; Cocomazzo, 2009). The other two trials were phase I case studies. The studies are presented here in chronological order to demonstrate how the treatment has developed through systematic phases.

The first published study on the Camperdown Program (O'Brian et al., 2001) was a phase I trial reporting pilot data from the first three participants to reach the maintenance stage of the program. These three participants, ages 32, 37, and 51 years, were all men recruited from hospital treatment waiting lists around Sydney. Two had previously received treatment for their stuttering, 8 and 24 years previously, whereas the third had never received treatment. This study suggested that the program was very effective for these three participants, with significant stuttering reductions for all of them both within and beyond the clinic. The mean pretreatment and posttreatment scores of percentage of syllables stuttered (%SS) for each participant were 6.1% and 0.5% (participant 1), 5.4% and 0.6% (participant 2), and 10.4% and 1.0% (participant 3), respectively. This was achieved in an average of 18 clinic hours with no associated reduction in either speech rate or speech naturalness. The mean NAT scores for each of the posttreatment samples were in the range of 1 to 3, which is within the range of normally fluent speakers. Their low level of stuttering was maintained for between 10 and 13 months. These favorable results indicated that further research involving a trial with a larger number of participants was warranted.

The second published study, O'Brian et al. (2003a), reported on a phase II trial involving 30 adult participants ranging in age from 17 to 58 years. A pretreatment assessment occurred 2 weeks before commencing the program. Posttreatment assessments occurred immediately after entry into the Maintenance Stage and at 6 and 12 months after entry into that stage. At each assessment, participants used portable audiotape recorders to record their speech in the following three situations outside the clinic: talking with a family member, talking with a friend, and talking on the telephone. Outcome measures were %SS and speech rate in syllables per minute (SPM). These were collected by an independent observer. Inter- and intrajudge reliabilities of these measures were reported and found to reach acceptable levels. Intra- and interjudge reliabilities for %SS were 1.0 and 0.99, respectively. Intra- and interjudge reliabilities for SPM were 0.99 and 0.93, respectively. Speech naturalness was also assessed with a 9-point scale (Martin, Haroldson, & Triden, 1984) and compared to that of control speakers with normal fluency matched for age (±2 years) and gender. Two additional outcome measures used in this trial were client self-report data and social validity data. The self-report inventory, which was given to participants 3 to 6 months after entering the maintenance stage, sought information about average daily stuttering severity and speech naturalness ratings, clients' satisfaction with their speech, and their use of and feelings about prolonged speech. Finally, the social acceptability of participants' posttreatment speech was assessed by comparing their posttreatment speech with their pretreatment speech and with the speech of matched controls. Unsophisticated listeners were instructed to choose which speech sample in each pair of samples they felt more comfortable listening to (for a discussion of listener comfort, see O'Brian et al., 2003b).

Results for O'Brian et al. (2003a) showed that the mean time for participants to reach the Maintenance Stage was 20 hours (range, 13 to 29 hours). At Maintenance, the group mean was 0.4%SS (standard deviation [SD] = 0.6%), and at 12 months after treatment, the group mean remained at 0.4%SS (SD = 0.6%). Speech naturalness scores for more than half the group were also within one score of their matched controls. This result was generally confirmed by the self-reports, although these were not quite as positive. The biggest problem with this study was an attrition rate of approximately 30% during the course of treatment, although this was an improvement compared with an earlier study of prolonged speech (Onslow et al., 1996). Reasons for discontinuing treatment included relocation, change to work commitments, discomfort with prolonged speech, and failure to meet program requirements. Unfortunately, one subject died during the maintenance period. Otherwise, the trial presented strong evidence for the efficacy of the treatment.

The efficacy of the Camperdown Program with adults prompted a pilot study to investigate its viability with adolescents who stutter. Hearne et al. (2008) reported the use of the Camperdown Program with three adolescent males who were 13, 14, and 16 years of age. These adolescents were all able to learn to use the prolonged speech technique from the exemplar during individual sessions with the clinician but were more resistant to using it in everyday situations than typical adult clients had been. Assessments were made before treatment, 1 month after intensive treatment, at entry to maintenance, and 6 and 12 months after intensive treatment. At each assessment, the participants were required to complete two 10-minute phone conversations to strangers. These conversations were tape recorded, and measures of %SS were obtained by independent observers (two experienced SLPs not associated with the study and blinded to the pre-post status of each participant). Daily treatment SR scores, using the 9-point scale described earlier, were also collected. These self-reported SR ratings closely tracked the objective %SS scores, increasing the apparent trustworthiness of the data.

Different outcomes were achieved with each of these three participants: one participant completed maintenance successfully, one participant withdrew during maintenance after some stuttering returned, and the final participant withdrew during treatment. The best outcomes were achieved for the oldest adolescent, and the worst outcomes were observed for the two younger adolescents. It was considered likely that the large problem-solving component of the program was either too difficult or too much effort for younger adolescents to deal with. It is difficult to draw conclusions from such limited data; however, the fact that two of the three adolescents were able to successfully reduce their stuttering both within and outside the clinic in the short term provided sufficient evidence to justify a phase II trial of the Camperdown Program with this population.

Although the Camperdown Program had been shown to be efficacious in reducing stuttering in adults, many Australians are unable to access this treatment due to distance and lifestyle factors. Therefore, the next study (O'Brian, Packman, & Onslow, 2008) was a phase II trial designed to investigate the viability of the program when delivered via a telehealth service delivery model. This clinical trial assessed the outcomes for 10 adult clients, age 22 to 48 years, who, for a combination of distance and lifestyle factors, were unable to attend the clinic for treatment sessions. These participants all underwent a modified version of the original program with treatment components carried out at home alone using written, audio or audiovisual material and in sessions conducted with the SLP over the phone. The general concepts of the original program were retained, but treatment was conducted with a combination of email correspondence and phone consultations. At no time did any of the participants attend the clinic for assessment or treatment. The intensive group day was dispensed with, and the instatement stage was completed at home. The SLP initially instructed the participant in how to perform the fluency cycles over the phone and gave subsequent assistance over the phone when required. However, the majority of this stage of the treatment was completed independently by the participant.

For this clinical trial, outcome assessments were conducted immediately before treatment, immediately after treatment, and 6 months after treatment. At each assessment, three 10-minute audio recordings were made over the phone—one talking to the SLP and two talking to strangers. Each phone call was initiated from the clinic at a time unknown in advance to the client. Participants received the calls at home, work, their university, a friend's or relative's house, or in some other everyday environment. Self-reported stuttering SR scores were also documented as follows: (1) a typical and a worst SR score for each day of the week leading up to the assessment, and (2) a typical SR score for each of five situations selected by the client as representative of their daily life, with at least one of these considered a difficult situation. These situations included talking to family members, talking in the work environment, ordering food or drink, talking in a university course, and talking to a supervisor at work.

Primary dependent measures were %SS and SPM. The samples were collected over the phone and rated by SLPs independent of the study and blinded to the pre-posttreatment status of the participants. Secondary measures were NAT and self-reported stuttering SR scores. Results demonstrated that the group as a whole had an 82% reduction in stuttering from before treatment to immediately after treatment and a 74% reduction in stuttering from before treatment to 6 months after treatment. Both results were confirmed by self-report data. All participants increased their speech rate from pretreatment to immediate posttreatment samples, with the group mean shifting from 184 SPM to 228 SPM. More than half of the group achieved posttreatment NAT scores in the range of nonstuttering speakers. The strengths of this study were the reliability of the outcome stuttering measures, the fact that outcome measures were independent of the treatment, and the fact that all participants were retained throughout the length of the trial. The most troublesome aspect of this study was that two or three participants

showed slight increases in stuttering at the 6-month posttreatment assessment. The participant with the most significant relapse had reduced his treatment gain from 82% to 56% by 6 months after treatment. However, the study confirmed the viability of the telehealth delivery model for the Camperdown Program. A recent randomised controlled trial of this telehealth version compared with the standard delivery (Carey et al., in press) confirmed these beneficial outcomes. Results from 40 participants assessed 9 months after beginning treatment showed a significant reduction in stuttering in both groups and no difference in %SS outcomes between the two groups. The treatment effects were maintained over a 12-month follow-up period. The telehealth group was more efficient in terms of clinician time, requiring almost 4 hours less clinician contact time on average than the standard delivery group.

Finally, Cocomazzo (2009) reported on a student-administered version of the Camperdown Program conducted at the La Trobe Communication Clinic at La Trobe University in Melbourne, Australia. Participants were 12 adults, age 21 to 47 years, treated by 24 final-year undergraduate speech pathology students and two supervising SLPs. The structure of the original program was modified so that it could be delivered within an academic semester at the university. This meant that each participant received a standard 20-hour program regardless of his or her individual progress.

Assessments for the purpose of measuring outcome occurred before commencing the program, immediately after completing the program, and at 12 months after treatment. At each assessment, a 10-minute video recording was made within the clinic and two 10-minute audio recordings were made outside the clinic. Self-reports were also collected from the participants, along with student reports of their experiences of the program.

Primary dependent measures were %SS and SPM. There was an 86% reduction in stuttering frequency from before to immediate after treatment and a 56% reduction from before to 12 months after treatment, without any reduction in speech rate. Unfortunately, two participants showed evidence of relapse at the 12-month posttreatment assessment. These results were generally confirmed by participant self-report. The strength of this study was that it was conducted at a site independent of where the treatment was developed and with independent student SLPs, under supervision.

In summary, there is reasonably strong evidence for the efficacy of the Camperdown Program presented in different treatment formats with adult participants. There is also some evidence for its efficacy with older adolescents. Further evidence of its long-term benefits and replication from independent sites are needed to strengthen these data.

PRACTICAL REQUIREMENTS FOR THE CAMPERDOWN PROGRAM

The original trial of the Camperdown Program (O'Brian et al., 2003a) in a group format required three SLPs and some dedicated infrastructure. However, it is possible for only one SLP to give this feedback once clients are familiar with the process. In this scenario, clients take over much of the responsibility for conducting the treatment in the same manner as was done in the telehealth trial (O'Brian, et al., 2008). When conducting the program in a group format, the other requirement is a room large enough to accommodate the required number of SLPs and clients.

Equipment requirements for the program are minimal, regardless of the service delivery model, and include the following: a copy of the prolonged speech exemplar recording and a means of playing it, the associated transcription, some form of speech recording device, and some means for clients to document their progress through the program. The exemplar recording can be an audiovisual or audio-only version of the exemplar. Depending on equipment available to the SLP and client, it may be presented on computer, television monitor, tape recorder, or any other modern digital medium in the clinic. The advantage of a computer version is reliable instant accessibility without the need for constant rewinding of a tape. Clients have often transferred the exemplar in audio or audiovisual format onto another recording device, such as an MP3 player or mobile phone, for playing and listening to outside the clinic. The exemplar text

is also useful, written in large font for those with limited vision, given that some clients do not commit it to memory particularly quickly. Clients also need some form of individual speech recording device so that they can record and listen to themselves for the purposes of self-evaluation. They also need such a device for recording situations and practice outside the clinic when possible. Again, clients have found a range of modern technologies for this purpose. Still, the SLP may choose to lend a small portable tape recorder to the client depending on circumstances. Simple pencil-and-paper record forms usually suffice to record progress at all stages of the treatment program. An individual chart or graph usually works best for clients to document SR and NAT scores when instating stutter-free speech (see Appendix 14.1). This way they can easily look back at scores across previous cycles when planning problem-solving strategies. Clients are required to document daily SR and NAT scores for specific situations each week. Usually a diary works best for this purpose. No other equipment is required for the operation of the program. Because measures of stuttering frequency and programmed instruction using target rates have been dispensed with during the program, no rating machines are required.

The procedures for the Camperdown Program were designed so that they could be implemented by SLPs with limited formal training. For example, teaching prolonged speech from the exemplar recording means that an SLP does not need to be proficient in using prolonged speech, only in giving feedback about how close the client's production is to the exemplar. Studies have also shown that acceptable reliability has consistently been achieved by groups of observers using SR scales even with no training or with little previous exposure to the scales (Cullinan, Prather, & Williams, 1963; Curran & Hood, 1977; Eve et al., 1995; Lewis & Sherman, 1951; Sherman, 1952; 1955; Young, 1961; 1969). Finally, Ingham et al. (1985), Ingham, Gow, and Costello (1985), and Ingham et al. (1989) all reported that the naturalness scale developed by Martin, Haroldson, and Triden (1984) could be used reliably by SLPs and clients without training. Therefore, there appears to be little training required for SLPs to be able to administer the program. The fact that the student SLPs in the Cocomazzo (2009) study administered the program successfully further suggests that little training is required.

In terms of time demands, individuals vary in the amount of time taken to reach the maintenance stage of the program. However, the mean is approximately 20 hours (O'Brian et al., 2003a). When the program has been conducted on an individual basis, the SLP time is reduced to a mean of approximately 14 to 15 hours per client. This is because a lot of the required "drill" work can be completed by the client at home rather than during the routine clinic visit. In the standard service delivery models, little SLP time is required outside the face-to-face contact with the client.

KEY COMPONENTS OF THE APPROACH

The Camperdown Program consists of four stages: *teaching sessions, within-clinic instatement of stutter-free speech, problem-solving sessions,* and *maintenance*. These stages, along with their primary speech goals and criteria (explained in the following sections), are shown in Figure 14.1. The program can be administered traditionally, with a combination of weekly individual and group-intensive face-to-face sessions, or as a distance intervention program with sessions conducted over the phone and tasks set for clients to carry out on their own away from the clinic. Regardless of the format, the concepts underpinning the program and the four stages remain largely unchanged, as do the aims for each stage.

STAGE I: TEACHING SESSIONS

In this stage, clients learn to (1) evaluate their stuttering severity using a 9-point SR scale, (2) produce the prolonged speech pattern by imitating the exemplar, and (3) vary and evaluate their speech naturalness using the 9-point NAT scale.

1. The 9-point SR scale is used by SLPs and clients both within and beyond the clinic instead of measures of stuttering frequency. With this scale, 1 = no stuttering, 2 = very mild stuttering, and 9 = extremely severe stuttering. Clients are taught to use the scale from the first clinic visit. Agreement between client and

SLP is established over the first few visits. Ratings from short within- and beyond-clinic speech samples are compared and discussed each week until there is reasonable agreement. "Reasonable agreement" is operationalized as SR scores obtained by the client and SLP differing by no more than one scale value. In this stage, clients also practice graphing typical and sometimes worst daily SR scores.

When reasonable agreement has been reached, clients are asked to select five situations representative of their daily life, with at least one being considered a difficult situation. Situations may include such activities as talking to family members, talking in the work environment, having a drink with friends, ordering food to go, speaking in a university tutorial, or talking to a supervisor at work. Clients then document a *typical* pretreatment SR score for that situation for comparison with SR measures made later in the program.

See Video Clip 2 for an example of a clinician teaching a client to use the SR scale.

2. While the participant learns the prolonged speech pattern, the SLP does not define or describe the specific features such as soft contact sounds, gentle beginnings to words, or the prolongation of vowel sounds. Instead, the client watches a video or listens to an audio recording of the prolonged speech exemplar, which consists of one of the authors (Mark Onslow) reading the Rainbow Passage in a slow and exaggerated manner in connected speech. As the client watches and/or listens to the reading, the associated written text is also available. The client then reproduces that speech pattern as closely as possible, first in unison with the video and then imitating it. The SLP gives feedback about the accuracy of the client's imitation of prolonged speech without reference to any specific descriptors. Feedback directs the client back to the demonstration video to try to imitate sections of the exemplar more closely. The SLP will usually break the text into small units for imitation and feedback.

See Video Clip 3 for an example of a clinician teaching a client to use prolonged speech.

After mastering the prolonged speech pattern while reciting the Rainbow Passage, the participant attempts to use prolonged speech in monologue and then spontaneous conversation, still in a slow and exaggerated manner. The aim of the client using prolonged speech consistently at this slow and exaggerated level is to completely eliminate stuttering. The client must be able to achieve completely stutter-free speech (although unnatural sounding, with NAT scores from 7 to 9) within the clinic for an entire session before progressing to stage II.

3. The SLP introduces and demonstrates the 9-point NAT scale. The SLP then facilitates production by the client of stutter-free speech at various naturalness levels. The aim is to remain stutter-free while experimenting with different features of prolonged speech. The NAT scale quantifies how acceptable the resulting speech sounds.

STAGE II: INSTATEMENT OF STUTTER-FREE SPEECH WITHIN THE CLINIC

During this stage, clients learn to:

1. Use natural-sounding consistently stutter-free conversational speech in the clinic
2. Refine their self-evaluation skills using the SR and NAT scales
3. Use basic problem-solving skills that they will then use in stage III to assist with generalization of stutter-free speech into everyday situations

This stage can be implemented in a group intensive format over 1 or more days; it may be spread over several sessions of individual treatment with an SLP, or it may be taught initially over the phone to a client with the client then left to complete most of this stage on his or her own at home. The basic processes in any of these formats will be the same.

When a 1-day intensive format is used, stage II takes place during an 8-hour group session. During this session, clients rotate through a minimum of 14 **fluency cycles**. The early cycles consist of three 5-minute phases. There are two speaking phases, the *Practice* and *Trial Phases*, and one *Evaluation Phase*. Figure 14.2 shows one complete cycle.

Appendix 14.1 shows a record form for the fluency cycles and phases. The Practice Phase consists of 3 to 4 minutes of SLP-supervised practice using exaggerated stutter-free prolonged speech similar to the video exemplar with or without the exemplar tape as a model. Reading with the exemplar recording every third or fourth cycle is useful, but often clients prefer just to use spontaneous speech at NAT 9 at the beginning of other cycles. The main requirement is stutter-free speech at NAT 9. Time should be allowed within the 5-minute period for feedback and discussion of prolonged speech with the SLP. Feedback by the SLP is given in the same manner as when teaching prolonged speech in the *Teaching Sessions*. No attempt should be made to experiment with more natural-sounding speech. The aim is to reinforce accurate imitation.

The Trial Phase consists of 3 to 4 minutes of SLP-supervised speaking in monologue, with the client instructed to use whatever features of the prolonged speech pattern are needed to control stuttering. During this phase, the client is instructed to attempt to achieve three goals in the following order of priority: (1) maintain an SR score of 1 to 2, (2) sound as natural as possible, and (3) match online self-evaluations of SR and NAT scores to those of the SLP.

Each Trial Phase is audio-recorded by the client. At the end of each Trial Phase, the SLP and client individually record an SR and NAT score for the client's speech. If the SR score for this trial (as determined by the SLP) is greater than 2, then the client is required to return to a Practice Phase during the next speaking phase because it is assumed that the client needs to use more or different features of prolonged speech to control stuttering and thus more practice is needed. Together, the SLP and client work out a strategy for the next cycle.

The Evaluation Phase is an opportunity for the client to listen to the recordings of the previous two speaking phases in order to: (1) re-evaluate stuttering severity offline (particularly if there was disparity between client and SLP scores), (2) evaluate the speech naturalness during that phase, and (3) decide on a strategy for using prolonged speech in the next phase. For example, if the SR score was too high (>2), then the client would consider either using different features of prolonged speech or introducing more consistent and exaggerated prolonged speech

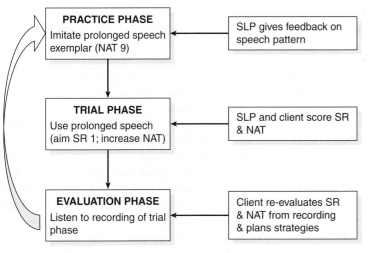

Figure 14.2. The stages of one fluency cycle.

generally. If the speech sounded unacceptably unnatural although stutter-free, the client might reduce the amount of prolonged speech during the next cycle. This establishes a procedure that will be encouraged as a technique during later Problem-Solving Sessions for assisting generalization of stutter-free speech.

See Video Clip 4 for an example of a fluency cycle.

For the first six of these Practice-Trial-Evaluation cycles, phases are each 5 minutes long. The Practice and Trial Phases are conducted individually with an SLP, and the Evaluation Phase occurs independently. For the remaining eight cycles, the Practice and Evaluation Phases remain 5 minutes long, but a 20-minute group conversation replaces the individual Trial Phase monologue with the SLP. Clients are encouraged to engage in conversation in the group rather than continuing to speak in monologue. The three goals for the group sessions remain identical to those of the individual Trial Phase. Each client is paired with an SLP for the Practice and Evaluation Phases. In the Practice Phase, the client practices prolonged speech and also plans strategies for using prolonged speech in the group. In the Evaluation Phase, the client evaluates and discusses with the SLP his or her speech in the last group session and plans a strategy for the next cycle.

Although the program contains no hierarchical progression through the day, the following guidelines apply to the speaking phases:

1. The Practice Phase is always followed by a Trial Phase during the next speaking phase.
2. A Trial Phase with an SR score of 1 to 2 leads to a choice of a subsequent Practice or Trial Phase during the next speaking phase.
3. A Trial Phase with an SR score greater than 2 is always followed by a Practice Phase during the next speaking phase.
4. Every third cycle begins with a Practice Phase regardless of previous outcomes.
5. After six cycles, if the client is consistently producing speech at NAT 6 or greater (that is, consistently using an exaggerated speech pattern), movement toward more natural-sounding speech will be facilitated by the SLP.

If this stage of the program is to be implemented by the SLP with an individual client in weekly sessions, the following adaptations need to be made. First, the SLP outlines and describes the aim of each phase. Then the SLP and client work together through one complete cycle of Practice-Trial-Evaluation, practicing exaggerated prolonged speech, experimenting with prolonged speech while remaining stutter-free, and then evaluating the SR and NAT scores achieved both after speaking and after listening to the recording. Scores are documented on a chart that also has questions after each phase to prompt the client to think through problem-solving strategies. Together, the SLP and client work out a strategy for the next complete cycle, taking into consideration the progression rules. Several cycles are conducted together, with the SLP assisting the client to form strategies for progression, dependent on the progression rules and the results of previous cycles. When the SLP is satisfied that the client understands the general procedure, the client is encouraged to practice the cycles at home until the next session. Progression to the next stage occurs when the client is able to consistently produce relatively natural-sounding (NAT score of 3 or less) stutter-free speech for at least five consecutive cycles or throughout an entire clinic visit. The form used for this stage of treatment can be seen in Appendix 14.1.

STAGE III: PROBLEM-SOLVING SESSIONS

In this stage, clients aim to generalize their stutter-free speech to everyday situations by (1) establishing appropriate practice regimens for stutter-free speech, (2) evaluating their stuttering severity and speech naturalness daily in everyday situations, and (3) developing strategies for reducing stuttering and/or maintaining fluency in everyday situations.

1. At the beginning of each session, the SLP confirms that the client is still able to produce stutter-free, natural-sounding speech in the clinic. If the SR score is greater than 2, the client is required to practice the prolonged speech pattern at a more unnatural level and then increase naturalness without increasing stuttering severity.
2. The SLP and client discuss and re-establish practice routines for speech technique for the coming week. It may be appropriate for the client to continue practicing the prolonged speech technique at NAT 7 to 9 for a number of weeks during the initial problem-solving sessions. However, for most clients, a practice level at NAT 4 to 5 is usually more appropriate once they are consistently controlling their stuttering most of the time in everyday situations.
3. The SLP and client discuss the typical and worst daily SR and NAT scores achieved during the previous week and the situations in which stuttering was not under control. They also discuss the ratings for various beyond-clinic speech tasks that may have been set. They listen to any recordings of speech tasks that the client has made.

4. The SLP and client discuss problem-solving strategies for further reducing stuttering in any specific everyday situations. This may involve the addition of simple cognitive behavioral strategies directed toward anxiety associated with stuttering. For example, clients may be encouraged to identify and modify negative thoughts associated with stuttering and to gradually confront anxiety-provoking situations. Progression to the next stage occurs when the client reports SR scores of 2 or less with associated NAT scores of 3 or less in everyday speech situations that are important and relevant to the individual client for at least 3 consecutive weeks. Clients may also progress if there has been no further reduction in ratings made outside of the clinic over four sessions without good cause. For example, if a client changes jobs or is undergoing excessive personal stress, it might be expected that progress will plateau for a short period.

See Video Clip 5 for an example of a clinician guiding a client through problem solving.

STAGE IV: MAINTENANCE

In this stage, sessions become less frequent as the client takes on problem-solving activities without the support of the SLP. The client is encouraged to document SR and NAT on a daily basis, particularly for problem situations, and to develop strategies for maintaining speech gains.

ASSESSMENT METHODS TO SUPPORT ONGOING DECISION MAKING

Measures used in the Camperdown Program are (1) SR and NAT scores by the SLP and client for documenting stuttering severity and speech naturalness in everyday situations before and after treatment, for recording progress throughout the treatment process, for informing treatment decisions, and for setting immediate and long-term goals; and (2) optional %SS calculated by the SLP for documenting stuttering frequency from recordings made outside the clinic both before and after treatment and for confirming client self-reports.

The following publications provide evidence supporting the use of the speech measures used in the Camperdown Program. O'Brian et al. (2004) reported a strong linear relationship between %SS scores and SR scores on the 9-point scale; that is, high %SS scores usually indicated high SR scores and vice versa. The only exception to this was in cases where there was either a small number of significant fixed postures (blocks) or a large number of innocuous repetitions in the speech sample. In the first scenario, the %SS would be low, whereas the SR score would be high, and in the second scenario, the %SS is likely to be high, whereas the SR score would be low. Therefore, the authors concluded that, in most cases, the two scores could be used interchangeably by SLPs. Both measures showed high inter- and intrajudge agreement when used by SLPs who had regular contact with stuttering clients. O'Brian, Packman, and Onslow (2004) reported good agreement between SLP and client for most clients for self-reported SRs on the 9-point scale when used during the treatment process. Finn and Ingham (1994) and Ingham et al. (1989) also reported that adults who stutter can reliably rate both the sound and feel of their own speech using a 9-point speech naturalness scale.

Assessment for the Camperdown Program involves the following actions by the SLP: (1) taking a case history and providing information about stuttering, (2) obtaining a speech sample in the clinic, (3) obtaining client measures of stuttering severity (SRs) in at least five self-selected everyday speech situations, and (4) obtaining two conversations recorded outside the clinic of the client talking to strangers (optional but useful if obtained). Diagnosis of stuttering is made conjointly by the client and SLP based on presenting symptoms at assessment and history of stuttering behaviors.

1. At assessment, the following case history information is taken: personal details, including name, street, email address, and phone number; occupation; client's first language; client's description of stuttering, including severity and known triggers; onset of stuttering and pattern since onset; detailed history of previous treatment, including whether programs were completed and their outcome; strategies used to control stuttering and their effectiveness; anxiety about stuttering and specific speech situations; family history of stuttering; what client wants to achieve from therapy; and general health and information about other communication problems. Information given to the client at assessment depends on the client's level of interest and understanding. It typically includes general information about stuttering, its nature and cause, and its relation to anxiety; evidence for different types of treatment and their effectiveness; and general information about time commitment and support if continuing with treatment. If requested, more specific information is given about published research findings.

2. During the assessment visit, a pretreatment SR measure is made during a 10-minute conversation with the SLP. This sample can also be given a %SS rating by the SLP, but this is not essential.

3. Clients are instructed to think of five different situations that are representative of their daily life, including at least one difficult speaking situation. Situations could include talking to a spouse (or family member), talking to friends at a social gathering, speaking during meetings at work, using the phone at work, talking to the boss or a teacher, talking to a preschool teacher, ordering food at a restaurant or takeaway, giving a tutorial or work presentation, and talking to strangers on the phone. The client then documents a *typical* (and often a *worst*) SR for that situation before beginning treatment.

4. Where possible, one or two pretreatment recordings made outside the clinic are obtained of the client talking. This may be organized by the clinic. Each phone call, with the client's approval, may be initiated by the clinic (usually by students or administrative staff) at a time unknown in advance to the client. Clients can receive these calls at home or work or in some other everyday environment. These are rated for SR by the SLP and used for comparison with similar posttreatment recordings. Alternatively, the client may make a recording of his or her speech in an everyday situation that is then used for the same purpose.

As described in previous sections, SR and NAT scores are used routinely during the treatment process. The 9-point SR scale is used by SLPs and clients both within and beyond the clinic to replace measures of stuttering rate. Clients are taught to use the scale from the first clinic visit. Agreement between client and SLP ratings is established over the first few visits. Ratings from short within- and beyond-clinic speech samples are compared and discussed each week during the Teaching Sessions until reasonable agreement occurs between the client's and SLP's scores.

The SR scale is used during the instatement of stutter-free speech to evaluate stuttering severity in the two speaking phases of each fluency cycle. The scale also forms the basis for evaluation of stuttering severity beyond the clinic during the problem-solving sessions. Clients can use the SR scale differently for different purposes. Clients can use the scale to report their stuttering severity both in terms of a global measure and for individual situations for which reliable measures of stuttering from recordings would be difficult to make. For example, ratings can be for particular situations, to indicate typical stuttering for a day, for best or worst situations for a given period, or for evaluating practice conversations. This feedback is used to foster discussion between the SLP and client about establishment and modification of appropriate generalization strategies. Finally, the scale is used to evaluate stuttering severity in relation to program criteria for the maintenance stage. The SR scale complements, but does not replace, stutter-count measures in the process of treatment research outcome evaluation.

Because the program involves speech restructuring, the 9-point NAT scale (Martin et al., 1984) is used by SLPs and clients to evaluate and document the clients' speech quality throughout the program. With this scale, 1 indicates extremely natural-sounding speech, and 9 indicates extremely unnatural-sounding speech. The ultimate aim is for clients to finally achieve a NAT score of 3 or lower, because this range has been shown in previous studies (Ingham, Gow, & Costello, 1985; Martin et al., 1984; Runyan, Bell, & Prosek, 1990) to be generally within the range found among normal speakers.

The NAT scale is introduced once the client has familiarity with unnatural-sounding speech during the teaching sessions. It is used in the problem-solving sessions to report on speech quality in situations outside of the clinic. Strategies are then discussed to address the balance between speech quality and stuttering severity. Whenever stuttering severity remains low, clients are encouraged to increase their speech naturalness. On the other hand, if a reported increase in stuttering severity seems related to an increase in speech naturalness (lower values on the NAT scale), clients are encouraged to experiment with more or different features of prolonged speech. In these sessions, clients also learn to identify and use different NAT levels as a strategy to assist generalization. For example, clients may decide to practice speech at a NAT of 4 or even 5 before attempting a particularly difficult phone call.

The NAT scale has been shown to be reliable for SLPs giving feedback to clients about their speech and also for clients' self-evaluation of speech quality (Finn & Ingham, 1994; Ingham et al., 1989; Ingham & Onslow, 1985). However, in our experience, most clients tend to rate their speech more according to how natural it "feels" than according to how natural it "sounds." Hence, online client ratings almost always report higher numbers (more unnatural speech) than SLP ratings, although client offline ratings are often comparable. This problem is best addressed by having clients regularly listen to and evaluate their speech quality using audiotape recordings. This reporting of higher numbers by clients is similar to the finding of Ingham et al. (1989). They reported that two of three participants rated their stutter-free speech as feeling unnatural despite listeners reporting that it sounded highly natural.

Clients move into the Problem-Solving Stage of the program when they are able to remain consistently stutter-free (SR score of 1 to 2) while sounding reasonably natural (NAT score of 3 or better) in the clinic throughout an entire clinic visit. They move into the Maintenance Stage of the program when beyond-clinic SR scores are typically 2 (preferably confirmed by one or two beyond-clinic recordings) or when no further reduction in stuttering has been achieved over a number of weeks (usually approximately 4 weeks) without cause.

TAILORING THE TREATMENT TO THE INDIVIDUAL CLIENT

The Camperdown Program is not a "one size fits all" treatment. The design of the program is such that in all stages (except the instatement of within-clinic stutter-free speech in group format), it accommodates individual client needs and expectations regardless of individual cultural or personal factors. Because the program is structured around treatment concepts and is mostly administered on an individual clinician-client basis, rather than a group model, it is easy to adapt all aspects of the program to any client's specific needs. The exception to this occurs when an intensive group day is used in stage II and clients follow a fairly rigid routine throughout the day. Any client with difficulties complying with this format would normally not be assigned to a group program but would have the entire treatment program conducted on an individual basis. Also, the program does not specify a particular number of treatment hours for each client. Therefore, a client with learning problems or difficulties achieving some goals will probably take longer to achieve maintenance criteria.

The program has been used with those for whom English is not their first language. For these clients, the treatment is conducted initially in English. Quite often it is the case that stuttering reduces for these clients in English but may remain a more significant problem in their other language. In these cases, treatment is then directed specifically at the other language. Usually all that is required is extra practice in the other language, first at unnatural-sounding NAT levels and then at more natural-sounding NAT levels.

APPLICATION TO AN INDIVIDUAL CLIENT

The following client was treated for research purposes, and therefore, %SS measures were collected before treatment began and at its completion. These measures are presented for validation purposes only and are not required in a routine clinic environment.

ASSESSMENT

Emilio presented as a friendly and easygoing 30-year-old man who had a fairly laid-back attitude to both his stuttering and his life in general. He was born in Italy but had moved to Australia with his family when he was about 8 years of age. Italian was his first language, but he was proficient in English, having learned it at a young age. He had recently married and had a

wide circle of friends and a strong family network. He had worked as an engineer for a security firm since graduation.

Emilio referred himself to the stuttering clinic at the Australian Stuttering Research Centre, The University of Sydney, complaining of moderate but persistent stuttering that he believed had been present since around the time he started school. He felt that the severity had been worse during his school years but that it had reduced a little during his adult years. He described his speech as mainly "getting stuck on words," particularly when he was anxious or over-tired. He also commented that it was usually worse in Italian, which he only used when talking to family members. He frequently scanned ahead for difficult words and used word avoidance and substitution on a regular basis. The only technique he had used in an attempt to reduce stuttering in the past was slowing down, but he reported that this had never been much help.

Emilio had never sought treatment for his stuttering in the past because, although the stuttering had been significant, he had never perceived it as a great problem. Close friends and family had always been accepting of his speech and rarely even commented on it. Even during his school years, his friends had just accepted him the way he was and defended him when he was teased. However, he now felt that his stuttering was beginning to have an impact on his promotional prospects at work. He had considerable difficulty talking to his boss and to clients, particularly as his work required him to communicate predominantly over the phone. In these situations in particular, he felt that his stuttering let him down. There was no known family history of stuttering.

Pretreatment measures were taken in the clinic at assessment. During a 5-minute conversation with the SLP, Emilio's speech was rated as 4.8% SS. The 9-point SR scale was explained and demonstrated. Emilio then gave this sample a rating of 4, whereas the SLP confirmed a rating of 5. Stuttering was characterized by some fixed postures of relatively short duration, with and without audible airflow, and by some repeated movements. There were minimal verbal and nonverbal superfluous behaviors. He described this speech as fairly typical of a "reasonably good patch" but nonetheless representative of his stuttering severity in some everyday situations.

The SLP gave Emilio basic information about the nature and suspected cause of stuttering and an outline of what would be involved in treatment with the Camperdown Program, as administered on an individual basis. He was also told that treatment could only offer a means for control of his stuttering and that long-term maintenance of treatment benefits was likely to be difficult. Emilio elected to begin treatment the following week. To get a better indication of the range of pretreatment severity, Emilio was informed that he would receive a couple of 5-minute phone calls during the week from university strangers. These would be recorded and rated for severity. He was also asked to make a couple of very short (1-minute) recordings of his speech in different situations that might demonstrate the variability of his stuttering in everyday situations. Possible situations were talking to his wife on the phone at work and speaking in Italian to his parents.

STAGE I: TEACHING SESSIONS

It took Emilio three visits to the clinic to complete the first stage of the program. This involved learning to use prolonged speech in an exaggerated manner to control his stuttering and learning to reliably use 9-point scales to evaluate the severity of his stuttering and the naturalness of his speech. Session 1 began with a short recorded conversation with the SLP. This was used to compare the SLP's SR score with Emilio's score. Both agreed that the sample should be rated at 5. If there had been some dispute over the rating or what constituted stuttering, the recording could have been used as a basis for discussion. Emilio had also made two short recordings of his speech during the week, which were played and evaluated for stuttering severity, along with segments of the two recordings made from the clinic strangers. Stuttering was discussed, and samples were rated according to the SR scale. All samples received client rat-

ings that were within one scale score of the SLP's ratings. %SS scores for the two clinic-initiated 5-minute stranger calls were 5.6% SS and 5.8% SS (see Table 14.2 for pretreatment %SS scores). Because the SLP and client SR scores agreed, Emilio was asked to choose five or six situations that reflected a cross-section of his daily life and then to assign a *typical* pretreatment SR score to each of these. His chosen situations and associated ratings are shown in Table 14.3. Comparison of within- and beyond-clinic (recorded) SRs by Emilio and the SLP continued over the next two sessions. Emilio's ratings were consistently within one scale score of the SLP's ratings.

In session 1, the SLP also introduced the prolonged speech technique to Emilio. He was directed to listen to the exemplar recording several times while following the transcript and to think of how he would describe the speech pattern he heard. He used the words "slow," "drunk-like," "monotonous," and "slurred." Then, he and the SLP read the text together along with the exemplar trying to sound "slow," "drunk-like," "monotonous," and "slurred." The SLP read the text as well, not to provide an additional model but to make the client feel more comfortable about using an unusual speech pattern. The passage was broken into smaller sections, and Emilio was given feedback to listen more closely to some parts of the recording and to make his speech sound more like the model. Finally, the SLP gave Emilio an audio copy of the exemplar and accompanying text and instructed him to practice the speech pattern at home until he felt he could make his speech sound just like the recording.

During the following week, Emilio frequently practiced reading and repeating the exemplar passage along with the recording. He had a CD player in his car and played the recording over and over while driving to and from work each day. Therefore, by the second session, he was able to consistently recite the Rainbow Passage

Table 14.2. *Pre- and Posttreatment %SS Scores for Emilio When Talking to the Speech-Language Pathologist and Talking to Two University Strangers*

Situation	Pretreatment %SS	Posttreatment %SS	Postmaintenance %SS
Within-clinic clinician	4.8	0	0
Beyond-clinic stranger 1	5.6	0.1	0.6
Beyond-clinic stranger 2	5.8	0.5	0.5

Table 14.3. *Pre- and Posttreatment Self-Reported Severity Rating (SR) Scores for Emilio's Self-Selected Representative Situations*

Situation	Pretreatment SR	Posttreatment SR	Postmaintenance SR
Talking with wife	4/5	2	1
Talking with friends	4/5	3	2
Work phone calls	5/6	2	2
Talking in Italian	5/6	2	2
Ordering food or drink	7/8	3	2/3

using unnatural-sounding, stutter-free prolonged speech that closely matched the exemplar. During the session and over the next week, he used this speech pattern while reading the newspaper and then in spontaneous monologue. By session 3, he was able to converse with the SLP for more than 20 minutes using this speech pattern and remaining stutter-free. Interestingly, after this practice, Emilio remained mostly stutter-free for the remainder of the session even when talking at a normal speech rate. He also commented that after practicing the model at home, his stuttering severity had frequently reduced significantly.

Emilio was then introduced to the 9-point NAT scale, where 1 indicates normal-sounding speech (like the SLP) and 9 indicates very unnatural-sounding speech, similar to that of the exemplar. The SLP then rated Emilio's speech at the beginning of the session as approximately NAT 7 and when he had just been talking to the clinician (with a small amount of prolonged speech) as NAT 3. Emilio was then instructed to use whatever features of prolonged speech he needed to control his stuttering while seeing if he could talk at approximately NAT 5.

By the end of the third session, Emilio had met the requirements to move to the instatement stage of the program (stage II). These requirements consisted of (1) conversing with the SLP consistently for at least 20 minutes at SR 1 and NAT 7 to 9, (2) obtaining plus or minus one scale score agreement with the clinician for within- and beyond-clinic SRs, (3) demonstrating familiarity with the NAT scale, and (4) being able to vary his use of prolonged speech at different NAT rating levels.

STAGE II: INSTATEMENT OF NATURAL-SOUNDING STUTTER-FREE SPEECH

Emilio continued to attend the clinic for weekly 1-hour sessions during the instatement stage of

the program. He took three sessions to complete this stage, the aims of which were to: (1) establish natural-sounding stutter-free speech consistently in the clinic, (2) practice self-evaluation skills, and (3) develop some basic problem-solving strategies.

He was introduced initially to the fluency cycles and phases—Practice, Trial, and Evaluation (see description earlier)—of the program and shown how to record data on his record form (see Appendix 14.1). Emilio and the SLP then worked through three complete cycles together in the first stage II session (clinic session 4), with the SLP explaining the rules of progression and prompting Emilio to decide on strategies for each cycle and to evaluate the results of these strategies according to the questions on the record form. He was advised that he did not have to complete a Practice Phase in every cycle as long as he achieved an SR score of 1 or 2 in the previous Trial Phase. However, every third cycle or whenever his SR was greater than 2, he needed to begin a cycle with a Practice Phase. For example (see record form in Appendix 14.1 for Emilio's progress), in his first Trial Phase, Emilio chose to attempt to speak at SR 1 and NAT 4. This was because he felt that he had already been successful at home talking without stuttering and sounding fairly natural. At the end of the phase, Emilio thought he had spoken at NAT 3 with minimal stuttering (SR 2), but in fact, after listening to the recording, he agreed that his speech was closer to NAT 2 and that was why he had stuttered a little. Therefore, his strategy for the next Trial Phase was to bring his stuttering severity back down to SR 1 by increasing his naturalness to NAT 5. By doing this in cycle 2, he once again brought his stuttering completely under control (SR 1). In cycle 3, after his Practice Phase, he elected to consolidate his control again at NAT 5. After listening to the recording of this phase, he decided that although he felt as though he was talking at NAT 5, he sounded more like NAT 4.

At the end of this session, Emilio was advised to continue with the cycles at home for the next week, making sure to think of a good strategy for how to practice in each cycle and to evaluate whether he had achieved his goal each time. He was advised to try to do at least a few cycles on his own each day and to record the results on his record form. He was told that the ultimate goal of this stage of treatment was to consistently achieve an SR score of 1 or 2 at the most, with a NAT of 2 or 3, and that this must be demonstrable on his record form for at least six consecutive trials. He was also reassured that there was no predetermined number of cycles required or expected to achieve this goal, so that it may take as few as one or two or as many as six or seven visits to achieve this.

Emilio returned the following week (clinic session 5) with his record form. He had managed to practice the cycles for approximately half an hour on each of 5 different days, completing 17 cycles in total. Appendix 14.1 shows the first eight of these home cycles and his decision-making process. In summary, Emilio practiced the prolonged speech technique and then experimented with how natural he could sound without stuttering. As he progressed through the cycles, he gained more control over his stuttering and made decisions about how much technique to use, depending on his recorded evaluations. The process was continued during the clinic visit, and different strategies were discussed with Emilio. By the end of the session, he had achieved an SR of 1 and NAT of 2 several times during the Trial Phase. Again, Emilio's instructions were to continue with the fluency cycles at home for the next week, making sure to think of a good strategy for how to practice in each cycle and to evaluate whether he had achieved his goal each time.

Emilio returned the following week (clinic session 6) having achieved his goal of at least six consecutive trials of SR 1 and NAT 3 or less. In total, he had completed 29 cycles before achieving this goal. He was able to remain completely stutter-free throughout the session while talking to the SLP at a NAT of 2 to 3. Therefore, he progressed to stage III of the program.

STAGE III: PROBLEM-SOLVING SESSIONS

During the same session (clinic session 6), the SLP first explained the goals of stage III to Emilio. These were to establish an appropriate regimen for practicing his new speech skill and to develop problem-solving strategies, based on data collected outside of the clinic, to assist the generalization of this skill into the real world. Together, Emilio and the SLP worked out a realistic practice routine. They decided that because it took Emilio about 40 minutes each day to drive to and from work, that this would be a good opportunity for him to practice his speech. He would relax and listen to the radio for the first 20 minutes of the journey and then practice his speech for the final 20 minutes, once in the morning and again in the afternoon. The routine would be to: (1) practice with the exemplar at NAT 7 to 9; (2) speak for about 5 minutes talking at NAT 7, describing what he saw as he drove along; and (3) speak for the rest of the time at NAT 3 until he arrived at work or at home.

Emilio and the SLP then worked out a system for collecting beyond-clinic data for discussion at the next session. He was to document (1) a *typical* SR for each day (the SR he achieved for approximately 70% of the day); (2) the *worst* SR for each day, the NAT score for that situation, and the situation in which it occurred; and (3) SR and NAT scores for each of the target situations identified in the first session. He was also encouraged to record his speech in situations as appropriate and to bring in examples of these recordings each week.

Emilio took seven further clinic sessions to move through stage III of the program. The structure of each session followed the same basic format. Each session began with Emilio talking for about 5 minutes to confirm his use of stutter-free speech. This was followed by self-evaluation of stuttering severity and speech naturalness. If a criterion of SR 1 and NAT 2 was not achieved, practice ensued until it did. Second, Emilio and the SLP discussed Emilio's practice routine across the week. He did most of his structured practice in the car each day but also scheduled a short time over breakfast each day of the weekend talking with his wife and covering the same routine as outlined earlier. Because all practice was scheduled into already existing routines, Emilio had no need to find extra time to do it, and it was not difficult for him to remember to do it.

Third, Emilio presented his beyond-clinic data for discussion each week. This technique was used to help him focus on his progress each week, to reinforce that he was stutter-free in various situations, to identify specific situations that needed more direct targeting, and to plan specific strategies to deal with these situations. Initially the SLP suggested strategies that Emilio might use to assist in these situations. However, over the 7 weeks, he was encouraged to think of strategies himself, test them out, and report the results to the SLP the following week. Ultimately, he learned not to wait for each clinic session to receive feedback and advice. Instead, he consistently evaluated his own speech and documented his ratings for various situations each day. Then he implemented and evaluated strategies himself. For example, initially Emilio had problems using the phone to talk to clients or the boss at work. Strategies devised by Emilio and the SLP included: practicing the speech technique and initial opening conversational content for a short period by himself before making the call, talking briefly to somebody with whom he was consistently stutter-free immediately before making the call, and starting the call at a higher NAT score and then gradually increasing naturalness.

Emilio was encouraged to record his speech as often as possible. This served three purposes. First, the recordings brought to the SLP each week lent support to the validity of Emilio's self-reported beyond-clinic data. Second, Emilio was able to listen back to recordings of his own speech immediately after speaking to verify whether his evaluations of severity and naturalness at the time of speaking were accurate. It was frequently the case that he overestimated how unnatural he sounded and was pleasantly surprised with the result. Also it reinforced to him that he could increase his use of prolonged speech when he needed to without sounding obviously unnatural. And finally, as mentioned previously, an audio recorder has a therapeutic purpose because it can frequently act as a discriminative stimulus, leading clients to practice stutter-free speech in situations in which they otherwise might have stuttered.

At the end of each clinic session, Emilio and the SLP formulated a plan for what he wanted to achieve over the coming week. Emilio's SRs gradually decreased in most everyday situations over the course of several weeks. However, after about 5 weeks, it became evident that this was not transferring as easily to situations in which he spoke Italian. Therefore, he was encouraged to practice prolonged speech in Italian during his usual practice sessions in the car. Within 2 weeks, his stuttering in Italian had also reduced.

After 7 weeks in stage III, Emilio met the criteria for moving into the maintenance stage of the program. Emilio's SR scores remained at approximately 2 in most everyday situations for most of the time. Table 14.3 shows the typical SR for each self-selected situation at the end of this period. At this time, the SLP arranged for two university strangers to again contact Emilio unexpectedly and record a 5-minute conversation with him to confirm his reported SRs. These two recordings were rated at 0.1% SS and 0.5% SS. Due to his low beyond-clinic ratings and the fact that he was problem solving satisfactorily on his own, Emilio was ready to move into the maintenance stage of the program.

STAGE IV: MAINTENANCE

Emilio remained in stage IV for approximately 6 months with clinic sessions becoming less frequent as he showed that he was able to problem solve to keep his SR scores at 1 to 2. Over this time, he had patches where his stuttering severity increased. However, when this happened, he could implement strategies to bring it back under reasonable control again—one of the strengths of the program.

FUTURE DIRECTIONS

At this stage, most of the evidence for the efficacy of the Camperdown Program has been collected by members of the research group who developed and initially studied the program. The exception to this is the student-administered program at La Trobe University (Cocomazzo, 2009). However, due to constraints of the academic term, this replication did not necessarily allow for clients to continue in treatment until reaching maintenance criteria. Therefore, replication of the program at an independent treatment site, preferably with generalist SLPs rather than experts in fluency disorders, is needed to show that the program is broadly efficacious.

Also of concern is that long-term outcome measures so far have been limited to 12-month posttreatment data collected in the initial trial. In none of the other studies have data been collected for this period of time after treatment. It may be that the more intensive nature of traditional programs leads to longer-term benefits, even though the problem-solving strategies integrated into this program were intended to give clients more control over the maintenance of treatment gains. Also there is no conclusive evidence yet as to whether this program may be more or less suited to those who have had previous treatment, although early reports (O'Brian et al., 2003a; O'Brian, Packman, & Onslow, 2008) show that previous treatment made no difference to outcome.

The results of the telehealth reports (Carey et al. 2009; O'Brian, Packman, & Onslow, 2008) also provide a reason to investigate other methods of delivery of the Camperdown Program. In Australia, as in some other countries, distances from service providers can be great, and regular face-to-face contact with a clinician is virtually impossible. Further, as mentioned previously, the majority of adult stuttering clients are of working age, many of whom find it difficult to take time off from their work to visit a clinic. With current advances in technology, it is exciting to consider the many possibilities for delivering any treatment program, or part of it, to this population.

CHAPTER SUMMARY

The Camperdown Program:

- was developed in accordance with preclinical laboratory evidence and has progressed to phase I and phase II clinical trials
- is a behavioral treatment based on prolonged speech, which is learned by imitating a standard exemplar
- includes SLP and client-administered rating scales for the measurement of stuttering severity and speech naturalness
- does not require stutter-count measures, and therefore, limited equipment is needed
- is concept rather than procedure driven and can therefore be administered in a variety of service delivery models and individualized according to client need

- requires approximately 15 to 20 SLP hours and is therefore more efficient than traditional treatments

CHAPTER REVIEW QUESTIONS

1. What are the four stages of the Camperdown Program? What are the primary goals for each stage?
2. Does it matter if an SLP or a client cannot produce a "soft contact sound"? Why?
3. Why is a weekly within-clinic %SS rating score by the SLP or client unnecessary in a routine clinic environment?
4. When would it be appropriate to expect a client to use his or her new speech pattern in everyday speech situations?
5. When attempting to transfer stutter-free speech into everyday situations, what are the two most important skills for the client to develop and routinely use?
6. How is client progress evaluated throughout the program and by whom? Are the same methods used for evaluating final outcome? What additional information might be useful?
7. What equipment is needed to conduct the program in a one-on-one weekly clinic visit model?
8. What modifications might need to be made to the program if the client is unable to attend the clinic on a regular basis in person?

SUGGESTED READINGS

O'Brian, S., Packman, A., & Onslow, M. (2004). Self-rating of stuttering severity as a clinical tool. *American Journal of Speech-Language Pathology, 13,* 219–226.

O'Brian, S., Packman, A., Onslow, M., & O'Brian, N. (2004). Measurement of stuttering in adults: Comparison of stuttering-rate and severity-scaling methods. *Journal of Speech, Language, and Hearing Research, 47,* 1081–1087.

Onslow, M., & O'Brian, S. (1998). Reliability of clinician's judgments about prolonged speech targets. *Journal of Speech, Language and Hearing Research, 41,* 969–975.

Packman, A., Onslow, M., & van Doorn, J. (1994). Prolonged-speech and modification of stuttering: Perceptual, acoustic and electroglottographic data. *Journal of Speech and Hearing Research, 37,* 724–734.

CHAPTER 15

The Fluency Plus Program: An Integration of Fluency Shaping and Cognitive Restructuring Procedures for Adolescents and Adults Who Stutter

Robert Kroll and Lori Scott-Sulsky

CHAPTER OUTLINE

KEY TERMS

Cognitive restructuring: the alteration of attitudes, feelings, belief systems, and emotions associated with the act of speech communication. This is accomplished by replacing faulty or irrational thought processes with more accurate and beneficial ones through supported self-realization and counseling.

Communication Mentality: the attitude or position of empowerment to speak to anyone, at any time, in any environment, efficiently and effectively, and with little more than a normal amount of negative emotion.

Covert Practice: the silent, mental rehearsal of targets providing a positive mental preparatory set with which to enter a speaking situation.

Establishment: the acquisition of new speech motor behaviors and attitudes through the systematic application of practice regimens based on proven principles of learning.

Maintenance: the continuation of the therapy program as the involvement of the clinician is gradually decreased involving a long, gradual process of consolidation and stabilization of skills and maturing of expectations by both the client and the clinician.

Transfer: the voluntary or conscious application of learned or acquired behaviors outside of the clinic situation.

INTRODUCTION

This chapter represents our attempt at outlining the Fluency Plus Program, our current intensive treatment program for people who stutter. The stuttering treatment program that we describe has evolved over a period of more than 25 years and has been administered to both adolescents and adults. During this period, we have continuously subjected our treatment methodology to laboratory experimentation in an attempt to determine both efficacy and efficiency. We have studied our clients' responses to treatment, listened to their feedback, and modified the program based on our observations and clinical discussions. We have followed the literature and engaged in countless dialogues with our colleagues at conferences and coffee shops in our quest to develop what we consider to be the most comprehensive stuttering treatment program.

To be sure, the picture seemed to be much clearer when we set about to do this work as young and eager clinician/scientists. The first author of this chapter completed his graduate studies in the mid-1970s just at the time when several stuttering programs were being developed and disseminated to the professional community as well-written, structured, and fairly easy-to-follow clinical procedures. All that was needed was the supplies budget to purchase the "package," and the clinician would be armed with clinician and client manuals, forms, handbooks, and a set of procedures to follow to administer the program. It all seemed so crystal clear back then.

As we began to administer these programs, we soon discovered the many "unwritten parts of the manual." Issues arose during the program that did not seem to be included in the program materials. So began the process of refining and modifying and supplementing the original program. This process is dynamic and ongoing, and what is summarized here will no doubt be further modified as our research and clinical efforts continue to enlighten us with additional information regarding the most effective treatments. Thus, we write this chapter with the following proviso: The procedures we describe here are the most practical and effective we have found for a large number of the clients seen at the The Speech and Stuttering Institute in Toronto. However, this type of treatment is not suitable for many clients, who will be discussed later in the chapter. Some clients, who we think are good candidates for this procedure, will not respond to the treatment as we would have expected for a variety of reasons. These too will be discussed throughout the chapter. In short, we are attempting to provide the reader with a realistic synopsis of what these procedures can and cannot do for people who stutter. Having said that, we will try to provide enough information for the reader to be able to apply the treatment methodology of the Fluency Plus Program in his or her own practice or agency.

Our task is indeed daunting. It is very difficult to cover all of the issues that arise during a program of treatment given the space limitations of a book chapter. Describing a treatment program for stuttering is almost like writing a complete book about the subject. Indeed, if all contributors to this text were to fully discuss each and every detail of their program rationale, methodology, and procedures, we would need an empty bookcase for the series of volumes that would result.

We have come to view the Fluency Plus Program as unique for a number of reasons. First, the program is based on a strong connection between empirical research and clinical observation. We have been fortunate to attract many talented clinician/scientists over the years who have contributed immensely to the continuing refinement of the program. Our research team has consistently investigated both client and program variables and their relationships to treatment outcome. Being affiliated with major hospitals and universities has allowed us to use the most current technology to peer into the cortical structures of our clients in order to observe changes during and after treatment. We will summarize this work later in the chapter.

Another identifying feature of the Fluency Plus Program is the way it is presented to the client. Both client and clinician roles are clearly outlined during a rigorous assessment procedure. Clients are informed about the intensive nature of the program and the many hours of drill and practice that are required. The success of the program is based in large part on the decisions made by the client and clinician during the assessment. Clients who seem likely to benefit from Fluency Plus are encouraged to begin the program as soon as feasible. For those clients who do not appear to fit the criteria for inclusion, we search for alternatives. Again, these criteria will be further elaborated upon later in this chapter.

Another one of the most valuable aspects of the Fluency Plus Program is the maintenance component. We will outline the evolution of the program and illustrate the importance of maintenance following intensive treatment. This is one of the most challenging areas to address. Having a structured maintenance program seems to have prevented countless individuals from experiencing partial or total regression of stuttering and has further allowed us to examine long-term treatment effects.

Fluency Plus deals with both the stuttering behavior as well as the many psychological factors that affect the individual who stutters. We have attempted to provide as comprehensive a program as possible in order to address much of what the person who stutters is experiencing. Perhaps the most distinctive part of this program relates to the honest messages that are received by the client as to what the program can and cannot provide. In essence, Fluency Plus demonstrates to the individual that he has a choice of how he communicates. By learning and applying a predetermined set of fluency skills and by approaching speech situations with a healthy mental set, high levels of fluency can be achieved. This of course requires a great deal of commitment and a lot of intensive training. In short, the client learns that the benefits derived from this behavioral treatment are directly related to his adherence to program elements and active involvement with it.

THEORETICAL BASIS FOR TREATMENT APPROACH

THE NATURE OF STUTTERING AND ITS TREATMENT

Many definitions and descriptions of stuttering can be found in the literature. Most reflect the author's particular bias or theoretical perspective. For the purposes of our discussion, we have selected one formal definition and one less formal description of stuttering.

One definition of stuttering characterizes the disorder as a complex multidimensional condition in which the flow of speech, or fluency, is disrupted by involuntary speech motor events (Bloodstein, 1995). There are two key words in this definition that deserve our attention. First, the term "multidimensional" implies that stuttering is the result of a number of coexisting factors which, when combined in a specific manner, result in the disfluent speech of the person who stutters. These multiple factors may include genetic, personality, psychosocial, physiologic, and emotional factors. It is not the purpose of this chapter to delve into the many theories and experimental studies that have addressed these dimensions of stuttering. Suffice it to say that the practicing clinician should be continually looking for clues in these areas to explain the onset, development, and perpetuation of the speech pattern.

The second key word in this definition, "involuntary," can be interpreted in a number of ways with regard to the speech motor events of stuttering. Although much has been written about the feelings of helplessness and sheer lack of speech control in stuttered speech, it is important to note that the purpose of the current program is to bring speech to the level of conscious control. Thus, although the act of stuttering may seem and feel totally involuntary to the untreated individual, the successful participant of our intensive treatment program will acquire the skills necessary to produce a conscious, volitional form of smooth, free-flowing speech.

Let us now turn to our less formal description of stuttering. This description acknowledges two fundamental aspects of the disorder: (1) the stuttering problem and (2) the stuttering behavior. The stuttering problem refers to stuttering as a life issue. Here we are looking at issues such as self-esteem and self-concept, confidence, peer interaction, attitudes, emotions, psychological factors, and quality of life. The stuttering behavior, on the other hand, refers to those maladaptive speech behaviors commonly referred to as stuttering. These specific behaviors, or disfluency types, include silent blocks; sound, syllable, and word repetitions; sound prolongations; and dysrhythmic phonations. Here again, the literature is replete with a myriad of classification systems for types of disfluency (Conture, 1990; Cordes, 2000; Johnson & Associates, 1959; Sander, 1961; Silverman, 1974; Young, 1961). An additional component of the stuttering behavior involves the secondary, accessory, or contingent behaviors associated with stuttering. These behaviors include mannerisms such as head jerking, eye blinking, foot stamping, facial grimacing, and a variety of other subtle and, at times, not so subtle, struggle behaviors. The third aspect of the stuttering problem is avoidance. Avoidance occurs when the individual anticipates stuttering and engages in behaviors designed to disguise or avoid overt stuttering. Avoidance behaviors include word substitution, phrase revision, and the use of starters or fillers, such as automatic phrases at the beginning of sentences.

Stuttering has been associated with numerous theoretical constructs and a myriad of clinical strategies designed to assess and treat it. North American speech-language pathologists have traditionally found themselves in one of two clinical camps with regard to the treatment of confirmed stuttering in adolescents and adults. The first of these groups views stuttering as representing patterns of avoidance and struggle behavior that have been learned as responses to motor breakdowns in speech. Treatment procedures focus on reduction of negative emotion in order to decrease struggle, avoidance, and anxiety. Moreover, specific techniques are taught to assist the individual in modifying the tension, blockage, and fragmentation of stuttered speech to achieve less effortful, tension-free, and more free-flowing speech patterns (Guitar, 2006).

The second group approaches the modification of the stuttering response to fluent speech by the systematic application of behavioral principles. In this framework, certain aspects of stuttering are viewed as essentially learned behaviors that can be altered through appropriate response-contingent stimulation (Brutten & Shoemaker, 1967; Flanagan, Goldiamond, & Azrin, 1958; Shames & Sherrick, 1963). More recent explorations of the stuttered speech response have begun to uncover some of the neural substrates of stuttering, explaining the disorder as neurologically based with consequent motor aberrations in speech output (Braun et al., 1997; De Nil & Kroll, 2001; Fox et al., 1996; Ingham, 2001; Kroll & De Nil, 1998; Wu et al., 1995). Given the neurologic substrates and the conditioned responses of the individual toward speaking as an explanation of stuttering, therapy procedures attempt to reconstruct the respiratory, phonatory, and articulatory gestures used in fluent speech production (Boberg & Kully, 1985; Kroll & Beitchman, 2005; Kroll & De Nil, 1995; Webster, 1974).

For many years, members of our discipline argued their respective positions concerning the treatment of stuttering. Those clinicians who were more oriented toward the psychodynamics of stuttering accused the pure behaviorists of being too superficial in their view of the disorder. They argued that the behaviorists were not getting to the "deeper" issues and that their therapy approaches were too simplistic and superficial. In a similar fashion, behaviorists accused their counterparts of not adhering to the rigors of scientific enquiry and methodology.

Given these two views of the nature of stuttering, it is safe to say that most traditional speech therapy programs for stuttering fall within two major categories. The first of these is stuttering modification, and the second is fluency shaping (Guitar, 1998). Stuttering modification deals more with the disorder as a problem. It deals with the psychological aspects and addresses the attitudes, feelings, and emotions resulting from stuttering. Related areas that are worked on include self-acceptance, avoidance and anxiety reduction, and attitude change. Reducing fear is a major goal of stuttering modification therapy. This type of therapy attempts to teach the individual to modify his moments of stuttering by eliminating the tension and struggle associated with the disfluent moment. Specific techniques include cancellations (the deliberate repetition of the stuttered word), pull-outs (modifying the moment of stuttering as it occurs), and preparatory sets (covert planning of appropriate motor sequences before speaking); all of these techniques were first advocated by Van Riper (1973). The ultimate goal for the individual with advanced stuttering is to change the stuttering pattern to speech that is more relaxed, easy, and open. It is important to note that the goal here is to stutter more fluently, not to speak with perfectly normal fluency.

Fluency shaping therapy techniques generally differ from stuttering modification mainly in terms of the end products or desired goals for the client. Whereas stuttering modification therapy attempts to modify the moment of stuttering to achieve easier, less effortful stuttered speech, the goal of fluency shaping is to replace stuttering with stutter-free speech. In this therapy, fluency is reinforced and gradually shaped to approximate normal-sounding speech. Therapy procedures attempt to reconstruct stuttered speech by training fluency skills at the respiratory, phonatory, and articulatory levels. There is little, if any, attention paid to fear and avoidance reduction or other psychological factors associated with stuttering. Strict adherents to fluency shaping therapy restrict their efforts to only those observable, "measurable" speech behaviors. Thus, it is considered essentially of no use to deal with such immeasurable phenomena as fears or emotional states. Once the new speech patterns are established within the clinic setting, fluency shaping programs address beyond-clinic transfer and generalization of skills.

The 1980s ushered in an era of intense activity of clinical research aimed at identifying key components of clinical procedures deemed to be effective at reducing or completely eliminating stuttering behavior (Boberg, 1976; Cooper, 1976; Ryan, 1979; Shames & Florance, 1980; Shine, 1981; Webster, 1979). Specific clinical procedures were subjected to empirical validation. Those deemed to be effective were maintained and incorporated into many published clinical programs, and those that were deemed ineffective were discarded. Research in stuttering began to emphasize the notions of accountability and treatment effectiveness as the literature began to be filled with early if somewhat flawed outcome studies (Gregory, 1979; Ingham, 1984a). Indeed, questions pertaining to treatment validity are still the major topics of current books and chapters as we have learned to more fully scrutinize our clinical treatment procedures for people who stutter (Cordes & Ingham, 1998; Ingham & Cordes, 1999).

TREATMENT EFFICACY AND EFFECTIVENESS

Even as advances in efficacy in controlled, laboratory-derived treatment settings were being documented and reported, treatment effectiveness in typical clinical settings lagged behind. In our experience, the format and scheduling of therapy in traditional programs for stuttering emerged as one of the factors precluding substantial gains in clinical treatment. Clients were most often seen once a week for hour-long sessions or, at most, twice weekly. This spaced learning resulted in protracted therapy durations, lasting in many instances for 2 to 3 years or even longer. This therapy format would inevitably lead to situations that would supplant

the therapy process. In some instances, the client would become extremely dependent on the clinician for advice concerning many aspects of his life. Issues pertaining to vocational, social, marital, or other concerns unrelated to the presenting stuttering problem would begin to be the predominant focus during therapy. Eventually the therapist would begin to question the client's commitment to speech improvement. Indeed a very common therapy scenario would pair a male client, age 25 to 35 years, with a female clinician of the same age or slightly younger. It is little wonder that in so many instances, this therapy process was extended!

Another major issue with older treatment formats involved the minimal demands they placed on the client. Issues of self-reliance and ownership of the therapy process were not built into the treatment programs. Most of the teaching and practice took place within the confines of the clinic. All too often the client would leave the session having been instructed to "think about what we discussed today" or else to engage in a minimal amount of home practice.

This in-clinic therapy approach created serious problems pertaining to transfer or generalization of speech skills. Nonetheless, after several months of therapy, speech fluency would inevitably increase as the client-clinician relationship grew more comfortable and secure. Unfortunately for the client, however, this increased fluency was primarily due to decreased communicative stress and familiarity with the listeners rather than to conscious and deliberate production of a type of fluency that would endure increased communicative stress in real-world situations. Clients would then agonize over why their speech differed so greatly between the clinic and "out there." Difficulty with generalization of speech skills to beyond-clinic settings would often prompt the client to question his progress in therapy. Here again, due to the protracted nature of the therapy as well as to those earlier-mentioned interfering factors, accurate and complete assessment of speech gain was often impossible. Clinicians would encourage their clients at this point, noting attitudinal and adjustment gains despite the absence of any observed changes in speech fluency.

Thus, a growing disconnect was observed between results reported from treatment studies and results observed within clinics. Empirical evidence from laboratory-derived experimentation was suggesting that stuttered speech could be effectively modified to more normal-sounding forms, yet clinical practitioners continued to engage in therapy programs and formats that were highly inefficient and often comprised of vague instructions and inadequately defined objectives. The need to intensify treatment as well as to assign greater responsibility to the client for the therapy process was built into many of the intensive programs first reported in the mid to late 1970s (Boberg, 1976; Webster, 1979).

At this point in our evolution as a profession, it is comforting to note that the largely nonproductive arguments and polarization among professionals regarding the most effective ways of treating stuttering are slowly giving way to programs that address both the stuttering problem and stuttering behaviors. More and more treatment programs describe themselves as comprehensive, inclusive, or integrative as clinical researchers demonstrate the benefits of multidimensional approaches. Clinicians and researchers who at one time expressed very strong and somewhat rigid views regarding their treatments are gradually incorporating new elements as they identify critical variables that had gone unaddressed in earlier versions. Indeed, the popular text, *Stuttering: An Integrated Approach to Its Nature and Treatment* (Guitar, 2006) reflects this trend (Kroll et al., 2006). It is with such an integrative treatment model in mind that we present what we hope is a thorough outline of our treatment, the Fluency Plus Program at The Speech and Stuttering Institute in Toronto, Canada.

EMPIRICAL BASIS FOR TREATMENT APPROACH

The purpose of this chapter is an attempt to summarize our efforts at (1) resolving the discrepancy between laboratory-derived procedures and clinical work with stuttering and (2) establishing an integrated treatment program addressing fluency establishment, skill transfer, and fluency maintenance while also addressing the critical psychological barriers to fluency attainment. Our model has evolved over a 30-year period, and what follows is a chronology of specific program phases and modifications.

EARLY STUDIES

One of the first Canadian intensive treatment program for adults who stutter was introduced at the Clarke Institute of Psychiatry in Toronto in the late 1970s by the first author of this chapter. The treatment was based on the Precision Fluency Shaping Program developed by Webster (1974) and was designed initially to be used in an intensive, daily format by adolescents and adults. Its basic premise was that the person who stutters inadvertently violates fundamental rules of speech mechanics and must be taught to replace stuttered speech with normal-sounding fluency. The program was administered during a 3-week intensive period wherein clients were seen daily for up to 5 hours of group and individual therapy. The establishment phase trained fluency skills related to speech rate, respiratory, voice, and articulatory control. The generalization phase involved practice of these skills in natural settings. The program was appealing to us for a number of reasons. First, the highly structured and organized nature of the program materials allowed for a logical and well-planned sequence of clinical activities. Second, the program techniques and procedures had been derived from laboratory experimentation. Finally, the program was intensive in nature, requiring a full-time commitment from the clients for a 3-week period. These factors, combined with the fact that basic principles of human learning were carefully incorporated throughout the approach, convinced us to introduce the program to our clinic.

Leibovitz and Kroll (1980) conducted an initial retrospective study on 100 randomly selected clients who participated in the Precision Fluency Shaping Program in Toronto. They reported on stuttering frequencies from pretreatment and posttreatment videotapes from their randomly selected sample of 78 males and 22 females ranging in age from 12 to 60 years. Additional pre- and posttreatment data were obtained using the Perceptions of Stuttering Inventory (PSI) (Woolf, 1967), an instrument designed to provide self-report data on struggle, avoidance, and expectancy behavior. This early study reported that greater than 90% of the subjects participating in the intensive program demonstrated significantly improved fluency counts in addition to positive attitudinal shifts, as reflected by reduced PSI

Table 15.1. *Number of Cases at Each Dysfluency Level in Conversation before and after Intensive Therapy*

% Disfluent Words	Pretreatment	Posttreatment
0%–3%	2	58
4%–10%	14	30
11%–26%	45	12
27%–41%	25	0
42%+	14	0

From Leibovitz and Kroll, 1980.

Table 15.2. *Number of Cases by Total Perceptions of Stuttering Inventory Scores before and after Intensive Therapy*

	Total Score	Pretreatment	Posttreatment
Normal Range	0–10	9	82
	11–20	16	15
	21–30	30	2
	31–40	26	1
	41–50	15	0
	51–60	4	0

From Leibovitz and Kroll, 1980.

scores (Tables 15.1 and 15.2). The authors cautioned, however, that these data represented only pre- and posttreatment scores and anticipated that many clients would be unable to adequately maintain these gains without supplemental counseling, support, and follow-up. The authors reported that the transition from participants' functioning in the highly structured and rigorous intensive treatment program to functioning essentially on their own often resulted in either partial or total regression of speech skills. Thus began the modification of the original program

with an additional maintenance component consisting of in-clinic group sessions designed to assist clients with fluency issues in the posttreatment environment.

FOLLOW-UP STUDIES

To further assess treatment effectiveness, Kroll, Gaulin, and Tammsalu (1981) reported on pretreatment, posttreatment, and follow-up data obtained from 23 former program participants attending a self-help meeting. The subjects for the study consisted of 21 males and 2 females, ranging in age from 15 to 59 years. The amount of time after treatment ranged from 1 month to 5 years, 11 months, with a mean of 2 years and 5 months. Results of this study again demonstrated significant improvement in speech fluency immediately after treatment. Follow-up data reported some regression from posttreatment levels, notably in conversation, but the levels were still well above pretreatment levels. Mean percent dysfluency scores in conversation were 28.5% before treatment, 3.7% after treatment, and 7.8% at follow-up. Maximal regression was found to occur 6 months to 1 year after treatment, followed by gradual further improvement that soon leveled off, resulting in fluency scores well above pretreatment levels (Table 15.3).

The authors of this study also collected self-report ratings of daily functioning from their subjects. Only 20% of the subjects reported satisfactory performance in everyday speech situations before treatment. By contrast, after various intervals after treatment, 86% of the subjects reported either little or no difficulty with daily speaking experiences.

In addition to the requirement for a formal maintenance component after intensive stuttering treatment, we identified many areas that

Table 15.3. *Mean Percent Disfluency Scores in Conversation for 23 Subjects Grouped According to Time Intervals after Treatment*

No. of Subjects	Interval After Treatment	Pretreatment Score	Posttreatment Score	Follow-Up Score
4	1–6 months	27.5	1.4	6.4
5	7–12 months	35.1	4.3	11.2
5	1.1–3.0 years	27.3	4.3	8.2
6	3.1–5.0 years	24.0	6.7	9.0
3	5.1–6 years	28.8	1.7	4.1

From Kroll, Gaulin, & Tammsalu, 1981.

needed to be addressed during the program that were not specifically targeted as goals in the original program. We discovered that we needed to devote many hours to a number of issues related to feelings of negativity concerning stuttering, acceptance of modified speech patterns, learning to cope with anxiety, establishing realistic expectations and goals, analysis of specific beliefs and attitudes, and a variety of other areas that will be discussed later in this chapter. We began to see the need to incorporate strategies designed to assist clients in altering their self-perceptions, attitudes, and overall belief systems. In other words, cognitive restructuring evolved as an integral part of our intensive therapy program. Indeed, the current literature contains several endorsements of supplementing behavioral techniques with cognitive or affective restructuring (Blood, 1995; DiLollo, Neimeyer, & Manning, 2002; Ladouceur, Caron, & Caron, 1989; Neilson, 1999). Very early on in our clinical efforts, we came to realize that behavioral change alone without modifications of attitude and other areas of cognition would inevitably lead to problems during treatment and most certainly in the posttreatment environment. These realizations were later confirmed by others administering intensive adult stuttering treatment programs (Andrews & Craig, 1988).

Our program was then modified to include specific cognitive restructuring goals in addition to the behavioral goals pertaining to the overt speech behavior. Moreover, we increased our efforts at strengthening our formalized maintenance phase. Following the intensive program, clients were enrolled for a maintenance program consisting of follow-up group sessions scheduled on a progressively fading basis and lasting for 1 year. *Manual of Fluency Maintenance: A Guide for Ongoing Practice* (Kroll, 1991) was written to assist program participants in developing a systematic home practice program and to establish both short- and long-term goals for fluency. Indeed, in the months and years following the establishment of intensive programs, fluency maintenance was identified as one of the most critical challenges facing clients in the posttreatment environment (Boberg, Howie, & Woods, 1979; Ingham, 1984b). We also established a number of support systems for past clients in addition to formal maintenance pro-

grams. These included refresher courses and focused self-help groups, both of which will be discussed later in this chapter. Thus, the Fluency Plus Program evolved to include the above components.

Subsequent follow-up studies of our intensive program confirmed the results of our early studies and shed additional light on the long-term speech performance of clients in the posttreatment environment. In general, these studies indicated that the majority of clients demonstrated an initial dramatic decrease in stuttering immediately after treatment with regression rates ranging from 5% to 20% 1 or 2 years following intensive treatment (De Nil & Kroll, 1995; De Nil et al., 2003; Kroll et al., 1997).

MEASURING TREATMENT EFFECTS USING NEUROIMAGING

Our seminal research using neuroimaging techniques added confirming data as to the speech processing of individuals who stutter and brain activation before and after treatment and 1 year after a maintenance program (De Nil et al., 2003; Kroll & De Nil, 2000; Kroll, De Nil, & Houle, 1999). Thirteen adults diagnosed with developmental stuttering, age 20 to 40 years, and 10 nonstuttering adults, age 19 to 34 years, completed silent and oral reading tasks and a verb generation task while functional images of their brain activation patterns were obtained using positron emission tomography (PET). The stuttering subjects were scanned at three separate times: before intensive therapy with Fluency Plus; immediately after the 3-week intensive portion; and 1 year later. Fluency counts and Stuttering Severity Instrument (SSI) scores (Riley, 1972) were obtained at the pretreatment, post–intensive treatment, and follow-up times. PSI scores were also obtained at these times (Table 15.4).

In addition to other findings, we have demonstrated that people who stutter, in general, demonstrate increased cortical activity when performing oral speaking tasks. This increased activity is observed before treatment and is thought to reflect increased effort during speech production. Interestingly, the subjects demonstrated a persistent pattern of cortical overactivation immediately following treatment, although this overactivation was more left lateralized.

Table 15.4. *Mean Percent Disfluencies for Reading and Conversational Speech and Mean Stuttering Severity Index (SSI) and Perceptions of Stuttering Inventory (PSI) Scores for Stuttering Subjects (n = 13) before a 3-Week Intensive Stuttering Reduction Therapy, Immediately after the Therapy, and 1 Year Later*

Subjects	% Mean Disfluencies Reading	% Mean Disfluencies Conversation	Mean SSI Score	% Mean PSI Score
Before treatment (n = 13)	6.07 (7.45)	7.07 (4.85)	15.3 (5.79)	48 (15.8)
After treatment (n = 13)	0.76 (0.83)	1.61 (2.72)	8.15 (2.07)	18 (11.9)
1 year later (n = 13)	1.07 (0.95)	3.46 (2.90)	10.3 (3.92)	21 (11.1)

From De Nil et al., 2003.

We interpreted this overactivation, even in light of very high levels of fluency immediately after treatment, as the result of the cognitive demand associated with the deliberate monitoring of fluency skills as per the Fluency Plus Program. What is most compelling is the pattern observed following a year of successful maintenance, where the cortical activity seen in the stuttering subjects begins to approximate those patterns seen in non-stuttering speakers, although not completely. We have interpreted this finding as suggesting that speech becomes more automatic for the speaker after a consistent program of fluency practice. This series of neuroimaging studies has strongly suggested the necessity of fluency maintenance programs following intensive treatment. Major changes in cortical activity from posttreatment to follow-up suggest that the formalized practice routine consisting of skill training and cognitive restructuring (Kroll, 1991) plays an important role in establishing speech patterns that are more easily accessed by the client (Fig. 15.1). Of course, additional studies will shed even more light on brain activation changes after treatment, thus allowing us to further tease out those critical elements of the maintenance program that are most responsible for the observed effects. Moreover, investigations of those clients who relapse during the maintenance period could potentially provide us with useful predictive information.

After more than 25 years of clinical and research experience with stuttering treatment for adolescents and adults, we can say with confidence that there are specific and fundamental principles that must be included for effective therapy. First and foremost, the program must be based on empirically tested procedures. This statement reflects the growing awareness of the importance of evidence-based practice that is discussed so frequently in our discipline (Cordes & Ingham, 1998). Second, the program must be comprehensive and include establishment, transfer, and maintenance stages of treatment. Third, although the program may deal initially with observable behaviors, attention must be paid to the attitudes, feelings, emotions, and other cognitive factors that could potentially impact an individual's response to any of the treatment phases. Fourth, the program must be administered on an intensive schedule. Finally, effective behavioral programs for stuttering must incorporate several fundamental principles of learning.

The following list of points reflect what we have found to be crucial in providing effective and complete treatment programs for individuals who stutter.

Speech Represents Complex Behavior

There are no simple solutions to stuttering, even in what appear to be milder cases. It is unlikely that simply teaching easy breathing or slow speech will be sufficient to modify the gamut of maladaptive speech behaviors that we see as stuttering.

Treatment Techniques Focus Primarily on Observable Behaviors

The primary focus of treatment must be to modify the physical aspects of the speech production process. This will involve working on the distorted respiratory, phonatory, and articulatory behaviors. The aim is to modify these speech behaviors via a series of exercises designed to retrain movement patterns for speech.

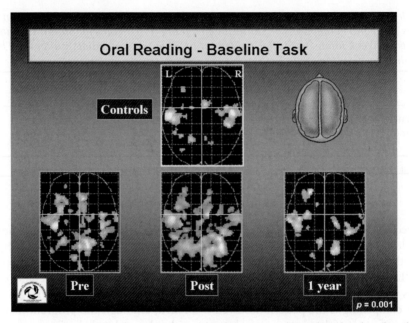

Figure 15.1. Positron emission tomography scans of control and stuttering subjects during oral reading illustrating widespread increased activation immediately after treatment and subsequent reduction after 1 year of maintenance therapy (Kroll, De Nil, & Houle, 1999).

Fluency Skill Training Is Supplemented by Cognitive Restructuring

Attitudinal and emotional factors must be addressed during treatment. Individuals presenting with confirmed, chronic stuttering often develop coping strategies that impact therapy progress. Comprehensive treatment programs will deal with self-talk strategies, coping with fear and anxiety, and eliminating avoidance behavior.

Treatment Must Be Intensive

Intensity of treatment can refer to the format of therapy (i.e., daily programs consisting of several hours of in-clinic sessions), but intensification can also refer to the performance expectations placed on the clients' home practice between sessions. For example, it is not sufficient to provide vague, non–goal-oriented instructions such as "Try this for a few minutes when you get home tonight." We have found that the client must be given specific instructional guidelines for home practice that are supplemented by printed materials at the end of each session. It is not uncommon for us to request several hours of home practice between clinic sessions.

Fluency Skills Must Be Overlearned and Exaggerated

During the initial stages of treatment, fluency skills are taught in a much exaggerated way to increase the client's awareness of the details of speech. These behaviors are taught individually and are practiced at each level until overlearning or ease of production is achieved. Then, they are transferred from simple speech responses to ongoing conversation.

Reduction of Response Variability

It is essential to provide the client with specific definitions of desired behaviors as well as ranges of acceptable speech responses. It is inappropriate to tell a client to "breathe easier" or "talk slower" without adequately specifying performance expectations for specific fluency skills. Home assignments should be assessed in a similar fashion using analysis of recorded practice sessions. During clinic sessions, the client should be provided with immediate feedback pertaining to the accuracy of his speech responses. This feedback may be provided by instrumentation such as timing devices, biofeedback units, or analysis of recorded speech and clinician feedback.

Fading and Client Self-Reliance

Therapy techniques, materials, and equipment (e.g., stopwatches) are introduced at critical times during treatment and then withdrawn as the client achieves performance criteria at each program step. In this fashion, the tendency for the client to become overly dependent on an intermediary program step or piece of instrumentation is avoided. The goal throughout the program is to achieve self-reliance for all aspects of both the behavioral and cognitive components of the speech process.

Transfer of Fluency Skills Must Be Addressed

The therapy program cannot take place solely in the clinical environment. Specific transfer activities must constitute an integral part of the overall treatment program. The timing and type of transfer activities must be scheduled to accommodate the client's needs and preparedness to incorporate newly learned fluency skills in the natural environment. The sequence of transfer activities must follow the same structured and logical progression as that used during initial training.

Maintenance Programs Must Be Incorporated

To complete all phases of comprehensive treatment, the client must be provided with a set of guidelines and procedures to follow independently in the posttreatment environment. These guidelines must be specific and provide the client with detailed instructions as to how to develop effective practice schedules to maintain fluency gains. Maintenance or follow-up sessions constitute part of the treatment program and should be conducted on a progressively fading basis.

Posttreatment Support Groups Provide a Bridge

These posttreatment groups represent a bridge between the structured program offered during the clinical program and the client's independent home practice routines. These posttreatment groups have been established as work meetings where former program participants gather on a regular schedule to focus on the original therapy skills acquired during the intensive program. Client feedback, dialogue, and problem solving are encouraged during these meetings. For the most part, they are run independent of professional intervention, and the group adheres to a formal organizational structure, including a slate of elected officers.

Refresher Programs Must Be Offered

Past program participants are never formally discharged from the program. Refresher programs are conducted twice yearly to allow individuals to reacquaint themselves with the details of the original program and to attend a 2-day seminar during which they can receive professional feedback and face the challenges of communication in large groups. Clients participate in these refresher programs voluntarily. We have found that these programs are especially beneficial for those clients residing at great distances from the clinic, which preclude them from attending the series of follow-up maintenance sessions.

PRACTICAL REQUIREMENTS FOR TREATMENT

LEVEL OF TRAINING REQUIRED

The Fluency Plus Intensive Adult Program should only be administered by qualified speech-language pathologists. Although we have attempted to include here sufficient detail to ensure replicability of the program, it is recommended that the clinician have significant background and experience treating and counseling people who stutter. Ideally, the clinician will have spent a number of clinic hours shadowing Speech and Stuttering Institute staff and developing accurate production of the eight target behaviors and familiarity with the program equipment and manuals.

TIME REQUIREMENTS OF TREATMENT

The Fluency Plus Intensive Adult Program consists of a 3-week intensive phase and an 11-month maintenance phase. The intensive phase consists of daily 4.5-hour sessions, Monday through Friday, with 2 to 4 hours of home assignments to be completed after clinic each day and on weekends. It is recommended that clients be free of work or school responsibilities for the duration of the intensive phase. During the maintenance phase, clients are required to dedicate approximately 1 hour per day to practice activities and record keeping. Clients are also required to attend 17 1-hour maintenance sessions, scheduled on a weekly, bimonthly, and monthly basis to complete 12 months of treatment. Clients who are unable to attend maintenance meetings in person are required to prepare and mail or email recorded samples of their speech and schedules of practice on or before each scheduled maintenance meeting.

EQUIPMENT REQUIRED

Equipment required by the clinician to replicate the Fluency Plus Program includes treatment manuals, analog stopwatch, video camera, videotapes, video monitor, audio recorder, and audiotapes. It is also required that each client have access to a voice onset biofeedback device throughout the duration of the intensive phase for in-clinic and out-of-clinic use. At the Speech and Stuttering Institute, we use two forms of voice onset biofeedback. The first is the electronic "voice monitor," which provides feedback with the lighting of a green indicator light if voice onset is performed within defined parameters of loudness and loudness change (Smith & Kroll, 1979). The second is the Dr. Fluency computer software program, which provides a graphic representation of the loudness and loudness changes of the voice onset across time (Friedman, 1992). Sufficient physical space is required to accommodate group lecture sessions and paired practice sessions. Clients are required to have an analog stopwatch, an audio recorder, and two audiotapes for use during and following treatment.

COST OF TREATMENT

The cost of administering the Fluency Plus Program is a reflection of the required clinical hours and available material resources. Accordingly, this cost will vary with region and healthcare setting. Practically speaking, one should allow for a minimum of 77 direct clinical hours, 12 clinical preparation hours, 16 clinical analysis hours, and 10 administrative consultation hours. Depending on group size and schedule flexibility, a co-clinician may be required to provide remedial sessions and clinical feedback in outside transfer activities. Materials costs include the reproduction of manuals and forms, and equipment costs include

biofeedback devices and computer software. Space requirements should also be taken into account.

KEY COMPONENTS OF THE APPROACH

TREATMENT GOALS

Ultimately, the treatment objective of the Fluency Plus Program is the achievement of the **Communication Mentality**. Communication Mentality is the ability to speak to anyone, at any time, in any place, effectively and efficiently, and with little more than a normal amount of negative emotion. To meet this objective, three basic treatment goals must be achieved:

1. Clients must gain control over speech muscle movement patterns through the **establishment** of fluency-facilitating target behaviors.
2. Clients must gain the ability to produce controlled speech in all relevant speaking contexts through the acquisition of **transfer** skills and the **cognitive restructuring** of attitudes, beliefs, and feelings.
3. Clients must acquire a skill set to support the long-term **maintenance** of treatment gains.

STAGES OF INTERVENTION

The Fluency Plus Program is comprised of three overlapping stages of intervention, which correspond to each of the three treatment goals:

1. *Establishment of Fluency-Facilitating Targets.* The motor-speech system is restructured through the establishment of eight fluency-facilitating speech behaviors called targets. A target may be defined as a specific muscle movement pattern performed within defined parameters. The establishment phase is supported by providing the client with a practical and relevant education about the anatomy and physiology of speech and stuttering.
2. *Transfer and Cognitive Restructuring.* Alongside the establishment of the physical mastery of target behaviors, the processes of transfer and cognitive restructuring are achieved. Transfer may be defined as the use of the newly acquired speech pattern outside of the clinical setting and in various speaking activities; and cognitive restructuring may be thought of as changes in the way a client

thinks and feels about stuttering and communication as well as changes in the mental set with which he enters into speaking situations. Clients are introduced to critical concepts to facilitate successful transfer throughout the program. Each of these concepts is supported by specific cognitive restructuring goals. In this way, transfer and cognitive restructuring may be considered codependent and are achieved simultaneously.

3. *Maintenance and Staying Connected.* Clients are introduced to critical concepts that are instrumental to the maintenance of long-term fluency gains. A detailed program of daily practice activities is introduced along with record keeping and goal-setting strategies. Clients are scheduled to attend a year-long series of follow-up sessions to support practice, assess skill maintenance, problem solve, and address ongoing attitudinal goals. They are also encouraged to become members of the Demosthenes Society, a volunteer-run support group of alumni of the program, and to participate in yearly refresher seminars.

PROGRAM PROGRESSION

In the following description of the Fluency Plus Program progression, we have attempted to outline the procedures and activities we use to establish the behavioral skill requirements of the program. In addition, we have indicated in bolded italics those sections addressing cognitive restructuring goals. Please see Figure 15.2 for a summary of the program sequence and clinical goals.

Intensive Phase

Day 1

Pretreatment Measures Each client participates in a videotaped interview and is asked to provide a videotaped reading sample as measures of speech fluency.

For an example, see Video Clips 1 and 2 for this chapter on thePoint.

For each of these measures, words spoken per minute and percent words stuttered are calculated, stuttering form type and frequency are analyzed, and secondary behaviors are noted. Each client also completes two pen-and-paper attitude scales to measure perceived communication competency, perceived presence of struggle and avoidance behaviors, and perceived awareness of expectancy of stuttering. The attitude scales used at the Speech and Stuttering Institute include the PSI (Woolf, 1967) and the Modified Erickson Scale of Communication Attitudes-S24 (Andrews & Cutler, 1974).

Introductions After a brief overview is provided regarding speech, stuttering, and the philosophy and format of the Fluency Plus Program, an informal group introduction activity is completed. *For many participants in the program, meeting and speaking with other people who stutter is a rare experience. One of the profound advantages of the group treatment model is the opportunity to achieve a most critical cognitive restructuring goal. By virtue of acceptance and positive regard for other group members who stutter, each participant's process of self-acceptance is begun. A mental shift from negative self-perception to positive acceptance is forged. Many clients express feelings of relief upon learning that others share their experiences and feelings. Comfort is found in the knowledge that they are not alone.*

Counseling A portion of each clinic day is devoted to group counseling through a variety of activities. Each activity serves as an opportunity to introduce and explore concepts critical to achieving specific cognitive restructuring goals. Clients are always encouraged to ask questions and bring forward points for discussion because we recognize that the most teachable moments are often those that arise from spontaneous inquiry. For this reason, the program must remain flexible enough to accommodate counseling needs as they arise.

Establishment of the Stretched Syllable Target The Stretched Syllable Target is introduced at the 2-second stretch rate.

See Video Clips 3 and 4.

Four rules defining the target are provided:

1. Each syllable is prolonged (or "stretched") for 2 seconds as measured by an analog stopwatch.
2. The first "stretchable sound" (vowel or voiced continuant) is prolonged for 1 second.
3. The remaining sounds of the syllable are prolonged for the remaining second.
4. A 1-second pause is inserted between syllables for inhalation.

	Day	Establishment Goal	Transfer Goal	Cognitive Restructuring Goal	Maintenance Goal
I N T E N S I V E P H A S E	1	Stretched Syllable Target (2 SS)	Home Assignments Self-Evaluation	Self acceptance	
	2		Feedback Self-Correction Practice on the Telephone	Addressing situational fears	
	3	Full Breath Target	Speech Making in 2-SS	Achieving an objective view of stuttering Acceptance of full-time speech modification	
	4	Gentle Onset Target	Covert Practice	Managing anxiety Achieving openness about speech modification	
	5	Slow Change Target Reduced Air Pressure Target			
	6	Reduced Articulatory Pressure Target Stretched Syllable Target (1 SS) Amplitude Contour Target			
	7	Full Articulatory Movement Target	Conversation Practice Taped dialogues out-of-clinic	Habituating the modified speech pattern	
	8		Speech Making in 1 SS Viewing pre-therapy tape	Desensitization to public speaking Habituating a positive preparatory mental set Viewing stuttering from a scientific view point Readiness to change Awareness of avoidance behaviors	
	9	Stretched Syllable Target (½ SS)			
	10	Stretched Syllable Target (New Normal)	Speech Making in ½ SS	Acceptance of modified speech	
	11		Monitored vs. Lucky Fluency Out-of-clinic conversation	Acceptance of full-time New Normal Viewing success in terms of control not fluency	Shaping
	12		Telephone Transfers	Desensitization to speaking on the telephone Familiarization with New Normal Increasing willingness to approach speaking situations	Structured Transfer
	13		Speech making – New Normal Out-of-Clinic Transfers	Objective evaluation of targets Managing negative self-talk	
	14				Spontaneous Transfer Mini Program
	15				Review Record Keeping Goal Setting
POST-INTENSIVE PHASE	1 year				Follow-up Meetings Refresher Seminars Alumni Support Group Toastmasters

Figure 15.2. Summary of the Fluency Plus Program sequence and clinical goals.

This target is established using single-syllable words initiated with stretchable sounds (e.g., ON, IN). Next, stretchable multisyllable words are introduced (e.g., NOR MAL, RE VERT) with close attention to accurate timing durations and awareness of the stable positions and movements of the articulators. Next, two "unstretchable" categories of sounds are defined. The voiceless fricatives (/h/, /f/, /s/, /ʃ/, /tʃ/, /θ/) and the plosives (/p/, /b/, /t/, /d/, /k/, /g/). When producing syllables beginning with these sounds, the unstretchable sound is produced briefly, and the subsequent stretchable sound is stretched for 1 second. Clients are best able to benefit from this stage of treatment if they are helped to understand the rationale for the extreme and unusual durations of the 2-second stretch. It is explained that the Stretched Syllable Target is required to decrease the force and acceleration characteristic of stuttered speech. It provides an opportunity to feel and notice the details of speech movements and make modifications to these details. The Stretched Syllable Target is the foundation for the establishment of each of the other targets. Furthermore, clients must understand that the extreme stretching of the 2-second stretch will be short lived and shaped toward a natural rate of speech through a progression to the 1-second stretch, the half-second stretch, and ultimately, a "New Normal" rate of speech within a range considered typical for natural and functional communication.

Home Assignments Home assignments are provided at the end of each clinic visit to reinforce skills and concepts acquired in clinic. The completion of home assignments begins the process of transfer of targets to the out-of-clinic environment, and thus, an overdependence on the clinic environment is avoided.

Self-Evaluation Clients are instructed to audio-record their home assignments each day and to review these recordings for target accuracy. Clients are instructed to self-evaluate consistently by monitoring accurate timing durations by stopwatch, feeling stable articulatory positioning and movements, and listening back to audio recordings.

Day 2
Feedback Audio recordings of home assignments are reviewed at the beginning of each clinic visit, and feedback is provided regarding target accu-

racy. Clinical feedback is gradually faded out as clients become increasingly able to self-evaluate and receive feedback from their fellow group members. Clients are encouraged to give one another objective and supportive feedback by commenting on the accuracy of target parameters. In the case of poor client performance or compliance, individual meetings are scheduled to address client needs.

Self-Correction Clients are introduced to a method of responding to target errors called self-correction:

1. Stop as soon as any missed detail of a target is noted and exhale any stored air.
2. Take a new breath.
3. Repeat the syllable on which the error was noted correctly and move on to the next syllable.

There are three significant benefits to performing self-corrections: (1) clients have the opportunity to independently evaluate and repair their own target errors without overreliance on clinical feedback; (2) inaccurate practice trials are replaced with accurate ones; and (3) the unproductive habits of forcing through blocks or restarting entire phrases following a moment of stuttering are replaced.

Two-Second Stretch in Continuous Reading When applying the 2-second stretch to continuous reading exercises, a short portion of text must be memorized and then produced aloud using the stopwatch to monitor accurate timing durations. Clients are instructed to audio-record their reading assignments, listen to their recordings, and note errors. If more than six errors per 50-word paragraph are noted, clients are encouraged to redo the assignment with greater accuracy.

Introduction to Transfer Transfer is defined for the client as taking the fluency skills learned in the clinic and applying them outside the clinic in a variety of speaking activities. It is explained that the transfer process actually began when home assignments were completed out of clinic.

Transfer Assignment on the Telephone To further the transfer process, clients are required to complete a reading assignment over the telephone. This assignment is initially completed with a fellow group member who is able to offer objective feedback. As treatment progresses, clients are encouraged to complete subsequent assignments with various group members and non-group individuals over the phone. *In this way, clients begin to address the critical cognitive restructuring goal of reducing the fear associated with speaking on the telephone. Many clients enter treatment with great difficulties and significant anxiety about using the telephone. Participating in successful transfer of clinical skills on the telephone begins the process of a mental shift in perception. The telephone becomes associated with control and success rather than tension and struggle.*

Day 3

Speech Physiology A detailed description of the physiology of speech and stuttering is given. *An understanding of the speech mechanism supports the acquisition of targets and also addresses a critical cognitive restructuring goal. Stuttering ceases to be viewed as a character flaw or failing. Instead, stuttering is viewed as a predictable result of faulty movement patterns of speech that can be corrected and controlled through the conscious application of targets.* Clients are also taught to classify speech sounds as vowels (Class I), voiced continuants (Class II), voiceless fricatives (Class III), or plosives (Class IV). Regardless of language, sounds may be classified in this way and categorized as stretchable or unstretchable. The sound class also determines the target sequence that must be applied. Multilingual clients are encouraged to complete a portion of each home assignment in each of the languages they speak.

Transfer to Conversation Level Simple questions and answers are modeled initially by the clinician. With gradual fading of the model, clients are required to produce longer and more spontaneous utterances while applying the Stretched Syllable Target accurately. At this stage, clients are encouraged to maintain constant adherence to the 2-second stretch during all in-clinic speech. Gradually, this requirement is extended to all speech activities in and out of the clinic. *We observe that when clients are required to consistently use targets in clinic from an early stage, they are more easily able to achieve transfer later in the program because a critical cognitive restructuring goal is addressed. Ultimately, clients must understand that the modified speech*

pattern must be applied in all speaking activities, not just those designated as practice or those perceived to be "difficult." Without full-time adherence to monitored fluency, clients fail to fully consolidate the new muscle movement patterns and run the risk of posttreatment regression.

Establishment of the Full Breath Target The Full Breath Target is introduced following a review of the anatomy and physiology of the respiration system and requires the establishment of the coordination of speech with diaphragmatic breathing. The introduction of the Full Breath Target is reserved until sufficient mastery of the Stretched Syllable Target is achieved. Without the establishment of the Stretched Syllable Target, many clients exhibit insufficient control over voice initiation to accurately practice the Full Breath Target with speech.

Video Clip 5 for an example of the Full Breath Target.

The three steps of the Full Breath Target are as follows:

1. *Take a slow, comfortably full breath in by feeling the abdomen move out.* Clients should monitor abdominal movements with their hand. Movements of the chest and shoulders should be limited.
2. *Consciously eliminate any pause or breath holding following inhalation.* This assures that the vocal folds are kept open prior to voicing to prevent hard glottal attack and laryngeal blocking.
3. *Passively exhale without force, feeling the abdomen return to rest.* Voicing is initiated on the exhaled breath stream. The Full Breath Target is established at the 2-second stretch rate at the word, sentence, paragraph, and conversation levels and maintained through the introduction of all other targets.

Day 4

Speech Making Clients present a prepared 3-minute speech at the 2-second stretch rate, with monitoring of the accuracy of the Stretched Syllable and Full Breath Targets by the other members of the group and the clinicians. Midway through the speech, clients are asked for a self-evaluation of target accuracy. Peer and clinician feedback is also provided. Throughout treatment, external feedback is faded, and a greater emphasis is placed on self-evaluation in order to foster greater self-reliance. *There is often significant anxiety leading up to the first in-clinic speech, yet performance is typically successful in the clinical setting. Clients are provided with an opportunity to reflect on their perceptions of the relationship between anxiety and stuttering and to comment on how anxiety was managed during their public speaking assignment. Consistently, clients are able to gain the insight that although they felt a level of anxiety, they were able to control their speech movements through active monitoring of targets. In this way, clients are able to achieve the cognitive restructuring goal of understanding that although anxiety can certainly impact their speech, it is not the cause of their stuttering. Stuttering can be managed through diligent adherence to target accuracy regardless of anxiety level.*

Establishment of the Gentle Onset Target At this stage, clients are prepared to accurately acquire control over voice initiation through the Gentle Onset Target.

Video Clips 6 and 7 demonstrate Gentle Onset at consonant-vowel and word level.

They have achieved the necessary decrease in the force and acceleration of their speech through the Stretched Syllable Target and have acquired skillful diaphragmatic breathing through the Full Breath Target, which will now serve as the first step of the Gentle Onset Target. The Gentle Onset Target is introduced following a review of the physiology of the voicing system. It is explained that the controlled initiation of voicing without hard glottal attack or laryngeal blocking requires a gentle initiation of vocal fold vibrations and a gradual increase in the strength of these vibrations. A graphic representation of loudness changes over time is provided in the form of a smooth, bell-shaped curve, and the five steps of the Gentle Onset Target are introduced:

1. Take a slow, comfortably full breath.
2. Initiate voicing very quietly and gently.
3. Increased loudness gradually.
4. Reach full conversational loudness.
5. Decrease loudness again in a gradual fashion.

The Gentle Onset Target is introduced at the syllable level for Class I sounds, and a series of exercises are completed to establish the Gentle Onset muscle movement pattern for controlled voice initiation. In addition to clinician feedback, a biofeedback device called a voice monitor is provided for use in and out of the clinic for the duration of the intensive phase of the program. The voice monitor is used to provide clients with information about the accuracy of their productions. Clients also use the Dr. Fluency computer software program, which provides a graphic representation of loudness changes over time. The Gentle Onset Target is established at the 2-second stretch rate at the syllable, word, sentence, paragraph, and conversation levels and maintained throughout the program.

Establishing Covert Practice **Covert Practice** is defined as the silent, mental rehearsal of target patterns. This skill is introduced and practiced on isolated Class I sounds. The objective is for the client to be able to invoke a mental image of the Full Breath, Stretched Syllable, and Gentle Onset Target patterns on demand. *This skill will become an essential component of a critical cognitive restructuring goal. Clients will establish a constructive rather than destructive mental set with which to enter into outside transfer situations. Clients will become able to occupy the mind with a mental image of what the target production sounds like, feels like, and would look like on a graph in order to block out distracting negative thoughts as they enter speaking situations.*

Transfer on the Telephone Following a discussion of the importance of openness and acceptance of stuttering in the treatment process, clients are instructed to complete a reading assignment over the phone with a nongroup individual. It is explained that this will necessitate a short introduction to the goals of the program and will provide an opportunity to include this member of their social circle in the therapy process. *This assignment is repeated throughout the program to facilitate the achievement of a critical cognitive restructuring goal. Clients achieve an increased openness with regard to their stuttering and speech therapy and broaden their circle of supporters. Freedom to actively demonstrate controlled speech replaces the pressure to hide the new speech pattern.*

Day 5 The Gentle Onset Target is extended to syllables beginning with Class II and Class III sounds.

Establishment of the Slow Change Target with Gentle Onset Class II The Slow Change (SC) Target is introduced together with the Gentle Onset Target for Class II syllables and requires the controlled movement of the articulators between stretchable sounds within syllables without the rapid or jerky movements characteristic of stuttered speech. The SC Target is established at the 2-second stretch rate at the syllable, word, sentence, paragraph, and conversation levels.

Establishment of the Reduced Air Pressure Target with Gentle Onset for Class III The Reduced Air Pressure (RAP 1) Target is introduced together with the Gentle Onset Target for Class III syllables and requires production of voiceless fricatives without excessive air flow such that the subsequent voiced sound can be initiated with an accurate gentle onset. The voiceless fricative is not stretched but produced so that it is audible but does not prevent controlled voice initiation on the subsequent stretchable sound. The RAP 1 target is established at the 2-second stretch rate at the syllable, word, sentence, paragraph, and conversation levels.

Day 6

Establishment of the Reduced Articulatory Pressure Target The Reduced Articulatory Pressure (RAP 2) Target is applied to Class IV syllables and requires production of plosive sounds without excessive pressure at the point of contact between the lips and tongue such that the continuation (as with /b/, /d/, /g/) or initiation (as with /p/, /t/, /k/) of voicing on the subsequent stretchable sound can be controlled with an accurate gentle onset. The RAP 2 Target is established at the 2-second stretch rate at the syllable, word, sentence, paragraph, and conversation levels.

Establishment of the 1-Second Stretch At this stage in the program, the rate of speech is increased, and syllables are joined for the first time. Each syllable is now prolonged for 1 second, and two syllables are produced in succession without stopping before the 1-second pause. Thus, the Stretched Syllable timing pattern of 2 seconds of speech and 1 second of breathing is maintained. At the 1-second stretch rate, the first stretchable sound of each syllable is prolonged for one-half second, and the remainder of the syllable is prolonged for the other one-half second. The 1-second stretch rate is introduced at the syllable level and established at the word, sentence, paragraph, and conversation levels through a series of practice activities.

Video Clip 8 demonstrates using the 1-second stretch at the single-syllable word level.

Establishment of the Amplitude Contour Target On progression to the 1-second stretch rate, the Amplitude Contour Target is introduced. The Amplitude Contour Target requires that constant voicing is maintained between joined syllables and that each syllable is produced with an accurate gentle onset curve. Thus, an amplitude contour, or "loudness curve," is produced for each syllable pair. The first syllable is initiated quietly; loudness is increased gradually to full loudness and then decreased gradually to a suitable starting point for the next syllable to begin with control. The Amplitude Contour Target allows voicing to continue between syllables without stopping or blocking. The Amplitude Contour Target is established at the 1-second stretch rate at the word, sentence, and paragraph levels.

Video Clips 9, 10, and 11 demonstrate this progression.

Day 7

Establishment of the Full Articulatory Movement Target The Full Articulatory Movement (FAM) Target requires the full and deliberate movement of the articulators from one sound to the next within syllables. Clients are cued to monitor their production of this target in a mirror to avoid the restricted or "clenched" articulatory movements characteristic of many people attempting to avoid or disguise overt stuttering. The accurate production of the FAM target results in a normal pattern of relaxed and free-flowing movements as words are formed and allows the client to more reliably monitor each of the other targets. The FAM target is established at the word and sentence levels.

Video Clips 12 and 13 show this.

One-Second Stretch—Conversational Level At this stage, clients participate in conversational activities in clinic at the 1-second stretch rate and incorporating all eight targets. These activities provide opportunities to reinforce target skills under more naturalistic speaking demands and in a more social context. *Engaging in social communication practice activities is critical to the achievement of the cognitive restructuring goal of habituating the modified pattern and being able to formulate language and apply targets simultaneously.*

Quiz Clients are given a short pencil-and-paper quiz on the skills and concepts covered. Clients who do not pass the quiz are scheduled for individual sessions to reinforce concepts.

Transfer to Out-of-Clinic Dialogue Clients are instructed to record a face-to-face dialogue out of clinic with a friend or family member using the 1-second stretch rate. This form of transfer activity promotes the cognitive restructuring goal of desensitization to the awkwardness associated with using a modified speech pattern. With experience, reactivity to the situation is decreased, and clients become able to focus more exclusively on the accuracy of their targets. This activity is repeated throughout the duration of the program, and clients are encouraged to vary their partners as much as possible to achieve a level of comfort with a greater circle of supporters.

Day 8

Speech Making—1-Second Stretch Clients give a prepared 3-minute speech to the group at the 1-second stretch rate. *Ongoing desensitization to public speaking is achieved, and anxiety management through the conscious application of targets is discussed. For many clients, public speaking is often avoided, and thus, experience may be significantly lacking. It often comes as a surprise for clients to learn that virtually all people, even people who do not stutter, experience a heightened level of anxiety in public speaking situations. A critical cognitive restructuring goal for these clients is to gain confidence in their ability to manage anxiety through conscious application of Covert Practice and targets. This goal is typically best addressed through repeated and supported opportunities to speak before an audience.* In-clinic speeches are regularly audio- or video-recorded to provide clients with an opportunity to objectively analyze their performance.

Establishment of Self-Monitoring Self-monitoring is defined as independently attending to the ac-

curacy of target behaviors. One way to effectively self-monitor is to choose two targets to attend to, or "monitor," prior to speaking. Clients are encouraged to vary the target pair chosen to gain accuracy on all targets. Although clients are attempting to accurately perform all targets, they will evaluate two targets in particular. *In this way, clients are cued to engage in Covert Practice prior to beginning to speak, and the cognitive restructuring goal of habituating this preparatory mental set is advanced.* Self-monitoring promotes the development of critical self-awareness and evaluation skills and fosters an independence from clinical reinforcement. Additional peer and clinician feedback is provided as needed and gradually faded out.

Videotape Analysis At this stage of treatment, we conduct a group counseling session around the viewing of a portion of each client's pretreatment videotape. The assignment is to identify the targets that are missing from the pretreatment speech sample. In this way, clients are encouraged to analyze their own particular patterns of stuttering and be able to identify how each target is related to the control of the speech mechanism. *This exercise facilitates the achievement of a number of cognitive restructuring goals. First, clients are able to view their stuttering from a scientific rather than emotional perspective. Moments of stuttering cease to be painful experiences of failure and become a logical set of muscle movement patterns to be analyzed and learned from. Second, clients are exposed to an objective view of their pretreatment speech pattern and rate. For many, it is this exposure that generates the acceptance and motivation needed for success in treatment. Finally, clients are given the opportunity to recognize the nonovert elements of their particular pattern of stuttering. Awareness is achieved with regard to avoidance behaviors such as word switching, circumlocution, the use of starters and fillers, and limited elaboration.*

Day 9

Establishment of the Half-Second Stretch The rate of speech is increased to the half-second stretch. Each syllable is now prolonged for a half second, and four syllables are produced in succession without stopping before the 1-second pause. Again, the Stretched Syllable timing pattern of 2 seconds of speech and 1 second of breathing is maintained. At the half-second stretch rate, the first stretchable sound of each syllable is prolonged for one-quarter of a second, and the remainder of the syllable is prolonged for the other one-quarter of a second. Because one-quarter of a second is difficult to accurately monitor on the stopwatch, clients are counseled to ensure that they are able to feel the stable position of the first stretchable sound in each syllable. The half-second stretch rate, integrating all targets, is established at the word level with voice monitor reinforcement and generalized to the sentence, paragraph, and conversation levels.

Video Clips 14, 15, and 16 demonstrate the half-second stretch at the multiword, paragraph, and conversational levels.

Day 10
Speech Making at the Half-Second Stretch Rate Clients present a 3-minute prepared speech at the half-second stretch rate. The accurate and deliberate application of targets, Covert Practice, self-monitoring, and self-correction are emphasized.

Speeches at many different stretch levels are shown in Video Clips 20 through 23.

Consolidation of the Half-Second Stretch Clients participate in a variety of reading and speaking activities to consolidate and integrate each of the eight targets at the half-second stretch rate.

Introduction to New Normal The final speech rate introduced is termed New Normal. At this stage, the client is no longer required to time and count syllables. Instead, rate of speech is now defined as the amount of stretch that allows the client to feel each of the targets being completed accurately, yet is natural enough to be transferred to all outside speaking situations. At New Normal, the natural pattern of syllable stress and vocal intonation is re-established while maintaining accurate production of each of the targets. New Normal is introduced through a series of contrast exercises at the word level. The word is produced at the half-second stretch rate until all targets can be felt and performed accurately. Next, the client is cued to reassign natural stress by lengthening the

appropriate syllable. Modifications to tone, rhythm, expression, and naturalness are discussed, modeled, and refined. The New Normal speech pattern is then generalized to the phrase level with a discussion of how word stress influences the expression of meaning. A series of audio-recorded exercises are used to provide feedback with regard to target accuracy and naturalness. *Clients are encouraged to constantly listen back to audio-recorded samples of their New Normal speech pattern to achieve and reinforce the critical cognitive restructuring goal of acceptance of the modified speech pattern. Listening to recordings promotes desensitization to the newness of the pattern and provides a more objective interpretation of how the pattern may be perceived by listeners. By listening to their recorded speech samples, clients are reassured that in contrast to internal perceptions, their New Normal pattern is quite acceptable to listeners and preferable to the fragmentation, struggle, fear, or avoidance characterizing their pretreatment pattern.* The New Normal speech pattern needs to be established as the client's full-time pattern of speech regardless of situation or listener through a thorough process of transfer. It is understood at this stage that the degree of prolongation defining New Normal is individual to each client and that this pattern changes and develops over time as accuracy and consistency of target production advances.

Examples of New Normal at the word, sentence, and conversational levels are illustrated in Video Clips 17, 18, and 19.

Day 11
Monitored versus Lucky Fluency At this stage, deliberate use of targets at the New Normal rate is required in all in-clinic speaking activities. With practice, many clients have achieved a near normal pattern that is characterized by a speech naturalness that is virtually indistinguishable from their spontaneously fluent pretreatment speech. Clients are cautioned not to fall into the trap of mistaking spontaneous or "lucky" fluency for accurately monitored targets. Throughout treatment, many clients report an increased frequency of spontaneous fluency. *We are able to address a central cognitive*

restructuring goal by counseling clients to avoid relying on lucky fluency because it tends to be unstable and can often deteriorate just when it is needed the most. By contrast, an emphasis is placed on Monitored Fluency, which is fluency that is earned and stabilized through conscious and deliberate application of targets. During break times, clients are encouraged to continue to monitor their targets and report a rating of their consistency on a 10-point scale (1 = very minimal monitoring of targets, 10 = extremely consistent monitoring of targets). *Successful completion of these transfer trials is based on the consistent application of targets and not speech fluency. In this way, we are able to address two important cognitive restructuring goals. First, clients must accept that fluency must be earned through conscious application of targets. Second, speech success is best evaluated in terms of the application of targets regardless of fluency.*

Maintenance Clients are introduced to the concept of Maintenance. Fluency maintenance is a long, gradual process of consolidation and stabilization of skills and maturing of expectations by both the client and the clinician. Maintenance is viewed as a continuation of the therapy program as the involvement of the clinician is gradually decreased. The Maintenance period is supported by a defined schedule of ongoing practice designed to promote lasting fluency and involves four types of practice introduced as (1) shaping, (2) structured practice, (3) spontaneous practice, and (4) review.

Introduction to Shaping The first form of Maintenance practice is called shaping and involves reading at increasing rates, starting with the 2-second stretch rate and ending with New Normal. This type of practice is best done at the beginning of the day to "set the stage" for speaking over the rest of the day. Shaping should be followed by a somewhat less structured activity in the form of a short monitored conversation to allow for transfer of the skills practiced. Shaping is completed with clinician feedback on each morning of the final week of the intensive phase of the program.

Day 12

Introduction to Structured Transfer At this stage, clients are given the opportunity to transfer their New Normal speech through the process of Structured Transfer. Structured Transfer is defined as transfer speaking activities that are done for the primary purpose of practicing fluency targets. Examples include making taped and evaluated telephone calls to businesses to ask for their hours of operation and going into stores to ask for the location of certain products. Clients are taught a three-step process to facilitate successful transfer exercises:

1. *Covert Practice* is defined as the silent, mental rehearsal of targets. In preparation for a transfer, the client selects two targets and brings to mind a mental image of their accurate production. Recall that Covert Practice was introduced early in the establishment phase and developed through structured assignments. Covert Practice is instrumental in creating a positive mental set with which to enter into transfer speaking situations. Any negative thoughts (e.g., "I can't do this" or "I will stutter for sure") are replaced so that the client is prepared to apply targets.

2. *Active monitoring of targets* is required during a speaking activity to constitute a successful transfer. Clients are encouraged not to rely on spontaneous or "lucky" fluency but to actively and deliberately produce speech within target parameters.

3. *Evaluation of target accuracy* is the final step of transfer in which the client is asked to identify those targets that were produced accurately and those that require more attention or refinement. Clients are advised not to frame their evaluations in terms of fluency or stuttering, and a critical cognitive restructuring goal is addressed. It is unhelpful for clients to continue to judge the quality of their speaking solely on fluency because a transfer evaluated as "fluent" may result from spontaneous fluency and be unrelated to target accuracy. Similarly, a transfer evaluated as "stuttered" provides no basis for improvements in subsequent trials. Conversely, transfers evaluated in terms of target accuracy promote positive opportunities for learning and skill development. Clients are provided with a Transfer Record template (Fig. 15.3) to promote consistent adherence to the three steps to transfer.

Once established, Structured Transfer becomes the second form of daily Maintenance practice.

FLUENCY PLUS PROGRAM
Transfer Record Sheet

Instances

	1	2	3	4	5	6	7	8	9	10
2 Targets to Monitor										
Situation										
Phone										
Face-to-face										
Nervous										
No										
Slightly										
Very										
Duration										
Short										
Medium										
Long										
Target Accuracy										
Excellent										
Good										
Poor										
Evaluation										
Covert Practice										
Stretching										
Full Breath										
Gentle Onset										
Slow Change										
RAP I										
RAP II										
FAM										
Amplitude Contour										

NOTES:

Figure 15.3. Client Transfer Record Sheet.

Telephone Transfer Practice Clients participate in supervised and supported telephone transfers. They are asked to choose two targets for Covert Practice, to evaluate their level of anxiety, and to exaggerate targets accordingly. In this way, clients are able to enter the speaking situation with a positive preparatory mental set. Clients are counseled to dial in a calm and controlled way and to breathe normally while the phone is ringing. The error many clients make is to anticipate

- "I hope they won't ask me to go to lunch because my speech will be terrible"
- "Maybe I'll just pretend I don't know the answer."
- "I hope they don't ask me to introduce myself."
- "Uh-oh! Here comes a word that starts with a "D". Let me pick another one-fast!"
- "I know they are going to laugh at me if I stutter."
- "I don't want to answer the phone, I might stutter."

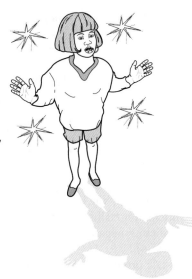

Figure 15.4. Negative self-talk.

their speaking turn and take their full breath too early, resulting in breath holding and blocking. Instead, clients are counseled to wait and breathe normally until the person on the other end of the line has answered and completed their greeting before initiating their speaking turn. Clients begin by completing transfers involving one short question. Following the completion of the call, clients are asked to evaluate their target accuracy. Any target that is identified for improvement is selected for Covert Practice in subsequent calls. Gradually, clients graduate to longer and more complex calls while maintaining a high level of target accuracy. *The process of completing this hierarchy of telephone transfers in the clinic and with supervision provides an irreplaceable opportunity for a number of cognitive restructuring goals to be addressed. First, desensitization to speaking on the phone with unfamiliar listeners is achieved as transfers become associated with control and success rather than tension and struggle. Second, ongoing familiarity with the new feeling of using the modified speech pattern is achieved. Third, transfer success is evaluated based on willingness to try and attention to targets rather than amount of stuttering. In this way, every transfer can be viewed as a success even when difficulties arise. This new perspective of success becomes a critical hallmark of successful long-term maintenance. Telephone transfers are regularly audio-recorded and reviewed for target accuracy and speech naturalness.*

Examples of telephone transfer are given in Video Clip 25.

Day 13

Speech Making in New Normal Clients present short prepared speeches in New Normal on each of the final 3 days of the intensive treatment phase. *These opportunities serve to reinforce many of the behavioral and cognitive elements of the program. Clients are encouraged to make audio recordings of their speeches. Not only is audio recording a key evaluation tool, but it also provides ongoing opportunities for the client to become accustomed to the newly acquired speech pattern.*

Video Clip 24 illustrates a speech using New Normal.

Outside Transfer Clients participate in two sessions of outside transfer at a local shopping mall. The objective of these outside transfer sessions is to gain skill and experience transferring targets to face-to-face speaking situations with unfamiliar listeners under the guidance of the clinician. The same three steps outlined for telephone transfers are followed.

Negative Self-Talk Prior to undertaking face-to-face transfers, clients are introduced to the concept of *negative self-talk* messages, how they are generated in the brain, and how they impact speech in a negative way. Negative self-talk

Figure 15.5. Covert practice.

- "Hey, here's a chance for me to use my targets!"
- "I think I'll use my breathing and gentle on set skills this time.
- "My opinion is important and I am going to make this point"
- "I know the answer and I am going to say it out loud in class."
- "I can almost feel my speech being so smooth and easy, even before I open my mouth."
- "This way of talking feels great, and my skills are the key!"

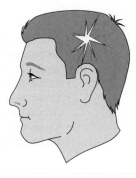

messages take the form of "the little voice inside your head" anticipating failure, recalling past failures, and predicting negative reactions from the listener (Fig. 15.4).

Negative self-talk promotes tension and nervousness. As a result, it becomes very difficult to use targets or even to remember that there are targets to be used. The concept of demands and capacities is introduced and related to how negative self-talk competes with the function of the motor, speech, and language centers and detracts from the accurate performance of targets. *A group counseling session is conducted in which each client contributes what they perceive to be their particular negative self-talk messages and the impact of those messages on their speech. To successfully transfer targets from clinic to everyday use, clients must achieve the cognitive restructuring goal of replacing negative self-talk with Covert Practice. In this way, clients achieve a positive mental set with which to enter into speaking situations by engaging in strict mental focus on target behaviors to the exclusion of distracting negative self-talk (Fig. 15.5).*

Day 14

Introduction to Spontaneous Transfer Spontaneous transfer is defined as the conscious use of targets in naturally occurring exchanges and conversations throughout the day. In the third week of the program, clients are asked to carefully monitor targets during all speaking in clinic and during defined periods out of the clinic. Clients are encouraged to rate their performance on a 10-point scale in terms of accuracy. In the Maintenance phase, together with Shaping and Structured Transfer, Spontaneous Transfer becomes the third form of daily Maintenance practice.

Mini Program During the final days of the intensive portion of the program, clients are instructed on how to produce a recorded sample of their speech demonstrating the targets at the syllable, word, sentence, and paragraph levels and at each rate of speech. This recorded sample is saved and reviewed frequently as a reference throughout the maintenance period.

Day 15

Introduction to Review The fourth form of Maintenance practice is *Review*. Initially following the intensive phase of treatment, Review consists of redoing each manual exercise to reinforce skills and concepts. During the intensive program, many details are discussed in a short period of time. It is to the client's advantage to review these details within the first 2 to 3 months after treatment. After this initial review of the program manuals, Maintenance Review consists of reflection activities to assess performance and set goals.

Record Keeping Clients are provided with a chart to use to track their plans and evaluations for each of the four forms of Maintenance practice on each day of the week. This Weekly Record serves as a reference for review and for reporting practice at maintenance follow-up meetings (Fig. 15.6). Clients are counseled that they will need to have available approximately 1 hour per day for the completion of Maintenance activities and record keeping.

Follow-Up Meetings Clients are provided with a year-long schedule of follow-up maintenance meetings.

Alumni Support Group Clients are encouraged to become members of our alumni support group called the Demosthenes Society. This volunteer-run self-help group was founded almost 30 years ago and provides a unique avenue through which clients are able to maintain contact with other

FLUENCY PLUS PROGRAM
Weekly Maintenance Record

	Shaping		Structured		Spontaneous		Review	
	Plan	Evaluate	Plan	Evaluate	Plan	Evaluate	Plan	Evaluate
Day 1								
Day 2								
Day 3								
Day 4								
Day 5								
Day 6								
Day 7								

Figure 15.6. Client Weekly Maintenance Record.

graduates of the program with a similar desire to maintain their speech gains. The Demosthenes Society meets once per month and is led by an executive committee. Meetings typically begin with a group shaping session and involve a number of transfer opportunities. Members who live far from Toronto receive the Blockbuster newsletter and are encouraged to become members of a tele-phone contact list in order to participate in phone transfers.

Posttreatment Measures On the last day of the intensive portion of the program, clients are interviewed and asked to provide a reading sample on videotape as a measure of speech fluency. Each client also completes two pen-and-paper attitude scales, the PSI (Woolf, 1967) and the S24 (Andrews & Cutler, 1974).

How to Measure Postintensive Progress Clients are counseled to view postintensive progress differently from the rapid, easily measurable changes in their speech fluency over the intensive period. It is important to understand that maintaining these initial gains is now the challenge and progress is defined by consistent adherence to New Normal pattern and speech practice over a period of weeks and months.

Guest Speaker A past participant of the program is invited to share his or her thoughts and experiences with the graduating group.

Postintensive Maintenance Sessions In the year following intensive treatment, clients are scheduled to participate in weekly, bimonthly, and monthly maintenance sessions. Maintenance sessions provide ongoing tracking of skill maintenance and progress, opportunities for practice, clinical feedback and guidance, and emotional support. Clients who attend follow-up sessions regularly demonstrate sustained motivation and commitment, develop a mature approach to long-term maintenance, and evolve successfully as their own best clinicians. A great many behavioral and cognitive goals are addressed in the maintenance year. Many of these goals are summarized in the third program manual, *Manual of Fluency Maintenance: A Guide for Ongoing Practice* (Kroll, 1991), and many others will arise. Each clinician will need to develop a range of counseling skills through time, experience, and a passionate interest in the treatment process. Additionally, it is important that clinicians demonstrate a shared commitment to the maintenance process. Consistent records of client progress should be maintained, and goals must be continually set and evaluated. Maintenance sessions should not be considered optional but instead promoted as an essential phase of the therapy process.

Weekly Maintenance (Four Sessions)
- Clients report on four forms of practice and record keeping.
- Clinician supports the individualization of practice schedules to fit client lifestyle and time demands.

- Clinician charts and provides feedback on in-clinic observations of target accuracy, client reports of target accuracy and situational speech fluency, consistency of target monitoring, and speech satisfaction.
- Clinician leads group discussions regarding reasonable fluency expectations, acceptance of the new speech pattern, and consistency.
- Clients are supported in generating realistic long-term goals to be achieved within 2 to 3 months (e.g., monitor Full Breath and Gentle Onset Targets on all phone calls at work) and the corresponding short-term goals to be achieved within 1 to 2 weeks (e.g., make three taped and evaluated telephone calls each day at work).
- Clinician identifies clients in need of additional support due to poor skill development or regression and schedules individual treatment sessions.

Bimonthly Maintenance (Four Sessions)
- Clinician continues to chart and provide feedback on speech performance and practice.
- Long-term goals are reviewed and revised.
- Posttreatment videos are reviewed and compared to present speech pattern.
- Attitude scales are reviewed, and ongoing attitude goals are identified (e.g., negative perceptions, situational avoidances).

Monthly Maintenance (Nine Sessions)
- In-clinic observations and client report of speech fluency are gathered.
- Regression is addressed through modifications to the practice schedule and individual sessions if needed.
- Suggestions for problem solving are shared or generated independently.
- Long-term and short-term goals are reviewed and revised independently.
- Individual practice schedules are tailored through a process of supervised trial and error such that clients become able to independently manage post-Maintenance practice.

Post-Maintenance
- Clients are instructed to continue with their modified schedule of practice and to contact the clinic to schedule individual sessions if regression is unmanageable.

- Clients are advised to continue to attend Demosthenes meetings.
- Clients receive information regarding yearly refresher seminars offered by the Stuttering Centre. Refresher seminars are held over 2 days and provide a review of the program basics as well as opportunities for supervised practice and transfer.
- In some cases, poor practice and extended periods of lack of contact with the clinic result in full regression. These clients are eligible to retake the intensive program.
- For most clients, a mature approach to long-term maintenance is achieved and refined over time. Clients are encouraged to stay in contact with the clinic and to stay mindful of the tools they have acquired to sustain skill maintenance (Fig. 15.7).

A 6-week posttreatment maintenance session is illustrated in Video Clip 29.

ASSESSMENT METHODS TO SUPPORT ONGOING DECISION MAKING

PRETREATMENT ASSESSMENT CONSIDERATIONS

Clients wishing to participate in the Fluency Plus Program are seen for an initial assessment to determine their suitability for daily intensive treatment. We will not deal with traditional fluency assessment strategies because much has been written on this topic (Guitar, 2006). The reader is referred to the summary of the first day of the program when specific speech and attitudinal measures are collected. We will discuss some of the critical client variables that ultimately will be used in determining candidacy for Fluency Plus. At the outset, it should be stated that the frequency of overt stuttering should not be considered a factor determining candidacy for treatment.

Obviously, the individual willing to participate in a full-time, 15-day intensive therapy program must have valid and legitimate reasons for seeking treatment. We like to refer to these as "bread and butter" issues. Often these are vocational issues and may refer to the potential participant's ability to gain employment in a chosen field or to

advance in a career path. Younger clients may express the need for improved communication skills so they can pursue specific courses in college or university. Furthermore, some clients express the need to become more active socially with friends or with community organizations. These clients relate feelings of isolation and, in many instances, frustration at not being able to participate fully in social activities.

The client wishing to participate in the program for "cosmetic" reasons is a puzzling one. These clients are not necessarily held back by the stuttering except for the fact that they view the condition as a blemish or negative mark that is embarrassing socially and affects their self image. One could argue that the client who sees his or her stuttering in this way may be willing to work very hard at improving communication skills. On the other hand, such clients may not have spent adequate time at developing their self-perceptions through introspection and discussion with family and friends. These clients may in fact require some additional form of therapy to modify or adjust self-perceptions.

Finally, the client who is brought to therapy by a spouse, parent, or significant other who is distressed by the stuttering may in fact be resistant to the notion of therapy. We see this often with adolescents who vehemently resist therapy either because they deny that their stuttering is a problem or because they are reluctant to relinquish a good chunk of free time to sit in a therapy group. These clients are typically counseled as to the inner motivation required to benefit from Fluency Plus or any other treatment for that matter.

The client's perceptions and expectations of the therapy program are probed during the initial assessment. Our program has received a fair amount of attention by the media and in the professional community due to its unique and specialized nature. Although one would assume that this attention is beneficial to both the providers and recipients of the program, the lay public is often left with a rather simplistic view of what the therapy can and cannot accomplish depending on the nature of the print or electronic story. As a result, clients often come to the Stuttering Centre with preconceived notions of what we can do for stuttering. We spend much time providing the client with a realistic synopsis of the therapy and trying to

FLUENCY PLUS PROGRAM
Tools for Successful Maintenance

Give yourself one point for each statement that is true of you.

Avoiding Relapse Tool #1 –
ACHIEVE MASTERY OF TARGET BEHAVIOURS
q I perform shaping accurately at all rates (including conversation)
q I transfer targets to all speaking situations
q I review my manuals and my mini-program regularly to the extent that I know, understand, and could explain all 8 targets to someone
q I monitor my speech in all speaking opportunities even when I don't think I need to

Avoiding Relapse Tool #2 –
DEVELOP TECHNIQUES WHICH SUPPORT POSITIVE PREPARATION FOR SPEAKING OPPORTUNITIES
q I realize and remind myself that optimal use of targets is not possible without positive mental preparation
q I use Covert Practice to block out negative thinking, decrease anxiety, and facilitate target use
q I monitor for any negative thinking as I enter speaking opportunities and can choose more helpful self-talk statements

Avoiding Relapse Tool #3 –
COMPLETE AND EVALUATE PRACTICE ACTIVITIES DAILY
q I plan and evaluate monitored speaking activities every day
q I purposefully place myself in situations to increase my chance for practice (e.g. pick up the phone, ask for the time, join a club etc.)
q I do shaping followed by a monitored conversation with evaluation

Avoiding Relapse Tool #4 –
SYSTEMATICALLY REDUCE FEARS AND AVOIDANCE BEHAVIORS
q I monitor myself for any avoidance behaviors such as word-switching, keeping quiet when I have something to say, "keeping it short", or staying away from a situation because it will require talking
q I purposefully place myself in talking situations I fear or feel anxiety about in order to overcome fears and avoidance behaviors
q I say all the words I want to say regardless of whether I perceive that they will be easy to say fluently
q I know how to design practice opportunities to help to overcome remaining fears

Avoiding Relapse Tool #5 –
ACCEPTANCE OF THE NEW SPEECH PATTERN
q I tape record myself often using targets in real situations and listen to it
q I have used targets consistently for a period of longer than 21 days to become accustomed to the new feeling and sound
q I discuss stuttering and speech monitoring openly with those close to me
q I participate in a variety of opportunities to hear others using targets (e.g. Follow-ups, Demosthenes meetings, Refreshers)

Avoiding Relapse Tool #6 –
SELF-CORRECTION AND EVALUATION OF TARGET ERRORS
q I realize and remind myself that stuttered speech results from inaccurate target performance
q I monitor for inaccurate targets in my speech (not just stuttering) and evaluate the inaccuracy
q I consistently perform a "self-correction" when I have missed a target in daily speech

Avoiding Relapse Tool #7 –
ESTABLISH A SUPPORT NETWORK
q I am in contact with other people who are following a speech maintenance program on at least a monthly basis
q I talk openly with friends and family about speech practice and maintenance
q I realize and remind myself that the emotional resilience required to succeed in maintenance can only be maintained with the support of others

Figure 15.7.   Client Maintenance Checklist.

Avoiding Relapse Tool #8 –
EXAMINE PERSONAL REASONS FOR WANTING TO MAINTAIN SPEECH GAINS
q I can list 5-10 reasons why adhering to a speech maintenance program is worthwhile for me
q I review these reasons on a regular basis
q I realize and remind myself that speech gains can not be maintained without active daily efforts

Avoiding Relapse Tool #9 –
WORK TOWARDS A LIFESTYLE THAT ACCOMMODATES CHANGE
q I make priority time in my schedule for maintenance practice and activities
q I take care of my well-being (i.e., positivity, energy) by exercising, doing things I enjoy, surrounding myself with positive people
q I take care of my health by sleeping well, eating well, and avoiding the excessive use of alcohol, nicotine, caffeine, and other drugs

Avoiding Relapse Tool #10 –
DEVELOP PROBLEM SOLVING AND SELF RELIANCE SKILLS
q I identify and record long-term goals for my speech performance
q I write down a list of measurable, action-based short-term goals, to be completed within two weeks, to help me to achieve my long-term goals
q I review, check-off, and revise these goals regularly

Less than 22 Points – You have lots of room for improvement. Use more of these tools to increase your likelihood of long-term maintenance.
22-27 Points – Well done. You are doing a lot of great things for your speech. Consult these tools for guidance should you wish to improve.
28-33 Points – Congratulations! You are taking a mature, well informed approach to maintenance. The sweet taste of fluency will be yours for years to come.

Figure 15.7. (*Continued*).

---

determine if, after the discussion, the client is still seeking the magic bullet to eliminate the stuttering completely. We also assess whether the client has grasped the concentrated effort required by the program and whether he or she is fully cognizant about his or her own roles and responsibilities during the program as well of those of the clinician. During the interview, we try to check for indicators of self-reliance and the ability to work independently. Moreover, we look for clinical signs indicating that the client possesses the ability and drive to change or modify his or her behavior. For example, during the assessment, the client may report on a specific self-development course or challenge that has successfully been completed.

We have determined that all of these indicators have clinical relevance. However, aside from one of our studies examining performance variables associated with treatment outcomes (Kroll & De Nil, 1995; Ulrich et al., 1992), there is little empirical evidence to corroborate the importance of these indicators. Even with our years of clinical experience with intensive programs, we continue to be positively or negatively surprised by client behavior during treatment.

Another area of concern pertains to the emotional stability and objectivity displayed by the client during the assessment. We discourage individuals from participating in our program if they are currently undergoing major life stresses or changes because we would predict that the communication issue may not be the priority at this point in time. Finally, we try to ascertain whether there are any reading or learning challenges that may interfere with participation in a rather fast-paced group environment. If we are uncertain as to the individual's potential to benefit from this treatment, we will devote a portion of the initial assessment to performing some trial probes. During these probes, we provide clients with some of the written program materials and observe the client working independently for a short period of time to determine comprehension, ability to grasp the concept being introduced, and overall accuracy of verbal and written responses to the presented instructional material.

ADVANCEMENT CRITERIA DURING TREATMENT

Given the structured format of the Fluency Plus Program, it is anticipated that most clients will progress through the sequence of therapy phases at a similar pace. It is for this reason that clients are carefully screened before they are considered for treatment in the intensive program (see previous section). Client progress is assessed on a daily basis via clinician analysis of recorded home assignments and clinician and peer evaluation during large and small group sessions. At each stage during the program, the clinician checks for skill mastery of target behaviors. Skill mastery is operationally defined as the ability to produce a given target behavior with 80% accuracy and without cueing or modeling by the clinician. Clinically, it is important to determine whether the client has cognitively incorporated the skill and is able to accurately produce the desired behavior with ease.

For those cases when a client is unable to reach satisfactory performance criteria for a given target or speech-related activity, supplementary individual sessions are provided until the client is able to satisfy the program requirements. In most cases, these supplementary sessions can be carried out with an additional therapist during the program hours or after normal clinic hours. Again, most individuals can reach a satisfactory performance level with a minimum of supplementary sessions. In extraordinary cases, clinical decisions regarding reducing or modifying performance goals may have to be made in order to provide the client with at least some experience of goal achievement.

TERMINATION (POSTINTENSIVE CONSIDERATIONS)

It is difficult to use the terms "termination" or "discharge" when we are dealing with chronic adult stuttering. Through evidence-based clinical programs, such as Fluency Plus, we are providing clients with management strategies that we believe are the most likely to result in more fluent-sounding speech and healthier cognitive attitudes regarding communication. The vast majority of our clients will require an ongoing, self-administered program of fluency maintenance, as well as potentially benefiting from our structured refresher courses and self-help group. We have seen individuals develop both improved speech skills and healthier attitudes in the months following intensive treatment. In some cases, these positive gains may not be fully realized for years, when they come to our attention during the refresher courses.

Having more or less discarded the notion of termination, let us turn to some of the postintensive issues that can serve to alert the clinician to areas that may have to be addressed during maintenance. Perhaps the single most frequently observed challenge facing postintensive program participants is the ongoing requirement that they continually and actively monitor speech targets while talking. Those clients who exit the intensive program unwilling to incorporate the target skills on a more or less full-time basis will inevitably experience difficulties with the maintenance phase. Another very common challenge for postintensive clients pertains to acceptance of their modified speech pattern and concern with listeners' reactions to this speech. Those who show high levels of concern with what the newly acquired speech pattern sounds like and whether or not these patterns are accepted by listeners will likely resist using newly acquired fluency skills on a full-time basis. These clients will need much additional guidance and direction during the maintenance sessions immediately following intensive treatment.

There are many other factors that need to be addressed during the postintensive phase before clients can be considered as possessing complete sets of speech management skills—in other words, before they are considered as having successfully completed a comprehensive treatment program. Clients must be able to constructively and objectively analyze speech patterns in the natural environment; they must demonstrate a willingness to continually and actively monitor their own speech performance, thereby accepting the cognitive challenge of focusing not only on what they are saying, but how they are saying it. This is especially relevant during communicatively stressful situations. Behavioral change brings on new challenges. Clients must accept new roles and responsibilities that accompany more fluent speech as well as attitudinal and psychological changes that arise from dramatic treatment effects. Many of these changes occur in a very short period of time, given the intensive nature of the treatment. Clients most often need a period of time to adjust to the change, set realistic long- and short-term goals, and learn to cope with the rather rocky road that lies ahead during the maintenance phase. These and many other issues preclude the clinician from prematurely "terminating" treatment.

TAILORING THE TREATMENT TO THE INDIVIDUAL CLIENT

Clearly, the first question that arises for many clients following their initial assessment pertains to the schedule and format of Fluency Plus. Many clients cannot immediately arrange to attend clinic sessions for the intensive 3-week block. Clients are given adequate time to prepare and, if deemed appropriate for the program, are given the schedule for the upcoming year of programming. If arrangements are made to commence treatment 6 months from the time of the assessment, clients will often be able to arrange leaves from their employment settings. Students can opt for programs conducted during the summer months when many are not in class.

Regardless of the efforts made to accommodate individual client schedules, there are still those whose work situation or other commitments simply preclude the opportunity to attend a daily treatment program. We are also fully aware that most clinicians may not be able to administer the Fluency Plus Program in its intensive format. Intensive programs are usually conducted in the relatively few specialized centers for stuttering scattered around the world. The vast majority of speech-language pathologists do not have the resources or time allocation necessary to implement daily, intensive treatment programs for stuttering. For these reasons, we have developed a version of the program that can be implemented on a nonintensive basis. Clients are seen in 1- to 2-hour group sessions once per week. It is important to note that the principle of intensification is still applied to this format. Rather than doing the practice drills in clinic, clients are requested to complete between 1 and 2 hours of home practice assignments per day between clinic sessions.

These assignments are once again recorded and reviewed by the clinician at the beginning of each weekly session. We have determined that clients are able to complete Fluency Plus in 28 weeks before entering the maintenance phase of treatment. It should be noted that all of the program details and procedures are retained, and other than scheduling alterations, no additional modifications are implemented.

It should also be stressed that the severity of stuttering, as determined by behavioral measures and additional assessment techniques, is not an indicator for program modification. Clinically, however, one might be tempted to administer a scaled down version of the program to the person exhibiting milder forms of stuttering. For these clients, it may seem reasonable to pick one or two key fluency skills rather than administering the entire program. Indeed we have attempted this strategy on occasion, but it has been largely ineffective.

The Fluency Plus Program for Children (Kroll & Scott-Sulsky, 2006) has been developed for use with school-aged children (ages 8 through 12 years). Although the program again retains all of the learning principles; the therapy material, language level, and terminology have been modified to accommodate a younger population. We have been administering this program in a nonintensive group format and have conducted a series of training workshops for clinicians who wish to implement this approach. We are currently in the process of collecting data on these programs.

For clients with challenges or special needs, further modification of the program is necessary. Some clients do not have the requisite language skills to fully comprehend either the written materials or verbal instructions provided by the clinicians. Other clients exhibit specific learning or reading challenges requiring special or supplementary instruction. Program modifications for these cases include altering performance expectations regarding the specifics of target behavior production. Such modifications include simplification of target details and replacing some of the information provided in the manual with concise verbal explanations by the clinician. When appropriate, small groups are formed if clients present with more or less similar profiles. In other instances, these clients are scheduled for one-on-one sessions.

APPLICATION TO AN INDIVIDUAL CLIENT

Susan B. is a 28-year-old bilingual speaker of English and Bengali who was assessed at the Speech and Stuttering Institute on May 2, 2006. At the time of her assessment, her speech was characterized by hard glottal attacks, sound prolongations, and laryngeal blocks. Secondary behaviors observed included eye blinks and lip tremor. Her stuttering was rated as severe with regard to frequency and moderate with regard to duration and struggle. She reported that she regularly used avoidance strategies such as starters, fillers, and word switching to avoid stuttering whenever possible in public. Susan also reported that she avoided speaking with unfamiliar listeners, speaking into microphones or tape recorders, and speaking in group situations. Susan reported that she had participated in treatment at the ages of 8 and 10 years with some success in structured settings but that her gains had been difficult to maintain. She reported that her goal was to be able to apply fluency-enhancing techniques consistently across settings and to be able to explore new career options.

Based on her assessment, it was recommended that she participate in the adult group intensive Fluency Plus Program in January of 2007. Susan was judged to be an excellent candidate for this model of treatment based on the following criteria. First, through her assessment interview and reading sample, she demonstrated that she possessed the intellectual capacity to manage the rigorous demands of the intensive nature of the program. Second, she demonstrated through her oral mechanical examination and trial therapy probe that she was capable of managing the physical demands of altering her motor movement patterns. Third, she evidenced the emotional readiness to benefit from group therapy and to address the cognitive restructuring requirements of the program. Specifically, Susan demonstrated insight with regard to her avoidance behaviors, she described a manageable level of concern regarding listeners' reactions to her speech, and reported realistic outcome goals of treatment. Fourth, she evidenced a high level of motivation to successfully complete treatment and participate in a long-term maintenance program. Finally, she was able to accommodate the logistical requirements of freeing herself from work, school, and social obligations for the 3-week duration of the intensive phase of the program.

Susan began her treatment program on January 15, 2007 with seven other group members. For 3 weeks, she attended daily clinic sessions and dedicated between 2 and 4 hours to the completion of home assignments each evening. For a detailed description of the program, please see the "Key Components of the Approach" section of this chapter.

Susan proved to be a dynamic and supportive member of the group. Because she had participated in speech therapy as a child, she was able to share with the group two critical insights. The first was that she had experienced significant relief by using fluency-enhancing techniques in clinical settings in the past. She could attest to the fact that targets could be effective tools to produce fluent speech. The second insight was that without diligent practice and maintenance, it had not been possible for her to effectively control her speech in out-of-clinic settings in the long term. Susan's experiences proved to be very valuable in putting a real face on the philosophy of the Fluency Plus Program: Real and lasting changes in both speech behaviors and speech attitude are possible only through a rigorous reconstruction of the speech system together with a systematic restructuring of the cognitive set, a thorough and supported period of transfer, and a long-term program of maintenance.

Throughout the establishment phase of treatment, Susan worked diligently and acquired the target behaviors successfully. One particular strength was her ability to self-evaluate. She was committed to tape recording and reviewing all of her assignments and to learning from errors. She developed a keen awareness for target accuracy and offered helpful feedback to other group members.

A second strength was Susan's sincere follow-through with regard to a critical cognitive restructuring goal of the program. She took to heart the suggestion that optimal success in treatment cannot be achieved without a genuine acceptance of one's self as a person who stutters. She gained a level of comfort and openness about stuttering by completing a number of assignments that required her to practice with a variety of partners outside of the group. This afforded her the opportunity to discuss her speech condition and therapy program with a number family members, friends, and coworkers. She gained the ability to move confidently into the transfer phase of the program without feeling self-conscious about using her modified pattern of speech. In essence, she was able to avoid a common pitfall experienced by many clients. She felt no pressure to conceal the fact that she was using a modified speech pattern and was able to recruit friends and family to help her to remember to monitor her speech consistently.

As the group moved into the transfer phase of the program, Susan successfully completed many assignments requiring her to use targets in a variety of speaking situations. Susan's success can be attributed to a number of factors. First, Susan consistently followed the systematic approach to transfer outlined in the Fluency Plus Program. She was very diligent about preparing herself mentally for transfer situations using Covert Practice. She consistently used her modified speech pattern across all transfer situations regardless of perceived difficulty to avoid relying on spontaneous fluency. She evaluated her performance in transfer situations consistently and often used a tape recorder to maximize her evaluation accuracy. Susan also worked very hard to consistently evaluate the success of her transfers based on her *target accuracy* and not on the fluency of her speech. In this way, she was able to see each transfer situation as successful, with opportunities to learn and improve. She was also able to avoid the pitfall of misjudging spontaneous or "lucky" fluency for target accuracy.

Susan is currently in the Maintenance phase of her treatment program. She has taken many positive steps to creating a lifestyle that supports her goal of long-term fluency maintenance. Susan carefully completes her daily schedule of maintenance practice. When she neglects her practice, she realizes the negative effect on her speech but manages these ups and downs with a positive attitude. She thoughtfully selects short-term goals at each follow-up meeting that will support her long-term goal of successful maintenance. She does a portion of her practice in Bengali to support full-time monitored fluency when speaking with her family. Susan began to participate in activities that support the mainte-nance of her new speech pattern including joining the Demosthenes Society and volunteering at the Speech and Stuttering Institute. Most recently, she revealed that she has been accepted to a Master's Program in speech-language pathology.

CASE STUDY

John G., age 25 years, was referred by his family physician for a speech assessment for stuttering. Analysis of his intake interview revealed stuttering on 4% of words spoken, characterized by brief silent laryngeal blocks and prolongations. His verbal responses were characterized as brief with reduced eye contact. His utterances were characterized by revisions, fillers, inappropriate pauses, and circumlocution. When asked if he was aware of using any avoidance strategies, he stated that he "didn't think so." He rated his speech problem as 10 on a 10-point scale (1 = minor influence and 10 = major concern). When asked to complete a reading sample, he refused.

1. What additional case history information would you, the clinician, need to determine this client's candidacy for an intensive group treatment program?
2. What are the counseling needs of this client? How may these needs affect this client's ability to benefit from treatment?

   After appropriate counseling, it was determined that John would be an appropriate candidate for a group, intensive treatment program.
3. What information will John need about the intensive, group treatment program to make an informed decision to consent to and benefit from treatment?

   With the appropriate information, John agreed to participate in the next available program. John excelled in establishing the fluency-facilitating targets and demonstrated excellent motivation and compliance with the in-clinic and out-of-clinic assignments with the exception of those assignments requiring him to recruit listeners from outside of the treatment group to participate in recorded dialogue assignments at the various stretch rates. Initially, John made excuses for not completing these assignments, but eventually, he admitted that it was "just too difficult to tackle."

4. What cognitive restructuring goals might you, the clinician, define for this client at this stage? How could these goals be addressed?

With the appropriate intervention, John was able to complete the requirements of the establishment phase of the program and was successful in adhering to the New Normal speech pattern consistently in clinic and with a small group of his close family members and friends. John demonstrated accurate adherence to the three steps of transfer and successfully completed many telephone transfers in and out of clinic. When faced with outside face-to-face transfers, however, John reverted to his pretreatment speech pattern of blocking and using avoidance strategies.

5. What behavioral and cognitive restructuring goals would you, the clinician, identify for this client? How could these goals be addressed?

With supplementary support, John was successfully able to transfer his New Normal pattern to a number of face-to-face speaking environments. John evidenced motivation to adhere to the prescribed schedule of Maintenance practice but was unable to commit to attending follow-up meetings due to his work schedule.

6. What alternative plan would you, the clinician, develop in order to support John throughout the Maintenance phase of the program?

FUTURE DIRECTIONS

It is truly exciting to have witnessed the dramatic changes in stuttering treatment since we implemented our first treatment programs for people who stutter. Through our research and clinical observations, we have consistently sought to refine and adjust our programs in order to provide the most effective and efficient treatment programs. The dramatic improvements in speech fluency and communication attitudes that so many of our clients have been able to achieve motivate and inspire us to continually scrutinize and improve our programs.

Fluency maintenance remains a central issue, especially for clients residing at great distance from the Speech and Stuttering Institute. These clients are unable to attend scheduled Maintenance sessions and, as mentioned, will correspond with the clinician via email or telephone. With advances in technology, we are working at developing easier and more effective ways of communicating with the clinic. Future work in this area will undoubtedly see the increased application of web cams, audio files of speech, and other forms of digitally transmitted communication.

We also need to collect efficacy data for our nonintensive programs. Although we have observed substantial clinical gains with these treatment formats, we do not yet have treatment efficacy data. It will be interesting to perform empirical comparisons between the intensive and nonintensive programs and to ultimately determine the relative benefits of each of these formats.

Our current efforts are geared toward training speech-language pathologists to administer the Fluency Plus Program for Children. We have published a series of studies examining the academic and clinical preparation of clinicians treating individuals who stutter (Klassen & Kroll, 2005; Kroll & Klassen, in press; Kroll & O'Keefe, 1990). Our Canadian data tend to confirm those obtained in other parts of the world (Kroll et al., 2006; St. Louis & Durrenberger, 1993; Yaruss & Quesal, 2002) and confirm that a high proportion of practicing speech-language pathologists do not rate their competencies or comfort levels very highly when called upon to treat stuttering. In many cases, these studies point to serious deficiencies in the number of formal practicum hours received during classroom training and during clinical placement opportunities. We have identified the need for postgraduate continuing education in stuttering treatment. We are presently testing a workshop model in which clinicians attend a 3-day training program to learn the principles, techniques, and therapy strategies incorporated in Fluency Plus for Children. We look forward to measuring the effectiveness of this training and to see whether we are ultimately reaching more clients through these efforts. As we strengthen and expand our techniques that assist clients in modifying their cognitive and attitudinal approaches to communication, we look forward to developing even more valid and reliable instruments to measure such change. Indeed, preliminary work in this area has already begun focusing on quality of life and its changes as a result of treatment for stuttering (Yaruss & Quesal, 2004; 2006). We plan to continue this work so that we can more fully measure the impact of treatment as we define progress from behavioral as well as affective and overall quality-of-life indicators.

CHAPTER SUMMARY

- Fluency Plus is a comprehensive treatment program for stuttering in adults. It combines fluency shaping techniques with cognitive restructuring strategies.
- The program is based on empirical research and clinical observation amassed over a 30-year period.
- The following essential principles are integral to the Fluency Plus Program: clinical procedures must address both behavioral and psychological aspects of stuttering; therapy must be intensive; fluency skills must be overlearned and exaggerated; response variability must be reduced; transfer must be addressed; maintenance must be incorporated; and postintensive support strategies must be offered.
- Fluency Plus is typically administered in a group treatment format consisting of a 15-day intensive schedule followed by a year-long series of postintensive maintenance meetings. The program can also be administered using alternate treatment schedules.
- Long-term maintenance is supplemented by such support opportunities as refresher seminars and program-specific self-help groups.

CHAPTER REVIEW QUESTIONS

1. List the identifying features of the Fluency Plus Program.
2. What does cognitive restructuring refer to? Provide an example of a cognitive restructuring goal.
3. How would you differentiate between the stuttering behavior and the stuttering problem?
4. What two treatment approaches are integrated in the Fluency Plus Program?
5. What is the communication mentality? Why is this concept important to treatment?
6. Why is it important to include a prolonged speech technique like stretched syllable?
7. What is the rationale for teaching Full Articulatory Movement?
8. Explain the steps of the transfer process.
9. Clients are asked to recruit family or friends as practice partners. What cognitive restructuring goals does this activity address?
10. How is the evaluation process carried out during transfer? How should a successful transfer be defined?
11. What is the relationship between anxiety and stuttering?
12. What are the four forms of maintenance practice?

SUGGESTED READINGS

De Nil, L. F., Kroll, R. M., Lafaille, S. J., & Houle, S. (2003). A positron emission tomography study of short and long term treatment effects on functional brain activation in adults who stutter. *Journal of Fluency Disorders, 28*, 357–380.

Guitar, B. (2006). *Stuttering: An Integrated Approach to Its Nature and Treatment* (3rd ed.). Baltimore: Lippincott Williams & Wilkins.

Kroll, R. M., & De Nil, L. F. (2000). Research using PET scans identifies neural bases of stuttering and its treatment. *Stuttering Foundation of America Newsletter, Summer edition*, 1–3.

Neilson, M. D. (1999). Cognitive-behavioral treatment of adults who stutter: The process and the art. In R. F. Curlee (Ed.), *Stuttering and related disorders of fluency* (pp. 181–199). New York: Thieme Medical Publishers, Inc.

Webster, R.L. (1979). Empirical considerations regarding stuttering therapy. In H.H. Gregory (Ed.), *Controversies about Stuttering Therapy*. Baltimore: University Park Press.

ACKNOWLEDGEMENTS

We wish to acknowledge the many talented speech-language pathologists, research colleagues, and students who have helped us in developing and refining our program since its inception. We have also learned a great amount from the insightful comments and suggestions offered to us by our clients, and for this, we are especially grateful. We also wish to thank Ms. Lauren Greenwood for her superb editorial skills and her invaluable assistance in preparing this chapter.

CHAPTER 16

Application of the SpeechEasy to Stuttering Treatment: Introduction, Background, and Preliminary Observations

PETER R. RAMIG, JOHN B. ELLIS, AND RYAN POLLAND

INTRODUCTION

The SpeechEasy is an inconspicuous, fully digital fluency aid marketed and distributed since 2001 by Janus Development Group, Inc. of Greenville, North Carolina. Identical in appearance to most hearing aids, the SpeechEasy is intended to help those who stutter through the mechanical alteration of auditory feedback. The device employs two simultaneous forms of altered auditory feedback (AAF): delayed auditory feedback (DAF) and frequency altered feedback (FAF). DAF involves reproducing an acoustic signal with a small time delay, typically between 20 and 200 ms, in effect producing an echo of the speaker's own voice. FAF increases or decreases the frequency of the acoustic signal, causing individuals to hear their voice at a pitch that is either higher or lower than normal. These two technologies have been shown over the years to increase fluency for many who stutter (Adams & Ramig, 1980; Andrews et al., 1983; Chase, Sutton, & Raphin, 1961; Howell, El-Yaniv, & Powell, 1987; Kalinowski et al., 1996; Stuart et al., 1996).

Prior to the introduction of the SpeechEasy in 2001, DAF was used in stuttering treatment programs to teach a variety of fluency-enhancing strategies within the confines of the therapy room (Craven & Ryan, 1984; Curlee & Perkins, 1973; Helliesen, 2006; Ryan, 1974; Ryan & Van Kirk, 1971; Shames & Florence, 1980; Van Riper, 1973). In contrast to the SpeechEasy, those machines were quite large and required cables and headphones to transmit the delayed signal to both ears. As a result, most clients were reluctant to use the units in their everyday speaking environments because they were conspicuous and cumbersome. More so, before the 1970s, DAF machines were so large and heavy that their use outside of the clinic was largely impossible. In contrast, the SpeechEasy is battery operated and small enough to be cosmetically pleasing, allowing the wearer to benefit from AAF without the drawbacks of earlier devices.

The SpeechEasy can only be dispensed by American Speech-Language-Hearing Association (ASHA)-certified speech-language pathologists (SLPs) who have received training by the manufacturer. In contrast to other treatments described in this book, a SpeechEasy client may or may not be enrolled in weekly, ongoing personal contact with an SLP. Although the manufacturer recommends, if possible, that traditional stuttering

Table 16.1. *SpeechEasy Clinical Principles*

First Principle	The SpeechEasy emulates the choral reading effect.
Second Principle	Combined passive and active inhibition maximizes fluency.
Third Principle	The SpeechEasy does not cure or eliminate stuttering.
Fourth Principle	Help clients have realistic expectations for the SpeechEasy.
Fifth Principle	Address internalized, emotional factors as indicated.

treatment be implemented in conjunction with use of the device, circumstances often preclude this recommendation. For example, due to factors such as travel distance, socioeconomic status, and work demands, some clients may only visit a certified SpeechEasy provider twice: once for an initial evaluation and then a second time when the client's custom-made device arrives from the manufacturer.

The primary population served by the Speech-Easy includes children and adults who stutter. Almost all of the clients we have served to date have been adults and teenagers, most of whom have been through one or more traditional stuttering therapy programs. Based on providers' experiences with the device, the manufacturer acknowledges the importance of previous stuttering therapy and client willingness to adapt to using the device as indicators of improved outcomes (SpeechEasy Professional Information Packet, 2006). Because the SpeechEasy appears to be more effective for clients who have a basic understanding and acceptance of stuttering, the manufacturer recommends a minimum age of 10 years, although younger children have been fit with success by some providers. The youngest client we have personally evaluated and fit was a 9-year-old girl. We agreed to evaluate and fit this child with a severe stuttering problem because she lived in an outlying area of Colorado where services for the treatment of stuttering were not available and because clinicians contacted by the parents said they did not feel comfortable in their knowledge of the disorder. Our preference, as stated and supported by the manufacturer, is to provide traditional treatment options for younger children who stutter before considering the SpeechEasy. We feel this device should be considered for young children only when traditional treatment is not available or has been demonstrated by itself to be ineffective.

The manufacturer has outlined several clinical principles that describe how the device works and

its relation to other forms of stuttering therapy (Table 16.1) (SpeechEasy Professional Information Packet, 2006). The first principle assumes that the SpeechEasy uses AAF to emulate the choral reading effect, which occurs when those who stutter become significantly more fluent while reading the same words in unison with another speaker. To reproduce this effect, shorter DAF delays are usually preferred to longer ones to provide the foundation for more natural-sounding speech. The second principle assumes that the SpeechEasy's combination of DAF and FAF *passively* inhibits stuttering, which is in contrast to traditional therapy techniques such as prolongations and easy onsets that presumably *actively* inhibit stuttering. This combination of passive and active effects constitutes the so-called dual inhibition hypothesis (Saltuklaroglu, Dayalu, & Kalinowski, 2002). The third principle simply states that the SpeechEasy is not a cure and does not completely eliminate stuttering. In other words, the SpeechEasy is not universally effective with all who stutter, and its individual effectiveness will also vary for each user. Consequently, the fourth principle reminds providers to help clients have realistic expectations for their Speech-Easy and to emphasize *relative* improvements in the frequency, duration, and physical struggle associated with stuttering. The final and fifth principle encourages clinicians to be mindful of lingering anticipation, fear, anxiety, and word substitutions experienced by clients that may need to be addressed concurrently with device use.

THEORETICAL BASIS

The use of AAF for treating stuttering has been in practice for years, although its application outside of the clinic was constrained by limitations in microtechnology. The first portable AAF device—the Derazne Correctophone—was developed as early as 1959, and since then, several devices have appeared on the market employing

DAF, FAF, masking noise, or some combination of the three. The SpeechEasy falls into the final category because it employs both DAF and FAF. The rationale for offering two simultaneous forms of AAF is that some believe such devices will better prevent the user from adapting to the feedback over time (Kalinowski et al., 1998). In fact, the manufacturer reports that, "FAF is believed to be the catalyst which keeps the effects of DAF from wearing-off over time" (Speech Easy Training Manual, 2006). Interestingly, a study testing whether DAF and FAF together would enhance fluency more than either condition alone failed to find an additive effect (Macleod et al., 1995). The explanation for these findings was that either no additive effects of AAF exist or a floor effect occurred in both singular conditions, such that further improvement in fluency could not be produced in the combined condition. In addition to potentially minimizing adaptation effects, others feel that combination AAF devices such as the SpeechEasy allow clients a greater degree of freedom in choosing the particular feedback mode they prefer (Molt, 2005).

The development of the SpeechEasy and other AAF devices was spurred by the well-established fact that the overt symptoms of stuttering can be immediately, often dramatically, reduced under certain conditions. Identified decades ago by Johnson and Rosen (1937) and later by Bloodstein (1950) and Andrews et al. (1982), these fluency-enhancing conditions include, for example, speaking with a metronome, whispering, singing, slow rate, talking while alone, choral speech, and the triad that includes DAF, masking noise, and pitch changes (now collectively called AAF). Fluency induction under AAF is particularly relevant because it indicates that the auditory system may function improperly in persons with developmental stuttering. More specifically, improvements in fluency under AAF conditions suggest a defective auditory monitoring system for sequential speech output. The inference, of course, is that altering auditory input may help correct the impairment. This hypothesis receives further support from studies showing that normally fluent speakers can be made to produce stuttering-like dysfluencies while under DAF (Black, 1955; Lee, 1951).

It should be noted that although the benefits of these fluency-enhancing conditions occur immediately upon application, they usually disappear with equal suddenness once the procedure is removed (De Nil et al., 2003; Ingham, 2001). Consequently, the SpeechEasy is currently marketed without reference to a carry-over effect. Although long-term, longitudinal research could potentially disprove this assumption, the consequences of using AAF over extended periods of time have not yet been satisfactorily determined. Therefore, until the research provides clearer answers, use of the device is considered a long-term endeavor for most clients.

If the issue of carry-over is somewhat opaque, the precise reasons why AAF induces fluency are even murkier. Although this phenomenon has been demonstrated repeatedly in the literature, there is little consensus regarding the underlying mechanisms for the effect. This uncertainty stems from several issues. First, there is the unresolved question of exactly what proportion of a given individual's stuttering can be attributed to auditory processing deficits. Next, these deficits may exist at both a higher, linguistic level and at a more rudimentary level in the auditory system. Hall and Jerger (1978), for instance, found that many who stutter do not show the normal right-ear advantage in dichotic presentation of meaningful linguistic stimuli. Others have demonstrated difficulties in sound localization in this population (Rousey, Geotzinger, & Dirks, 1959). The aggregate results of these and other studies (Blood & Blood, 1984, Curry & Gregory, 1969; Hannely & Dorman, 1982; Toscher & Rupp, 1978) have pointed toward a subtle abnormality of central auditory function in at least some individuals who stutter. It is not yet understood, however, how such defects related to the auditory feedback of speech may contribute to stuttering episodes. Finally, there are potentially many types of distortion intrinsic to the feedback systems used to monitor speech (Mysak, 1960; Quinn, 1972; Van Riper, 1982). Possible sources of distortion could include asynchronous signals between hemispheres; delays in bone, tissue, and air conduction of sound waves; and interference between auditory feedback and proprioceptive feedback. Although these distortions presumably exist in all individuals, those who stutter may be more vulnerable to even the smallest asynchronies or overloads. Whatever the central cause of the deficiency or breakdown in auditory self-perception, the different forms of AAF that appear to momentarily correct the error likely do so through different means. Unfortunately, a thorough examination of the means through which each mode of AAF may operate is beyond the scope of this chapter. Here we feel it sufficient to detail two tenable hypotheses for the causal mechanisms operating under DAF and FAF because those are the technologies that the SpeechEasy employs. Before we examine potential neurologic mechanisms, however, we will first survey briefly some of the past peripheral explanations for the effectiveness of AAF.

For much of its time as a therapeutic tool, the benefits of DAF in particular were thought to derive from a reduced rate of speech. Along with many other experts (Goldiamond, 1965; Ryan & Van Kirk, 1974; Shames & Florence, 1980; Stager & Ludlow, 1993), Wingate (1970; 1976) attributed the fluency-enhancing effects of DAF to a slower rate and viewed such speech as a motoric byproduct of matching one's speech to the delay. Although it is true that speech rate often decreases under DAF, the view that fluency improvement is due solely to using a slower rate has since been challenged. More recent studies have demonstrated that a slowed speech rate is in fact not a necessary antecedent for increased fluency—not only under DAF, but also under FAF and masking conditions as well (Kalinowski et al., 1993; 1996). These data support the notion that it is the altered auditory signal itself, rather than incidental changes in the speech mechanism, that plays the central role in fluency induction in these cases. Another popular belief was that stuttering decreased under DAF because the delay caused the speaker to elongate the syllables in each word, a technique long known to improve fluency (Van Riper, 1973). This does occur with many who use the technology, but according to Kalinowski et al. (1993; 1996), extended syllable durations per se do not appear necessary to induce fluency. Relatedly, Perkins (1979) and other researchers have noted that the technique of syllable prolongation can be learned without the use of DAF. Consequently, instead of a necessary component of treatment or, in some cases, a treatment unto itself, they considered the technology merely an instrument to aid clients in learning syllable prolongation, and perhaps a superfluous one at that.

The question remains, then: What are the basic mechanisms through which AAF produces its effects? For those who believe that some constitutional impairment of neuronal activation or timing may be partially corrected through these procedures, how is this achieved? With the advent and continued refinement of modern neuroimaging techniques, researchers have begun to approach these questions in increasingly sophisticated ways. The results have been intriguing, albeit somewhat frustrating. As certainly as AAF improves fluency in many who stutter, it is equally clear that the effects are variable across individuals, speech tasks, and/or communicative settings (Armson & Stuart, 1998; Bloodstein & Bernstein Ratner, 2007; Ingham et al., 1997). Our own research, which provided custom-fit SpeechEasy devices for subjects to wear daily for 4 months, bears this out as well (Pollard et al., 2009). It can be inferred from these findings that some individuals who stutter rely more on auditory feedback than others when attempting to achieve greater fluency. This in turn results in a priori heterogeneous samples that are routinely grouped together for the purposes of statistical analyses, potentially obscuring within-subject effects that can be quite noteworthy.

Despite such limitations, what the literature does tell us is that the response patterns and anatomy of the auditory cortices of persons who stutter differ in significant ways from their fluent controls (Braun et al., 1997; Foundas et al., 2001; 2004; Fox et al., 1996; Salmelin et al., 1998). For instance, Foundas and colleagues have explored the theory of a defective speech monitoring system through a series of experiments using magnetic resonance imaging (MRI). MRI is a noninvasive technique that allows one to view the structure of living tissue within the body. The impetus behind their research was to test the hypothesis that those who stutter have anomalous anatomy in cortical speech-language areas, including portions of auditory cortex. The supposed differences in brain anatomy could be reflected through aberrant gyral patterns, atypical size, or interhemispheric asymmetries that are reduced or reversed. With regard to DAF, it was found that subjects with atypical rightward asymmetry in a region of auditory temporal cortex called the planum temporale became more fluent under DAF than those subjects with typical leftward asymmetry in this area (Foundas et al.,

2004). The explanation for this finding comes from the two-loop timing theory of speech output (Nudelman et al., 1989; 1992). This theory posits two main feedback loops working in synchrony to coordinate speech production: an outer "linguistic" circuit and an inner "phonatory" circuit. The outer linguist circuit is thought to be involved in certain language functions and lower level processing of auditory verbal information, such as selecting and monitoring speech sounds. The inner phonatory circuit, by contrast, is thought to be involved with the motor programs of the vocal apparatus. Stuttering is modeled as a transient instability in these systems caused by mistiming between or interrupted activation of the two circuits (Foundas et al., 2001; 2004). In other words, "a defect at any point within either of these distributed neural networks could induce stuttering by disrupting the flow of information, which in turn would induce asynchronous activation of the paired muscles that mediate speech production" (Foundas et al., 2004, p. 1645). From this view, DAF may work by resynchronizing the two circuits.

An alternative to the two-loop timing hypothesis is the dual premotor systems model of stuttering put forth by Per Alm (2005). This theory is grounded in Goldberg's (1985; 1991) dual premotor systems hypothesis, which argues that the human brain has two parallel systems for the planning and execution of movements. The lateral system (e.g., lateral premotor cortex, cerebellum) is thought to be active when movement is controlled relative to external sensory input, for instance when speaking with a metronome or during choral speech. The medial system (e.g., supplementary motor area, basal ganglia) relies on automatized, internally generated programs in the absence of external feedback, for instance during spontaneous speech. This model holds that stuttering is caused primarily by disturbed functioning of the medial system, particularly the basal ganglia. More specifically, the model describes speech as a motor sequence and suggests that the basal ganglia send impaired "go signals" to trigger the next motor segment in the sequence. Many conditions that induce fluency are thought to work either by providing an external timing cue (e.g., metronome effect, choral effect, singing) or through de-automatization of speech control

(e.g., FAF, MAF, accent imitation) (Alm, 2005). These conditions allow control of the speech output to momentarily bypass the impaired medial system in favor of the intact lateral system. Alm suggests that FAF may de-automatize the control of speech, facilitating a shift to increased control from the lateral system during the presence of the altered feedback. This theory is of course speculative at the moment, but it receives credence from recent neuroimaging research demonstrating increased activity in the superior temporal cortex bilaterally while speaking under FAF (Watkins et al., 2008).

EMPIRICAL BASIS

Although numerous studies dating back to the 1930s have examined the effects of AAF, we will limit our discussion to reviewing recent work bearing more directly on the SpeechEasy. A body of literature leading to the release of the SpeechEasy was published during the 1990s by researchers primarily associated with the East Carolina University Stuttering Research Laboratory, many of whom were responsible for the device's development (Armson & Stuart, 1998; Hargrave et al., 1994; Kalinowski et al., 1993; 1996; Macleod et al., 1995; Stuart, Kalinowski, & Rastatter, 1997; Stuart et al., 2002). The group effects from this research have collectively shown that all modalities of AAF produce immediate reductions in the overt symptoms of stuttering in controlled laboratory environments. As mentioned previously, these researchers also demonstrated that a slowed speech rate and/or extended syllable durations may not be required for an individual to benefit from these conditions. Consequently, these researchers argue that speech naturalness can be maintained while using the SpeechEasy. Furthermore, the fluency-enhancing effects of AAF have also been documented while persons who stutter talk in front of audiences of varying sizes (Armson et al., 1997) and engage in scripted telephone calls (Zimmerman et al., 1997).

In light of the fact that the SpeechEasy is intended to be worn during activities of daily living, the results from the Armson et al. (1997) and Zimmerman et al. (1997) studies are of some interest. These results have been cited as evidence that "the robust effects of altered auditory feedback occur outside the laboratory environment" (Stuart et al., 2003, p. 233). Although this is not untrue, closer scrutiny of those studies reveals that although significant group effects were found for DAF and FAF conditions, there was conspicuous variability within the samples. In the Zimmerman et al. (1997) study, two of the nine subjects showed no appreciable reduction in stuttering during DAF, whereas another subject had no response to either DAF or FAF. In Armson et al. (1997), two of the nine subjects showed no response to FAF with audience sizes of two or four people, and one subject appeared to become more dysfluent under FAF. Although these results do not pertain directly to the SpeechEasy, they support our own observations from having fit the device on numerous clients. That is, variation in how clients respond to the device both inside and outside of the clinic is the norm.

The immediate effects of the SpeechEasy in a laboratory setting have also been measured. A recent study found that the device produced group reductions in stuttering ranging from 30% to 74%, depending on the speech task and whether SpeechEasy fitting protocols were followed (Armson et al., 2006). Fluency improvement during monologue speech was also shown for approximately half of the participants. This is significant because it conflicts with the FAF results of Armson and Stuart (1998), who found much poorer effects during monologue. Another noteworthy finding from this study was that, as with much previous AAF research, response to the device was idiosyncratic. In the authors' words (Armson et al., 2006, p. 149):

> [T]he degree and pattern of benefit varied greatly across participants. Although a few participants exhibited both a dramatic reduction in stuttering and relative freedom from stuttering in the device conditions, others showed a modest or minimal reduction and continued to exhibit a relatively high level of stuttering.

While much work has been done to document the immediate efficacy of AAF, far less is known about the long-term effects of the SpeechEasy itself. Although data have been collected by our team as well as by others in a handful of ongoing studies, there is relatively little published research on the subject. The largest survey of SpeechEasy

wearers thus far was conducted by Rainmaker & Sun Integrated Marketing in 2004. Of the 2,548 people who were contacted, 19% responded. Of those who responded, more than 80% had owned a SpeechEasy for 12 months or less. Several "key findings," as highlighted by the manufacturer (SpeechEasy Consumer Information Packet, 2006), are as follows:

- More than 80% of SpeechEasy customers were satisfied with their decision to obtain a SpeechEasy device.
- More than 90% would recommend that those who stutter consider SpeechEasy devices as a treatment option.
- On a scale of 1 to 10, with "10" being fluent and "1" being extremely disfluent, more than 65% rated themselves a "5" or less prior to obtaining a SpeechEasy device. After obtaining a SpeechEasy device, 75% rated themselves a "7" or higher.
- Two out of three reported that their fluency continued to improve the longer they wore the device.
- Two out of three reported that results from the device met or exceeded their expectations.
- Approximately 80% would still purchase a SpeechEasy device if they had the choice to make over again.
- More than 80% of those who had received speech therapy both before and after having a SpeechEasy device reported improved satisfaction with their progress towards fluency during speech therapy sessions when wearing their device as compared to their progress in speech therapy sessions prior to having the device.
- More than 85% reported a heightened sense of confidence, freedom, and/or self-reliance, as well as an improvement in social and professional relationships.
- Three out of four reported a positive to very positive impact in their lives.
- Two out of three reported a good degree to a dramatic improvement in fluency.
- Whether improvements in fluency were moderate or significant, benefits were reported in:
  - Day-to-day conversations
  - Reading aloud
  - Presentations and speaking in front of audiences

- Business meetings
- Telephones calls

In our experience to date, we have seen a percentage that is less than the 80% satisfaction rating reported by Rainmaker & Sun. Of the clients we have evaluated, approximately one-third responded with substantially improved fluency, one-third responded with some improvement, and one-third experienced no noticeable change. An important caveat is that our percentages also include clients who were evaluated but did not purchase the device. Whereas Rainmaker & Sun surveyed clients who had purchased and were users of the SpeechEasy, our data are based on a broader sample of individuals who stutter. It is important to consider this distinction because subject population differences can influence the overall picture that is presented. Also, other than a study recently conducted at the University of Colorado (Pollard et al., 2009) we have not previously given formal surveys to our clients after they have been wearing the device for more than 2 months. Again, it bears repeating that our percentages include clients who were evaluated but did not purchase the device.

Very few studies have examined the long-term effects of AAF as used during everyday speaking situations. Of those that have, Dewar et al. (1979) reported equivocal findings from a study of the Edinburgh Masker, a wearable electronic device that delivered binaural masking noise. More recently, Van Borsel, Reunes, and Van den Bergh (2003) had subjects wear a headphone DAF device during a series of daily and weekly speech tasks (e.g., telephone calls, monologue, conversation with an acquaintance) for a period of 3 months. After 3 months of exposure to DAF, the percentage of stuttered words had decreased by 50% across tasks for the group, and carry-over fluency was observed without the device in place.

For several years after its introduction, the only published studies measuring the long-term effects of the SpeechEasy itself were conducted by the team who developed the device. Stuart et al. (2004) had eight participants wear custom-fit devices for a period of 4 months. They found that, while reading aloud and giving a monologue in quiet therapy rooms, stuttering rate was significantly reduced with the device in place at the initial fitting and remained so 4 months later. In a later publication, the same cohort of subjects displayed maintained fluency enhancement and speech naturalness with the device at 12 months after fitting (Stuart et al., 2006). Unfortunately, no individual speech data were reported in either study.

Several recently completed or ongoing studies are relating more equivocal findings than those obtained by Stuart and colleagues. For instance, a recent multiple single-subject study followed subjects for several months to measure SpeechEasy effects during situations of daily living (O'Donnell et al., 2008). Although statistical analyses of group data were not performed, their findings are comparable to ours in that variable between subjects effects were seen. Also, similar to our sample, many of their subjects' response patterns changed over time, with some showing an adaptation effect after prolonged use. Molt (2006a; 2006b; 2006c), reporting interim data on a relatively large sample of subjects (n = 20), found that reductions in stuttering and improvements on qualitative measures held for the majority of subjects after 3 months of use. Similar to our data, Molt also reported that some subjects demonstrated an incongruity between attitudinal measures and objective fluency scores. Overall, he reported that, "very few subjects experienced virtual elimination of stuttering behavior when using the device, and several had experienced a diminishing of the device's effectiveness. However, virtually all participants continued to give high satisfaction ratings" (Molt, 2006c). These variable and occasionally discrepant findings are echoed in other research beginning to come forth. For example, Runyan, Runyan, and Hibbard (2006) reported that although five out of nine subjects no longer wore their device at 2 to 3 years follow-up, all of their subjects would elect to purchase the SpeechEasy again. Interestingly, a consistent finding emerging across studies is that use of the device appears to provide an increase in perceived confidence for many subjects, often resulting in reductions in reported anxiety and avoidances (Cook & Smith, 2006; Molt, 2006a; Runyan, Runyan, & Hibbard, 2006; Pollard et al., 2009). This boost in confidence may, in part, account for the curious discrepancy sometimes seen between an individual's still fairly high stuttering levels and his or her favorable opinion of the device.

Since the SpeechEasy is a relatively new fluency aid, it is understandable that evidence for its effectiveness when worn in everyday life is inconclusive at present. It seems promising, however, that research currently being carried out, as well as future inquiries, will help provide more definitive conclusions.

PRACTICAL REQUIREMENTS

It is the corporate policy of the manufacturer that only ASHA-certified SLPs are eligible to dispense SpeechEasy devices after completing a 1.5-day training course (SpeechEasy Professional Information Packet, 2006). Although these training sessions were originally provided at various locations, Janus has recently required that all training, which is offered free of charge, take place at its headquarters in Greenville, North Carolina. As such, SLPs interested in fitting the device are responsible for costs related to transportation and accommodations. During training, representatives from the manufacturer discuss their vision for the device and its intended use as an adjunct to, rather than a replacement for, traditional stuttering therapy. Trainees are also introduced to the detailed evaluation procedure and gain experience operating the equipment used to calibrate the device.

The typical SpeechEasy kit includes demonstration devices with disposable foam comfort tips, mock shells of model variants (e.g., behind-the-ear [BTE], in-the-canal [ITC], completely-in-the-canal [CIC]; Fig. 16.1), a Comfort Fit (CF) device with eartubes, cleaning instruments, AudioPro hardware, SpeechMaster software, and various cables needed to manipulate and program device settings. It should be noted that the AudioPro hardware interfaces with a computer via a serial port connection, so a serial-USB adaptor may be necessary when connecting to some computers, especially many laptops. Although the equipment can take time to comfortably master, in our experience, the manufacturer provides rapid, effective customer support when needed. We recommend that potential providers thoroughly familiarize themselves with SpeechEasy fitting procedures (beyond those skills gained during official training) before working with clients. This is not to imply that procedures are overly taxing—rather, in our opinion, better clinical outcomes are invariably gained when fitting and programming are as effortless as possible.

Because the SpeechEasy is a custom-fit device, clients visit an audiologist for a hearing evaluation (including air conduction and tympanometry) and to obtain an ear impression. We strongly urge SLPs to liaise closely with audiologists to ensure the best possible outcomes. In our view, the audiologist's role in the fitting process goes well beyond taking an ear impression. For example, an individual who stutters may in some cases exhibit a concomitant degree of hearing loss; in these cases, all three parties will need to work together to find the most appropriate solution. In

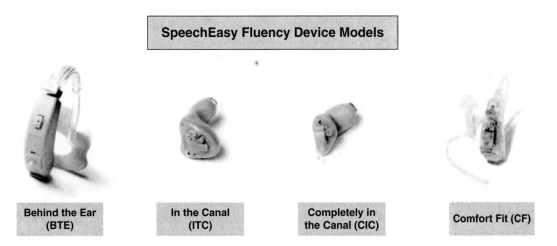

SpeechEasy Fluency Device Models

Behind the Ear (BTE) In the Canal (ITC) Completely in the Canal (CIC) Comfort Fit (CF)

Figure 16.1. SpeechEasy fluency device models.

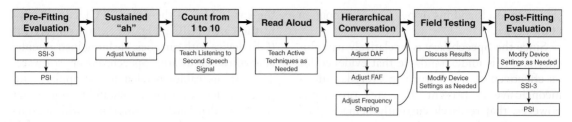

Figure 16.2. SpeechEasy evaluation protocol.

other cases, younger SpeechEasy wearers will need to be monitored so that updated shells can be manufactured in response to developmental growth; incidentally, the SpeechEasy retail price includes a one-time complimentary refit. Clients may also need to be briefly educated about cerumen management in relation to frequent SpeechEasy use. For these reasons, good interprofessional communication will help to make the entire process better for all clients. Although the majority of Speech-Easy fittings are of the "plug-and-play" variety in terms of the ear impression and shelling process, SLPs and audiologists working together can more effectively find solutions when atypical cases are presented.

KEY COMPONENTS

The SpeechEasy fitting protocol involves several steps (Fig. 16.2). During first contact, brochures and other materials can be shared, and a fitting appointment can be scheduled. It is recommended to plan at least 2 to 3 hours to comfortably complete the fitting process (SpeechEasy Training Manual, 2006). Case history information may be obtained at this time or through mail prior to the initial fitting. At the fitting itself, 300-syllable reading and conversation samples should be taken for baseline purposes. Next, the demonstration device is inserted using a foam comfort tip, typically into the ear opposite the one used when speaking on the telephone. The delay is initially set to 60 ms, and the frequency shift is set 500 Hz above the client's voice. Once the demonstration device is securely placed, the client should find the second speech signal audible yet unobtrusive. To determine an appropriate volume setting and begin the process of acclimatization to the signal, the client produces a series of prolonged /a/ sounds and then counts to 10. The overall device volume is then adjusted in response to client feedback. Because

the SpeechEasy is assumed to emulate the choral reading effect, providers are encouraged to instruct and remind clients to actively listen to the signal produced during speech.

Clients next read a passage aloud while attending to the feedback, as the clinician notes the frequency and duration of stuttering, speech naturalness, accessory behaviors, and overall ease of speech. Depending on the nature of the stuttering observed and feedback solicited from the client, the SLP either progresses to hierarchical conversation tasks or introduces one of several active techniques to augment performance. These techniques include easy vocal onsets, starter sounds (e.g., initial /m/ or schwa), fillers (e.g., /m/ or schwa inserted between words), prolongations, and continuous phonation (SpeechEasy Professional Information Packet, 2006). When necessary, these modifications are introduced to help initiate voicing and/or enhance responsiveness to the second speech signal and may be reduced if the client finds that choral effects and naturalness stabilize. Personally, we do not stress the use of starters or fillers to help generate voicing because we feel that these are not desirable contributors to normal speech production and could potentially develop into maladaptive accessory behaviors. We instead teach clients how to gently move into and prolong the first sound of a word. This strategy offers an alternative to the client's typical blocking behaviors and provides a signal for the SpeechEasy to reproduce.

Although there is currently a lack of research on the topic of SpeechEasy use combined with concurrent stuttering treatment, we have observed that some SpeechEasy users may additionally benefit from ongoing stuttering therapy that incorporates traditional, active stuttering management techniques. For instance, we report one case in which a college-aged individual received traditional stuttering therapy while wearing the device (Pollard et al., 2007). He reportedly found easy onsets to initiate voicing to be the most helpful therapeutic technique, while desensitization exercises to decrease more covert stuttering behaviors were viewed as being beneficial as well. He also described how, as therapy progressed, he came to restrict the use of his device to only periodic, higher stress situations such as classroom presentations and involvement in large study groups. At other times, he reportedly maintained a satisfactory level of fluency solely through the use of active techniques learned during treatment. Although limited in scope, this single example illustrates how SpeechEasy use can change over time as mastery of stuttering management techniques increases.

During the initial fitting, longer or shorter delays can also be tested and finalized before trying higher or lower frequency shifts. Although retaining acceptable levels of speech naturalness is important, longer delay times can be used in some cases to encourage a slower speaking rate. To this end, longer delay times may be beneficial for those clients who also exhibit cluttering.

In our experience, it can be helpful at this time to have parents, caregivers, or partners present to provide opinions about speech naturalness at different delay times. These reactions can sometimes be more meaningful to the client than clinician/provider-based judgments alone. Because the technology employed by the SpeechEasy shifts the entire speech signal up or down in 500-Hz increments, alternate frequencies (e.g., 1,000 Hz up or 500 Hz down) can also be sampled before finalizing a setting based on client preference. Finally, the SpeechMaster software includes a 16-band equalizer to boost specific frequencies (up to 20 dB each). This fine tuning may be helpful in accentuating speech-related frequencies.

Additional tuning to adjust DAF, FAF, or volume settings can take place during subsequent visits. Typically, clients returning for follow-up have used their SpeechEasy for some time in various speaking environments and want to try another AAF setting or perhaps have the device volume or frequency shaping adjusted. All of these adjustments can easily be made in the clinician's office by reconnecting the unit to the programming hardware. These sessions also allow the SLP time to review strategies for tuning into the second speech signal, improving voice initiation, and coping with background noise. We have found that these efforts often result in improved client satisfaction with the SpeechEasy.

To increase the appeal and versatility of the device, all BTE and ITC models currently incorporate dual memory settings, whereas CIC devices can do so at an extra cost. These dual controls permit wearers to toggle between two distinct settings using a button located on the device's exterior. In many cases, the second memory setting is programmed with no frequency shift and no time delay for those instances when clients wish to listen to others without filtering. Other settings have also been encouraged more recently to facilitate use of the device in noisier backgrounds. In other cases, clients include a longer time delay with the second memory setting to temporarily encourage a slower speaking rate. Incidentally, because the SpeechEasy is built on a digital platform, occasional firmware updates for the device are made available to providers by the manufacturer. This allows individuals who have previously purchased a SpeechEasy to visit a provider to have their devices reprogrammed. In the past, these firmware updates have attempted to attenuate levels of background noise, for example. The manufacturer of the SpeechEasy has also recently developed an additional model, the Comfort Fit, which was designed to permit more natural sound passage and reduce background noise relative to CIC, ITC, and BTE variants.

The SpeechEasy, similar to more traditional forms of stuttering therapy, is a costly investment. At this time, devices range between $4,100 to $4,900, excluding options such as an external volume control for CIC models ($200) and a soft custom ear mold on BTE models ($100) (SpeechEasy Professional Information Packet, 2006). Other expenses include initial fitting and audiologic fees, which may cost $300 to $500 total. Clients can typically expect to receive their custom-fit devices 3 to 4 weeks from the order date. After the final fitting, the manufacturer recommends that two 30-minute follow-up sessions and two phone contacts be scheduled during the device's 60-day trial period (SpeechEasy Training Manual, 2006).

Although the SpeechEasy may be returned during this 60-day trial for a 90% refund, the compounded cost of personally trying and then returning the device during this period may approximate $1,000, when partial nonrefunded fitting and audiologic fees are included. In some cases, additional stuttering therapy may be needed to optimize outcomes, which can further increase the final bill.

Fortunately, the manufacturer provides an array of payment options, including CareCredit, HELPcard, and credit card purchases. The Care-Credit option offers no-interest payment plans (up to 18 months), as well as longer term (i.e., 24 to 60 months) 9.9% annual percentage rate payment plans (CareCredit brochure; in SpeechEasy Policy and Procedures Manual, 2006). Other possible payment options include Veteran's Administration coverage, Vocational Rehabilitation funding, and insurance reimbursement. As providers, we have experienced some success in dealing with Vocational Rehabilitation in the past. Additionally, the manufacturer is currently working with Healthcare Reimbursement Solutions, Inc. to increase the probability of insurance coverage for the device. At this time, however, insurance coverage for the SpeechEasy is undoubtedly the exception rather than the rule.

Throughout this process, from the moment of first contact onward, clinicians will need to help clients separate fact from fiction regarding the potential benefits of a SpeechEasy. One point to clarify is that although true choral reading has been proven to be effective in enhancing fluency, the SpeechEasy, in contrast, attempts to *emulate* the choral reading effect. As such, the device emulates true choral reading imperfectly, although not without benefit, and the magnitude of these benefits appears to be individually based. In other words, some individuals who stutter are helped by the SpeechEasy significantly, others somewhat, and some not at all. In response to the amount of publicity the SpeechEasy has received in the national press, providers need to help clients see the device in its proper perspective; although the SpeechEasy may produce dramatic results for some, it is not a cure, and some degree of active stuttering management on the part of the client is invariably needed to produce the best results. To this end, the manufacturer itself trains providers to gently minimize the client's expecta-

tions when first trying the device (SpeechEasy Training Manual, 2006). Ultimately, although the national press and certain SpeechEasy wearers may herald the device as "miraculous," we as clinicians and researchers should refrain from such descriptions.

When setting realistic expectations, the issue of background noise is one that providers should disclose and discuss with prospective Speech-Easy clients during the evaluation process. Although efforts have been taken by the manufacturer to minimize the reproduction of ambient noise, including the development of the Comfort Fit model, background noise remains one of the most frequent drawbacks we hear from SpeechEasy users, research subjects, and potential clients. In our initial exposure to the Comfort Fit device, background noise appears to be reduced relative to other SpeechEasy models. However, intolerance to noise in some situations (e.g., restaurants, bars, social gatherings, etc.) can inevitably interfere with effective SpeechEasy use. In such settings, clients may use a null second memory setting (i.e., DAF: 0 ms; FAF: 0 Hz), turn off the device, or temporarily remove it. Therefore, SpeechEasy users will need to have a communication back-up plan in these environments that is not reliant on the device.

ASSESSMENT METHODS TO SUPPORT ONGOING DECISION MAKING

Clients' personal experiences with how the SpeechEasy impacts their stuttering during the initial 2- to 3-hour evaluation are the determining factor as to whether or not they will purchase the device. To date, we have observed that approximately 20% to 25% of those evaluated chose not to purchase a device primarily because they felt it was of little or no help. Of the remaining 75% who purchased a device, approximately 8% returned it for a refund within 60 days. Ultimately, the decision is client based. This is a crucial point for the clinician to understand because inconsistencies between observed outcomes and the client's final decision are possible. For instance, we have met clients who did not exhibit quantitative increases in fluency but who nevertheless desired to purchase the device.

Conversely, others who demonstrated measurable fluency enhancements were not swayed. This peculiarity has been a most interesting eye opener for us throughout our experience with the SpeechEasy and raises interesting questions regarding prevailing conceptualizations of evidence-based practice.

As mentioned in the Introduction, clinicians may have a limited degree of exposure to many who are interested in the SpeechEasy. Clients often travel from long distances to seek an evaluation because the number of certified providers in many states may be few and dispersed. This diminishes opportunities for regular contact during which additional therapy strategies can be taught that may augment the client's use of the device. Others are not able to afford additional therapy or may opt out of the opportunity because they have tried other treatments in the past and have found these experiences frustrating and unsuccessful. For these reasons, contact with a client may only occur once during the evaluation and another time weeks later when the custom-made unit arrives for the final fitting. After this, some clients may never be seen again. Although this is not the case for all or even most clients, it is nonetheless a common occurrence. We feel it is important to state that the SpeechEasy may be the only reasonable and potentially effective option for those living in outlying areas. These individuals are unable to attend the regularly scheduled sessions necessary for most traditional treatments, leaving the SpeechEasy as one of their only viable alternatives. Despite these less-than-optimal circumstances, we have worked with such clients who nonetheless appeared to be helped substantially by the device alone.

For those clients for whom direct contact is not an issue, the likely result will be better support, more time spent practicing the initiation of air and voicing, and the opportunity for the SLP to collect outcome data over time. Stuttering severity can then be monitored using the Stuttering Severity Instrument-3 (SSI-3), Perceptions of Stuttering Inventory (PSI), Overall Assessment of the Speaker's Experience of Stuttering (OASES), or other stuttering assessment tools. However, regardless of whether the client is seen only twice or several times, probably the most important outcome measure will be client self-report—the information gathered from the client about his or her SpeechEasy and its effectiveness. We have long regarded the client's perspective as being at least as meaningful for treatment decision making as counting overt stuttering behaviors, which only reflects the client's speech at a given moment and may not be representative of typical speech performance.

TAILORING THE TREATMENT TO THE INDIVIDUAL CLIENT

Because of the short time that the SpeechEasy has been available, our exposure to fitting persons from diverse cultural backgrounds is limited. Although our evaluations are straightforward and mostly noninvasive, we are aware of the importance of considering cultural differences when interacting with clients. For example, the test device can be more quickly inserted into the preferred ear of the client if we assist in that process. With clients who may feel uncomfortable with the physical contact often needed to seat the device, we can verbally direct them to properly place it themselves. This accommodation may take a bit longer, but it can alleviate client uneasiness in any instances where cultural differences proscribe close person-to-person contact when first meeting. The interested reader is referred to a chapter written by Cooper and Cooper (1998) for valuable suggestions for respecting diversity when interacting clinically with persons who stutter. Many examples are given of culture-dependent variables that SLPs should be sensitive to in serving the needs of fluency clients.

By its inherent design, the SpeechEasy evaluation is tailored to the client's needs. It is the client's response to the DAF, FAF, frequency shaping, and volume settings that directs the evaluation. Any necessary adjustments thereafter are based on what works best for the individual, and desired settings that work for some clients may be very different than for others. Thus, essential to the prescribed design of conducting a SpeechEasy evaluation is flexibility to meet individual client needs.

Other factors can also influence the need to modify what we recommend as a result of the client's response to the SpeechEasy. Some clients experience better results by using a longer DAF delay and adjusting their speaking rate accordingly to talk in unison with the auditory feedback. This results in a slower speaking rate. If the client and clinician discover and agree that this strategy works best, more emphasis and time can be spent on maximizing the benefits of this option. For others, slowing their speaking rate is less critical to fluency enhancement. Some of these clients prefer to match a normal speaking rate to a shorter delay. Others prefer to talk at a normal rate while ignoring or speaking over a longer DAF delay. Whether such clients speak to the delay or speak over it, we have found that clients may need a great deal of additional practice initiating air and voicing to gain maximum benefit from the SpeechEasy.

Flexibility in working with the client after the final fitting is also an example of individualizing the experience. That is, once they have used the device for a period of time, many will call to ask if we can change the AAF settings, volume, or frequency shaping in hopes of improving their response to the device. Some may also decide to pursue any variety of traditional stuttering treatments while using the SpeechEasy. The intervention plan will then be determined based on what the client and SLP feel would be most beneficial. For some, it may focus more on either fluency shaping or modification of stuttering. For others, a combination of both may be needed.

APPLICATION OF THE TREATMENT TO AN INDIVIDUAL WHO STUTTERS

Of several successful clients we have fit with the SpeechEasy, we have chosen to report on a middle-aged female we will call "Linda." Linda attended a prestigious law school and graduated near the top of her class. Since earning a law degree, she has been working as a tax attorney for a large legal firm in Colorado. She came to us stating that she had not been enrolled in stuttering intervention since she completed a 2-year stint with airflow therapy while in high school. She reported that she worked on this technique with a clinician who was understanding and supportive but felt that "it worked much better in the room with the therapist than it did outside of the therapy room." As a result, within a few years after treatment, she had all but abandoned airflow techniques and, instead, had increased her use of deliberate pauses and hesitations in an attempt to minimize her worsening overt, audible stuttering. She indicated that this worked "fairly well" through law school and for many years as a working attorney when speaking one-on-one. She estimated her stuttering severity during this period to be mild. However, about 7 years ago, her law firm required her to present courses on tax law to groups of attorneys and accountants. At that time, she felt her confidence diminish and her anxiety increase at the thought of talking, not just to groups, but in her everyday interactions as well. In her words, "My stuttering seemed like it skyrocketed. The silent pauses became longer and ineffective. It got to the point I was afraid to go to work." She reported that her stuttering had "become more audible with visible struggle."

Linda's experience with increased stuttering and apprehension led to her desire to contact us about the SpeechEasy. After a 20-minute phone consultation, wherein Linda exhibited substantial dysfluencies, an evaluation was scheduled for the following week. Based on the SSI-3, Linda's stuttering severity at the assessment and prior to inserting the device was severe (Table 16.2). Her stuttering patterns consisted of long silent pauses, physical struggle, and word avoidances. After proceeding through the testing protocol, she preferred a DAF setting of 48 ms and an FAF shift of +500 Hz. The second memory setting included a 65-ms delay and +1,000-Hz frequency shift.

Table 16.2. *Stuttering Severity Before and After Initial and Final SpeechEasy Fittings*

Condition	SSI-3 Score	Stuttering Severity
Baseline without device	34	Severe
Initial fitting	22	Mild
Final fitting	22	Mild
29 months after final fitting	12	Very Mild

SSI-3, Stuttering Severity Instrument-3.

Consistent with SpeechEasy protocols, practice with initiating air and voicing was conducted with some success during the evaluation. We felt that Linda would benefit from more sessions to perfect this strategy, but she was unable to attend these because of her work commitments. During the evaluation, she reported that it was helpful to slow her rate as a result of talking in unison with the SpeechEasy. Linda appeared excited by the improvement in fluency that she experienced with the device in the therapy room, as well as during her 1-hour trial outside of the clinic. The SSI-3 was administered again at the end of the evaluation and at the final fitting 3 weeks later. On both occasions, her stuttering with the device in place was rated as mild (Table 16.2). Of course, these initial improvements in fluency would not necessarily indicate how Linda might respond over time in her everyday speaking situations.

Linda spoke with us by phone 6, 14, and 29 months after her final fitting. Although the first two follow-up calls were brief, Linda reported on both occasions that she stuttered much less than she had for many years prior to purchasing her SpeechEasy. The 29-month follow-up included contact in the clinic where the SSI-3 was once again administered (Table 16.2). At this time, Linda recounted a very successful past and ongoing experience with her SpeechEasy. She stated that she "wore the device for at least eight to ten hours a day for the first eight months" and typically only used the first memory setting (DAF: 48 ms; FAF: +500 Hz). In contrast to some other clients, she reported that she found little use for the second memory setting. During this approximately 2.5-year period, Linda "felt a huge surge in confidence" because she "felt more stutter-free in all speaking situations" and was reportedly "able to conduct her seminars with 90% improved speech." She also reported that, except when teaching her seminars, she had reduced her wearing time to 4 to 5 hours per day over the past year and further stated that, "I almost never wear it after work hours anymore because my stuttering is so much better now." In addition, Linda said that:

Easing into the stuttering with voicing and talking in sync with the faster [DAF: 48 ms], not slow delay setting, helps me more

than anything. My confidence has been high for the past two years. My slower talking seemed odd way back when, but now I'm comfortable with it and so many people tell me how great I sound. Not only that, but I feel more relaxed in my whole life.

In Linda's experience, wearing the unit for a few hours in the morning often enabled her to be more fluent for the rest of the day. As such, this case provides anecdotal support for a carry-over effect resulting from prolonged, regular use of AAF. There is little doubt that Linda is a successful case. At last contact, she had reported significant success using the SpeechEasy for almost 2.5 years.

INTRODUCTION TO VIDEOTAPED SAMPLES

We filmed a sampling of clients who reported success with the SpeechEasy. These brief interviews with three adults who stutter were filmed at different times after being fit with the device. These clients decided to purchase the device either after receiving a detailed SpeechEasy evaluation described in this chapter or after participating in a 6-month longitudinal research project that tracked SpeechEasy use (Pollard et al., 2009). All three decided to purchase their devices because they felt it helped them speak more fluently.

As you watch these clips, note that the first two subjects initially talk without the SpeechEasy. After a short period of time, they place the device in their ear and continue talking with the clinician. Despite the difference in the amount of stuttering between the two conditions, we caution viewers to consider each client's subjective impressions regarding the usefulness of their SpeechEasy within naturalistic speaking environments. Making efficacy-related judgments about any form of treatment should include measurements of everyday speaking experiences that extend beyond an artificial clinical environment. For this reason, subjects were asked to share their opinions of the SpeechEasy as an aid for fluency enhancement.

Subject 1 is a young adult male who has worn the SpeechEasy for only a few weeks. In the first section of his video clip, he is talking with the clinician without the device in his ear. After a few minutes, he then inserts the SpeechEasy and continues with the conversation. The frequency and severity of his stuttering are clearly reduced while using the device. In a subsequent interview, taken 6 months after filming, he reports continued success with the SpeechEasy but states that the fluency benefits derived from its use are "now a little less when compared to the first couple of weeks."

Subject 2 is a 60-year-old male who has worn the SpeechEasy for approximately 2 years. Similar to Subject 1, he is initially speaking with the clinician without using the device. After several minutes, he places the SpeechEasy in his ear and continues conversing. He reports that the device continues to be helpful since he first purchased it but to a lesser degree as compared to the first few months. Since his retirement a few months prior to filming, he reports wearing the device less because he no longer gives oral presentations. Although he reports that he wears the device more intermittently now, he feels it continues to be helpful in certain situations.

Subject 3 is a 57-year-old male who is mildly cognitively impaired. Formerly a person with a very severe stuttering problem, he improved his fluency dramatically through conventional stuttering modification treatment prior to acquiring the SpeechEasy. However, he later volunteered to participate for several months in a SpeechEasy research study and felt his fluency was improved even more. This experience led him to continue to wear the device after completion of the study. At the time of filming, he had been using it for approximately 8 months. Unlike Subjects 1 and 2, he chose to wear the device during the entire filming session. As a result, his segment with the clinician shows only conversation with his device inserted. This subject's fluent but slower speaking rate is indicative of how he presently speaks in all situations, whether or not he wears the device. Based on our experience with this client over many years, his speaking rate in the video clip is not an artifact of the clinical setting or the filming.

FUTURE DIRECTIONS

As we indicated in the "Empirical Basis" section of this chapter, available evidence has demonstrated that AAF can be effective at improving

fluency for many—but not all—who stutter (Armson & Stuart, 1998; Hargrave et al., 1994; Kalinowski et al., 1993; 1996; Macleod et al., 1995; Stuart et al., 2002). We have personally witnessed SpeechEasy success cases similar to Linda, as well as other instances when the device ultimately proved ineffective. These different outcomes can likely be explained in part by what past research has suggested; namely, that fluency improvement under AAF is not universal and may not reliably generalize outside of the clinical environment (Armson & Stuart, 1998; Bloodstein & Bernstein Ratner, 2007; Ingham et al., 1997; Pollard et al., 2009). The frequent inconsistencies between results obtained in the laboratory and those reported in naturalistic settings are likely influenced by the mercurialness of the disorder. That is, the nature of stuttering is such that the overt stuttered speech patterns as well as the covert struggles of those who stutter often fluctuate dramatically in relation to speaking environment, listener identity, speaking task, speech content, and levels of internal and external stress (Bennett, 2006; Guitar, 2005; Van Riper, 1982). Therefore, the context-dependent nature of the disorder becomes an issue when one considers how its symptoms have commonly been measured in the literature. When subjects speak under any fluency-inducing condition, they usually have their speech recorded in a quiet laboratory setting, often while reading a passage out loud (Andrews et al., 1982; Bloodstein, 1950; Johnson & Rosen, 1937; Kalinowski et al., 1993). The ecologic limitations of research findings obtained under such conditions are apparent and can be addressed by more naturalistic sampling procedures.

More longitudinal inquiries into the effects of the SpeechEasy are also needed. Individuals who stutter do not live their lives in a laboratory or a clinic, and being able to read a passage aloud fluently may be of little practical utility to them (Pollard et al., 2009). Thus, it would be valuable to measure how the clients respond to the device in real-life speaking situations over time. If the fluency-enhancing effects of the SpeechEasy are to have substantive value, they must be shown to be both durable and robust across the kinds of situations that persons who stutter encounter in their daily lives. There remain numerous additional questions to be further addressed, including:

- Why is the SpeechEasy's effectiveness both within and across users less than universal?
- What are the neurologic mechanisms underlying changes in fluency due to DAF and FAF as used by the SpeechEasy?
- How do clients' responses to the device change over time in their daily lives?
- Does the SpeechEasy facilitate generalization of fluency after prolonged use?
- What factors (e.g., prior therapy experiences, stuttering pattern, degree of use) best predict success?
- Are their noteworthy effects (either positive or negative) of SpeechEasy use in younger clients?
- In what types of speaking environments does the device work best?
- In what settings does it function poorly or produce no benefit?
- How is daily use of the device affected by background noise?
- Is there an initial period of adapting to the device before optimal fluency enhancement occurs?
- What additional fluency techniques will optimize one's response?

From the perspective of practicing SLPs who may be providing or coming into contact with the SpeechEasy, we feel that two particular issues warrant consideration. First is the notion of changes in frequency of stuttering versus overall severity of stuttering. For whom it is effective, the Speech-Easy may decrease the sheer number of disfluencies exhibited, but it may also decrease the duration or the amount of tension underlying those disfluencies, or perhaps provide the client with a feeling of confidence that allows him or her to communicate more freely. It would be worthwhile to describe these response patterns. Unfortunately, such nuanced measures of fluency improvement have by and large not been reported in the AAF literature.

Second, client variables that may predict success with the device are not well understood. Correlational research in this direction may therefore be helpful. Such characteristics as one's unique stuttering pattern or previous experiences with and opinions of past treatment, among other factors, may be reliable indicators of a particular client's candidacy for the device. Considering the costs involved even if one

eventually returns the device, this would be valuable information for clinicians and clients to possess. We should note here that at least one lab has conducted investigations along these lines (Molt, 2007a; 2007b). The early results are encouraging insofar as they indicate that reliable, practical means for screening SpeechEasy candidates are within reach.

MEDIA PORTRAYAL OF THE SPEECHEASY: INITIAL REACTIONS AND CONCLUDING THOUGHTS

We would like to conclude this chapter with our personal reasons for including the SpeechEasy as a potential treatment option within our clinical practice. Sadly, devices said to cure stuttering have been falsely touted for decades. As a result, many SLPs and stuttering researchers were understandably leery in 2002 when numerous reports about the device were aired on popular television programs and in newspapers and magazines. Much of the initial skepticism stemmed from how the SpeechEasy was portrayed by the media as being a new and revolutionary treatment for curing chronic stuttering. Almost without exception, some of America's most popular television programs depicted the device as immediately eradicating severe, disabling stuttering. Many television viewers who saw the device hailed it as a "miracle" because they witnessed a dramatic drop in stuttering, along with emotional testimonials from clients, families, and one of its developers. Given these portrayals, many did not understand that the immediate fluency improvement was not representative of all who stutter and may not have persisted across various environments. Although we now know there are clients who do experience long-term, life-changing benefits while using the SpeechEasy, most of the public did not appreciate the fact that some individuals who stutter experience little or no benefit from AAF devices.

Sensationalistic reporting on the SpeechEasy attracted the interest of persons who stutter, parents of disfluent children, and other interested parties, while initially turning many SLPs against its use as a potential therapy tool. As a result of the slanted media blitz, many professionals knowledgeable of the nature and treatment of stuttering questioned the credibility of both the device and the manufacturer. Some saw it as yet another gimmick, something that gave false hope to people who stutter. Others assumed it merely provided a temporary distraction and questioned the long-term effects of the device. Still others felt that the dramatic media cases were not an accurate representation of all who stutter.

We received scores of telephone calls and emails requesting our opinion of the Speech-Easy and how to purchase the device that "cures" stuttering. Unfortunately, we could respond with little authority at that time because we had not had the opportunity to examine it. Despite several studies attesting to the fluency-enhancing effects of AAF in general, no efficacy data about the SpeechEasy were then available. Our lack of experience with the device and inability to provide unbiased, factual information spurred us to receive training from the manufacturer. As certified SLPs who stutter, we had a special interest in the treatment and research of fluency disorders. We were initially doubtful of the worthiness of the SpeechEasy as a treatment tool and felt that the only way to learn firsthand about the device was to examine it while keeping an open mind.

Based on our experiences during SpeechEasy training, we agreed that the device had a positive effect on our fluency and thought that it could be of potential benefit to some of our clients. Therefore, we felt comfortable becoming providers and including it as one of many viable options for the treatment of stuttering. Subsequently, we were able to provide an informed, even-handed perspective to potential clients and families that differed from what was portrayed in the media. The aim of this chapter was to afford that same perspective in a written form so that clinicians working with clients who stutter may have a credible resource as well. We hope we have effectively done so.

SUGGESTED READINGS

Armson, J., Kiefte, M., Mason, J., & De Croos, D. (2006). The effects of SpeechEasy on stuttering frequency in laboratory conditions. *Journal of Fluency Disorders, 31,* 137–152.

O'Donnell, J. J., Armson, J., & Kiefte, M. (2008). The effectiveness of SpeechEasy during situations of daily living. Journal of Fluency Disorders, 33, 99–119.

Pollard, R., & Ellis, J. B. (2008). The SpeechEasy: Emerging evidence for interested clinicians and prospective buyers. 11th International Stuttering Awareness Day Online Conference (ISAD11). Available at http://www.mnsu.edu/comdis/isad11/papers/pollard11.html.

Pollard, R., Ellis, J. B., Finan, D., & Ramig P. R. (2009). Effects of the SpeechEasy on objective and perceived aspects of stuttering: A six-month, Phase I clinical trial in naturalistic environments. *Journal of Speech, Language and Hearing Research, 52,* 516–533.

SpeechEasy Consumer Information Packet. (2006). Available from Janus Development Group, Inc. 112 Staton Road, Greenville, NC 27834. Phone: 866-551-9042. http://www.speecheasy.com/

CHAPTER 17

The Physiologic Basis and Pharmacologic Treatment of Stuttering

GERALD A. MAGUIRE, GLYN RILEY, DAVID L. FRANKLIN, AND ERGI GUMUSANELI

CHAPTER OUTLINE

INTRODUCTION
THEORETICAL BASIS FOR TREATMENT
   APPROACH
EMPIRICAL BASIS FOR TREATMENT
   APPROACH
   Risperidone
   Olanzapine
   Other Neurotransmitter Systems Including
     GABA
PRACTICAL REQUIREMENTS
KEY COMPONENTS

ASSESSMENT METHODS TO
   SUPPORT ONGOING DECISION
   MAKING
TAILORING THE TREATMENT TO THE
   INDIVIDUAL CLIENT
APPLICATION OF TREATMENT TO AN
   INDIVIDUAL WHO STUTTERS
FUTURE DIRECTIONS
CHAPTER SUMMARY
CHAPTER REVIEW QUESTIONS
SUGGESTED READINGS

KEY TERMS

Dopamine: a neurotransmitter.

Gamma-aminobutyric acid (GABA): a neurotransmitter.

Pagoclone: an investigational partial GABA agonist medication being studied for stuttering.

Risperidone and olanzapine: two novel dopamine antagonist medications that have been studied in stuttering but approved for the treatment of schizophrenia and bipolar disorder.

INTRODUCTION

Pharmacologic treatments have evolved tremendously over the years and are prescribed as therapy for multiple central nervous system disorders. However, studies in a variety of different psychiatric disorders have shown that the effects of medications are augmented by psychotherapy. For example, the standard treatment for major depressive disorder includes medication and cognitive behavior therapy (Kim, 1996). A similar approach involving speech therapy and pharmacotherapy has been used for patients who stutter. However, the focus of this chapter is on the single approach using medications to treat stuttering. These modalities will likely never cure stuttering, but emerging pharmacologic treatments have demonstrated promising potential for patients. Although a given medication may benefit some patients more than others, the medications described here reduced stuttering significantly in a group of participating patients. This group had reductions in their behavioral measures such as stuttering severity and percent syllables stuttered; however, they still may have benefited from cognitive behavior therapy to address avoidance, locus of control and related issues, and further reductions in stuttering severity. Further research is warranted to investigate this potential combined therapy in stuttering. The pharmacologic studies of stuttering in recent years have been conducted in randomized, double-blinded, placebo-controlled designs and have demonstrated clinically and statistically significant differences between treated and untreated stuttering groups. Therefore, these approaches deserve review in a book designed to document established and emerging interventions for people who stutter.

THEORETICAL BASIS FOR TREATMENT APPROACH

Stuttering is a common speech disorder classified by the *Diagnostic and Statistical Manual of Mental Disorders–Fourth Edition* (DSM-IV) as an Axis I disorder (American Psychiatric Association, 2000). The DSM-IV is the diagnostic manual for psychiatric disorders, and stuttering is listed in Axis I, defining it as a major disorder that affects patient functioning. It is characterized by frequent sound prolongations, recurrent word and syllable repetitions, broken speech, and substitutions or omissions of problematic words. By definition, stuttering interferes with social, academic, or occupational function. As a result, individuals who stutter often develop high levels of social anxiety, fear, and even avoidance of social situations altogether (Maguire et al., 2000b; Stein, Baird, & Walker, 1996). Although no single therapy has been developed to cure stuttering, speech therapy and pharmacologic treatments designed for alleviating stuttering symptoms have yielded promising results. These therapies, combined with cognitive behavioral therapy and treating other comorbid conditions such as social anxiety, offer a comprehensive approach that is likely to be beneficial to patients who suffer from stuttering.

Stuttering is thought by many to be a developmental disorder, with most cases beginning in early childhood (Yairi & Ambrose, 2005). There are a few rare cases of acquired stuttering presenting in adulthood; however, these cases are most often associated with recent events, such as brain trauma, stroke, or changes in medication (Ludlow & Dooman, 1992). Most current approximations forecast that stuttering affects 1% of the adult population (Andrews et al. 1983) and 4% of children (Yairi & Ambrose, 2005). Nearly 80% of developmental stuttering begins by 4 years of age (Yairi & Ambrose, 2005); 74% of those cases spontaneously remit within 4 years of onset. Nevertheless, many cases persist into adulthood, and early recognition and treatment should not be avoided given that encouragement of communication is essential in education and blossoming development of children (Riley & Ingham, 2000).

Stuttering has long been recognized throughout history and in every culture. One of the earliest known individuals with the disorder was Demosthenes, the famous Greek orator. Adoring tales of perseverance describe Demosthenes' determination to improve his own stuttering. It has been written that he practiced speaking and reciting poems against the crashing waves of the ocean with his mouth full of pebbles and spent limitless hours analyzing the best debaters of his time. Descriptive tales illustrate Demosthenes' courage and dedication to finally overcome his stuttering and become one of the finest speakers of ancient Greece. Our understanding of stuttering has evolved remarkably since the description of these romantic tales. For centuries, it was thought that stuttering was related to anatomic aberrations within the tongue or larynx. Aggressive surgical interventions and other manipulations of these organs failed to improve stuttering symptoms. The pioneering work of Orton and Travis in the early part of the 20th century led to a significant change in the understanding of stuttering (Orton, 1927; Travis, 1931). They postulated that stuttering arose from abnormal cerebral activity, signaling a significant paradigm change in the etiology of stuttering from the tongue and throat to abnormalities in the brain. Despite the insights of Travis and Orton, psychoanalytical views prevailed for the next few decades without much treatment success, and neurologic research on stuttering was largely ignored (Ingham, 1984).

The majority of stuttering treatment practiced today involves speech therapy (Manning, 2001). These treatments have been successful in alleviating many of the stuttering symptoms observed in young children under 6 years of age, while the brain is still in development (Riley & Ingham, 2000). These observations open the door for the exploration of other treatment modalities in adolescents and adults for the treatment of stuttering. However, in considering comprehensive guidelines for the treatment of stuttering, not only should the clinician take into account DSM-IV diagnostic criteria, but the clinician should also bear in mind all features of the disorder including fluency enhancement, improving social anxiety, and cognitive restructuring. Although the assessment of the latter two components necessitates a more subjective approach by asking patients how their stuttering influences their daily activities, objective measures that rate speech and fluency have been commonly used in studies.

Recent functional positron emission tomography (PET) studies of the brain showed that individuals who stutter revealed decreased cerebral activation within the cortical speech areas and striatum (Maguire, Riley & Yu, 2002; Pool et al., 1991; Wood & Stump, 1980; Wu et al., 1995; 1997). Also, similar research has shown that the left hemispheric speech areas are hypoactive compared to the right hemisphere. Sommer et al. (2002) described that the increased activity within the right hemisphere in stuttering individuals may represent a counterbalance for decreased left hemispheric function. Furthermore, they also suggest the possibility of timing defects between the left frontal cortical areas, a region thought to be involved in the planning of language, and central areas involved in speech as determined by magnetoencephalography (MEG) scans. In the early 1980s, Van Riper (1982) hypothesized that stuttering was a disorder of timing defects within the brain. Salmelin et al. (2000) used MEG scans to investigate cortical timing sequences between individuals who stutter and fluent controls. In their studies, the control group exhibited an activation of the left frontal cortical region before the central speech region, a rather reasonable expectation, because people are believed to plan their speech before speaking. However, in the stuttering group, there was no discernable pattern, and in many cases, the central cortical areas involved in speech were initiated before the frontal cortical areas involved in planning.

In addition to functional imaging studies evaluating metabolic function, research has also been done on morphologic differences in the brains of individuals who stutter (Jancke, Hanggi, & Steinmetz, 2004). In a sophisticated study where 10 adults with persistent developmental stuttering were matched against 10 control adults with similar age, sex, education, and hand preference, gray and white matter differences were compared with high-resolution magnetic resonance imaging scans. Their results demonstrated statistically significant increases in white matter volumes within the right superior temporal gyrus, inferior temporal gyrus, precentral gyrus, and anterior middle frontal gyrus. Their studies also demonstrated a larger volume of white matter in the left auditory cortex compared with the right auditory cortex in

the *control* group, whereas those in the stuttering group had symmetrical white matter volumes bilaterally. The constellation of these findings is consistent with the suggestions of Sommer et al. (2002) that stuttering is related to an abnormal development of left hemispheric areas with compensatory contribution from the right hemisphere. One fascinating observation frequently made in stuttering research is that individuals who suffer from stuttering symptoms can be induced to have fluent speech through methods such as singing or reading in chorus (Ingham, 1984). These techniques, which are known as "induced fluency" tasks, have been used alongside imaging studies to better understand areas within the brain that are affected in individuals who stutter. In functional PET imaging studies, induced fluency states specifically normalized cerebral metabolism of the cortical speech centers, Wernicke's and Broca's areas, without having any effect on the metabolism of the striatum, a basal ganglia structure postulated to act as the timing and initiation center of motor movement (Wu et al., 1995).

To explain these findings, we turn to the work of Nudelman et al. (1992) who postulated the involvement of two "loops" for speech, an inner (medial) system and an outer (lateral) system (Fig. 17.1). The lateral system is preserved in stuttering and can be activated through singing and reading in chorus. However, the inner loop, which may be mediated by the striatum and under the influence of dopaminergic and GABAnergic neurons, remains impaired. A comprehensive explanation for our findings (Wu et al., 1995) may be that induced fluency tasks activate the lateral system, bypassing the abnormally underactive striatum (the medial system). Current theories suggest that the general phenomenon underlying timing and initiation defects observed in stuttering may be striatal hypofunction, and recent investigations also provides support for this concept (Neumann et al., 2003).

Dopamine is the principal naturally occurring neurotransmitter identified within the basal ganglia (Gerfen, 2000). Alm (2004) has suggested that dopamine is an inhibitor of striatal metabolism, indicating an inherent connection between striatal hypometabolism in stuttering

Proposed Neurologic Pathway of Stuttering

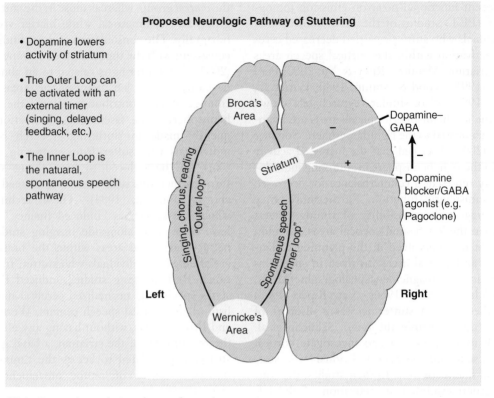

- Dopamine lowers activity of striatum

- The Outer Loop can be activated with an external timer (singing, delayed feedback, etc.)

- The Inner Loop is the natuaral, spontaneous speech pathway

Broca's Area

Striatum

Singing, chorus, reading "Outer loop"

Spontaneus speech "Inner loop"

Wernicke's Area

Left

Right

Dopamine–GABA

Dopamine blocker/GABA agonist (e.g. Pagoclone)

Figure 17.1. Proposed neurologic pathways of stuttering.

patients and a hyperdopaminergic state. Alm and others have also postulated that a peak increase in dopamine receptors during childhood development may be associated with stuttering onset, and the natural decrease in receptors over time may explain why some cases of stuttering remit and why others persist into adulthood. Over the course of the last few years, much evidence has surfaced linking abnormal elevations of cerebral dopamine activity to stuttering (Maguire et al., 2000b). Stimulant medications involved in increasing dopaminergic activity have been shown to exacerbate or even initiate stuttering symptoms (Maguire et al., 2000a). As will be described in greater detail, dopamine antagonists have also been shown to decrease symptoms of stuttering. Stuttering also shares many obvious similarities with Tourette's syndrome, a disorder of known dopamine abnormality. Both Tourette's syndrome and stuttering have their onset in childhood, follow a waxing and waning course, present with motor and vocal tics, affect males to females in a 4:1 ratio, and respond at least partially to treatment

with dopamine antagonists (Maguire, Riley, & Yu, 2002).

The striatal hypometabolism in stuttering seen from previously described PET imaging studies seems to be straightforwardly related to an excess of dopamine. Wu et al. (1997) further investigated the "dopamine hypothesis of stuttering" and found that there was higher presynaptic dopamine levels in stuttering patients compared to controls. 6-Fluoro-dihydroxyphenylalanine (6-FDOPA) is an indirect measure of presynaptic dopamine levels. Huang et al. (1991), using PET, showed that 6-FDOPA uptake was measured to be higher within the medial prefrontal cortex, deep orbital cortex, insular cortex, and auditory cortex. With elevated presynaptic dopamine levels being an indication of a hyperdopaminergic state, this study supports the hypothesis that dopaminergic tracts within the mesocortical and limbic systems may be elevated in individuals who stutter. Alm (2004) has shared these thoughts and vastly contributed to the theory that a hyperdopaminergic state within the basal ganglia may lead to stuttering.

EMPIRICAL BASIS FOR TREATMENT APPROACH

Many pharmacologic treatments have been tested for stuttering, but only a few have shown clinically significant efficacy in controlled trials. Furthermore, only a small handful of pharmacologic studies used placebo controls and objective measurements of stuttering severity. Even a smaller subset of these involved procedures that followed the patients over a sufficient period of time. However, the one historical component firmly established within these pharmacologic studies is that therapies aimed at lowering cerebral dopaminergic activity improved stuttering fluency (Brady, 1991). Quinn and Peachey (1973) and Goldman (1996) demonstrated that dopamine-blocking medications such as haloperidol and thioridazine improved fluency in stuttering patients. Unfortunately, these medicines presented with the risks of extrapyramidal symptoms, tardive dyskinesia, and sexual dysfunction, making long-term compliance difficult. Nevertheless, these studies demonstrated promising potential for the testing of newer line dopamine antagonists in clinical trials.

Numerous medications have been studied in stuttering that shed light on other neurotransmitter systems that may or may not be involved in this disorder. The neurotransmitter other than dopamine that is likely involved in stuttering is **gamma-aminobutyric acid (GABA)**. Benzodiazepines and barbiturates have not been shown to be effective for the treatment of stuttering, despite acting on GABA, but may lessen apprehension and nervousness through their anxiolytic and sedative qualities (Brady, 1991). Selective serotonin reuptake inhibitors have not demonstrated success thus far for the treatment of stuttering, but this type of medication may also benefit patients who suffer from anxiety or depression related to their stuttering (Costa, 1992). Calcium channel blockers have been reported to have mild antidopaminergic effects, but limited research with verapamil showed inadequate effectiveness in treating stuttering (Brady, Mcallister, & Price, 1990). Recent research with the partial agonist of GABA, **pagoclone**, has shown promising results in the largest pharmacologic trial of stuttering ever conducted (Indevus Pharmaceuticals, 2006).

RISPERIDONE

In a randomized, double-blind, placebo-controlled study (Maguire et al., 2000a), the efficacy of **risperidone** was assessed for the treatment of developmental stuttering in adults. Risperidone is a novel dopamine antagonist that is approved for the treatment of schizophrenia and bipolar disorder. Unlike first-generation dopamine antagonists such as haloperidol, it has a much lower risk of motor system side effects. Eligibility for the study involved having a developmental form of stuttering (not an acquired type by head trauma, stroke, infection, medication, etc.). Subjects were also excluded from the study if they had major medical problems, had been previously treated with antipsychotic or other psychoactive medications, or had a history of drug abuse. Sixteen patients (12 men and 4 women), between 20 and 74 years of age (mean age, 40.8 years), were enrolled onto the study, and they were all initially followed for 2 to 4 weeks for baseline assessment, during which their stuttering severity was rated twice. In a double-blind manner, patients were then randomly assigned to receive 6 weeks of treatment with either risperidone or an identically appearing placebo tablet. The patients in the experimental arm started with an initial dose of 0.5 mg once daily at night and had their dosage increased by 0.5 mg/day every 4 or more days, as tolerated, up to a maximum of 2.0 mg/day. All of the patients were closely followed during the course of the study.

During the 6-week treatment period, stuttering severity, adverse events, tolerability, and compliance with the medication regimen were rated every 2 weeks. Extrapyramidal symptoms and symptoms of tardive dyskinesia were also measured at baseline and every 2 weeks by means of the Simpson-Angus Scale (Simpson & Angus, 1970), the Barnes Akathisia Scale (Barnes, 1989), and the Abnormal Involuntary Movement Scale (Smith et al., 1979). Stuttering was assessed through standardized conversations with the same interviewer who asked each subject to describe a recent movie, vacation, or other non–emotionally charged event. Subjects also read from standardized passages containing 500 syllables. All of the sessions were audio- and video-recorded, and the following four variables were measured: percentage of syllables stuttered (%SS); duration of longest stuttering events;

time spent stuttering as a percentage of total time speaking (%TS); and overall stuttering severity as measured by the Stuttering Severity Instrument-3 (SSI-3) (Riley, 1994).

In a speaking and reading sample, the SSI-3 measures the duration of the three longest stuttering events, percentage of syllables stuttered of syllables spoken, severity of related tic motions, and a global score of these components using a Computerized Scale of Stuttering Severity (Bakker & Riley, 1997). When considering the assessment of a patient who stutters, the clinician should also inquire about the patient's fluency of speech in all sorts of different social environments. The severity of stuttering may change with variations in social settings, and appreciating and recognizing diverse speaking environments is crucial in the assessment of stuttering (de Kindkelder & Boelens, 1998). Furthermore, because stuttering presents with a waxing and waning presentation, a longitudinal assessment over a period of months is desirable for the most accurate evaluation of a patient's stuttering symptoms (Wu et al., 1995).

At the end of the double-blind phase, patients in the active medication group experienced mean reductions in all four categories of stuttering severity (Maguire et al., 2000a). The active medication reduced %SS by 50% versus 28% for placebo. The SSI-3 was reduced by 31% with risperidone and 15% with placebo. Furthermore, the decreases in the risperidone group were statistically significant for %SS, %TS, and SSI-3, with confidence level of $p < .01$ for all three. Six of the eight patients on risperidone also experienced a small decrease in stuttering duration, although these results were not statistically significant. However, the changes in stuttering severity were not statistically significant in the placebo group. Figure 17.2 depicts the changes in the two groups.

These results demonstrate a potential role for risperidone in the treatment of developmental stuttering. Risperidone was tolerated well overall, especially compared to previously investigated dopamine antagonists such as haloperidol and thioridazine. The patients in this trial did not exhibit extrapyramidal symptoms (motor stiffness), akathisia (motor restlessness), or tardive dyskinesia (abnormal muscle motions.) However, three subjects in the experimental group complained of sedation, which resolved with maintaining a lower

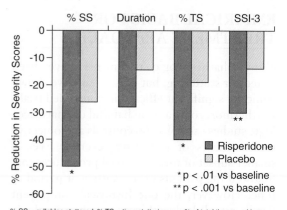

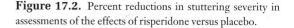

% SS = syllables stuttered; % TS = time stuttering as a % of total time speaking. SSI-3 = Stuttering Severeity Instrument, Third Edition (measured overall stuttering severity). Maquire GA, et al. *J Clin Psychopharmacol.* 2000;20(4):479-482.

Figure 17.2. Percent reductions in stuttering severity in assessments of the effects of risperidone versus placebo.

dose of risperidone. One female patient also reported galactorrhea (breast milk secretion) and amenorrhea (lack of menses) during the trial, which were likely related to this compound's potential side effect of raising the levels of the hormone prolactin. She was able to successfully complete the trial, and these unpleasant events resolved spontaneously 2 months after the risperidone was discontinued.

The risperidone data offer promising prospects for patients who suffer from stuttering. Further research is warranted for determining the effectiveness of risperidone in the treatment of stuttering. In particular, investigation on a larger scale and for a longer interval of time would be especially valuable for determining a better gauge of tolerability, value, and effectiveness.

OLANZAPINE

Given the promising direction set forth by the risperidone data and also the historical recognition of dopamine antagonists in the treatment of developmental stuttering, other atypical antipsychotic agents offer promise in the advancement of stuttering research and treatment. **Olanzapine** is a unique atypical antipsychotic agent because it demonstrates broader neurotransmitter effects, including dopamine blockade, serotonin blockade, acetylcholine release, and glutamate modulation. In addition, olanzapine has a lower potential for motor system side effects such as Parkinson's disease and tardive dyskinesia compared with older dopamine antagonists. Furthermore, it is thought to have minimal influence on prolactin levels, one of the unwelcome side effects observed in risperidone and other antipsychotics (Maguire, 2002).

In a 12-week, double-blind study, the efficacy and tolerability of olanzapine were compared with the efficacy and tolerability of placebo in the treatment of developmental stuttering (Maguire et al., 2004b). Subjects were excluded if they had a history of substance abuse, major medical or neurologic condition, or another Axis I psychiatric disorder as determined by the DSM-IV. Twenty-four adults between the ages of 18 and 56 years were randomly assigned to a treatment or placebo group. All of the subjects had onset of stuttering prior to 8 years of age, and their stuttering severities ranged from mild to severe as assessed by the SSI-3. Twenty men and three women with a mean age of 33 years completed the trial, and one subject in the placebo group was dropped from the study due to the onset of recurrent major depressive disorder, which was discovered during the trial to have been a pre-existing condition. All subjects began with a dosage of 2.5 mg/day of olanzapine or identical placebo for the first 4 weeks, and then dose was increased to 5.0 mg/day for the last 8 weeks.

Keeping in mind that stuttering severity varies over time in individuals, patients were rated twice, as in the risperidone trial, over a 4-week baseline period prior to randomization. The patients were rated from multiple perspectives, including an objective measure of stuttering severity (SSI-3), the Clinical Global Impression (CGI) (Smith et al., 1979), and the subject-rated Subjective Screening of Stuttering Severity, Locus of Control, and Avoidance (SSS) (Riley, Riley, & Maguire, 2004). In addition to a physical examination and review of systems, the patients were also monitored for potential side effects using the Simpson-Angus Scale, Barnes Akathisia scale, and the Abnormal Involuntary Movement Scale. Another variable that was measured was fasting blood glucose because novel dopamine antagonists have been reported to be associated with hyperglycemia (Haupt & Newcomer, 2001).

In this study, olanzapine was found to be statistically superior to placebo in all three rating systems (SSI-3, CGI, and SSS), with levels of significance of $p < .05$. Stuttering severity on the SSI-3 improved by 33% on olanzapine compared

with 14% with placebo. The patients in the olanzapine group also showed an average change on the CGI of 3.0, which represents moderate improvement, whereas patients in the placebo group demonstrated essentially no improvement. The SSS revealed an improvement of 22% on olanzapine and of <1% in the placebo group. Figure 17.3 shows the results for both groups. Fortunately, no patients experienced any dopamine-related neurologic side effect such as Parkinson's disease, akathisia (motor restlessness), or tardive dyskinesia. Olanzapine treatment was also not associated with prolactin-related side effects, unlike risperidone. However, mild sedation and weight gain were observed in this clinical trial. Patients on olanzapine gained an average of 3.5 kg (7.7 lb) versus 0.35 kg (0.77 lb) on placebo, but no elevations in fasting blood glucose were observed. All participants in the study elected to take olanzapine voluntarily at the end of the trial, indicating patient satisfaction with treatment of their stuttering.

In one case report, olanzapine was reported to worsen stuttering symptoms (Bär, Häger, & Sauer, 2004). However, the six patients in this study had multiple pre-existing psychiatric conditions, and the majority of patients were previously on typical antipsychotic therapy such as haloperidol for management of their psychotic symptoms. Long-term typical antipsychotic therapy leads to dopamine blockade and the potential for an increase or upregulation of receptors in the basal ganglia. Discontinuation of typical antipsychotic

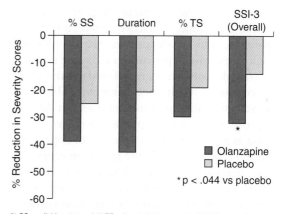

% SS = syllables stuttered; % TS = time stuttering as a % of total time speaking. SSI-3 = Stuttering Severity Instrument, Third Edition (measured overall stuttering severity). Maquire GA, et al. Annals of Clinical Psychiatry.

Figure 17.3. Percent reductions in stuttering severity in an assessment of the effects of olanzapine versus placebo.

therapy can result in a relative hyperdopaminergic state and potentially trigger or exacerbate stuttering. In this case series, such a mechanism is likely, especially given that stuttering ceased in the patients weeks after the initiation of olanzapine despite receiving increasing doses.

The olanzapine study demonstrating efficacy in stuttering provides a strong foundation for further pharmacologic investigation. Although the study was larger and longer than the risperidone studies, it was still limited with a small sample size of 23 patients and a duration of 3 months. It does, however, open the door for longer term, multicenter studies where the safety and efficacy of olanzapine can be better appreciated in the treatment of adult developmental stuttering. The weight gain and precautions of hyperglycemia are noteworthy reservations that must be appreciated. Patients during this study were warned of possible increases in appetite and weight gain, and it is imperative for clinicians to warn any patient on an atypical antipsychotic about these side effects.

OTHER NEUROTRANSMITTER SYSTEMS INCLUDING GABA

Olanzapine was highly efficacious in reducing stuttering symptoms over a relatively short period of time. Olanzapine likely exercises its effects through dopamine blockade, given that this is its primary mechanism. However, olanzapine influences other neurotransmitter systems. Many studies have attempted to expand on the theory that a hyperdopaminergic state is associated with stuttering. Stager et al. (1997), in a small study, compared pimozide, a selective dopamine antagonist, to paroxetine, a selective serotonin reuptake inhibitor. This study demonstrated a positive clinical response in patients on pimozide therapy, whereas the paroxetine group failed to exhibit any improvement in stuttering symptoms. This study suggests that altering serotonin does not directly improve stuttering symptoms. However, serotonin as a potential adjunct therapy to dopamine-blocking agents in stuttering treatment cannot be discounted based on this limited study. Recent studies have offered new insights into why individuals stutter concerning a connection between dopamine and GABA.

The connection between dopamine and GABA provides new explanations and insights into the physiology of stuttering. By selectively acting on the neurotransmitter GABA, one may be able to affect the dopamine system without inducing many of the side effects of direct dopamine antagonists. Theophylline, a pharmacologic agent used for the treatment of asthma and chronic obstructive pulmonary disease, has improved our understanding of the relationship between GABAergic and dopaminergic neuronal transmission. Theophylline has been postulated to lead to a type of acquired stuttering in a minority of patients, and its mechanism is thought to result from an inhibition of GABA receptors (Sugimoto et al., 2001). GABA is the primary inhibitory neurotransmitter in the central nervous system. GABA has many roles in physiologic inhibition, but one of the interesting neuronal pathways within the basal ganglia involves the inhibition of striatal dopaminergic neurons. Movsessian (2005) describes a mechanism of theophylline-induced stuttering via inhibition of GABAergic neurons leading to a reduction in the activity of the inhibitory dopaminergic nerve channels. Thus, inhibiting GABA neurons can lead to disinhibition within the basal ganglia, leading to a hyperdopaminergic state and potentially a state of stuttering.

Theoretically, if GABA blockade inhibition could lead to a form of acquired stuttering, one can postulate that a GABA agonist, or partial agonist, could be of therapeutic benefit for individuals who stutter. On the surface at least, GABAergic transmission can lead to an inhibition of dopaminergic transmission, resulting in decreased dopamine levels within those parts of the brain thought to be responsible in stuttering. Current clinical trials are underway exploring such hypotheses.

Indevus Pharmaceuticals (2006) recently announced encouraging phase II clinical data for pagoclone in the treatment of persistent developmental stuttering. Pagoclone is a novel GABA-A selective receptor modulator that does not act at sites occupied by benzodiazepines. The potential benefit of a nonbenzodiazepine GABA modulator is that it is free of some common benzodiazepine side effects such as sedation, withdrawal, and addiction. Examples of benzodiazepines include diazepam and alprazolam. Concerns with the benzodiazepines include tolerance, addiction, and sedation.

Although the exact mechanism of action is unknown, data from animal studies suggest that the in vivo characteristics of pagoclone are likely mediated by an active metabolite that acts as a partial or full agonist depending on the subunit composition of the GABA receptor (Atack et al., 2006). By selectively acting on a subunit of the GABA receptor, pagoclone should be void of many potential side effects of the older GABA agents such as the benzodiazepines.

The clinical trial of pagoclone (Maguire et al., submitted for publication), the largest pharmacologic study ever conducted in stuttering, consisted of 132 patients participating in an 8-week, double-blind, placebo-controlled, multicenter study. Eighty-eight patients received increasing doses of pagoclone, ranging from 0.3 to 0.6 mg/day, and 44 patients received placebo. Changes in stuttering severity were measured using SSI-3, Stuttering Severity Scale (SEV) (O'Brian et al., 2004), SSS, Clinician Global Impression-Improvement (CGI-I), the Liebowitz Social Anxiety Scale (LSAS) (Liebowitz, 1993), and the Speech Naturalness Scale (SNS) (Martin, Haroldson, & Triden, 1984).

Preliminary data from the study reveal that pagoclone produced a statistically significant difference ($p < .05$) compared with placebo in five measures (Indevus Pharmaceuticals, 2006). An added benefit observed in the study, as illustrated by the LSAS, is that pagoclone improved social anxiety in individuals who stuttered. Furthermore, unlike many forms of speech therapy where fluency is improved at the expense of disrupting the natural flow of speech (i.e., compromising speech quality via inducing excessive enunciation or monotone-like speech), pagoclone improved stuttering while improving the naturalness of speech as determined by the SNS.

Pagoclone was demonstrated to be safe and well tolerated, and no serious or harmful side effects occurred during the study. The most common side effects were headache (12.5% for pagoclone vs. 6.8% for placebo) and fatigue (8% for pagoclone vs. 0% for placebo). Given the promising results with pagoclone and the high patient satisfaction, nearly 90% of individuals in the study participated in the open-label phase of the clinical study. In this study segment, all patients received pagoclone. Preliminary data suggest that patients originally on placebo and switched to pagoclone have begun to show signs of improvement in their stuttering symptoms, and patients originally in the active treatment arm continue to demonstrate improvement. The company has announced plans to meet with the U.S. Food and Drug Administration (FDA) to pursue further clinical development of pagoclone for the treatment of stuttering. However, one should review the peer-reviewed publication that has been submitted at the time of this book's release before making broad conclusions about this study.

As indicated earlier, pagoclone has shown promise as a medicine that treats stuttering through modulation of GABA. GABA has also been shown to be affected directly by some antipsychotics in animal studies. Marx et al. (2003) demonstrated that olanzapine and clozapine, but not risperidone or haloperidol, caused elevations in cerebral cortical allopregnanolone levels. Allopregnanolone is a potent modulator of GABA-A receptors with anxiolytic and anticonvulsant properties. As an outcome of these studies, it is very likely that atypical antipsychotic therapy in the treatment of stuttering may have multiple mechanisms of action that include dopamine blockade within the striatum and modulation of GABA receptors. Figure 17.4 depicts where some of these actions may take place. An emerging link between dopamine and GABA is developing in stuttering research, and further investigations on how these two neurotransmitter systems are interrelated is warranted.

PRACTICAL REQUIREMENTS

A speech-language pathologist (SLP) who plans to provide treatment that addresses the medical aspects of stuttering needs to practice in association with a medical doctor (MD). Because the studied medications are active in the central nervous system, a psychiatrist or neurologist may be the best-trained professional to evaluate these treatments. The psychiatrist may have added expertise in performing cognitive behavioral therapy, which may be of benefit in stuttering treatment. Medications have side effects and interactions with other medications that require careful evaluation by a physician specialist.

Any professional who is engaged in treatment planning and delivery for this population needs to understand all of the assessment measures. We envision a collaborative network between SLPs and physicians as these treatments emerge. In this manner, the physicians and SLPs should be aware of literature in both disciplines.

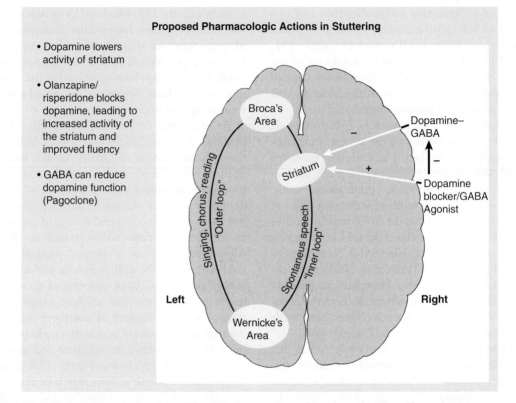

Proposed Pharmacologic Actions in Stuttering

- Dopamine lowers activity of striatum

- Olanzapine/ risperidone blocks dopamine, leading to increased activity of the striatum and improved fluency

- GABA can reduce dopamine function (Pagoclone)

Broca's Area

Dopamine– GABA

Striatum

Dopamine blocker/GABA Agonist

Singing, chorus, reading "Outer loop"

Spontaneus speech "Inner loop"

Left

Right

Wernicke's Area

Figure 17.4. Proposed neurologic activity of dopamine in stuttering and how it may be affected by medications.

KEY COMPONENTS

The description of treatment involves the compliance with pharmacologic therapy. The first stage is obtaining an adequate medical examination and history. One should be mindful of medical comorbidities (e.g., liver disease, diabetes) that may need to be addressed before beginning pharmacotherapy. The families/caregivers should be used to gauge the potential improvement or lack thereof with the pharmacotherapy. One should educate the patients and families that the medication will at best lead to a partial reduction in stuttering and that one should not discount the potential of other stuttering therapies.

ASSESSMENT METHODS TO SUPPORT ONGOING DECISION MAKING

We use standard measures of stuttering severity; self-reports of severity, locus of control, and avoidance; and ratings by the attending physician or clinician to assess a wide spectrum of

behaviors and attitudes. The measures are taken during a 4-week baseline period, during the medication/placebo treatment period (8 to 24 weeks), and during a 12-month follow-up period. The effects of medication vary between individuals, so we need a profile of the effects to determine the value of the medication and, if it is effective, the types of other treatments required for a comprehensive treatment plan.

Listener judgments of stuttering severity are made from a video-taped sample of at least 500 syllables of conversation or monologue and 200 syllables of reading using the SSI-3) (Riley, 1994). Scaled scores representing the *frequency* of syllables stuttered (%SS), average *duration* of the three longest stuttering events, *physical concomitant* ratings, and *total SSI-3* score are noted.

Severity instruments other than the SSI-3 may be selected. The use of %SS as the only measure of severity results in a loss of information because it only correlates loosely ($r = .74$) with the SSI-3 total score.

Self-reports by the persons who stutter are required during baseline, medication, and follow-up conditions to understand how they view the effects of the medication. We use the SSS (Riley, Riley, & Maguire, 2004). The Perceptions of Stuttering Index (PSI) (Woolf, 1967), the Locus of Control of Behavior (LCB) (Craig, Franklin, & Andrews, 1984), and the Overall Assessment of the Speaker's Experience of Stuttering (OASES) (Yaruss & Quesal, 2006) may also be useful.

The treating physician will likely not have the requisite background to use advanced speech assessments. We suggest using the CGI to provide a way to report any changes in stuttering during the treatment conditions. The CGI measures a global view of change associated with therapy.

Clinical significance refers to any change that improves the client's communication in a useful way. We propose that a change on any of the previously mentioned measures of 30% or more constitutes a clinically significant change.

TAILORING THE TREATMENT TO THE INDIVIDUAL CLIENT

The potential of weight gain and metabolic abnormalities (lipid and blood glucose increases) associated with certain dopamine antagonist medications should be addressed with each individual patient. One should follow the FDA package insert prescribing information for each agent used. Novel dopamine antagonists such as olanzapine have been implicated in cases of new-onset diabetes mellitus. Therefore, one should exercise caution in prescribing this medication and related compounds in individuals with risk factors for diabetes.

APPLICATION OF TREATMENT TO AN INDIVIDUAL WHO STUTTERS

We present two examples of stuttering reduction following medication. The speaking and reading samples made before and after medication are available on the DVD that accompanies this textbook.

The first case was a man who took olanzapine in the trial described earlier (Maguire et al., 2004a) for 12 weeks (Table 17.1). He had a substantial reduction in stuttering severity as demonstrated by a reduction in the SSI-3 score from 26 (moderate) before medication to 6 (subclinical) after treatment, a change of 80%. Frequency was reduced by 86%, and duration was reduced by 67%. The SSS Severity subtest showed a reduction of 24% in his self-reported evaluation. The Locus of Control and Avoidance subtests showed very little change, with reductions of 9% and 7%, respectively. Overall, this person reached dismissal criteria for stuttering severity but still needed systematic treatment to increase his internal locus of control and reduce avoidance techniques. See Table 17.1 for further details.

The second case was a man who took pagoclone at the dose level described earlier for 8 weeks. His SSI-3 score was reduced from 30 (moderate-severe) to 18 (mild). Frequency was reduced by 58%, and duration was reduced by 68% (Table 17.2). His self-reported changes indicated by his scores on the SSS showed substantial changes in Severity (74%), Locus of Control (67%), and Avoidance (75%). The only treatment given was the pharmacotherapy. Overall, his stuttering severity needed further treatment to reduce the 3% SS and the 1.8-second

Table 17.1. *Changes after Medication in a Person Who Stutters Who Responded Well to Olanzapine*

Measure	Percent Change	Before Medication	After Medication	Difference
SSI-3	80	26	6	20
Percent syllables stuttered	86	12.1	1.7	10.4
Mean duration of the longest stutters	67	2.1	0.7	1.4
SSS Severity	24	17	13	4
SSS Locus of Control	9	32	29	3
SSS Avoidance	7	29	27	2
SSS Total	12	78	69	9

SSI-3, Stuttering Severity Instrument-3; SSS, Subjective Screening of Stuttering.

Table 17.2.   *Changes after Medication in a Person Who Stutters Who Responded Well to Pagoclone*

Measure	Percent Change	Before Medication	After Medication	Difference
SSI-3	40	30	18	12
Percent syllables stuttered	58	6.5	3.0	3.5
Mean duration of the longest stutters	68	5.6	1.8	3.8
SSS Severity	74	23	6	17
SSS Locus of Control	67	54	18	36
SSS Avoidance	75	24	6	18
SSS Total	70	101	30	71

SSI-3, Stuttering Severity Instrument-3; SSS, Subjective Screening of Stuttering.

duration of his longest events. Also, internal locus of control needed further improvement.

Medication worked differently in these two cases. Olanzapine seemed to have possibly improved the motor speech programming, resulting in more fluent speech. Pagoclone had less of this motor effect but seemed to reduce the effort to remain fluent and the avoidance behaviors. These two people were among the best responders to the medications in the respective studies. Each would have likely benefited from additional stuttering therapy.

FUTURE DIRECTIONS

At this time, the most promising treatment for developmental stuttering should incorporate a multidisciplinary approach consisting of long-term follow-up with physicians, speech therapists, and family members. Given the overwhelming consequences that stuttering can have on development, all children who stutter should be evaluated by an SLP. In very young children between the ages of 2 and 8 years, the primary treatment should include speech therapy. Keeping in mind that more than half of the cases of developmental stuttering resolve during childhood or adolescence, stuttering severity should be closely monitored in these individuals. Pharmacologic research may be warranted for children who fail to respond to speech therapy. Although no pharmacologic agent has been approved for the treatment of stuttering in adults, let alone children, many studies support the use of psychiatric medications off-label for numerous conditions (Kim, 1996). Pharmacologic studies delineating the efficacy and tolerability in child and adolescent stuttering would

be of great benefit. Speech therapy and cognitive and behavioral therapies have individually demonstrated some efficacy for the treatment of stuttering in some adults and adolescents (Boberg & Kully, 1994). Researching the combined efficacy of medication with speech therapy is indicated given the results with either treatment in monotherapy. These techniques may very well work in a synergistic fashion.

When considering any type of therapy for the treatment of stuttering, the clinician should also take into account whether other secondary medications or substances exacerbate the clinical presentation. As described earlier, theophylline is one medicine that can induce stuttering in patients. Other medications that may exacerbate stuttering include methylphenidate, dextroamphetamine, bupropion, anti-Parkinsonian agents, and sertraline (Maguire et al., 2004b). Furthermore, any substances of abuse that elevate dopamine levels, including cocaine and methamphetamine, have a likely potential of initiating or exacerbating stuttering. Thus, it is imperative for the clinician to be aware of a wide variety of factors when assessing and deciding on a treatment strategy for stuttering.

In addition to anxiety and depression, social phobia has been associated with stuttering as a frequent comorbid condition (Stein, Baird, & Walker, 1996). According to the DSM-IV diagnostic criteria, social phobia is a strong, persistent fear of situations where embarrassment can take place (Sadock & Sadock, 2000). Stuttering is thought to elicit social phobia via causing a sense of impeding fear or anticipatory anxiety in circumstances when speech is obligatory. As a result, many individuals may withdraw away from social settings where verbal communication occurs and, unfortunately, often find themselves at a disadvantage in multiple facets of their lives. This social phobia is more likely to be related to self-perception of dysfluency and not necessarily related to the pathologic degree of stuttering (Stein, Baird, & Walker, 1996). An all-inclusive treatment plan including cognitive and behavioral therapy could address avoidance issues and may be valuable for the treatment of social phobia in individuals who stutter.

During recent times, new thoughts and novel methods of research have improved our understanding of stuttering and provided optimism and expectation for improved therapeutic opportunities. New information about the neurologic and genetic basis of stuttering and expanded treatment modalities is emerging at a breathtaking pace. Collaboration between physicians and SLPs is essential as these new treatment modalities emerge. Psychiatrists will likely be the physicians treating most stuttering, given the utility of cognitive behavioral psychotherapy and the knowledge of neurotransmitters that affect behavior and cognition. It is likely that, in the near future, studies will show that speech therapy and cognitive behavioral psychotherapy are enhanced through proper use of adjunctive pharmacotherapy.

Pharmacologic, neurophysiologic, and functional imaging studies have unearthed many of the mysteries suggesting why individuals stutter. These series of studies have suggested that increased dopamine activity with a resultant hypometabolic state within the striatum is a principal neurologic correlate of stuttering. Dopamine antagonist medications have been demonstrated to be efficacious in the treatment of stuttering. However, significant promise is held with pagoclone, a selective GABA modulator that has recently been shown in the largest pharmacologic trial of stuttering to date to be an effective, well-tolerated treatment for stuttering, and further research is warranted.

To obtain further information regarding pharmacotherapy in stuttering, more research is needed in large randomized controlled trials. Pagoclone holds significant promise as a potential agent for stuttering therapy as part of a comprehensive treatment program and may result in the first medication to be approved by the FDA for the treatment of stuttering. Future research should also continue to investigate why some patients respond well to medication and others do not. Testing genetic differences in response to medication (pharmacogenetics) and brain imaging studies hold promise as techniques in describing such heterogeneity.

CHAPTER SUMMARY

- Because stuttering is a speech disorder with significant neurologic underpinnings, medications that affect brain physiology are of increasing interest.
- Recent research has shown that medications that alter dopamine and/or GABA may have beneficial effects in reducing stuttering.
- Further research will be needed to assess the effects of combining speech therapy with pharmacotherapy.

CHAPTER REVIEW QUESTIONS

1. The prevalence of stuttering in the adult population is approximately:
   a. 0.3%
   b. 0.5%
   c. 1%
   d. 8%
   e. 15%
2. The timing and initiation center of speech in the brain that has been postulated to be involved in stuttering is:
   a. The occipital cortex
   b. The hippocampus
   c. The corpus callosum
   d. The striatum
   e. The medulla
3. Which of the following medications has been shown to improve stuttering?
   a. Pagoclone
   b. Risperidone
   c. Olanzapine
   d. All of the above
   e. None of the above
4. Which of the following neurotransmitters has been implicated in the pathophysiology of stuttering?
   a. Dopamine
   b. GABA
   c. Serotonin
   d. All of the above
   e. A and B only

5. Pagoclone has which of the following effects on speech?
   a. Worsens speech naturalness
   b. Improves speech naturalness
   c. No difference

6. Which of the following medications has been shown to improve the social anxiety associated with stuttering?
   a. Pimozide
   b. Risperidone
   c. Haloperidol
   d. Pagoclone
   e. Olanzapine

7. Which of the following medications may worsen stuttering symptoms?
   a. Bupropion
   b. Dextroamphetamine
   c. Sertraline
   d. Methylphenidate
   e. All of the above

8. Which of the following characteristics of stuttering is false?
   a. Typical age of onset is in childhood.
   b. It has a male-to-female ratio of 1:4.
   c. It has a weak genetic component.
   d. Right hemispheric speech areas are underactive.
   e. None of the above

9. Which of the following "loops" of speech functions abnormally in spontaneous speech in a person who stutters?
   a. The outer loop
   b. The inner loop

10. Which medication is FDA approved for the treatment of stuttering?
    a. Olanzapine
    b. Risperidone
    c. Pagoclone
    d. None of the above
    e. All of the above

SUGGESTED READINGS

Maguire, G. A., Riley, G. D., Franklin, D. L., Maguire, M., & Brojeni, P. (2004). Olanzapine in the treatment of developmental stuttering: A double-blind, placebo-controlled trial. *Annals of Clinical Psychiatry, 16,* 63–67.

Maguire, G. A., Riley, G. D., & Yu B. P. (2002). A neurological basis of stuttering? *The Lancet Neurology, 1,* 407.

Maguire, G. A., Yu, B. P., Franklin, D. L., & Riley, G. D. (2004). Alleviating stuttering with pharmacological interventions. *Expert Opinion Pharmacotherapy, 7,* 1565–1571.

Wu, J. C., Maguire, G., Riley, G., Lee, A., Keator, D., Tang, C., Fallon, J., & Najafi, A. (1997). Increased dopamine activity associated with stuttering. *Neuroreport, 8,* 767–770.

CHAPTER 18

The Roles of Evidence and Other Information in Stuttering Treatment

ANNE K. BOTHE, ROGER J. INGHAM, AND JANIS COSTELLO INGHAM

CHAPTER OUTLINE

KEY TERMS

"4S" hierarchy: sources of information for evidence-based practice, from Straus et al. (2005); in descending order of importance, the 4Ss are systems, synopses, summaries, and studies.

Clinician-based and client-based information: factors that, in addition to evidence, contribute to clinical decision making.

Evidence: in evidence-based medicine and evidence-based practice, as those terms are currently defined, evidence is equated with valid and important research findings.

Single-subject time-series experimental designs: a standard approach to clinical research in psychology, education, and other disciplines, including speech-language pathology, that uses rigorous scientific methods to identify functional relationships between experimental or clinical conditions and the behavior of individual clients or participants.

Systematic review: a comprehensive review of the literature conducted as a piece of research in itself, according to established methods intended to control the influence of possible biases in the selection, evaluation, and summary of literature.

INTRODUCTION

The view that one should base clinical practice on research results has not always been central in medicine, allied health, or education. Nevertheless, this view has a long history in these and related professions. Crilly (2001), for example, described clinical research conducted in the 18th century about bloodletting. Clinical psychology, similarly, was founded in the 19th century on the notion that "science and practice were considered inseparable" (Hayes, Barlow, & Nelson-Gray, 1999, p. 1). So-called "research-based" practice is also not new to speech-language pathology (McReynolds, 1990; Ventry & Schiavetti, 1980) or to stuttering (Costello, 1975).

What is new to stuttering, however, and to speech-language pathology and many other disciplines, is the prominence or even predominance of ideas related to research-based practice models. New journals, new accreditation and certification requirements, the structure of conferences, and even books such as the present volume all reflect a discipline and a profession that are focused on what might be termed *meta-practice* issues, or the larger issues that define not what we do but how we should determine what we should do. In this context, the present chapter is intended primarily to address one important theme from the current meta-practice literature about stuttering treatment: the definition and specification of the research-based "**evidence**" and the other relevant "**clinician-based and client-based information**," which can be used to support stuttering treatment. Our goal is that readers might be able to appreciate (1) the types or sources of evidence and information that exist; (2) the strengths and weaknesses of each; and (3) the activities that researchers, practitioners, and clients might undertake if the goal is to be able to combine all available research evidence plus clinician- and client-based information to create an evidence-based, client-centered, and outcomes-focused (Bothe, 2004b) approach to stuttering treatment.

RESEARCH-BASED EVIDENCE IN STUTTERING TREATMENT

Evidence-based medicine (EBM) has been defined in its very influential current form by several authors (Guyatt & Rennie, 2002; Sackett et al., 2000; Straus et al., 2005). More inclusively, adaptations of EBM for allied health and other applications may be referred to as evidence-based practice, or EBP (the more general term to be used throughout this chapter to refer to EBP, EBM, and the case where a distinction cannot easily be made). In this current form of EBP, "evidence" refers to research findings, and the goal of clinical practice is to find and implement the treatment that represents the best combination of information from three sources: (1) research (i.e., evidence), (2) physician or clinician expertise, and (3) patient or client preferences. In discussing the first source, research evidence, Straus et al. (2005) described a four-level hierarchy referred to as the "**4S hierarchy**": systems, synopses, summaries, and studies. They also suggested that clinicians should rely on the highest level of research evidence possible, as the following sections discuss for stuttering.

SYSTEMS AND PRACTICE GUIDELINES

At the top of the hierarchy, the first "S" is an "evidence-based clinical information system"

which, ideally, "would integrate and concisely summarize all relevant and important research evidence…and would automatically [electronically] link…a specific patient's circumstances to the relevant information" (Straus et al., 2005, p. 34). In other sections of the textbook by Straus et al., the related notion of a practice guideline is defined as a "systematically developed" (p. 165) statement that includes at least two parts: an up-to-date summary of the relevant evidence, followed by a detailed set of instructions for clinical practice based on that summary. Practice guidelines differ from the idealized evidence-based clinical information system in that the former are based on currently available evidence, whereas the latter are not developed, by definition, until sufficient good evidence is available. If all possible research about a particular topic had been completed, leaving no subtopics or subgroups of clients for which the available evidence was imperfect or incomplete, the conclusions reached by practice guidelines and by clinical information systems would overlap completely. Because such an ideal is almost impossible to achieve, and in recognition of the fact that clinical practice does not have the luxury of waiting for complete and ideal evidence, practice guidelines exist to translate the currently available evidence into the current best suggestion. Moreover, because the currently available evidence in any area is likely to be of mixed and variable quality, the initial summary section of a practice guideline is expected to include objective evaluation of all evidence, using a grading system such as the "levels of evidence" developed by a Canadian task force in the 1970s (see Straus et al., 2005) and now often described as the Oxford System (Phillips et al., 1998/2006).

There is no ideal clinical information system currently available for stuttering; there are also no practice guidelines that fit the description of Straus et al. A document entitled, "Guidelines for Practice in Stuttering Treatment," was composed by the Special Interest Division for Fluency and Fluency Disorders and published as an official statement of the American Speech-Language-Hearing Association (ASHA, 1995). This document was not designed in concert with EBP principles, however (see Ingham & Cordes, 1999), in part because of the time at which it was developed. Instead, it begins by asserting that "both common practice and published data should be considered" (ASHA, 1995, p. 26) in developing practice guidelines, and the document itself does not include the evaluation of treatment research and associated recommendations that EBP would suggest. Instead, it is formatted as an exhaustive list of all possible goals and approaches that have been used or that could be used for the assessment and treatment of stuttering. Because it provides no supportive reasoning for any of the information included or excluded and because it neither recommends nor rejects any of the many possible treatments it lists, it is less useful for practitioners seeking specific evidence-based guidance than practice guidelines based on current EBP recommendations might be.

SYNOPSES

Given that the highest level of systematic evidence-based clinical information is not available for stuttering, the clinician's next choice would be to look for synopses, Straus et al.'s second level in the 4S hierarchy. A synopsis is a brief summary meant to combine information from all available individual studies and from available systematic or other reviews (summaries) of those studies. Examples of synopses of the stuttering treatment literature include Conture's (1996) brief review of "the state of the art regarding treatment efficacy for stuttering" (p. S18) and the even briefer "Treatment Efficacy Summary" prepared by Conture and Yaruss (not dated) as part of a series provided by ASHA. Conture's (1996) synopsis included approximately three pages of text about stuttering treatment. It drew on previous summaries (Andrews, Guitar, & Howie, 1980), well-known textbooks (Bloodstein, 1995; Van Riper, 1973), and individual research studies to provide a few general recommendations about treatment with preschoolers, school-age children, teenagers, and adults. The summary by Conture and Yaruss (not dated) drew on reviews only to make a few general statements about treatment. Both pieces were apparently intended more to provide general information about stuttering treatment for a general audience than to provide specific treatment recommendations for clients or practitioners. Therefore, clinicians searching for evidence-based guidance regarding stuttering treatment must move on to the next level of Strauss et al.'s (2005) hierarchy of sources of evidence.

SUMMARIES

The state of knowledge in stuttering is such that there are multiple summaries, or reviews of the literature, available about the many individual studies that have been published (Andrews et al., 1980; Bloodstein, 1995; Cordes, 1998; Herder et al., 2006; Ingham, 1984; St. Louis & Westbrook, 1987; Thomas & Howell, 2001). Unfortunately for practitioners seeking specific advice, the conclusions reached in these reviews vary widely and are often in direct conflict with each other. It is therefore quite difficult to find a consensus among the reviews or to find recommendations for practice that appear to be supported by multiple sources.

One important point to recognize, however, is that some of the differences across reviews can be attributed to the methods used to conduct those reviews. Andrews et al. (1980) and Herder et al. (2006), for example, conducted meta-analyses of 29 and 19 studies, respectively, and among the most important features of both studies was the authors' use of an inclusion criterion that admitted only group-design research. Andrews et al. (1980) summarized results of studies that had at least three participants, and Herder et al. (2006) summarized only studies that had involved random assignment to treatment and no treatment or treatment and comparison treatment conditions. These decisions are justified on many methodologic grounds for the types of mathematical meta-analyses completed by these authors, but they also have important implications for the decisions reached. By requiring studies to have at least three participants, for example, Andrews et al. (1980) excluded studies by Martin, Kuhl, and Haroldson (1972) and Reed and Godden (1977), among others, that had used **single-subject time-series experimental designs** to study response-contingent approaches to stuttering treatment. Given that those papers had shown the effectiveness of response contingencies in reducing children's stuttering, excluding them substantially reduced the accuracy of Andrews et al.'s (1980) conclusion that "prolonged speech and gentle onset techniques appear the strongest treatments" (p. 297). Herder et al. (2006), in contrast, concluded that "no one treatment approach for stuttering demonstrates significantly greater effects over another treatment approach" (p. 61). Again, however, this conclusion was a function of the studies they included in their review.

These and similar problems caused by the methods used to summarize literature in any area have led to the development of relatively standard methods for conducting what are known as **systematic reviews** of the literature (see Chalmers, Hedges, & Cooper, 2002; Cooper & Hedges, 1994; Haynes et al., 2006; Littell, 2005). A systematic review of the literature evaluates both the methods and the results of a set of publications in a way that is recognized as research in itself (Chalmers, Hedges, & Cooper, 2002; Haynes et al., 2006; Littell, 2005). Methods for identifying and selecting papers for review are specified in the report of the review, for example, in a manner analogous to the specification of how human participants are defined and recruited for a study of human participants. Analyses of papers are completed using defensible and complete criteria, as well as such procedures as multiple raters or written data extraction instruments to reduce the influence of rater bias. All papers are also evaluated against all criteria, rather than each paper being subjectively described with no common standard (see Carlberg & Walberg, 1984; Cooper, 1982; Cooper & Hedges, 1994; Feldman, 1971; Jackson, 1980; Moncrieff, 1998). Current recommendations for systematic reviews in medicine and allied health, in particular, also include a growing awareness that clinical research conducted poorly tends to report better treatment results than clinical research conducted more stringently (Linde et al., 1999; Schulz et al., 1995). In general, therefore, it is widely accepted that systematic reviews need to be based on only the better designed and better executed studies, either by weighting the results from such studies more heavily or by excluding more poorly designed studies from the final review (de Craen, van Vliet, & Helmerhorst, 2005; Meade & Richardson, 1997).

The most recent and most comprehensive systematic review of the stuttering treatment literature, as of this writing, was recently published in two papers by two of the present authors and colleagues. The first paper focused on behavioral, cognitive, and related treatment approaches (Bothe et al., 2006b); the second paper focused on pharmacologic treatment approaches (Bothe et al., 2006a). Both papers were based on five

methodologic criteria, developed from multiple interdisciplinary (Chambless & Hollon, 1998; Cook et al., 1995; Guyatt & Rennie, 2002; Moher, Schulz, & Altman, 2001; Moscicki, 1993; Schiavetti & Metz, 2006) and stuttering-specific (Bloodstein, 1975; 1995; Conture & Guitar, 1993; Curlee, 1993; Ingham & Riley, 1998; Ingham & Cordes, 1997; Ingham & Costello, 1984; 1985) recommendations (Davidow, Bothe, & Bramlett, 2006). In general, the studies included in both of Bothe and colleagues' systematic reviews were required to meet any four of the following five criteria: (1) random assignment to groups or single-subject time-series experimental designs; (2) blind or independent observers; (3) pretreatment and posttreatment data; (4) beyond-clinic data; and (5) controls for the influence of speech rate, speech naturalness, and judge agreement if the study had measured stuttering frequency or severity.

Using those criteria, Bothe et al. (2006b) identified 39 studies of behavioral, cognitive, and related treatments for stuttering for in-depth analysis from among 162 total papers assessed. The results of that analysis are summarized in the following sections by age group.

Summary of the Literature for Preschool Children

First, for preschool children, the only studies that met at least four of the five methodologic criteria and reported maintained reductions in stuttering lasting 6 months or more were from response-contingent treatments, in which children were given immediate feedback concerning moments of stuttering and occasions of fluency (Harrison, Wilson, & Onslow, 1999; Lincoln & Onslow, 1997; Martin, Kuhl, & Haroldson, 1972; Onslow, Costa, & Rue, 1990; Reed & Godden, 1977; Ryan & Ryan, 1983; Wilson, Onslow, & Lincoln, 2004). The clinical use of response-contingent stimulation, especially for young children, evolved out of a classic series of studies conducted by Martin, Haroldson, Siegel, and colleagues at the University of Minnesota in the 1960s and 1970s (Martin, Kuhl, & Haroldson, 1972; for reviews, see Ingham, 1984; 1990). The immediate feedback provided to children about their speech production in these treatments either took the form of a specific comment (such as "that was good talking" as a child is finishing a nonstuttered utterance or "uh-oh, you got stuck" immediately upon an occasion of stuttering) or the form of some nonverbal consequence (such as a raised hand telling the child to stop talking when a stutter occurs).

The best developed and most extensively researched form of response-contingent treatment for children is Onslow and colleagues' Lidcombe Program (Onslow, Packman, & Harrison, 2003). This program is described in further detail elsewhere in this volume, and clinicians interested in applying response-contingent principles with young children who stutter might also want to read some of the original studies of using response contingencies to treat children's stuttering (Martin, Kuhl, & Haroldson, 1972; Reed & Godden, 1977; Ryan & Ryan, 1983) as well as some of the earlier reviews of these procedures for clinicians (Costello, 1983; Ingham, 1999). As these several publications suggest, there are many effective ways that response contingencies can be arranged for children's stuttering, from the classic puppet study by Martin, Kuhl, and Haroldson to many other adaptations.

Summary of the Literature for School-Age Children

For older children, Bothe et al.'s (2006b) systematic review identified several possible treatment approaches that had been supported in research that met the review's methodologic criteria. These included electromyographic feedback (EMG) (Craig & Cleary, 1982; Craig et al., 1996); gradual increase in length and complexity of utterance (GILCU) (Ryan & Ryan, 1983; 1995); prolonged or smooth speech (Craig et al., 1996; Onslow et al., 1996; Ryan & Ryan, 1983; 1995); regulated breathing, especially if a parent-administered homework schedule is also incorporated (de Kinkelder & Boelens, 1998; Ladouceur & Martineau, 1982); response contingencies (Ryan & Ryan, 1983); and a unique "programmed traditional" treatment package (Ryan & Ryan, 1983). Many of these approaches are reviewed in other chapters in the present volume.

Craig et al.'s (1996) and Hancock et al.'s (1998) reports of EMG and prolonged speech treatments are perhaps the most thorough or best designed of these papers. An attempt by other researchers (Block et al., 2004) to replicate

Craig et al.'s findings was not successful, however—something that raises an important point for stuttering treatment research and for stuttering treatment in general. Specifically, the difference between the results of Craig et al. (1996) and Block et al. (2004) suggest that variables related to the structural foundations of a treatment may be as important to a treatment's effectiveness as the core treatment technique. Bothe et al. (2006b) referred to these variables as the "infrastructure" of a treatment, or all the elements that support, surround, and potentially alter the effectiveness of a treatment. These elements might include scheduling details (intensive vs. weekly), the presence of self-evaluation components, the use of homework activities, or the use of explicit transfer programs, among others. In the case of the Block et al. results, and as they discussed, their replication of Craig et al.'s procedures did not incorporate Craig et al.'s response cost programs (a response-contingent component of the treatment). This omission may have been mainly responsible for the EMG program's reduced effectiveness, given that response cost and other response contingencies have been frequently demonstrated to influence stuttering frequency (Costello, 1983; Martin, Kuhl, & Haroldson, 1972; Reed & Godden, 1977; Ryan & Ryan, 1983). Similarly, the articles reviewed by Bothe et al. showed better results for prolonged speech treatments when those techniques were learned and used in a context that also provided contingencies for stutters, intensive or daily practice opportunities, work at home, and/or programmed structures that allow progression through treatment steps or phases only when specific performance-contingent criteria are met. Clinicians working with school-age children who stutter might therefore be well advised to focus on these programmatic or "infrastructural" variables, especially including providing children with as much self-managed and self-evaluated practice as possible in using fluent speech in multiple real-world speaking situations.

Summary of the Literature for Adolescents and Adults

For adolescents and adults who stutter, Bothe et al.'s (2006b) systematic review supported the use of prolonged speech–type procedures, which had also been identified in previous reviews of the literature as among the best options for improving stuttering speech (Andrews et al., 1980; St. Louis & Westbrook, 1987). Again, however, the support for these treatments suggested the importance of a comprehensive treatment framework that includes initial intensive work, practice in front of groups, specific beyond-clinic transfer or generalization tasks, self-evaluation of speech and/or self-management of program steps, feedback regarding speech naturalness, and an active, performance-contingent maintenance program that continues to address not only stuttering but also speech naturalness and self-evaluation skills. Self-management may be among the most critical of these elements, given the reports by James (1981) that self-delivered consequences following moments of stuttering can, by themselves, reduce stuttering (see also James's critique of later claims by Hewat et al., 2006: James, 2007). Self-management or self-evaluation is also among the key features of several other reports of successful treatments (Craig et al., 1996; Howie, Tanner, & Andrews, 1981; Ingham, 1982; Ingham et al., 2001; O'Brian et al., 2003; Onslow et al., 1996), a finding that is also consistent with Finn's (1997) investigations of self-managed recovery among adults who stutter. Again, therefore, the stuttering treatment research literature suggests not only specific treatment techniques (prolonged speech) but also, perhaps more importantly, several programmatic or infrastructure elements (e.g., self-evaluation) that can improve treatment effectiveness and the maintenance of treatment gains.

It is also important to note, especially for adults, that the Bothe et al. (2006b) review was organized to address both of the two categories of dependent variables that are often viewed as important to stuttering treatment outcomes. The first is speech-related variables, such as percent syllables stuttered and other measures of stuttering frequency. The second is nonspeech variables, including social, emotional, and cognitive (SEC) measures. Both types of variables are seen as important to greater or lesser degrees by various authors, researchers, clinicians, and clients, and both were addressed throughout the systematic review. Moreover, as part of their analyses, Bothe et al. also considered the links between treatment types and treatment outcomes, in terms of the two categories of variables. Treatments focused on speech (such as

response contingencies and prolonged speech) were found to be substantially more effective than treatments focused on SEC variables (such as counseling or other cognitive or emotional approaches to treatment) at improving speech variables (73% of 140 speech-focused treatments met an outcome criterion for stuttering frequency, whereas only 31% of 19 SEC-focused treatments met the same criterion). In addition, treatments focused on speech were almost as effective as treatments focused on SEC variables at improving SEC variables (88% of 34 speech-focused treatments and 92% of 14 SEC-focused treatments met an outcome criterion for SEC measures). Thus, the well-designed studies identified by Bothe et al. did not support the choice to use treatments focused solely on SEC variables, except perhaps in the case where clients request help with SEC variables only and specifically do not want to change their speech. Even more intriguing was that claims that treatments must address both types of problems directly were not supported for the same reason—the finding that speech-focused treatments such as prolonged speech can improve both speech and SEC variables.

Summary of the Pharmacologic Treatment Literature for Stuttering

In a separate article, but following the same systematic review methods, Bothe et al. (2006a) reviewed 31 articles that had investigated the effectiveness of a pharmacologic treatment for stuttering. Only 11 of those 31 articles met three of the five methodologic criteria described earlier (as slightly revised for pharmacologic research); none met more than three. On the basis of those 11 studies, plus four other relatively well-designed studies (which met three modified criteria), Bothe et al. (2006a) were unable to identify any uncompromised positive findings. Specifically, one study of haloperidol reported positive results (Wells & Malcolm, 1971), but this report was contradicted by four others reporting poor outcomes (Andrews & Dozsa, 1977; Prins, Mandelkorn, & Cerf, 1980; Rantala & Petre-Larmi, 1976; Swift, Swift, & Arellano, 1975). One study met the systematic review's outcome criterion for stuttering frequency (Maguire et al., 2000, for risperidone), and three met the outcome criterion for SEC variables (Gordon et al., 1995; Harvey et al., 1992; Stager et al., 1995). In all four of those reports, however, the results were complicated by placebo effects, lack of comparison groups, or both.

This lack of clearly demonstrated effectiveness for the pharmacologic agents tested to date for stuttering was further complicated by several safety concerns and interaction effects, as Bothe et al. (2006a) also discussed in further detail. As but one example, Maguire et al. (2004, p. 66) recently concluded from their study of olanzapine that it is a "useful, well-tolerated medication" for stuttering. However, Maguire et al.'s results met none of the very lenient outcomes criteria defined for the Bothe et al. systematic review, and their report also did not mention that olanzapine is marketed under the trade name Zyprexa. This detail is important because the manufacturer of Zyprexa, Eli Lilly, has noted that Zyprexa may result in "hyperglycemia, in some cases extreme and associated with ketoacidosis or hyperosmolar coma or death" (U.S. Food and Drug Administration, 2004). Such complications are unusual in speech-language pathology and, as such, represent a large set of important new issues for speech-language pathologists to consider.

In summary, as this discussion of the Bothe et al. (2006a; 2006b) systematic reviews of the stuttering treatment literature has shown, systematic reviews can provide clinicians with summaries of the information they need to be able to develop treatment plans in an evidence-based framework. Many questions remain, but, as Bothe et al. concluded, evidence is available in their systematic review papers and elsewhere that can help clinicians and clients identify evidence-based, client-centered, and outcome-focused approaches that have been shown to achieve speech-related and/or SEC-related goals in stuttering. Equally important, systematic reviews such as the Bothe et al. (2006a) review of pharmacologic approaches to stuttering treatment can help clinicians and clients eliminate from further consideration those options that do not appear to have documented promise of success in improving either speech-related or SEC-type variables.

STUDIES

Following systems, synopses, and summaries, Straus et al.'s (2005) final "S" refers to individual studies, which are also available as a source of evidence for practitioners in stuttering. Studies serve

a critical purpose as the basis for systems, synopses, and summaries, but Straus et al. suggest that reading individual research reports should actually be a last resort for practitioners. The reasoning behind such advice stems primarily from the large number of publications and the small amount of time available to clinicians; requiring every practitioner to spend time finding, reading, evaluating, and applying every article would obviously be among the most inefficient ways possible to organize a profession or a discipline (Bothe, in press).

Nevertheless, in stuttering, and for most practice settings in speech-language pathology (e.g., acute care hospitals or elementary schools), the number of new treatment research publications appearing in a given month or year is not large. Reading at least some of them is probably a worthwhile goal for most evidence-based practitioners. It is also important to note, for stuttering, that there are a few key studies that provide a disproportionately large amount of the treatment research base. Perhaps the need is not for clinicians to find time to read all articles, or even all new articles, but for graduate classes or continuing education courses to be structured on the general model of a "great books" course, presenting all of the relatively few well-designed articles that are especially important to the stuttering treatment research literature. The present authors suggest, as a starting point, the review papers and chapters listed as Suggested Readings at the end of this chapter, plus perhaps as few as 10 reports of original research (Boberg & Kully, 1994; Craig et al., 1996; Hancock et al., 1998; Ingham, 1982; Ingham et al., 2001; Lincoln & Onslow, 1997; Martin et al., 1972; Onslow, Andrews, & Lincoln, 1994; Ryan & Ryan, 1983; 1995).

CLINICIAN-BASED INFORMATION IN STUTTERING TREATMENT

Having addressed research-based sources of evidence for stuttering treatment, it is also important to acknowledge some terminological complexities. The primary problem is simply that most authors in current versions of EBP equate "evidence" and "research" (Straus et al., 2005). This practice was intentional for the areas of medicine within which EBP was developed, but it should not be overinterpreted to mean that no other information is seen as important. In fact, clients' preferences and clinicians' expertise, as well as the outcomes obtained during treatment with an individual client, are explicitly recognized within EBP as central, or as providing information that must be considered and that can be as important in an individual case as information from the research literature (see Haynes et al., 1996). EBP sources tend not to refer to this information as evidence, however, instead equating evidence with research and referring to information held by clinicians, or gathered from clients, using other terms. The terminological details are unfortunate, for several reasons, including that they leave the door open for inaccurate criticisms such as that EBP does not value clinicians' knowledge or clients' wishes (see Bothe, 2004a; Straus et al., 2005; Trinder, 2000). The important point is that EBP begins with research evidence and requires research evidence, but nevertheless also recognizes that both clinicians and clients usually have knowledge and skills that are relevant to treatment decisions. For the purposes of this discussion, therefore, such knowledge and skills might be referred to as clinician-based and client-based sources of information, to differentiate them from the research-based evidence discussed earlier.

Clinician-based information, then, resides in the knowledge and skills that individual clinicians have about their own settings, resources, schedules, populations, skills, and abilities (Haynes et al., 1996). Again, EBP recognizes and values such knowledge and skills, despite the complaints to the contrary raised by some critics (Trinder, 2000). Within EBP, the key to judicious use of clinicians' expertise simply lies in the sequence of events. First, the available research is reviewed and evaluated to identify an empirically supported possible treatment, and second, the clinician assesses that possibility in light of other information and makes a final decision with the client. Clinical expertise remains in the "clinical art of making small (not wholesale!) adjustments to the proven treatment so that the benefits are optimized for an individual client's circumstances" (Ingham, 2003, p. 201), or in "clinicians' on-going attempts to balance everything they know and everything that occurs during treatment to their clients' benefit" (Bothe, 2003, p. 250).

One of the points that must be acknowledged about clinicians' knowledge, however, is that

clinical experience and clinical decisions have their limitations. Groopman (2007) has recently discussed this issue for physicians (in a very readable book intended for general audiences), building on well-established heuristics and biases that are known to affect essentially all human decision making (Kahneman, Slovic, & Tversky, 1982; Tversky & Kahneman, 1974). Within stuttering in particular, Finn (2004) addressed the importance of confirmation biases, or human thinkers' tendency to acknowledge, accept, and incorporate into their future thinking any evidence that confirms their initial beliefs while not accepting, acknowledging, or in some cases even noticing evidence that would contradict an initial belief. Our tendency as clinicians, in this context, is to see evidence that supports the initial belief that the treatments we select work, something that becomes a problematic cognitive bias if it leads us to ignore, avoid, or explain away any evidence to the contrary. Human beings also tend to reason based on an "availability heuristic," or the tendency to place substantial cognitive weight on examples that come easily to mind. If examples of clinical success or treatment options come easily to mind because they were dramatic examples from the mass media, however, then the potential problem is that comparatively dull examples from a research article might be overlooked.

Confirmation biases and the other problematic heuristics that tend to control human reasoning and decision making are not insurmountable, but they are fascinatingly difficult to overcome (Kaheman & Tversky, 1996; Tversky & Kahneman, 1974). Therefore, EBP acknowledges the importance of clinicians' information, but it simultaneously attempts to mitigate the potentially negative effects of using only clinical experience as the basis for decision making by recognizing the primary and central importance of research-based evidence.

CLIENT-BASED INFORMATION IN STUTTERING TREATMENT

Finally, with respect to what might be termed "client-based" sources of information, one of the many strengths of EBP, as presented by Guyatt, Sackett, and colleagues, is that it takes patient preferences very seriously. One of the many difficulties in translating the notion of patient preferences to stuttering treatment, however, is that true "preferences" data, as that term is used by EBP authors to refer to economic utilities (Straus et al., 2005; Torrance, 1987; von Neumann & Morgenstern, 1947), are not available in stuttering. Utilities represent the strength of an individual's preference for particular outcomes or health states when faced with uncertainty, measured on a scale from 0.0 to 1.0 using specific standard procedures and with 0.0 defined as the value placed on death and 1.0 defined as the value placed on perfect health. Bramlett, Bothe, and Franic (2006), to which interested readers are referred for explanations, recently introduced these measures to speech-language pathology, but it will be some time before true preference data, in the sense that the word is used in some of the medical outcomes literature, are available for stuttering treatments.

In the meantime, of course, there are many ways to incorporate individual clients' goals, needs, and desires more generally into stuttering treatment, and the complete practice of EBP requires that clinicians do so. Decision making starts with the research evidence, as discussed earlier, but EBP differs from attempts to identify "empirically supported treatments" (Chambless & Hollon, 1998) in an abstract sense; EBP focuses on one clinician-client pair at a time. Application of these principles is as simple as the examples provided by Straus et al. (2005), in most basic clinical textbooks, in many discussions of shared decision making in healthcare (Gurmankin et al., 2002; Schulpher, Gafni, & Watt, 2002), and even in the current version of the American Speech-Language-Hearing Association's (2003) code of ethics: a clinician explains the available research about possible treatment options to a client, and the pair then uses that information to make a decision that they believe will address the client's goals within the confines of the clinician's expertise. Given the availability of research support for more than one possible treatment approach, for example, clients might have different views of the costs associated with each, the time typically required to complete the programs, or the kinds of tasks required during each program. In some situations, there will be research evidence that suggests a course of action. If such research is not available or does not isolate a single course of action, the evidence-based clinician relies on information of

another sort to assist the client in making a decision. Such information might include the clinician's knowledge about resources or equipment (clinician-based information) or, in this context, might include such client-based information as a preference for a summer intensive treatment format or a preference for treatments that would be helpful toward a personalized goal of public speaking.

An additional and equally important way of including client-based information into treatment was suggested some time ago by Baer (1988; 1990), in his notion that treatment should ultimately be directed toward relieving the client's "source of complaint." This idea was echoed by Ingham and Cordes (1997), who concluded their consideration of the role of self-measurement in stuttering treatment by noting that the "most critical components of stuttering treatment outcome evaluation…might be the self-judgments or self-measurements made by the speakers themselves" (p. 423). This shift toward using clients' self-judgments of performance in treatment and in evaluating whether a personalized goal of stuttering treatment has been achieved has now become an integral part of some programs for adults (Ingham et al., 2001). It is also consistent with many larger recommendations in the health outcomes literature more generally and indeed may serve as an important link between stuttering treatment and other health outcomes methods and models (Franic & Bothe, 2007). As that literature makes clear, through such notions as the need for clients' self-assessment of their own health-related quality of life (HRQL), client-based information is an essential and necessary constituent in EBP. The process and the goal of EBP, in other words, are not only evidence based but also, and equally importantly, client centered and outcomes focused.

COMBINING ALL AVAILABLE EVIDENCE AND INFORMATION: EVIDENCE-BASED, CLIENT-CENTERED, AND OUTCOMES-FOCUSED CLINICAL PRACTICE IN STUTTERING

Among the many interesting features of EBP, as it is currently being discussed in stuttering and in speech-language pathology more generally, is that it is based on principles borrowed from medicine (EBM) (Straus et al., 2005). As a result, the versions of EBP emerging in our discipline (Dollaghan, 2004) have brought with them an emphasis on group-design research and, especially, random assignment group trials (randomized controlled trials [RCTs]), which characterizes much of the thinking and research in medicine, pharmacology, and other realms. Treatment research approaches and principles from sources or traditions other than medicine might arguably be more applicable to the practice of speech-language pathology, including principles from psychology, education, and other areas. One advantageous outcome of the current meta-practice discussions about EBP in speech-language pathology, therefore, might be a renewed or more widespread adoption of clinical research ideas from multiple traditions.

The principles of single-subject time-series experimental designs, to take one obvious example, were developed in experimental and applied psychology and education (Barlow & Hersen, 1984; Kazdin, 1982). These designs are known by several names, including single-subject designs, within-subject designs, and time-series designs. The main principles of single-subject time-series experimental designs, by any name, include the repeated observation of one participant, or in some variations a few participants, in both baseline (nontreatment) and experimental (treatment) conditions. Conclusions about the influence of an experimental condition are drawn by assessing changes in the level and the trend of well-defined behaviors (the dependent variables) as carefully controlled independent variables (such as the presence or absence of a treatment) are introduced or withdrawn. These designs have been part of stuttering treatment research since the 1960s, and they constitute an integral part of the decades-long history of research and practice in our profession (McReynolds & Kearns, 1983; Ventry & Schiavetti, 1980) and in many others. They were also important to a previous, and now almost forgotten, "accountability movement" in our field (Caccamo, 1973; Mowrer, 1972; Siegel, 1976), which posited, on ethical grounds, both that clinicians should be accountable for the methods they use and that those methods need to be justified (or,

in today's terminology, evidence based; see Ingham, 2003).

For several reasons, however, principles from single-subject time-series experimental designs have not been fully incorporated into research or treatment activities in speech-language pathology, even though a larger interpretation of the goals and principles of EBP would seem to indicate that the inclusion of these ideas might serve as the best possible means for achieving success with clients. The first four steps of EBP, as described by Sackett, Guyatt, and colleagues (Straus et al., 2005), require an evidence-based and client-centered decision-making process based on the three sources of information described earlier: (1) treatment procedures identified as effective via research findings; (2) the clinician's expertise; and (3) the client's preferences. Once a reasonable possible treatment has been selected, then the next step is to administer the treatment. The final step in many presentations of EBP, however, including the one by Straus et al., focuses not on evaluating the treatment but on evaluating the practitioner and the previous steps of the process.

In combining the best of all these traditions, then, one could select a treatment using EBP ideas and then use the principles of the scientist-practitioner or single-subject time-series experimentation to determine whether that treatment is working for an individual client and, most importantly, to create a data-based context in which to monitor the treatment's effects and to make changes if the data indicate the treatment is not working. For current stuttering treatments in particular, because the highest levels of the evidence hierarchy (systems, synopses, and even multiple meta-analyses and systematic reviews) are not yet widely available, it becomes the responsibility of the clinician to carefully assess the effectiveness of the selected treatment with each client. This point, which has also been discussed recently for EBP in speech sound disorders (Kamhi, 2006; Tyler, 2006), was exemplified for stuttering by Costello (1975) and has been described by the authors in a number of previous papers (Costello & Ingham, 1984; Ingham & Cordes, 1999, p. 213):

1. Because stuttering may show dramatic levels of variability over time, repeated evaluation

of speech performance is necessary before, during, and for a clinically meaningful period of time after treatment has ceased.

2. Because measures of speech performance in clinic conditions may have neither relevance nor resemblance to measures of speech performance in nonclinic conditions, repeated evaluation of speech performance is necessary within and beyond clinic conditions.

3. In order to prevent claims of changes in stuttering being confounded by measurement error, changes in speech rate, or unusual speech quality, reliable and independent measures of stuttering, speech rate, and speech quality must be made during spontaneous speech (see also Bloodstein, 1995; Curlee, 1993).

These points were phrased with a focus on speech measurement and stuttering frequency, but the same principles hold for any speech-related or social, emotional, or cognitive treatment target, as discussed throughout the Bothe et al. (2006b) systematic review of the stuttering treatment literature. Regardless of the dependent variable selected, treatment outcomes measurement in stuttering must take account of variability across time, variability across conditions, and the potentially confounding effects of other changes.

In general, for any dependent variable, the point is that one of the most fundamental principles of single-subject time-series experimentation, repeated measurement, can help clinicians determine if there are performance trends that suggest the need to begin, continue, or change treatment. The finding of a group trend of untreated recovery in young children, to take one relevant example (Yairi & Ambrose, 1999), gives clinicians no information as to whether or when treatment should be introduced for a particular child. As Ingham and Riley (1998) demonstrated, however, repeated measures data about a particular child can show, often within weeks, whether treatment is necessary or whether the child is recovering. The only caveat is that obtaining data before and during treatment, as important as that is, does not take the place of the thoughtful initial selection of a research-based treatment approach.

CONCLUSIONS AND RECOMMENDATIONS

One of the most contentious meta-practice issues raised in current discussions of EBP for stuttering involves the relative worth of research findings, clinicians' expertise, clients' preferences, and obtained treatment outcomes for individual clients as the "evidence" upon which treatment should be based (Power, 2002; Yaruss & Quesal, 2002). Such questions are reasonable, and this chapter has attempted to address some of the many questions that deserve thoughtful answers. Among the most important points to recognize in all such discussions is that all four types of information must be included, by definition, in EBP, and critics of EBP who claim otherwise are often arguing with inaccurate straw men (Bothe, 2003; 2004a; Trinder, 2000). Nevertheless, it is an error to underemphasize the importance of research in EBP, even in a well-intentioned effort to acknowledge the importance of other types of information. The application of research evidence is shaped by clinicians and clients, but EBP starts with, and must remain based in, rigorous research evidence about a treatment's efficacy and effectiveness.

The review of evidence and information provided in this chapter suggests that combining principles from EBP and principles from single-subject time-series experimental designs can lead to both a reasonable starting point (a research-supported treatment, personalized for a clinician-client pair) and reasonable methods for determining whether a selected treatment is working (repeated measures of relevant dependent variables in relevant settings). Both the methods used for selecting a treatment and the methods used to document its effects are critical to the ultimate goal of successful evidence-based, client-centered, and outcomes-focused treatment of stuttering.

CHAPTER SUMMARY

- Attempts to base clinical practice on research are not new to speech-language pathology, but there is a new emphasis on meta-practice issues including the nature of the evidence base that supports clinical practice.

- One version of evidence-based medicine is based on the "4Ss" of evidence: systems, synopses, summaries, and studies.

- In stuttering, the available systems, practice guidelines, and synopses do not provide specific useful information for clinicians or clients attempting to select a treatment.
- In stuttering, there are several summaries of the research literature available, each resulting in different recommendations because of the different methods used.
- A recent systematic review in stuttering (Bothe et al., 2006b) identified research-based options for treatment in children and adults that result in success for speech-related as well as social, emotional, and cognitive variables.
- Clinician-based and client-based information serve important roles as ways to modify and personalize treatment or management options first identified through consideration of research-based evidence.
- Group-design research methods common in medicine have served as the basis for the development of evidence-based medicine, but principles adapted from single-subject time-series experimental designs may be equally appropriate for developing, testing, and applying treatments in speech-language pathology, especially for assessing the effectiveness of an evidence-based treatment selected for use with an individual client.

CHAPTER REVIEW QUESTIONS

1. Is the view that one should base practice on research new to speech-language pathology and stuttering?
2. The chapter refers to an emphasis on evidence as a current "meta-practice" issue for speech-language pathology. What other meta-practice issues are currently important in speech-language pathology?
3. What are the "4Ss"? Which of the four would you most like to be able to find, and why?
4. Are there useful practice guidelines available for stuttering, as practice guidelines are defined within evidence-based medicine?
5. Why are the methods used to complete a review of the literature relevant to the conclusions drawn from that review?
6. Which types of treatments were reported in Bothe et al.'s (2006b) recent systematic review to be the most effective for preschool children?

7. Provide an example of an "infrastructural" variable that seems to be relevant to stuttering treatment for school-aged children, adolescents, or adults, and explain how that variable might influence treatment results.
8. Did the Bothe et al. (2006b) systematic review of the stuttering treatment literature address speech-related variables; nonspeech variables, such as social, emotional, or cognitive issues; or both? Why is this a relevant feature of their paper?
9. Have recent summaries of the literature supported the use of pharmacologic treatments for stuttering?
10. Do the authors of this chapter believe that practitioners should read original research studies?
11. Are the knowledge, skills, and expertise of an individual clinician relevant to EBP?
12. How can clients' desires and values be incorporated into EBP, in the absence of true economic "preferences" data?
13. How can the principles of single-subject time-series experimental designs be incorporated into EBP?

SUGGESTED READINGS

Bothe, A. K., Davidow, J. H., Bramlett, R. E., Franic, D. M., & Ingham, R. J. (2006). Stuttering treatment literature 1970–2005: II. Systematic review of pharmacological approaches. *American Journal of Speech-Language Pathology, 15,* 342–352. [a current review of stuttering treatment research]

Bothe, A. K., Davidow, J. H., Bramlett, R. E., & Ingham, R. J. (2006). Stuttering treatment literature 1970–2005: I. Systematic review of behavioral, cognitive, and related approaches. *American Journal of Speech-Language Pathology, 15,* 321–341. [a current review of stuttering treatment research]

Costello, J. M. (1983). Current behavioral treatments for children. In D. Prins & R. J. Ingham (Eds.), *Treatment of Stuttering in Early Childhood: Methods and Issues* (pp. 69–112). San Diego, CA: College-Hill. [a still-timely introduction to the principles and methods of operant treatments for young children, ideal for readers unfamiliar with this area]

Ingham, R. J. (1984). *Stuttering and Behavior Therapy: Current Status and Experimental Foundations.* San Diego, CA: College-Hill. [see especially Chapter 9, Operant Methodology and Stuttering, pp. 195–272, and Chapter 10, Prolonged Speech, Its Variants, and Stuttering, pp. 273–390]

CHAPTER 19

Neuroimaging and Stuttering

KATRIN NEUMANN AND HARALD A. EULER

CHAPTER OUTLINE

INTRODUCTION

A malaise with no real cure begets many remedies. What is true for the common cold is also true for stuttering. Until the 19th century, all kinds of naïve cures for stuttering were suggested (Appelt, 1945). These typically included treatments for a "weak tongue" or apparatuses like tongue weights or mouth prostheses as crutches for a deficient articulation apparatus. Speech exercises were on the list of remedies, but also moderate amounts of wine and even tongue surgery were tried. Maneuvers and tricks to make the speech fluent survive until today, but the 20th century brought new general theories of human behavior that were invoked to explain the ontogenetic onset (distal cause) and the immediate (proximate) cause of stuttering. Psychoanalysis and behaviorism were taken as models for psychogenetic theories of stuttering, with childhood trauma, repressed needs, or deficient speech learning as attributed causes. These kinds of theories are of little interest here because they could not muster sufficient empirical evidence for the explanation of the ontogenetic origin of stuttering. The neurologic bases for trauma and learning have remained obscure, although 19th century psychiatry already taught that there is "no psychosis without neurosis," meaning that each behavior has a neurologic substrate. The models most relevant in our context are those derived from brain anatomy and physiology, and they see stuttering as dysfunctional speech motor control. The advent of

modern brain imaging techniques has added salience to these theories, with an auxiliary thrust provided by behavioral genetics that showed a solid heritability for stuttering.

In this chapter, we will present a brief history of the neurologic theories of stuttering together with the parallel history of brain imaging methods. Inventions of new technologies, even those at first distant from theories of behavior, tend to stimulate theories of behavior. The steam engine was the model for psychoanalysis ("libidinal pressure"), the telephone was the model for behaviorism ("connectionism"), and the computer is the model for modern cognitive theories ("mind as wetware"). Thus, the new technologies developed for neuroimaging may give rise to new theories related to the behaviors of stuttering.

After a short general discussion of brain imaging, we will describe the findings of neuroimaging stuttering research and their implications for theories of stuttering. The brain is a complex organ, no longer a mystery, but still poorly understood. At best, the relations between brain and mind are only partly unraveled. The reader should, therefore, not expect final answers or that all terrains will be well illuminated. The last part of the chapter, a discussion of implications for the treatment of stuttering, is the most speculative, but this topic is the one of most interest for those hoping for better therapies of stuttering, who long for a cure and not just a treatment or remedy.

An overview of the various techniques of brain imaging used in stuttering research can be found in Appendix 19.1.

HISTORY OF NEUROLOGIC RESEARCH AND THEORY OF STUTTERING

Neurologic theories of stuttering appeared early in the 19th century, after Italian physiologists, whose names—Galvani, Volta—we know from high school physics, had experimented with the electrical stimulation of frog nerves. In this zeitgeist, an old explanation of stuttering by Hippocrates—too many ideas in mind for immediate expression—showed up in neurologic terms: stuttering as "exaggerated hastiness" of cerebral impulses (Freund, 1966).

The origin of structural brain imaging started with postmortem autopsy. Since the famous findings of the 19th century French physician and anthropologist Paul Broca and the German neurologist Carl Wernicke, it has been known that the left side of the brain controls expressive and receptive language, at least in right-handed persons. Cerebral laterality, handedness, and speech soon became connected in prevailing theories. Which brain side leads and which one follows must be clear; undue interferences between the brain halves lead to problems with speech and "correct handedness"—that is, right-handedness. Stier (1911) had observed that left-handedness and ambidexterity (both-handedness) occurred remarkably often among persons who stutter, and he thus attributed stuttering to a lack of one-sided cerebral dominance. These and related observations led to one of the most influential theories of stuttering, the Orton-Travis theory of muscular coordination disturbance due to insufficient cerebral dominance (Orton, 1927; Orton & Travis, 1929; Travis, 1931). The theory became popular because it appeared straightforward and simple and many hypotheses and explanations could be derived from it.

In their theory, the neurologist Samuel Orton and the psychologist Lee Travis reasoned that the problem of lacking cerebral dominance in stuttering was not primarily one of central processing, but of peripheral control. The right and the left side of the speech apparatus received their nerve impulses from their respective brain

side, and the dominant side gave the lead timing rhythm so that the subordinate side got synchronized. Failed peripheral synchronization resulted in stuttering. Children who were prone to ambidexterity or were made ambidextrous by an enforced shift to right-handedness, either by explicit training or implicit instigation through tools like scissors, were especially at risk for stuttering. To no longer teach kids that only the right is right and the left is wrong was considered emancipatory and bolstered the popularity of the theory.

Empirical evidence for the Orton-Travis theory, however, did not fulfill the expectations: (1) for each study that showed more stutterers among left-handed and ambidextrous persons, another study found no difference in handedness between stuttering and nonstuttering groups; (2) handedness is no longer considered a reliable indicator for interhemispheric speech processing; (3) children whose handedness is deliberately changed do not begin to stutter; (4) persons who stutter do not have a history of enforced handedness shift more often than persons who do not stutter; and (5) strengthening strict unilaterality in persons who stutter does not reduce stuttering (Bloodstein, 1995; Fiedler & Standop, 1994). The Orton-Travis theory of cerebral dominance fell into disrepute and is now considered obsolete. The problem with the theory of stuttering due to asynchrony of nerve impulses to the bilateral articulatory musculature, however, is not primarily the issue of cerebral laterality; instead, its problem is its theoretical connection with handedness and peripheral motor control. The role of cerebral laterality remained important and has even been revitalized with the advent of new methods and findings, for example, the dichotic listening task (Curry & Gregory, 1969), the Wada test (Jones, 1966; 1967), split-brain research, and modern brain imaging techniques, as we will discuss later. The concept of cerebral laterality and dominance can be found in various forms of new theories, particularly in those gathered by Bloodstein (1995) under the label of Breakdown Hypotheses.

Interest in cerebral laterality and other brain function led to the first studies of the electrical brain activity by electroencephalography (EEG), which was first applied to humans in the 1920s. It comes as no surprise that Travis tested the cerebral dominance theory of stuttering with this new technique (Travis & Knott, 1936; 1937), with many studies to follow in the next decades. The yield of these studies, however, was not copious (Bloodstein, 1995). EEG is prone to movement artifacts and is a complex, rough, and locally unspecific indicator of brain activity. In addition, the EEG recordings were typically read by visual inspection rather than by an automatic algorithm. Sometimes abnormal EEGs were detected in persons who stutter, but replicability was often disappointing, whether recordings were made from silent or from speaking stutterers. Nevertheless, there have been two kinds of findings first reported with EEG research. First, whereas nonstuttering speakers tend to activate the left (dominant) hemisphere during speech and language tasks, stutterers more often activate the right hemisphere when they speak (Moore, 1986; Moore & Haynes, 1980). Such increased right hemisphere activation during linguistic tasks in stutterers had also been demonstrated in dichotic listening tasks (Cimorell-Strong, Gilbert, & Frick, 1983; Curry & Gregory, 1969) and in early regional cerebral blood flow studies (Pool et al., 1991). Second, after stuttering-reducing therapy, the brain activity (alpha waves) shifted to more left hemispheric regions during speech tasks (Boberg et al., 1983; Moore, 1984).

Whereas the EEG can be considered a kind of pooled output of innumerable, simultaneously ongoing singular brain processes, event-related potentials (ERPs) are temporal EEG responses to specific external or internal stimuli. ERPs have been used to demonstrate atypical language processing in persons who stutter (Cuadrado & Weber-Fox, 2003; Weber-Fox & Hampton, 2008).

In the context of brain activity associated with stuttering, two additional techniques may be mentioned; these are direct intervention into the brain by electrical stimulation or by drugs. Direct electrical stimulation of the cortex has little effect except for maybe a twitch or an isolated sensation, but stimulation of deeper brain areas may elicit more salient and complex responses, including a change in verbal disfluencies. Stimulation of the supplementary motor area (SMA) and the ventral lateral thalamic regions has been shown to produce stuttering-like behavior in nonstutterers (Ojemann &

Ward, 1971; Penfield & Welch, 1951), whereas thalamic stimulation has also been shown to reduce stuttering (Bhatnagar & Andy, 1989). These findings imply that a well-known pathway, the cortico-striato-pallido-thalamo-cortical loop, is involved in language production and that disfluent speech may reflect some kind of dysfunction of that loop.

A pill to cure stuttering would sell well. Therefore, it is no wonder that all kinds of pharmacologic agents have been tried. Tranquillizers were the first ones, but the effects were not convincing, and the side effects, especially of permanent use, were unacceptable. Anxiety-reducing drugs, beta-blockers, calcium channel blockers, and, most prominently, neuroleptics used to treat psychotic symptoms are all drugs that have been tried for stuttering (Bloodstein, 1995). Neuroleptics do seem to have some effects, at least for some persons who stutter, but the benefits do not outweigh the negative side effects. The U.S. Food and Drug Administration has not approved any drug for the treatment of stuttering.

However, there are some research benefits to the study of the effects of neuroleptics because they have antidopaminergic effects and thus point to the role of the dopaminergic system in the control of movement and to a possible common cause for both stuttering and Tourette syndrome (Comings et al., 1996), a disorder characterized by involuntary movements (tics) and vocal sounds. The disfluency-reducing effects of drugs that block dopamine receptors confirmed a link between stuttering and the subcortical basal ganglia. The basal ganglia had already been associated with stuttering by German theorists almost a century ago (Freund, 1966). That idea was revisited and elaborated upon by Alm (2004), who saw the core dysfunction in stuttering as an impaired ability of the basal ganglia to properly produce timing cues for the next motor segment in speech. In the basal ganglia, which are a set of interconnected nuclei, input converges from most of the cortex, especially the sensorimotor and frontal cortex, via the striatum as a way station, and output descends to the brainstem. The basal ganglia thus are part of extensive basal ganglia-thalamo-cortical circuits, which modulate the activity of the frontal cortex by inhibiting potentially competing motor programs with inhibition and disinhibition effects due to dopamine release. The implications of this model and of our own model for findings from brain imaging research are detailed in the section of this chapter on neuroimaging findings.

Due to neural plasticity, cerebral activation patterns may change with short-term and long-term motor experiences—whether these experiences are unrelated to stuttering in adults with fluent speech (Mikheev et al., 2002) or are speech motor experiences gained in fluency-shaping therapy in adults who stutter (Neumann et al., 2005). Motor control is central to stuttering but, nevertheless, only part of the complex picture. Somatosensory and auditory areas are involved, as is the cerebellum (De Nil, Kroll, & Houle, 2001). In addition, brain activation differences between persons who stutter and non-stuttering persons may remain even when the former do not stutter during a speech production task or when they perform nonspeech oral movements. More recent theories of the cerebral control of stuttering try to move beyond the straightforward lateral dominance theory in order to integrate the various brain imaging findings into a theory of stuttering as a sensorimotor disorder, as has been done, for example, in the work of Max and his coworkers (Max, 2004; Max et al., 2004).

Max et al. (2004) try to integrate feedback and feedforward models of motor control in general. A motor plan is constructed and executed by a feedforward controller, and the execution is adjusted by a feedback controller that integrates in real time both afferent (sensory) and efferent (motor) signals. Persons who stutter have to deal with aberrant motor control processes and an overreliance on afferent (especially auditory) feedback because they cannot acquire stable and correct mappings between speech motor commands and sensory consequences, which in turn results in inaccurate computation of the feedforward commands. Max et al. (2004, p. 113) state: "If incorrectly prepared motor commands are executed, their sensory consequences do not match the desired consequences. This could result in an increased need for feedback-based corrections, including interruptions or resets of the feedforward commands that give rise to sound/syllable repetitions and sound prolongations." To minimize

the mismatch between predicted (feedforward) and actual (feedback) consequences of motor commands, the control system of persons who stutter tends to prefer longer movement durations. Stutterers show a variety of average reaction time differences when compared with persons who do not stutter, such as slower initiation of phonation and articulation and longer durations of stop-gaps, vowels, and consonant-vowel transitions (Bloodstein, 1995). These longer durations are not simply the result of treatment because they have also been found in stutterers who have never received any explicit treatment. Max et al. (2004) emphasize that these considerations are not specific to speech movements because the differences between stuttering and nonstuttering individuals are not confined to sensorimotor processes in speech production or even to movements of the orofacial system, but pertain to durations of certain goal-directed movements (e.g., opening/closing of lips, flexion-extension of finger, finger tapping) across the motor system (Brown et al., 1990; Max, Caruso, & Gracco, 2003; Smits-Bandstra, De Nil, & Rochon, 2006; Smits-Bandstra, De Nil, & Saint-Cyr, 2006). This theory, then, accounts for the fluency-enhancing effects of diverse speaking conditions (e.g., slowed speech, delayed auditory feedback, chorus speaking, gentle voice onsets, disfluency reduction with repeated readings of the same text, etc.) and is compatible with most of the findings from brain imaging studies, which are described in detail later in this chapter after the description of neuroimaging methods. In addition, the theory tries to explain life history phenomena of stuttering, like age of onset (i.e., the age at which new complex fine and gross motor skills have to be acquired), treatment efficacy with young children, spontaneous recovery, and genetic factors.

NEUROIMAGING

Neuroimaging includes a set of techniques that enables the direct or indirect imaging of the structure and function of the brain. It is a relatively new discipline with a large and still growing importance in neuroscience, medicine, and psychology. Two main categories of neuroimaging can be distinguished: structural and functional imaging.

Structural imaging examines the morphologic structure of the brain. In clinical applications, it is mostly used for the diagnosis of intracranial pathologies, such as tumors, trauma, or vascular diseases. The techniques used most are computed tomography (CT; or computer-assisted tomography [CAT]) and magnetic resonance imaging (MRI). In research, structural imaging is used for morphometrics, for example, to determine the size and shape of brain structures. In this chapter, structural imaging is only referred to when brain structures implied in stuttering are involved.

Functional neuroimaging enables the visualization of the brain activity associated with planning or executing a specific task. Whereas structural imaging is extremely valuable for detecting morphologic changes in the living brain, brain activity involves electrical and chemical changes that can be visualized by functional imaging methods.

Noninvasive functional brain imaging techniques can be divided into (1) methods that directly measure the electrical activity associated with neuronal firing, that is magnetoencephalography (MEG) and—in a liberal definition of neuroimaging—EEG; and (2) methods that measure neuronal activity indirectly by analyzing brain metabolism, such as positron emission tomography (PET), single-photon emission computed tomography (SPECT), functional magnetic resonance imaging (fMRI), and near-infrared spectroscopy. The most frequently used functional imaging techniques are PET and fMRI. Both techniques measure neural activity indirectly by detecting the locally specific changes in the blood flow and composition induced by neural activity. Areas with increased regional cerebral blood flow or metabolism "light up" on the scan.

Prior to the neuroimaging era, the main source of data on mechanisms underlying language came from the lesion-deficit model. Damaged sites of the brain were associated with a compromised function. Compared with this approach, neuroimaging offers a great advantage. Measurements can be conducted noninvasively in subjects with normal psychological and physiologic responses. Moreover, because neuroimaging is not limited to a region that has been damaged but is able to explore "normal" or compensatory cognitive, sensory, and motor

processing functions, it can identify functional specialization in regions that are not or are only rarely damaged or that preserve functionality due to cognitive or neuronal reorganization (Price, 2000).

Functional brain imaging methods are mostly used to determine when and where neural activity in the brain is associated with the ability to perform a particular cognitive task, to measure the activation of the brain during emotional states, and to study the function of certain brain areas of neurologic or psychiatric patients (Huesing, Jaencke, & Tag, 2006). There are two experimental approaches to study the brain activation in the context of cognitive processes. The first approach, the subtraction design, is based on the assumption that the difference in brain activation between the active, task-related processing condition and a baseline condition reveals the specific activation for the processing task. Both conditions should differ in as few factors as possible, optimally in only one. Second, parametric designs use correlation analyses performed on individual or group data in which clinical factors (e.g., reaction time or percent syllables stuttered in stuttering research) are correlated with activities in distributed brain regions.

NEUROIMAGING FINDINGS IN STUTTERING

Neuroimaging experiments in stuttering research started in the 1990s. Several groups are especially active in neuroimaging in stuttering research at the following locations: San Antonio (e.g., Fox, Roger and Janis Ingham), Bethesda (e.g., Ludlow, Braun, Loucks, Chang), Toronto (e.g., De Nil, Kroll, Houle), Düsseldorf/Helsinki (e.g., Salmelin, Schnitzler, Biermann-Ruben), Salt Lake City (e.g., Blomgren, Nagarajan), Hamburg/Göttingen (e.g., Sommer, Büchel), London (e.g., Watkins, Howell, Au-Yeung), and Frankfurt (e.g., Neumann, Giraud, Euler, Kell, Preibisch). Note that we will sometimes refer to work by the Frankfurt group as "our work" because of our participation in that group.

We will now give an overview of neuroimaging findings, first on structural findings and then on functional findings. Finally, we subsume both structural and functional findings under an integrated view. Brain regions that are relevant for speech-language processing and stuttering in particular are depicted in Figure 19.1.

NEUROMORPHOLOGIC FINDINGS

Recent neuromorphologic examinations provided evidence for some structural differences between the brains of stuttering and nonstuttering persons. The first findings came from Anne Foundas and her group (Foundas et al., 2001) at Tulane University. With high-resolution volumetric MRI, they detected that individuals who stutter have some abnormalities in speech-language areas. In particular, they found that stutterers have a larger planum temporale. The planum temporale is the retral upper superficial part of the superior temporal gyrus, which belongs to the temporal auditory cortex. It is a strongly lateralized and thus asymmetric structure of the brain that is involved in language functions, in particular language perception. Additionally, Foundas and her group described a reduction of the normal right-to-left hemispheric asymmetry of the planum temporale in stutterers compared with nonstutterers. Moreover, abnormal patterns of gyri (cortical folding) have been identified in frontal speech and language regions above the Sylvian fissure (depression between frontal and temporal brain). These abnormalities consisted of anatomic variants of the diagonal sulcus of the inferior frontal gyrus and additional gyri along the superior bank of the Sylvian fissure (Foundas et al., 2001). Other researchers have also reported similar right-hemispheric abnormalities (Cykowski et al., 2007). Because the development of gyri is a complex process, abnormalities in it can be indicative of a developmental disorder. In 2003, using volumetric MRI in adults with developmental stuttering, Foundas and her group showed that these subjects had atypical prefrontal and occipital lobe asymmetries, whereas nonstuttering control subjects had the expected larger right than left prefrontal and larger left than right occipital lobe volumes. Hemisphere and brain volumes did not differ between the stutterers and the controls (Foundas et al., 2003). Later the authors described the perisylvian region to be anatomically more heterogeneous in people who stutter than in control subjects (Foundas et al., 2004). Support for this statement came from voxel-based morphometry (VBM; see Appendix 19.1) findings in stutter-

ing and recovered children, who had—compared with nonstuttering children—reduced gray matter volume in the left inferior frontal gyrus and bilateral temporal regions (Chang et al., 2008). Moreover, in a diffusion tensor imaging (DTI; see Appendix 19.1) analysis, the children who had persistent stuttering showed the same reduced fractional anisotropy in the left white matter tracts underlying the motor regions for face and larynx as Sommer et al. (2002) had shown for adults who stuttered. Additionally, the children with persistent stuttering had a greater gray matter volume than the recovered group in the left and right superior temporal gyrus.

Using VBM, Jäncke, Hanggi, and Steinmetz (2004) detected in stuttering adults, compared with nonstuttering subjects, right-hemispheric enlarged volumes of white masses in the superior temporal gyrus, including the planum temporale; in the frontalis inferior gyrus; in the precentral gyrus adjacent to regions that represent the face and mouth; and in the frontal anterior medial gyrus. Additionally, the authors described a reduced asymmetry in stutterers compared with nonstutterers between left- and right-hemispheric auditory areas. The authors concluded that stutterers have anomalies not only in perisylvian speech and language areas, but also in prefrontal and sensorimotor areas. However, these reported results must be interpreted cautiously because of the current view that VBM is not the most appropriate method to investigate white matter. Also, Beal et al. (2007) demonstrated significant differences between stutterers and nonstutterers in localized gray matter and white matter densities of left and right hemisphere regions involved in auditory processing and speech production.

Recently, the London group (Watkins et al., 2008) detected with DTI a number of fiber tract differences between stuttering and nonstuttering persons in language and motor areas and in their homologues in the right hemisphere. The differences were seen in the following areas, among others: bilaterally in the precentral gyrus, the ventral premotor cortex, the inferior frontal gyrus, the supramarginal gyrus, the cerebellum, and the right corticospinal tract and the medial lemniscus.

Because no increases of right-hemispheric speech-language regions and no reduced right-left asymmetries of the brain have been detected

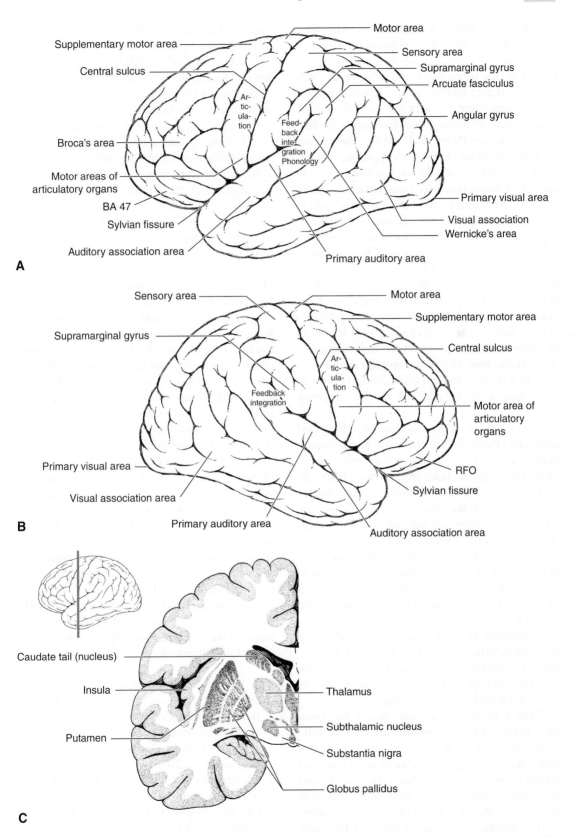

Figure 19.1. Brain regions involved in speech and language processing. **(A)** Brain from the left side. **(B)** Brain from the right side. **(C)** Basal ganglia and insula in a coronal section.

in stuttering children or in children who have recovered from stuttering, enlargements of right-hemispheric structures in adults could be caused by lifelong stuttering. Gray and white matter volume differences emerge in the left hemisphere speech areas compared with the right during the development of hemispheric dominance for language (Dorsaint-Pierre et al., 2006). Also at later ages, plastic brain changes are possible. Alterations in behavior and brain function result in changes in brain anatomy. Thus, enlargements of right hemisphere regions in stuttering individuals relative to the left could be analogous to increases in gray matter seen after motor training and after lifelong practice by musicians. These enlargements suggest the possible role of neuroplasticity in transforming neural structures in individuals because they could indicate the transition from beginning, potentially transient stuttering to persistent stuttering (Chang et al., 2008). It should be mentioned that postmortem and volumetric MRI studies have also found atypical anatomy of frontal, temporal, and parietal cortical regions in individuals with dyslexia and specific language impairment.

The question as to whether the described anatomic alterations are the cause or the consequence of stuttering is not completely solved. However, some cautious implications from the findings can be made. Changes in gray matter density, cortical thickness, gyral folding, or white matter integrity, compared with control populations, can be either pathologic or adaptive in nature (May & Gaser, 2006). A negative deviation of these parameters from the norm could indicate a primary lesion, whereas an addition of functioning brain substance might reflect an adaptation.

Reductions of brain tissue in the following left-hemispheric regions could count for a primary pathology in these areas and establish probably the most important and consistent structural correlates of stuttering.

First, a reduction of gray matter has been detected in the left frontal inferior gyrus in stutterers and in subjects who had recovered from stuttering in adulthood. According to our own recent results, these reductions correlated positively with severity of stuttering. Also, stuttering and recovered children had reduced gray matter in this region, as well as in bilateral temporal regions (Chang et al., 2008). Song et al. (2007) found reduced gray matter volume of the bilateral cerebella and medulla in adult stutterers, but this finding has not yet been replicated.

Second, with DTI, a disturbed integrity of white matter has been detected below the left-hemispheric sensorimotor representations of face, larynx, and articulation organs in the Rolandic operculum in stuttering adults (Sommer et al., 2002) and in stuttering children 9 to 12 years of age (Chang et al., 2008). These fibers belong predominantly to the arcuate fasciculus and connect temporal regions with frontal speech-motor-planning (including Broca's area) and motor regions. Additionally, Chang et al. (2008) identified abnormal white fibers in stuttering children in the corticospinal/corticobulbar tract bilaterally (which is involved in speech motor control) and in a posterior-lateral region underlying the supramarginal gyrus (rostral portion of the inferior parietal lobe that is connected to the classic frontotemporal language areas). Watkins et al. (2008) reported similar DTI findings in a study with young stuttering individuals. They found a disturbed integrity of the white matter underlying functional underactive areas in ventral premotor cortex. The authors mentioned that the white matter tracts in this area, because of connections with posterior-superior temporal and inferior parietal cortex, provide a substrate for the integration of articulatory planning and sensory feedback. White matter tracts that may be deficient in stutterers are also involved in speech production because of connections with primary motor cortex, a substrate for the execution of articulatory movements.

Increases in functioning brain substance that might indicate a more variable adaptation, dependent on stuttering severity, have been found in the following studies.

1. A VBM-detected increase in gray matter in those who stutterer, compared with nonstuttering individuals, in bilateral basal ganglia regions indicates a structural adaptation to a basal ganglia dysfunction in stuttering (Giraud et al., 2008).
2. An increased gray matter volume has also been detected with VBM in temporal, parietal, and frontal brain regions of stutterers (Song et al., 2007).

Table 19.1. *Summary of the Structural Findings in the Brains of Individuals Who Stutter*

Persistent Stuttering

Disturbed white matter integrity underlying the:

- sensorimotor representation of articulation organs like larynx, pharynx, and tongue in the left Rolandic operculum (adults and children)
- corticospinal/corticobulbar tract and supramarginal gyrus (children)
- ventral premotor cortex (young people)

Reduced or atypical right-left asymmetry in speech-language regions (adults)
Enlarged planum temporale, right more than left (adults)
Cortical folding variants (adults)
Other anatomic anomalies in perisylvian and other language areas (children, adolescents, adults)
Increased gray matter in the basal ganglia (adults)

Recovery from Stuttering

Reduced gray matter in the left inferior gyrus (adults and children) and in bilateral temporal regions (children)

3. Increases in white matter in stutterers, compared with nonstuttering individuals, have been found with VBM below left-hemispheric frontal regions, in interparietal regions, and in right-hemispheric temporal and frontal speech planning, speech motor, and auditory regions (Jäncke, Hanggi, & Steinmetz, 2004).

In sum, we agree with other authors who suggest that persistent stuttering is related to two anomalies in the left hemisphere: (1) deficits in the development of white matter tracts underlying the oral-facial motor regions; and (2) reduced gray matter growth in the inferior frontal region, including Broca's area. Both regions belong to the anterior portion of the perisylvian language center and are functionally related during speech production. Anomalies in the substrate for the integration of articulatory planning and sensory feedback and for the execution of articulatory movements seem to establish a primary lesion associated with stuttering. Compensatory, variable regions show increases in gray or white matter such as frontal, parietal, and temporal regions.

NEUROFUNCTIONAL FINDINGS

EEG studies have revealed much about stuttering (Boberg et al., 1983; Moore, 1984) but have not been able to provide precise localization of cerebral activations (De Nil & Kroll, 2001a). The appearance of neuroimaging techniques in the 1990s has greatly extended our knowledge of neurophysiologic processes underlying stuttering. Although most of these studies have used PET, increasingly, fMRI has proven useful.

In the beginning, fMRI was rarely used for the investigation of overt speech because motion artifacts impair its sensitivity to task-related activation (Preibisch et al., 2003b). Such artifacts are caused by magnetic field variations caused by movements of the head and pharyngeal space during speech. Recently, the temporal delay of the hemodynamic response has been exploited to suppress speech-related artifacts by temporally segregating speech-related motion from task-induced activation. The Frankfurt group developed an event-related design that allowed using fMRI for the investigation of brain function during overt production of full sentences in stuttering participants (Preibisch et al., 2003b). Prolonged stimulus durations and repetition times of 3 seconds allowed both an effective suppression of speech-related artifacts and the investigation of natural-sounding sentences in a familiar speaking situation. Another method for minimizing motion artifacts and the interference of scanner noise with stimulus presentation or subject performance is sparse sampling fMRI, where a silent gap is inserted between two successive image acquisitions (Amaro et al., 2002).

Previous neuroimaging studies have shown distributed neurofunctional correlates of stuttering in frontal and prefrontal speech motor planning and executive areas and in additional language, auditory, limbic, and subcortical regions (Braun et al., 1997; De Nil, 1999a; 1999b; De Nil & Bosshardt, 2001; De Nil, Kroll, & Houle, 2001; De Nil et al., 2000; 2008; De Nil & Kroll, 1995; 2001a; 2001b; Fox et al., 1996; 2000; Ingham, 2001; Ingham et al., 2000; Kroll et al., 1997; Pool et al., 1991; Salmelin et al., 1998; 2000; Watkins et al., 2008; Wu et al., 1995). Disfluent speech was mainly associated with widespread overactivation—especially predominant in the right hemisphere—of the motor system in both the cerebral and cerebellar hemispheres; a lack of normal activation in left-hemispheric language and auditory areas, in particular in anterior, superior temporal phonologic circuits; and a deactivation of a circuit between the left frontal and temporal cortex (Braun et al., 1997; De Nil & Bosshardt, 2001; De Nil, Kroll, & Houle, 2001; Fox et al., 1996; 2000; Kroll et al., 1997; Pool et al., 1991; Wu et al., 1995). Overactivations in the SMA, anterior insula, and anterior cingulate cortex (ACC) and deactivations in temporal regions have occasionally been reported (Braun et al., 1997; De Nil, Kroll, & Houle, 2001; Fox et al., 1996; Ingham et al., 2000; Salmelin et al., 1998). Induced fluency largely diminished the cerebral activation differences between stuttering and nonstuttering persons, although right-sided overactivations in motor cortices persisted (Braun et al., 1997; Fox et al., 1996). During the passive listening condition, stutterers were also reported to have greater activation than nonstuttering subjects in the left temporal regions, the right insula, the primary motor cortex, and the SMA (De Nil et al., 2008).

Not all functional neuroimaging studies were of the same high scientific quality. To search for generalizable findings, a meta-analysis of functional neuroimaging studies on stuttering was performed for those studies that compared cerebral activations of stuttered speech production in stutterers with fluent speech production in nonstuttering control subjects (Brown et al., 2005). This analysis revealed the following results. Similar brain areas are involved in stuttered speech as in fluent speech of the control subjects, predominantly the primary motor cortex, the premotor cortex, and the SMA, but with some differences: (1) some motor areas are overactivated in stuttering, including the primary motor cortex, SMA, cingulate motor area, and cerebellar vermis; (2) the frontal operculum (orbitofrontal cortex, Brodmann's area 47/12), Rolandic operculum, and anterior insula show an anomalous right laterality; and (3) auditory activations, due to hearing one's own speech, are mostly undetectable.

MEG experiments demonstrated a disturbed cortical sequencing of speech production in stutterers. In nonstuttering participants, the left inferior frontal cortex, which is responsible for articulatory planning, activates before the left motor cortex, which drives the articulatory motor execution. In contrast, this sequence has been shown to be reversed in stutterers (Salmelin et al., 2000). The most probable explanation for this phenomenon is a deficiency in the left hemisphere of the fiber connection that links these two regions (Sommer et al., 2002; Chang et al., 2008). Accordingly, right hemisphere overactivations could reflect compensation (Büchel & Sommer, 2004; Neumann et al., 2003; 2005; Preibisch et al., 2003a). Fluency induction might normalize the synchronization among language regions (Braun et al., 1997; Fox et al., 1996; Giraud et al., 2008; Neumann et al., 2003; 2005).

To investigate the hypothesis that right-hemispheric overactivation in stutterers reflects compensatory mechanisms, our group performed two fMRI studies with male adult stuttering and nonstuttering subjects (Preibisch et al., 2003a). One task was designed to tap speech motor processes by overt reading of short sentences. Overactivation in stutterers (compared to nonstutterers), which was consistent across all subjects, was detected in the right frontal operculum (RFO; Brodmann's are 47/12), reflecting an effect specific to stuttering (Fig. 19.2).

Because responses in the RFO were negatively correlated with the severity of stuttering, we hypothesized that the overactivation in the RFO reflects a compensation process rather than a primary dysfunction. Because the RFO is almost the right homologue of Broca's area, it seems plausible that it compensates for a deficient signal transmission between Broca's area and left-sided articulatory motor representations, as suggested by the previously described structural findings. Alternatively, the RFO may compensate for the dysfunctional left frontal speech-language regions by automatically taking over the disturbed functions. The phenomenon of shift of a compensatory function into a homologue region in the opposite hemisphere is a well-known phenomenon in cortical reorganization in cases of a brain lesion (Grafman, 2000). Specifically, this interpretation is supported by observations that the RFO is involved in a variety of corrective, self-monitoring, repair, and compensatory language functions in nonstuttering subjects—for instance,

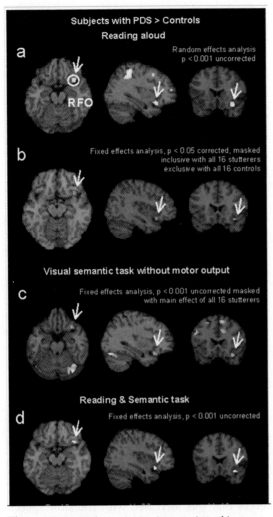

Figure 19.2. Higher activation in stuttering subjects compared with nonstuttering subjects. **(A)** Reading sentences versus viewing meaningless signs. Random effects analysis, $p < .001$, uncorrected. **(B)** Reading sentences versus viewing meaningless signs. Fixed effects analysis, $p < .05$, corrected, masked with the conjunction of all 16 stuttering subjects (each contrast $p < .05$, uncorrected). **(C)** Semantic decision task: synonym decision versus color decision. Fixed effects analysis, $p < .001$, uncorrected, masked with main effect of 16 stuttering subjects. **(D)** The right frontal operculum (RFO) is the only common activation in the reading and semantic decision task. (Modified from Preibisch et al., 2003a.)

in recovery from aphasia after frontal injury (Heiss et al., 1999; Rosen et al., 2000), compensation for dysfunction of the left frontal cortex in dyslexia (Pugh et al., 2001), evidence of response inhibition during dual task performance (Bunge et al., 2001; Herath et al., 2001), and by evidence for a "repair mode" for anomalies of speech and language that operates when normally functioning subjects have to notice and repair grammatical errors in auditorily presented sentences (Meyer, Friederici, & von Cramon, 2000).

In another task used in our studies, silent semantic judgments of synonym words were contrasted with color decisions to investigate cognitive and linguistic speech processing steps, while excluding speech motor execution. The RFO was the only region that was overactivated in stutterers across both tasks. This activation was not a correlate of stuttering because stutterers spoke fluently during reading in the scanner or did not speak at all during the semantic task. A compensation mechanism during early processing steps of speech production was therefore assumed to act independently of speech motor output demands. Initiation of articulatory routines may take place even when there is no need for speech and possibly already before critical early stages of speech production (e.g., at the level of phonology). This view would be consistent with the inversion of speech production steps in stuttering such that articulatory routines are initiated prior to activation of phonologic output codes (Salmelin et al., 2000).

FUNCTIONAL NEUROIMAGING FINDINGS BEFORE AND AFTER STUTTERING THERAPY

General Findings

After having described cerebral activation changes in untreated stutterers, we will describe evidence related to changes in brain activation patterns due to successful stuttering therapy. EEG studies had already revealed a shift of overall brain activity to more left-hemispheric regions (Boberg et al., 1983; Moore et al., 1984). With functional neuroimaging methods, specific cerebral activation changes due to fluency-shaping therapy have been investigated (De Nil, 1999a; 1999b; De Nil et al., 2003; De Nil & Kroll, 1995; 2001a; 2001b; Kroll et al., 1997; Neumann et al., 2003; 2005). If stuttering is caused by a disturbed neuronal synchronization during speech processing, the replacement of the automatized speech pattern of stuttering with a new one due to the therapy could be expected to cause a shift in cerebral activation patterns affecting the timing of the steps leading to speech production, thus reflecting compensation. If, alternatively, the fluency-shaping effect occurs solely due to decreased demands on the speech motor system secondary to rhythmization and prolongation of speech, reduced neuronal activity could be expected after fluency treatment.

The PET studies of the Toronto group showed initially higher activation in the ACC during silent reading in stuttering subjects compared with nonstuttering subjects, a difference that was reduced after therapy. During overt reading, those studies also showed a posttreatment increase in activation and more left-sided motor activation. These findings were interpreted by the authors as signs for an increased level of automaticity during speech production, reduced anticipatory needs to scan words for potential stuttering, increased emphasis of online self-monitoring, and optimized sequencing and timing of articulatory, phonatory, and respiratory movements gained through fluency-shaping therapy (De Nil & Kroll, 2001a; 2001b; Kroll et al., 1997).

To investigate the changes of cerebral activation patterns attributable to therapy-induced fluency, we compared the fMRI activation of stutterers before and immediately after a 3-week intensive fluency-shaping therapy course and additionally compared these activation patterns with those of nonstuttering subjects. In addition, five of the stutterers underwent fMRI after 2 years of continued practicing of the new speech pattern (Neumann et al., 2003; 2005). During overt reading, more distributed neuronal overactivations were detected in stuttering versus nonstuttering subjects. These overactivations were located mainly in precentral sensorimotor and frontal motor regions, whereas before therapy, the overactivations were mainly restricted to the right hemisphere. After therapy, the overactivations were even more widespread and more left-sided. The pretreatment overactivation of the RFO was markedly reduced after treatment. Another change after treatment was that stutterers showed more activation in the left precentral, middle frontal, ACC, insula, and putamen regions and bilaterally in the temporal cortex (Fig. 19.3).

Frontal cortex regions are implicated in speech motor planning and execution processes, and temporal areas are involved in auditory processes. The ACC is a nonspecific higher order region that shows activations, varying with task difficulty and load, in a variety of processes such as motor control, articulatory, attentional, and emotional processes (MacLean, 1993; Paus, 2001). Thus, whereas the Toronto authors interpreted a posttreatment reduction of a pretreatment increased ACC activation during silent reading as a sign for enhanced automaticity during speech production (De Nil & Kroll, 2001a), we regard posttreatment ACC effects to be rather a nonspecific therapy effect. Both the basal ganglia and the cerebellum are implicated in timing and coordination processes of sensorimotor actions during stuttering (Alm, 2004; De Nil, Kroll, & Houle, 2001; Giraud et al., 2008). The putamen overactivation in stutterers that was increased with the slow speech rate immediately after therapy together with a cerebellar activation after therapy may reflect

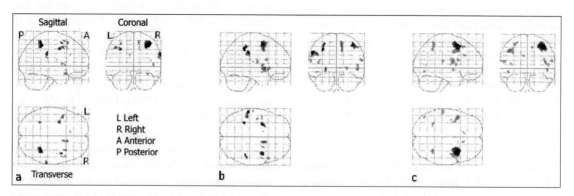

Figure 19.3. Regions where stutterers, during functional magnetic resonance imaging (fMRI), activate more than nonstuttering subjects while reading aloud **(A)** without any therapy (predominantly right-hemispheric activation), **(B)** immediately after a successful fluency-shaping therapy (more widespread activation than before with a shift of activity to the left hemisphere), and **(c)** 2 years after therapy (persistently more activation than before therapy, with a partial shift back to more activations in the right hemisphere). (From Neumann et al., 2003.)

the interplay between these regions in speech timing and motor control processes, as indicated also by other fMRI studies (Wildgruber, Acker-mann, & Grodd, 2001). Consequently, the rate at which a stutterer speaks after therapy could determine the region of motor control. Bilateral temporal activations seen after, but not before, therapy concur with reports that fluency-induc-ing maneuvers increase temporal activation (Fox et al., 1996) and confirm that temporal regions are part of a cortical and subcortical fluency-generating system (Jäncke et al., 1998; Pool et al., 1991). The left insula, in particular the anterior insula, has also been reported in other studies (Ingham et al., 2000) to be part of the dysfunctional left-hemispheric perisylvian net-work of stutterers. This region integrates audi-tory feedback into speech motor programs. It is activated in overt, but not in covert, speech (Ackermann & Riecker, 2004; Christoffels, Formisano, & Schiller, 2007).

In the semantic task, increased activation after, rather than before, therapy in the left inferior frontal cortex was detected (Neumann et al., 2003). This, together with the overactiva-tion in the RFO during semantic decision mak-ing (Preibisch et al., 2003a), indicates that successful compensation for stuttering may also recruit processing steps upstream from speech motor execution.

Consistent decreased activations in stutterers were observed in our and other studies during overt reading in left precentral regions (articula-tory processing) and during semantic decision making in left inferior frontal regions, that is, regions involved in auditory semantic and pho-nologic processing, supramodal visual process-ing, and motor programming of articulators (Heilmann, Voeller, & Alexander, 1996; Jäncke et al., 1998; Neumann et al., 2003). These observations agree with findings about deactiva-tions in stutterers in speech, language, and audi-tory regions (Fox et al., 1996; 2000; Ingham et al., 2000; De Nil & Bosshardt, 2001). The deac-tivations are likely to be the functional corre-lates of underlying deficient fiber connections between left frontal motor planning, motor exe-cution, and temporal regions (Sommer et al., 2002; Chang et al., 2008). This hypothesis is confirmed by the fact that the deactivations were unaffected by therapy, even after 2 years of

follow-up and despite controlled, continued prac-tice of the new speech pattern. The deactivations even remained unchanged when the stutterers spoke more slowly using their new speech pattern immediately after therapy. Hence, they are likely to reflect constitutional abnormalities.

An indirect comparison of the activation dif-ferences between the oral speech and the lin-guistic tasks in stutterers suggests that higher activations were restricted to overt speech and were not evident in the covert semantic task. Deactivations, however, were task specific but insensitive to therapy. The pre- to posttreat-ment differences between the patterns of over-activation were much more marked in overt reading than in semantic decision, but a shift to-ward more left-sided activations was common to both tasks. We conclude that compensation recruits more speech motor processes but may also engage cognitive-linguistic functions and that enhanced compensation after a successful therapy engages both systems to a larger extent than before therapy. This view is supported by studies of the Toronto group that revealed no differences between stutterers and nonstutterers in a silent verb-generation task compared with significant differences during speech produc-tion. This was interpreted as an indication of a deficiency in motor planning and speech execu-tion, rather than a deficiency at the cognitive-linguistic level (De Nil & Kroll, 2001a; 2001b; Kroll et al., 1997). In addition, the Bethesda and San Antonio groups emphasized repeatedly that abnormal cerebral activations and deactivations during stuttering are mainly associated with un-usual speech motor activity. Furthermore, they concluded that because these abnormal activa-tions and deactivations also involve premotor regions like the SMA and the right lateral Brod-mann's area 6, the preplanning phase of speech motor production is also implicated in stuttering (Braun et al., 1997; Ingham et al., 2000). The latter is a central assumption of the integrated motor control theory of stuttering of Max et al. (2004), which was outlined at the beginning of this chapter and which assigns a decisive role to feedforward and to feedback control mecha-nisms. This assumption is supported by the brain imaging findings concerning imagined stuttering. For instance, in PET scans during overt and imagined oral reading tasks, stutterers showed the same differences in activations and deactivations as fluent control subjects, regardless of whether they stuttered overtly or only imagined they were stuttering (Ingham et al., 2000). The activations were seen in regions implicated in motor control or in sensorimotor integration (i.e., anterior insula, prefrontal cortex, SMA, and cerebellum).

Poor timing skills during sequential finger-tapping tasks (Max, Caruso, & Gracco, 2003; Webster, 1993) and unusual saccades during silent reading tasks (Bakker et al., 1991; Brutten & Janssen, 1979) confirm the hypothesis of Max et al. (2004) that stuttering involves motor functions beyond simply the speech motor system. For example, the auditory system, which shows anomalies during stuttering, interacts with the motor system. Furthermore, the link between stuttering and cortical and subcortical systems that was found in neuroimaging studies shows that not only motor areas are involved (Giraud et al., 2008; Watkins et al., 2008). To sum up, cerebral motor and motor planning networks, together with their sensory, cerebellar, and subcortical integrates, are involved to a larger extent in stuttering than linguistic systems, and successful therapy may engage not only the motor system more than before, but also the linguistic system. This view is not uncontested, as we show later, but is shared by more and more researchers.

We assume that the overactivations seen in functional neuroimaging reflect compensation mechanisms in response to a permanent deficit in stutterers. The existence of the functional deficit could be indicated by the deactivations, and its permanence could be indicated by the continuation of deactivations despite therapy. The stable deactivations contrast with comparatively variable, task-specific overactivations after therapy. The dysfunction remains stable while compensation mechanisms may change and might depend on speech pattern and tempo, severity, and idiosyncrasies of stuttering. On the other hand, the complete absence of stuttering symptoms during fluency-shaping maneuvers like chorus reading, auditory masking, and whispering may support the view that stutterers are not inherently deficient in speech motor control regions (De Nil & Kroll, 2001a). The higher activation levels after therapy may indicate a higher degree of control and compensation, with still insufficient automatization of speech production. Furthermore, an expected therapy-induced increase in activity, which should include more left-hemispheric regions, was indeed observed and included not only speech, language, and auditory areas but also regions usually implicated in complex articulatory and motor timing demands (i.e., ACC, basal ganglia, cerebellum).

Our data (Neumann et al., 2003; 2005) suggest that overactivations indicate a particular compensation network including a variety of regions that are active already in untreated stutterers (Preibisch et al., 2003a). The compensation network appears to be recruited to a higher degree and with more success after fluency shaping (Neumann et al., 2003; 2005). This view is supported by the following findings: subjects who stuttered only moderately before treatment showed more distributed overactivations than those who stuttered severely; and subjects who stuttered moderately activated the very same regions that were activated in all stutterers after therapy.

Right-sided or bilateral overactivations of speech motor areas during overt speech, deactivations in the left frontal cortex regions, higher pretreatment versus posttreatment activation in the right hemisphere, and more distributed and increasingly left-sided overactivation in frontal regions after therapy agree with neuroimaging findings of other authors (Biermann-Ruben, Salmelin, & Schnitzler, 2005; Blomgren et al., 2003; De Nil & Kroll, 2001a; 2001b; De Nil et al., 2008; Watkins et al., 2008), which confirms the generality of these findings.

Reduced brain activity in stutterers was reported when task familiarity increased (Ingham 2001). Indeed, we observed that 2 years after therapy, when the new speech pattern either had become more automatized or was used less and thus became less available for use, the activation was slightly reduced compared with immediately after therapy (Fig. 19.3). However, a relatively high activation level persisted even after 2 years of practice, indicating a higher attentional and motor control demand for the new speech pattern that possibly can never become completely automatized.

In the overt speech task and in the covert semantic task, increased posttreatment activity was detected adjacent to the regions of persistent deactivation (Neumann et al., 2005). Most interestingly, areas with increased activation after therapy were seen in the direct vicinity of the areas where decreased white matter anisotropy was detected by other groups (Sommer et al., 2002; Chang et al., 2008) and by us (Fig. 19.4). Thus, an increased compensation very close to a dysfunctional region (e.g., a takeover of the functions by neighboring regions) can be assumed, instead of a repair of the dysfunctional region.

Implications of the General Therapy-Related Functional Neuroimaging Findings

It is a long-standing question in clinical neuroscience whether plasticity after a cortical lesion relies on neighboring areas or on regions distant from the lesion (Nudo, 2003). Stuttering could hence be a case of neuronal reorganization, with spontaneous compensation of a structural deficit (left-sided white and gray matter abnormality) by remote contralateral networks. However, because the examined stutterers had disfluency symptoms before therapy, the large-scale spontaneous compensation in untreated stutterers obviously only imperfectly takes over the impaired function. The therapy seems to shift the compensation for left-hemispheric deactivations from right homologue areas into left-hemispheric regions that are physiologically recruited for speech production in nonstuttering

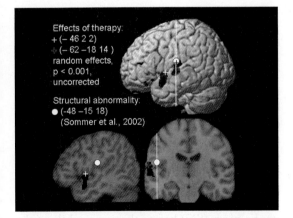

Figure 19.4. Left-hemispheric increase of activation after therapy (dark blotches). Some of the increases are located in the direct vicinity of the recently detected structural abnormality (white point). White lines indicate the respective positions of the depicted coronal and sagittal slice. (From Neumann et al., 2005.)

subjects. Thus, a more efficient compensation permitting accuracy of timing processes in speech production may require the restoration of a left-sided network. As is the case in poststroke recovery, where "normal-like" brain activations indicate good functional recovery but more activations outside the networks involved in control subjects signal poor outcome (Ward et al., 2003), in stuttering, the functional takeover by cortical regions that do not normally participate in the impaired process seems to be limited and bound to be insufficient (Neumann et al., 2005).

These findings suggest a compensation mechanism for a deficient synchronization of language production steps (Biermann-Ruben, Salmelin, & Schnitzler, 2005; Salmelin, et al., 1998; 2000). In particular, there is evidence that the deactivated regions in the left frontal cortex could be associated with a pathology in the left-hemispheric frontal gray matter and white matter connections and thus be responsible for an abnormal processing sequence between motor preparation and articulatory planning (Chang et al., 2008; Watkins et al., 2008). Moreover, the white matter abnormality underlying the premotor cortex (Watkins et al., 2008) probably disrupts tracts, which—via connections with posterior-superior temporal and inferior parietal cortex—provide a substrate for the integration of articulatory planning and sensory feedback and—via connections with primary motor cortex—for the execution of articulatory movements.

The London group took the earlier mentioned timing problem into consideration in Howell's EXPLAN theory of fluent speech control (Howell, 2004; Howell & Au-Yeung, 2002). In agreement with the results of the meta-analysis of Brown et al. (2005), the London group authors assumed that both motor and language-related brain areas would be abnormal in stutterers. If both language (PLAN) and motor (EX) processes are involved in speech control, the linguistic system should produce serial output in correct order. Normally, the motor system produces an output, and after finishing it, the next linguistic output is prepared and will be produced. If an element in the sequence is difficult for the linguistic system to generate and a delay occurs, speech fluency might be disturbed. This may happen by either repeating speech already produced or by pausing, allowing the speaker to complete the linguistic plan or to continue with the part of the plan available and then trying to complete the remainder as the planned portion is executed. If there is not sufficient time, prolongations, repetitions, or pauses will arise (Watkins et al., 2008). However, as mentioned earlier, stuttering seems to involve more cerebral speech motor processes than linguistic ones (Braun et al., 1997; Brown et al., 2005; Max, 2004; Neumann et al., 2003; De Nil & Kroll, 2001a; 2001b; Kroll et al., 1997). On the other hand, it has been shown that the more demanding a linguistic task is, the more differing brain activation patterns can be observed in stutterers, compared with nonstuttering individuals, in functional neuroimaging and in electrophysiologic studies (Blomgren, McCormick, & Gneiting, 2002; De Nil et al., 2000).

Fluency-inducing techniques might work as an external "clock generator" and reduce stuttering by providing a pacer that synchronizes the disturbed signal transmissions occurring between auditory, speech motor planning, and motor areas. Thus, deficiencies are not erased by therapy but are compensated for or functionally bypassed by artificial pacing that establishes an internal automatism. Indeed, posttreatment overactivations conspicuously occur in regions that are involved in timing processes, namely frontal speech motor planning and execution areas, temporal regions, and the basal ganglia.

Although most functional neuroimaging studies have been performed with males, there are indications that the cerebral activation differences between male and female stutterers might not be large (Watkins et al., 2008). Such differences were reported specifically for correlations with stuttered speech rather than with fluent or stutter-free speech. Stutter-free speech is usually observed in the fMRI scanner due to the masking effect of the loud scanner noise. Regions in which brain activity correlates with the latter have been described as "very similar for both sexes" (Ingham et al., 2004).

Findings Concerning the Basal Ganglia

For some years, the involvement of the basal ganglia in stuttering has been emphasized (Alm, 2004; Giraud et al., 2008; Maguire et al., 2000; Riley, Maguire, & Wu, 2001; Watkins et al., 2008). In an early neuroimaging study, basal

ganglia (left caudate) hypometabolism was demonstrated in stutterers (Wu et al., 1995; 1997). The neuronal connections between premotor cortex, motor cortex, and basal ganglia, which are involved in speech motor processing, indicate the association between a basal ganglia dysfunction and stuttering. Disfluencies typical for stuttering, together with tic-like involuntary movements, resemble focal dystonia that may arise from basal ganglia disturbance. Moreover, speech fluency–enhancing effects of dopamine antagonists (e.g., haloperidol, risperidone, olanzapine) and fluency-worsening effects of L-DOPA give indirect evidence for a dopaminergic dysfunction in stutterers presumably due to a hyperdopaminergic state (Maguire et al., 2000; Wu et al., 1997; Giraud et al., 2008).

The Frankfurt (fMRI) and London (fMRI and diffusion imaging) groups examined the involvement of the basal ganglia in stuttering, for example, the dysregulation within the cortico-striato-thalamico-cortical loop. In our study, brain activations during fluent reading were correlated with stuttering severity during everyday speaking situations (Giraud et al., 2008). To investigate the potential reorganization of the basal ganglia function after successful stuttering therapy, we additionally correlated the fMRI activations during reading aloud with the initial stuttering severity before and after therapy, which reduced the average percent syllables stuttered from 10% to 1%.

Before therapy, stuttering severity correlated positively with activations of the bilateral caudate nuclei and with the left medial superior-posterior parietal/postcentral region (Fig. 19.5). This pattern was no longer detected after therapy (Giraud et al., 2008). Stuttering severity before therapy correlated negatively with bilateral activation in inferior temporal areas. After therapy, this association had disappeared almost completely. Additionally, a negative correlation between the initial severity of stuttering and the posttreatment activation of the precuneus, the anterior nucleus of the thalamus, the left substantia nigra (SN) before therapy, and the right SN after therapy was observed. A bilateral activation in another part of the basal ganglia, the putamen, had been described after fluency-shaping therapy in a previous study (Neumann et al., 2003).

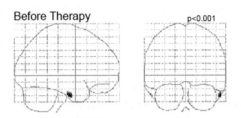

B Negative correlation with stuttering severity

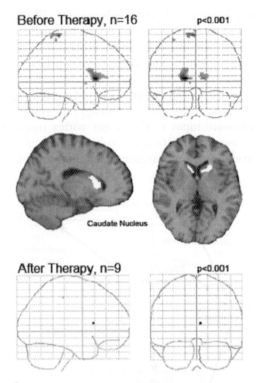

A Positive correlation with stuttering severity

Figure 19.5. Functional magnetic resonance imaging (fMRI) activations of the basal ganglia of stuttering subjects. **(A)** Brain activations during fluent reading that positively correlate with severity of stuttering before and after fluency-shaping therapy. **(B)** Brain activations during fluent reading that negatively correlate with stuttering severity before fluency-shaping therapy. After therapy no effect was detected. (From Giraud et al., 2008.)

Stuttering severity was associated with bilateral activations of the caudate nucleus (positive correlation) and of the left SN (negative correlation). The caudate, which is a part of the striatum, and the SN, which belongs to the pallidum, act antagonistically; that is, when activity in the caudate is high, activity in the SN is low (Gerfen et al., 1990). The positive correlation with stuttering severity and activations in the caudate and the negative correlation with activations in the SN are in accord with this functional antagonism. In particular, the subjects with more severe stuttering showed an increased activation in the caudate and a decreased activation in the SN, a feature that usually characterizes L-DOPA–induced dyskinesia (Rajput et al., 1997). The higher inhibitory feedback from the striatum to the pallidum may initiate a strong thalamic disinhibition and a subsequent hyperactivation in the speech motor cortex. In stutterers, such an unbalanced situation might occur transiently and undergo a

subsequent regulation of the motor output by the inferior prefrontal cortex (Giraud et al., 2008).

Figures 19.6A to 19.66D depict a functional model of stuttering based on our neuroimaging findings that includes cortico-striato-cortical loops (Giraud et al., 2008). For nonstuttering subjects, such a loop implies positive feedback between Broca's area and speech motor regions. For stutterers, the model involves the structural disconnection between Broca's area and speech motor cortex regions as described earlier. Because these neuronal speech circuits are organized in loops, the model may hold even if the white matter disconnection were the consequence of a dysfunction situated elsewhere in the loop. In this case, an altered sequencing between prefrontal and motor activations, as described by Salmelin et al. (2000), would result nevertheless. The input the striatum receives from the motor cortex would then be inaccurate both in timing and its phonologic nature. This could result in a diffuse activation of the striatum and possibly in a reduced suppression of competing phonologic motor patterns (Mink, 2003). A diffuse striatal hyperactivation could then lead to an imbalance in striato-cortical feedback and to an inadequate excitation of the motor cortex that would further maintain or amplify the imbalance. An imprecise motor input to the striatum fits with the observation that stuttering corresponds neither to a hyperdopaminergic nor to hypodopaminergic state but, instead, to a kind of dysregulation in the dopaminergic system (Goberman & Blomgren, 2004). Stuttering symptoms such as syllable repetitions and blocks could be explained by a lock into repetitive abnormal cortico-striatal loops (Giraud et al., 2008).

Subsequently, stutterers would engage a spontaneous compensation strategy to restore an adequate input to the motor cortex (upper fat arrow in Fig. 19.6C) by involving those right prefrontal and motor regions that are typically found

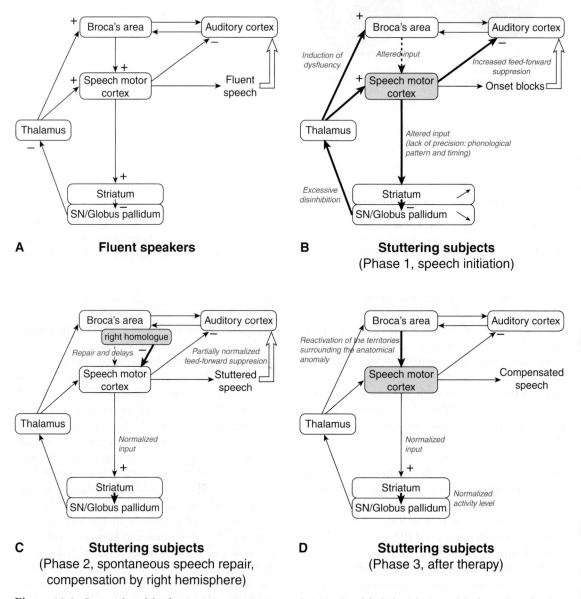

Figure 19.6. Proposed models of stuttering, compensation, and repair. Simplified physiologic model of speech production in **(A)** fluent speakers, **(B)** stuttering speakers during speech initiation, **(C)** stuttering speakers during spontaneous speech compensation, and **(D)** stuttering speakers after relateralization by fluency-shaping therapy. (From Giraud et al., 2008.)

to be overactivated in functional neuroimaging studies (De Nil et al., 2000; Fox et al., 1996; Ingham, 2001; Neumann et al., 2003; 2005). This hypothesis is consistent with our previous findings that the RFO, which is involved in self-monitoring and language repair, is consistently overactive in stutterers compared with nonstuttering subjects while performing language or verbal tasks (Preibisch et al., 2003a). Compensation by the RFO might be necessary if control by Broca's area is not possible due to a disconnection between left prefrontal and motor regions, as indicated by both the structural lesion (Sommer et al., 2002; Chang et al., 2008; Watkins et al., 2008) and an abnormal sequence of speech processing steps in stutterers (Salmelin et al., 2000). Thus, when stutterers use the RFO instead of Broca's area, a partial restoration of an appropriate input could be achieved, leading to more fluent speech but also to delays in speech production because of the distance between the RFO and the left speech motor cortex.

Successful stuttering therapy may relateralize speech processing to the left motor cortex by reactivating the regions surrounding those with structural anomalies (Neumann et al., 2005) and, hence, might remove the delay and normalize the input to the motor cortex and the striatum (Fig. 19.6D). Our model also easily accommodates findings of deactivations in the Broca's and Wernicke's areas during stuttering and globally normal patterns with only deactivations in the left caudate and increased activation in the SN during fluent chorus reading (Wu et al., 1995).

We also detected a positive correlation between stuttering severity and activation in the left medial posterior-superior parietal/postcentral region (Brodmann's area 4/5/7). A bidirectional neuronal connection of this region with the caudate nucleus is known based on experiments with primates (Leichnetz, 2001) and from Huntington's disease (Kassubek et al., 2004) and its therapy with fetal striatal allografts (Gaura et al., 2004). This neuronal connection, therefore, could explain the association between hyperactivity in the caudate in severely stuttering subjects and hyperactivation in the superior postcentral region.

Some findings suggest that more moderately stuttering individuals are better than more severely stuttering individuals in processing the meaning of spoken speech conveyed by their own auditory feedback. These findings include: (1) strong negative correlations between stuttering severity and activation in bilateral, predominantly right-hemispheric, anterior-inferior temporal cortices in our study (Giraud et al., 2008); (2) the known involvement of the right anterior ventral temporal regions in processing of semantic information of auditory origin (Marinkovic et al., 2003); and (3) the influence of the basal ganglia on late language-related evoked potential responses (Frisch et al., 2003). This generalization about the processing of auditory feedback information in stutterers fits well with the hypothesis that a deficiency in speech motor planning should directly alter auditory feedback processing (Brown et al., 2005; Max, 2004; Watkins, et al., 2008). In stutterers, the efference copy that parallels speech motor output could abnormally suppress auditory processing of subsequent utterances, which could also affect later processing steps such as processing of sound meaning (Giraud et al., 2008).

In our 2005 fMRI study, successful fluency-shaping therapy relateralized speech and language networks in all stutterers, with increased activation predominantly in left auditory and motor cortices, but also in the putamen (Neumann et al., 2005). This finding suggests that this therapy acts directly and markedly on basal ganglia function. Therapy corrected the abnormal activation of the caudate, which characterized the most severely affected stutterers. Only a small positive correlation in the right caudate and a negative correlation in the right SN remained. Because subjects did not stutter during scanning, a genuine normalization of speech production circuits involving the basal ganglia might have occurred, although the input to the basal ganglia might be transiently "abnormal" in stutterers whose "normal" state is a compensated one with increased right-sided motor activations (Giraud et al., 2008). The posttreatment reduced speech rate does not explain the disappearance of abnormal caudate activation because a low speech rate is normally associated with *increased* basal ganglia activity (Ingham et al., 2004).

If an anomaly in the gray and white matter in the left frontal cortex, prefrontal, and sensorimotor regions is typically associated with stuttering (Sommer et al., 2002; Chang et al., 2008; Watkins et al., 2008), then an activation pattern in other left-sided motor regions, such as the anterior insula or basal ganglia structures, could indicate associated left-hemispheric deviant motor and sensorimotor integration functions—congenital or following the structural deficits. Alternatively, it could reflect compensation. One could wonder how small structural anomalies are able to induce a large-scale cerebral reorganization. Obviously, the structural deficit is functionally potent enough to drive significant cortical and subcortical reorganization (Giraud et al., 2008).

Stuttering may not only be caused by cortical structural deficits and underlying fiber deficiencies, but also, more directly, it may be caused by a basal ganglia dysfunction that would interfere with the timing in speech production (Alm, 2004). One argument for this hypothesis is that activity in the caudate nucleus is correlated with stuttering severity before, but not after, therapy. Giraud et al. (2008) reported that, depending on the pretreatment activity level, therapy had different effects on the caudate; posttreatment activity decreased in case of a high initial activity level before treatment and increased in the opposite case. This finding fits with the observation that the impact of motor learning on the basal ganglia depends on the extent of automaticity achieved for the processes that are being learned. During initial stages of motor learning, decreased brain activity has been reported, while an already acquired motor sequence, which only had to be maintained as speed of execution increased, was associated with increased activity (Lehéricy et al., 2005). Possibly, the most severely stuttering subjects had to learn completely new motor sequences during therapy, while the less affected subjects had already achieved an advanced stage of training (Giraud et al., 2008).

The London group also detected cerebral overactivity in stutterers in the midbrain at the level of the basal ganglia (Watkins et al., 2008). Using fMRI, the London authors found lower activity in stutterers in the left ventral premotor cortex, in the right Rolandic operculum, bilateral in the sensorimotor cortex (face representation), and in the left primary auditory cortex. Furthermore, they identified overactivations in the left cingulate sulcus, bilateral in the anterior insula, and in a midbrain region at the level of the SN, the pedunculopontine nucleus (PPN), the subthalamic nucleus (STN), the red nucleus, and the cerebellum. Most of these overactivated

nuclei are part of the basal ganglia circuitry. The PPN is involved in the initiation and modulation of stereotyped movements, principally gait, and is, together with the STN, a target for therapy in Parkinson's disease, which may also include speech disfluency (Watkins et al., 2008). Activity in the red nucleus was also reported to increase after stuttering therapy (Neumann et al., 2003).

Watkins et al. (2008) performed their fMRI experiment during normal, delayed, and frequency-shifted feedback conditions. Delayed or frequency-shifted feedback revealed increased activity bilaterally in the superior temporal cortex in both stuttering and nonstuttering subjects and delayed feedback in the right inferior frontal cortex.

Functional Neuroimaging Findings in Stuttering Related to Brain Plasticity in General

To explain the brain changes that may take place in stuttering, we need to consider neuroplasticity in general. Two major forms of functional neuroplasticity can be observed in stuttering: homologous area adaptation and map expansion. The first means that particular cognitive processes are taken over by a homologous region in the opposite hemisphere. The second, map expansion, means that a performance-based increase of a functional brain region takes place (Grafman, 2000). The cerebral overactivations in stutterers indicate an expansion of regions recruited in speaking overtly, probably compensating for a primary lesion. The recruitment of the RFO is an adaptation of a homologous region. This spontaneous compensation seems, however, to be ineffective because the person continues to stutter. An effective therapy, therefore, shifts the compensation of the left-hemispheric deficits from the right-sided homologous areas to left-hemispheric regions close to the area of deficit. Thus, an effective compensation seems to require the restoration of left-hemispheric networks (lesion-compensation theory) (Neumann et al., 2005). Fluency-enhancing techniques, which involve practicing a slow, regular speech meter, may work as an external pacer and thereby restore and synchronize the disturbed signal transfer between auditory, speech planning, and execution areas.

Depending on whether activity levels in brain regions with abnormal activity in stutterers show a positive or negative correlation with stuttering severity, they can be considered pathologic (positive correlation) or compensatory (negative correlation). In other words, the regions that are more active when an individual stutters more severely (positive correlation) probably indicate primary pathology, whereas those regions that are more active when an individual stutters more moderately (negative correlation) should be of compensatory nature. However, structural defects are more likely to indicate the origin of a disorder rather than adaptation. These distinctions may help us to identify brain regions that are mobilized to compensate for stuttering as well as those associated with a long-lasting recovery. The overactivation that we found in the RFO correlated negatively with the severity of stuttering, indicating a compensation function of this region. However, cerebral activation and stuttering severity correlated positively in left-hemispheric perisylvian regions, in the auditory cortices, and in basal ganglia structures (e.g., the more somebody stuttered, the more he or she activated this regions in our study), suggesting a causal pathology in these regions, which are affected by the structural abnormalities mentioned earlier.

Recently, a superimposition of the statistical maps of the comparisons between stuttering and nonstuttering subjects makes it possible to demonstrate the relationship between the functional and structural differences. For example, the London group (Watkins et al., 2008) demonstrated that the reduced functional activations in the left ventral premotor cortex and the more ventrally located right premotor cortex in the stutterers lay directly above regions of white matter with reduced integrity.

IMPLICATIONS AND FURTHER DIRECTIONS

With improved neuroimaging techniques and data analysis procedures, functional and structural data become more and more consistent across studies. They allow an integrated view of both structural and functional anomalies in the brains of stutterers that can be now be pieced together. Functional neuroimaging studies identified more right hemisphere or bilateral neuronal activation in speech-language regions in stuttering individuals compared with nonstuttering individuals during overt speech. We assume that the right-hemispheric findings reflect a spontaneous but not very effective compensation for primary, left hemisphere lesions and resulting dysfunctions in the speech and language system of stutterers.

Compensation is enhanced and improved after fluency-shaping therapy but, if stuttering has persisted into adolescence and adulthood, does not result in fluent and completely spontaneous (automatic) speech in most cases. Although the right-sided overactivations largely persist after treatment, activation substantially increases in

Table 19.2. *Summary of the Functional Findings in the Brains of Individuals Who Stutter*

Without Therapy

More activation compared with nonstuttering subjects in frontoparietal motor and speech-language areas, predominantly in a right-hemispheric dorsal frontoparietal network and in left cerebellar regions

More activation in particular in the RFO (right frontal operculum, Brodmann's area 47/12); negative correlation with stuttering severity indicates compensation function

Less activation than in nonstuttering subjects in auditory regions during stuttering, more activation there than in nonstuttering subjects during fluent speaking

After Successful Fluency-Shaping Therapy Where Some Stuttering Continues

More and more widespread activation in regions associated with speech and language than before therapy

More activations in left-hemispheric areas, in particular in regions surrounding the lesion

Refunctionalization of the basal ganglia and the cortico-striato-thalamico-cortical loop

Persistent positive correlation between stuttering severity and activation in the left primary motor region of articulation (Rolandic operculum) indicates primary pathology

More activation in auditory regions than before therapy

Spontaneous and Therapy-Induced Recovery (Adults)

Activation in left frontal regions and in bilateral auditory regions left-hemispheric regions. This compensatory increase in activation involves regions adjacent to deactivated regions—deactivations that reflect underlying permanent structural white and gray matter deficiencies. Activity increases especially in auditory and frontal speech motor planning and execution areas, but also in regions that are recruited for articulatory complexity and timing demands (basal ganglia).

These findings lead us to the following implications: (1) the success of fluency-shaping stuttering therapy may be related to its effectiveness in mobilizing well-functioning cortical substrates located in the vicinity of functionally impaired neural tissue; (2) restoring left motor activation should be associated with an improved communication between Broca's area and the speech motor cortex and, therefore, should correct the temporal ordering of steps leading to speech production.

What we are searching for, however, are therapy approaches with (life)long-lasting effects. Could this be realized by automatizing a paced speech with an altered pattern? To find the most effective methods for therapy, one might want to examine adults who have completely or nearly completely recovered from stuttering. Our recent fMRI study with such male adults showed the expected overactivations in the RFO and in auditory regions in stuttering subjects and identified a region in the left frontal cortex as being the only area that was more activated in recovered stutterers than in persistent stutterers and in nonstuttering persons. The fact that recovered former stutterers expressed the core characteristics of stutterers, such as overactivation in the RFO and less gray matter in left inferior frontal cortex, indicates that they never lose their etiologic affiliation to the group of stutterers. However, the activation of the left frontal cortex region suggests that former stutterers show a characteristic way of compensating. This region is implicated in linguistic tasks (e.g., lexical/semantic tasks, such as covert picture naming, verb-generation tasks, word retrieval, and representing morphologically complex words) (Badgaiyan, Schacter, & Alpert, 2002; Dapretto & Bookheimer, 1999; Preibisch et al., 2003a, Thompson-Schill, D'Esposito, & Kan, 1999), as well as in motor tasks like point-to-point reaching movements, complex sequential movements, and motor planning (Schaal

et al., 2004). Anatomic and functional data from nonhuman primates and from humans indicate that this region executes a top-down control on perisylvian regions, such as the anterior insula, the planum polare, and the basal ganglia (Mesulam & Mufson, 1982; Petrides & Pandya, 2002), which are involved in the top-down control of sensory integration (Hashimoto & Sakai, 2003; Vuust et al., 2006). Vuust et al. (2006) showed a bilateral activation of the previously mentioned frontal cortex region if a musical rhythm had to be maintained in a countermeter but not during keeping time with an isometric rhythm. Efficient integration of a countermeter with a main meter was localized in the left orbitofrontal cortex and also involved the supramarginal gyrus and the insula, which are regions that are overactivated by persistent stutterers in our and other studies (Neumann et al., 2003; Watkins et al., 2008). This finding points to the role of speech meter processing in stuttering. Together, these findings suggest that the engagement of left frontal cortex regions and of the left insula in recovered stutterers could obviously eliminate stuttering by successfully merging discrepant speech meters into an adapted motor program. Thus, the training of speech meter (as tried in some therapy approaches) could potentially enforce long-lasting therapeutic effects in stutterers. Future therapy concepts should thus focus on the refunctionalization of this frontal cortex region and of the auditory and basal ganglia regions.

So far, neuroimaging has only been used to investigate fluency-shaping therapies. It would also be of interest to examine therapy effects of other therapies like stuttering modification or therapies specially designed for childhood, such as the Lidcombe program. However, it is critical to obtain reliable measures of stuttering before and after stuttering modification treatment that can then be correlated with the cerebral activation data. It would be particularly valuable to study the successful, therapy-induced brain plasticity processes of preschool children who are able to completely recover from stuttering. However, at this time, functional neuroimaging procedures are not suitable for use with young children (they would have to lie motionless in the scanner and perform cognitive tasks for at least 45 minutes; standard brain maps are not available).

Many other questions are worth addressing in neuroimaging research on stuttering. For instance, which differences in cerebral activity can be observed in subjects who relapse within a defined period after therapy compared with those who remain fluent? Would brain stimulation by repetitive transcranial magnetic stimulation (rTMS) be useful? Can the described neuroimaging findings help us to find target areas for such a therapy? So far, no successful rTMS therapy for stutterers has been reported, possibly because of the limited accessibility of the regions in question for this therapy, which is known to cause long-term plastic cerebral changes. Could deep brain stimulation (DBS) in extremely severe cases of stuttering that are resistant to other therapies be helpful? Which region would be a target area—the STN or another basal ganglia structure? As of now, there are no indications that DBS can enhance speech fluency. To the contrary, treatment for Parkinson's disease with deep brain stimulation of the STN has been reported to worsen stuttering severity (Burghaus et al., 2006).

However, study of neural plasticity has expanded rapidly in the past decades and has demonstrated the remarkable ability of the developing, adult, and aging brain to be shaped by environmental inputs in both healthy individuals and in individuals who have experienced a lesion (Rossini & Dal Forno, 2004). From studies of recovery from stroke, we know that neuronal networks adjacent to a lesion in the sensorimotor brain areas can progressively take over the function previously played by the damaged neurons. Such a reorganization effectively modifies the interhemispheric differences in somatotopic organization of the sensorimotor cortices.

Formerly, the prepubescent years were regarded as the golden age of motor learning, and beginning in middle age, it was thought that motor learning capacity diminished. Now, however, it is known that there is also a continual plastic remodeling in adults and that plastic changes in motor cortex occur during the acquisition of new motor skills in a matter of days or even minutes (Classen et al., 1998). Posttraining changes in the brain that have been demonstrated with neuroimaging methods include decreases in activity with brief training and testing soon after training and increases and shifts in activity after extensive training or therapy (Desmond & Fiez, 1998). PET and fMRI studies have shown that the plastic remodeling of brain regions involved in speech motor and linguistic processing may occur during fluency-shaping therapy of stuttering (de Nil & Kroll, 2001a; 2001b; De Nil, et al., 2003; Kroll et al., 1997; Neumann et al., 2003; 2005). Now, with the help of neuroimaging methods, we know a lot of key regions in which such changes may occur. We also know that the problem of articulatory planning and sensory feedback integration, and especially their relative timing, has to be solved in stuttering therapy for it to be even more effective. Targeting these key regions and problems is probably possible using a variety of therapies in addition to the fluency-shaping therapy studied so far, and neuroimaging may give further feedback about the nature of brain organization that can be achieved with these therapies.

ACKNOWLEDGMENT

We thank Luc De Nil for his constant stimulation and encouragement for writing this chapter and Yevgen Zaretsky for helping us to prepare the manuscript.

CHAPTER 20

Summary and Future Directions

REBECCA J. MCCAULEY AND BARRY E. GUITAR

CHAPTER OUTLINE

In this final chapter, we summarize the book as a whole by taking several steps back to get a big-picture view of similarities and differences and then the levels of research evidence supporting treatments within each age group and overall. Next, we will address the individual audiences for whom we wrote this book, adding to the comments we made to each in the very first chapter; in particular, we will offer some exercises and make further suggestions about how information contained here—and information like it that can be found elsewhere—can help groups of readers make decisions about stuttering treatment. Finally, we will close by addressing a new audience, readers who may actually come from the ranks of almost any of the other audiences—that is, future and current researchers whose efforts are sorely needed to continue the advancements chronicled here in helping people who stutter and their families.

SIMILARITIES AND DIFFERENCES

As you have seen over the course of reading this book, there is a wide array of interventions for stuttering intended to address basic goals ranging from reduction of stuttering to near-zero levels to improved attitudes about communication. Interventions vary not just in terms of their basic goals, but also in terms of how they are delivered, who participates in the treatment process, their activities, and even in the degree to which clients are asked to understand the treatment process and how they can contribute to it. Often, differences in treatments reflect varying perspectives about the causes and major influences on stuttering, as well as what treatment demands are realistic for clients who stutter and their families. Thus, it may be the differences between interventions that first attract our attention.

Nonetheless, shared features of stuttering treatments pique our interest as well. To the extent that the treatments demonstrate some level of efficacy, similarities may signal critical treatment elements capable of mitigating the development or continuation of stuttering. On the other hand, some similarities may simply highlight trends, or even fads, in how treatments have been developed and studied for stutterers of different ages. Thus, although considering the significance of similarities is challenging, it is potentially critical to optimizing treatment outcomes.

When treatments are compared across the three age groups—preschoolers, school-age children and adolescents, and adults—similarities within groups can be seen in their attention to age-related communicative demands, their assumptions about the likelihood that stuttering will be chronic, and the degree to which clients are viewed as able to engage cognitively in their treatment (and therefore the degree to which they are seen as autonomous partners in their treatment). Because of these age-related differences, it seems useful to take each age group in turn.

INTERVENTIONS FOR PRESCHOOL CHILDREN

In Chapter 4, the overview chapter for this group of interventions, we noted strong similarities across the three interventions. This might be unexpected, given the wide gulf that has historically separated advocates of indirect versus direct approaches to treatment of stuttering in preschoolers (Guitar, 2003). Researchers who favored indirect approaches focused their efforts on changing the child's environment (Conture, 2001; Van Riper, 1973), whereas those who favored direct approaches focused their efforts on modifying the child's behavior (Costello, 1983; Onslow, Packman, & Harrison, 2003). Nonetheless, the three interventions described here shared several common features that cross this theoretical divide. These shared features include **intensive parent involvement and support, praise of the child, and systematic assessment of progress**.

First, all three of the interventions incorporate parent involvement that includes setting aside one-on-one time with the child as well as other types of support for the child, including the use of direct praise. In the Palin Parent-Child Interaction program (Chapter 5), praise is used for any positive behavior; whereas in the Lidcombe Program, praise is used as a contingency for fluent speech. However, despite this difference in the focus of praise, it is considered an important element of all three approaches.

Second, each intervention incorporates support of the parents in their roles as interventionists. Parent counseling is treated as an integral component of both the Palin Centre program and the Stuttering Prevention and Early Intervention Program. Although this will include helping parents with work that is done at home, it is also intended to bolster parents' confidence and lessen their anxiety about their child's fluency. In contrast, in the Lidcombe Program,

interaction with parents focuses on home treatment and progress. Although more conventional counseling may occur informally within these discussions, it may also be that a focus on techniques and data constitutes sufficient parental support for many families.

Finally, all three interventions also incorporate systematic assessment of progress in which parents actively participate by offering out-of-clinic ratings or less formal observations about a variety of variables that often extend beyond the child's stuttering levels. Assessment variables may also include variables related to the parents' comfort with their own performance as well as their concerns about the child's speech.

In addition to these similarities, each of the three programs is based on an assumption that most of the children being treated have the potential to attain normal or near-normal fluency, no matter what the level of their risk factors or the degree of severity at the onset of treatment. Although this perspective may have always influenced clinicians working with preschoolers, until recently, that upbeat perspective may simply have been based on the high rate of natural recovery that can be expected in children (Yairi & Ambrose, 1999).

INTERVENTIONS FOR SCHOOL-AGE CHILDREN

Differences in goals and methods are quite evident across the four interventions described in this section. One apparent reason for these differences is the declining expectation that young people who continue to stutter will eventually recover and attain unmonitored fluency (either through natural recovery or intervention) (Johannsen, 2000; Seider, Gladstien & Kidd, 1983; Yairi & Ambrose, 1992; Yairi et al., 1996). This means that treatments increasingly address some of the affective issues associated with stuttering as part of mitigating the effects on communication and social interaction. In fact, Comprehensive Treatment (Yaruss, Pelczarski, & Quesal) dispenses with normal fluency as a goal, aiming for effective communication and quality of life instead, and Smooth Speech Treatment (Craig) is directed toward management of stuttering and improved social interaction and communication skills. The Lidcombe Program (Harrison et al.) and Fluency Rules (Runyan &

Runyan) continue to address goals related to natural-sounding and fluent speech, but also target younger school-age children.

Another reason for the degree of variability in treatments for this age group is likely to be that the increasing abilities of children to participate actively in their treatment makes direct teaching of specific techniques increasingly possible. In fact, the two interventions intended primarily for younger school-age children (i.e., the Lidcombe Program for school-age children and Fluency Rules program) most closely resemble interventions included in the section for preschoolers. In contrast, the two interventions that include adolescents as intended clients (i.e., Smooth Speech and Cognitive Behavior Therapy and the Comprehensive Treatment) incorporate elements seen in interventions for adults, such as the use of prolonged speech to instantiate fluency and modification of disfluencies to contend with residual stuttering.

In the overview chapter for this group of interventions, we noted that "even [their] similarities have differences." However, because here we have decided to focus on the bigger picture, we will reiterate the similarities recounted there, but in broader strokes. Three shared features relate to the **use of reinforcement, treatment hierarchies, and family involvement**. Reinforcement, although changing in form and degree of systematicity, is used by all four interventions. Verbal praise of fluency or other targeted behaviors is used by all of the interventions but is supplemented by other verbal contingencies (request for correction in response to stuttering) in the Lidcombe Program and by financial incentives in the Smooth Speech approach.

All four treatments also incorporate a hierarchy intended to bolster learning and promote generalization of newly learned skills beyond the home or clinic room. Whereas the Lidcombe Program uses a hierarchy that is more loosely structured, the remaining three treatments use more structured hierarchies, with the two interventions that include adolescent clients using the highest degree of structure. Hierarchies designed to slowly escalate task difficulty are widely used in speech-language interventions and may be required for successful fluency in the face of older children's years of experience with maladaptive speech patterns

Finally, families, especially parents, and more widely disbursed members of the child's communicative world, such as teachers, are involved in all four treatments, although the extent and timing of their involvement varies more than it did in the interventions we described for preschoolers. Parents are viewed as intervention agents only in the Lidcombe Program and an in-home version of the Smooth Speech program. Otherwise, their involvement is confined to homework activities designed to promote generalization (Smooth Speech); or they are viewed as team members who remind the child to use newly learned techniques (Fluency Rules) or simply as accepting listeners, along with peers and teachers, who can help the child improve communication skills more broadly. The changing, even lessening involvement of parents, along with the increasing involvement of others including peers probably reflects little more than the growing independence of developing children and adolescents. It can also be seen, however, as reflecting the continuing value of parents and increasing value of peers for their abilities to contribute to higher levels of treatment effects—those associated with communication and social roles facilitated by effective communication.

INTERVENTIONS FOR ADOLESCENTS AND ADULTS

In addition to two behavioral interventions, the section of the book on treatments for this age group describes two very different and controversial interventions—drug treatment of stuttering and an intervention involving a device, the SpeechEasy. Finding similarities across this entire group was obviously difficult; in fact, in our overview, we highlighted just one—each of the interventions indicates that subsequent to initial, more intense contact, the stutterer will continue to require at least periodic contact with knowledgeable professionals. We interpreted this as acknowledging the likelihood that none of these methods can assure adults who stutter a future completely free of stuttering. Although some readers will consider this an accusation of weakness on the part of these interventions, a default expectation of additional contact may be preferable to one in which relapse is seen as failure by either client or clinician. As Chapter 19 indicates, the ongoing presence of brain differences among people who stutter, regardless of their recovery, suggests that relapse may be a biologic default that can be responded to with unending vigilance or, alternatively, with calm resolve once it asserts itself.

An additional similarity across these interventions occurred to us, namely, that interventions for this group are the most pressed to fit in very busy lives that include work, relationships, and many challenges as large as stuttering—or larger. In fact, the appeal of the two more controversial interventions may come primarily from their apparent ease of use, although it is hoped that readers now appreciate the range of time as well as other demands entailed by each. Development of intensive and telehealth delivery versions for the more conventional interventions reflect responses to clients' time limitations that are available within the strictures of behavioral interventions.

RESEARCH EVIDENCE FOR INTERVENTIONS

Awareness of the strengths and weaknesses of the research supporting each intervention should sharpen the judgments of the clinicians and clients (or clients' parents) as they choose a treatment and plan their work together as a team. Similarly, once a treatment is chosen, awareness of the strengths and weaknesses of the research on which it is based can help support ongoing decision making. For example, more well-studied and substantiated elements of a treatment or treatment package may be viewed as less open to modification than those that have been less well studied. In addition, knowing that no treatment has been shown to work for every participant transforms the tasks of ongoing assessment from something that can be likened to tedious bookkeeping to something that can be more readily seen as navigation in uncharted waters.

INTERVENTIONS FOR PRESCHOOL CHILDREN

Thus far, the strongest research evidence supporting the efficacy of the Palin Parent-Child Interaction, the indirect treatment approach used at the Palin Centre, is a single-subject experimental design (Millard, Nicholas, & Cook, 2008). Although this type of design is not yet

fully incorporated within widely used hierarchies of evidence quality (see Chapter 18), its importance in communication disorders is widely acknowledged and is increasingly valued for the role it can play in evidence-based practice (Beeson & Robey, 2006; Dollaghan, 2007). The specific single-subject design used by Millard, Nicholas, and Cook (2008) consisted of a 6-week baseline, a 12-week period of treatment, and follow-up contact for up to a year with less frequent visits over that period. The design was replicated across six children. Four of the children reduced their stuttering significantly by the end of treatment in conversations with both parents, whereas another child did so with one parent only. The sixth child showed a similar improvement in fluency by the end of the follow-up period. This study, then, represents a good beginning for establishing the efficacy of the Palin Parent-Child Interaction and is supported by other studies demonstrating that particular intermediate goals identified within the treatment program are also effective (e.g., changes in parent communication).

The hybrid intervention, Stuttering Prevention and Early Intervention (Chapter 6), is supported by a number of pre- and posttreatment studies (Gottwald & Starkweather, 1999; Starkweather, Gottwald, & Halfond, 1990) as well as additional pre- and posttreatment data presented in Chapter 6. These provide some support for the value of this intervention for young children at risk for persistent stuttering. In her closing comments about the intervention, Gottwald acknowledged the need for additional work on the Stuttering Prevention and Early Intervention at other research sites and by other therapists as a means of addressing the ever-present potential concern of observer bias. As an equally crucial aspect of research quality, we would recommend incorporation of research design elements (e.g., single-subject design methods or random group assignment with a control group) that demonstrate control over extraneous variables (e.g., natural recovery).

The Lidcombe Program of Early Stuttering Intervention has been tested using a randomized controlled trial (Jones et al., 2005). In that study, greater improvement, as demonstrated through a very large effect size and statistically significant difference, was seen for the children who received the treatment than in the untreated children who served as the control group. Thus, the Lidcombe Program has stronger support than the other two preschool interventions described in this volume. However, demonstrating that a treatment for stuttering is better than no treatment is a low bar to clear, especially in light of the high natural recovery rate expected for this condition, which should require particularly precise measures and long-term follow-up. Still needed, therefore, are studies that compare the Lidcombe Program to other treatments, studies that increase the follow-up times to strengthen further claims regarding the persistence of children's gains, and studies that examine the role of specific elements of the program (e.g., the use of negative verbal contingencies for stuttering) as a means of making it more effective and/or more efficient.

It would be premature to say that the level of evidence provided for the Lidcombe Program means that the hybrid or indirect approaches should revisit, much less abandon, their attempts to modify the child's environment as a way of addressing beginning stuttering and the theory on which these are based. However, a direct comparison of the Lidcombe Program with one of these other interventions and a control group would provide important evidence about the relative effectiveness of direct and indirect approaches and the extent to which these approaches make contributions to children's fluency beyond those that occur naturally with time for many children. In addition, such a study or series of studies might help identify factors (child or parent) pointing to the most appropriate treatment choice for individual children and their families in terms of efficacy and/or efficiency.

INTERVENTIONS FOR SCHOOL-AGE CHILDREN

The Lidcombe Program for school-age children has presented pre-post data for a total of 23 children, ages 6 to 12 years, in two studies. Although substantial gains in fluency were shown, there were several design weaknesses. First, no control group was used in either study, so that the effects of natural recovery (rarer at this age) could be assessed. Second, posttreatment assessments were made relatively soon after fluency was established, during the maintenance phase of the program.

This makes it difficult to know whether fluency would have lasted after the maintenance phase ended. Third, four of the 11 participants in one study dropped out during the maintenance phrase, so it is not known whether these children relapsed and, if included in the data, would make the group averages less impressive.

The evidence for the Fluency Rules Program is also essentially pre-post data, which are reported in three cited studies. No control groups were used, and reliability of measurements was not reported. The Stuttering Severity Instrument data were reported for one of the groups of clients, and this provided more information about recovery than simple frequency of stuttering. However, in the other two groups, it was only noted that most clients were dismissed with normal fluency, but some continued to stutter. Another caveat about the evidence for Fluency Rules is that a majority of the clients in the studies were preschool children or very young school-age children. Thus, the findings with Fluency Rules treatment do not provide support for its use with older children.

The design of studies of outcome for Smooth Speech and Cognitive Behavior Therapy included a no-treatment control group as well as two different versions of the treatment: intensive and home-based nonintensive. For ethical reasons, the control group was denied treatment for only 3 months, but their lack of improvement during this time at least indicated that there was no placebo effect from being in the study. Outcome measures included frequency of stuttering—not as much information as severity ratings, but still quite adequate—as well as percent change and effect sizes. Moreover, pre- and posttreatment measures of anxiety were made, as well as parent ratings of the extent of relapse that occurred. Outcome measures were made for as long as 5 years after treatment—an unusually rigorous measure for treatment. A few participants were lost during the 5-year interval, as might be expected. Decreases in stuttering, effect sizes, and reductions in anxiety were all substantial for the participants who were tracked throughout the entire study.

The final treatment for this age group, Comprehensive Therapy, does not present research evidence for this relatively new treatment package. In the section in Chapter 12 on future directions, the authors indicate: "The most pressing need related to this treatment approach is empirical documentation that it is effective in helping children who stutter improve their fluency, minimize negative reactions, and reduce the negative impact of their disorder on communication in daily activities and participation in life" (p. 241). Although they have not yet assessed outcomes of this treatment, two of the authors have developed an instrument for assessment of all of the areas they deem important to address in treatment.

INTERVENTIONS FOR ADOLESCENTS AND ADULTS

Data on outcomes for the Camperdown Program have been collected in a series of five clinical trials, including a pilot study, a clinical trial involving 30 adults, an assessment of outcomes with adolescents, an assessment of outcomes when delivered via telephone and videotape, and a trial of the program conducted at an independent site by students. Outcomes of the initial large clinical trial were assessed at 6 and 12 months after the beginning of treatment. Frequency of stuttering, speech naturalness, self ratings of severity, and speech rate were assessed with adequate reliability. Results demonstrated substantial long-term changes in the variables of interest. It was noted, however, that almost a third of the initial participants dropped out before finishing the program.

The most recent outcomes for the Fluency Plus Program were assessed by comparing pretreatment, immediate posttreatment, and 1-year posttreatment frequency of stuttering and Stuttering Severity Instrument scores. It appears that all assessments were made in the treatment environment and that 1-year posttreatment measures were made immediately after the year-long maintenance phase of treatment, including cognitive therapy. Stuttering severity scores were reduced by almost half immediately after the intensive part of the treatment, but some regression occurred during the maintenance program, and the 1-year posttreatment severity scores showed only a one-third reduction from pretreatment scores.

The third and fourth interventions for adolescents and adults are quite different from the other two, and thus, the research support for the interventions is different. The chapter describing the SpeechEasy device notes that not all clients demonstrate a reduction in stuttering when tested for the effects of the altered feedback it provides. Thus studies of the outcome of this intervention may appropriately be limited to those who would find benefit. Because of these and other problems in using the device, outcome studies on the effectiveness of SpeechEasy have not been easy to carry out. Putting aside the potentially biased surveys conducted by the manufacturer and the developers of device, a few survey studies show that many users express satisfaction with the device despite the fact that they still stutter to some extent and the fact that many of them do not wear the device regularly. Valid and reliable data on SpeechEasy's long-term effectiveness are, as yet, unavailable.

The fourth intervention, pharmacotherapy, has research evidence from a number of clinical trials involving control groups receiving placebos, blinding of both the client and the clinician as to whether drug or placebo was given, and randomized assignment of participants to groups. This research has assessed not only changes in stuttering, but also changes in associated problems, such as feelings of helplessness, avoidance, and social anxiety. The drugs olanzapine and pagoclone appear to be the most promising, and results suggest that many individuals benefit from each of these. However, the authors noted that greater benefit would have been likely if pharmacotherapy was accompanied by speech therapy.

RECOMMENDATIONS FOR FURTHER WORK

In this section of the chapter, we will end as we began, with comments directed to specific groups of readers—students in speech-language pathology, adolescents and adults who stutter, parents of children who stutter, and finally, professors who teach students about stuttering. Here we will offer brief exercises and recommendations about how these groups may make further progress toward their own goals.

STUDENTS IN SPEECH-LANGUAGE PATHOLOGY
Where You Are Now

Among other things, we hope that you are at point where you understand the excitement that many of us feel about the current state of treatments for

Table 20.1. *Web-Based and Other Resources on Stuttering for Students (Potential Future Clinicians and Researchers)*

Sources for accessing web resources on stuttering and stuttering treatment
- **The Stuttering Homepage:** http://www.mnsu.edu/comdis/kuster/stutter.html
  This award-winning website, which was created and updated frequently by Judith Kuster, offers a universe of links.
- **SpeechBITE.com:** http://www.speechBITE.com/
  This website facilitates searching the web for information about Best Interventions and Treatment Efficacy. Most studies are rated for quality using a widely respected system. Single-subject experimental designs are currently included but as yet unrated; they will eventually be rated for quality using a system developed for such research.

Organizations that provide training opportunities and media resources on stuttering. Both of these include some information about research
- **Stuttering Foundation:** http://www.stutteringhelp.org/
- **National Stuttering Association:** http://www.nsastutter.org/

For future reference
- **Specialty Board on Fluency Disorders:** http://www.stutteringspecialists.org/ This organization allows certified speech-language pathologists to work toward recognition as specialists in the clinical management of fluency disorders.
- **List of Ph.D. programs with faculty experts on stuttering**, available as a link on the **Stuttering Home Page**
- **Information about current research projects in stuttering**, available on the **National Stuttering Association** website in the area for researchers. Approved researchers can recruit participants through this site; therefore, you can use it to identify active programs of research in stuttering

---

stuttering. Clinicians, researchers, and the clients who have worked with them have accomplished much in understanding the varieties of problems associated with stuttering and how these change over time. Those involved in stuttering treatment have also done much to generate ideas about what might help mitigate or remove the unique challenges facing stutterers in each different age group. Further accomplishments have ensued when clinician/researchers have used theories and less well-formed insights, or both, to shape treatments, and then begun the process of testing them to see *if* they work and for whom they work.

Despite big advances, big challenges remain. In their descriptions of the work done on their interventions, most of the authors in this volume recognize the big gaps in evidence associated with their intervention—in fact, some must admit that their only empirical support is at best indirect, consisting of support for one or more element of their multi-element approach. Such challenges as these can be nearly overwhelming to older clinicians and researchers when they consider themselves the sole contributors to future efforts. But this dilemma also suggests a wonderful niche for future work, however,

that might be yours to do—as a clinician, a researcher, or both.

As a prospective stuttering clinician, your future work is favored by the increasing accessibility of cutting edge information about research and contact with others who share a special interest in stuttering. Table 20.1 lists several resources that can help you find out information about existing and emerging interventions for stuttering, as well as ways to connect with others who may help you with reflections, recommendations, and even joint problem solving about issues in stuttering.

Your work is also aided by access to methods by which you can be encouraged, guided, and rewarded for your efforts to become proficient. In particular, the Specialty Certification in stuttering through the American Speech-Language-Hearing Association provides an important avenue for such work.

As a potential researcher of stuttering treatments, you are on the threshold of exhilarating times. The potential to examine stuttering and its various manifestations (physiologic, psychological, communicative, etc.) has never been better; for example, increasingly sensitive neuroimaging techniques and measures targeting effects of stuttering on quality of life will lead to richer descriptions than previously possible. Refinements of theories about the nature and treatment of stuttering should arise from efforts to provide coherent explanations across these different types of data. In addition, use of multiple outcome measures may help researchers understand better how treatments work (or do not work) and even what clients want from treatment.

Regardless of which of these or other futures you have in mind for yourself, we will close our specific comments to you with some suggested exercises. These, we hope, may take you a little further in your thinking about the specific treatments shared in this book, about what needs to be done to further all treatments in stuttering, and possibly, about your own role in all of this.

Four Exercises to Take You Further

1. Identify a treatment approach that you believe has weaker evidential support than some of the others. What steps might you take to provide evidence that the treatment is working for an individual client? What outcome measures would you use, considering both those recommended in the chapter on that treatment and those recommended in other chapters? What time frame would you recommend for revisiting the choice of treatment? And how would you discuss that decision with the client or his or her parents, or both?

2. Imagine that a young time-pressed client you are working with has decided to undertake a drug trial for treatment of her stuttering. She is a 26-year-old law student who wants you to fill her in on the pros and cons of such a step. Consider evidence summarized in Chapters 17 and 18 and in more recent sources concerning this controversial intervention. On those grounds, what would you tell her?

3. One of the fascinating aspects of expert decision making is that it is not as completely rationale as we would like it to be. Now, you may not be an expert yet, but what is true of experts is also true of those on their way to becoming experts. Keeping that in mind, identify a treatment that, in the course of your readings and discussions, seemed either especially valuable or especially problematic. Then identify two steps you might take to collect evidence *contradicting* your opinion.

Methods you might consider could include re-reading the chapter that describes the treatment while making an active attempt to consider the other side, finding critics or supporters in outside literature, or seeking that perspective from individuals in a chat room. Carry out at least one of these activities and see how your initial impression is modified.

4. Authors of each chapter on treatment were asked to address the question of future research. Choose one of the interventions and re-examine that chapter's section on future research. Take one of the ideas put forward there or one idea of your own and begin to draft a plan for a research project. To do that, you will want to be sure to consider what question your study would attempt to answer, who you would study, and what variables you would measure and manipulate or just measure. Then talk to someone else about your ideas and see what happens next—you might just have some research to conduct!

INDIVIDUALS WHO STUTTER
Where You Are Now

As an adolescent or adult who stutters and who chose to read this book, or even sections of this book, you are clearly sophisticated in your information gathering. Further, you may be quite intrigued by what this book has suggested to you about any previous treatment you have had or what future treatment you might want to consider. At our most optimistic, we hope that the information and opinions offered in this book have helped you identify a treatment option you think can further your own stuttering-related goals. More realistically, we hope that you have gained some information that you have found helpful in understanding your stuttering and how clinicians think about addressing it with you.

If the holes in empirical support you have read about have engendered any feelings of the "emperor has no clothes," that may not be such a bad outcome because recognizing the imperfections of existing treatments could instill sentiments of equality that could only further your developing a strong, or stronger, alliance with a good clinician. Squarely facing the likelihood that stuttering may always be a problem for you and that even some of the most well-studied interventions cannot assure success can put you in a particularly strong position from which to

Table 20.2. *Web-Based and Other Resources on Stuttering for Adults and Teens Who Stutter*

Information that can help you find a speech-language pathologist
- **Specialty Board on Fluency Disorders:** http://www.stutteringspecialists.org/consumers.html
  This is the consumer site for the **Specialty Board on Fluency Disorders**, which recognizes speech-language pathologists who are certified by the American Speech-Language-Hearing Association and have also demonstrated their expertise in fluency disorders.

Materials on stuttering
- Podcasts, brochures, and many links are available for teens and adults on the **National Stuttering Association** website (http://www.westutter.org/) as well as on the **Stuttering Foundation** website (http://www.stutteringhelp.org/).

Obtaining reimbursement for stuttering therapy
- Information about this topic is available under the topics listed for adults on the **Stuttering Foundation** website (http://www.stutteringhelp.org/) and on the **National Stuttering Association** website (http://www.westutter.org/).

Handling tough speaking situations
- **Using the telephone**
  Information on this topic is available under topics listed for adults on the **Stuttering Foundation** website.
- **Mastering the job interview**
  A booklet on this topic is available under topics listed for adults on the **National Stuttering Association** website.

Support groups
- **National Stuttering Association:** http://www.westutter.org, http://www.nsastutter.org/
  This organization's website provides access to group membership, annual conventions, newsletters meant for stutterers and their families, and information tailored for you, your employer, and others. Membership is $40 annually.
- **Teens Who STutter (TWST),** associated with the National Stuttering Association.

Material on self-therapy
- **"Self-Therapy for Stutterers"** is a book-length publication that can be read online or purchased from the Stuttering Foundation website (http://www.stutteringhelp.org/).

make a decision about what you want to do. For example, you may decide to accept the resources and ongoing commitment required by a behavioral intervention, accepting them in the way that advocates of meditation accept the demands of meditative practice—not ever easy, but worth the ongoing effort. Or, you may let yourself off the hook and recognize that trying a controversial option with its different set of risks and demands is something that, for the moment or the foreseeable future, is the route you would prefer. Or you may simply decide to follow your own way.

Regardless of your future plans, we hope that the ways in which the clinicians and researchers who authored the 12 treatment chapters discussed their treatments suggest that a speech-pathologist may have something to offer you. Notice that we say "a" speech-language pathologist rather than "any" speech-language pathologist. Finding a speech-language pathologist who you

can view as a colleague may be a first step toward changing the status quo of how you are handling your stuttering.

Table 20.2 lists some resources beyond those listed in Chapter 1 for collecting information about stuttering and stuttering treatments and for finding allies with whom to consult. In the following section, we close with three exercises that you may decide could further your thinking about future steps.

Three Exercises to Take You Further

1. First, choose an intervention that appealed to you; list those aspects of it that would be hard for you to live with—is it the time, the expense, the risk that it entails, or its basic goals? Whatever element you view as any sort of obstacle fits the bill. Next, brainstorm how you might work around each obstacle, giving first priority to ways in which you might

comply with the treatment as it has been planned, but find allies or resources that can make it doable. Then, if you cannot find ways to fit within the standard treatment, consider what modifications might make it more palatable, even if they fall outside regular treatment procedures. Finally, how might you talk about both sets of ideas with a clinician? Despite the fact that you can always take or leave treatments or refuse to comply with their procedures up to a point, the more brainstorming you have done ahead of time, the more likely you are to find a receptive audience who can work with you to tailor the treatment to meet your needs.

2. Although not addressed in this book, evidence exists to support realities already suspected by individuals who have sought professional help on any sort of issue: The clinician–client fit is hugely important to success (Zebrowski, 2007). Factors you may want to consider in identifying a therapist include his or her knowledge of the treatments you are interested in, knowledge of other treatments (since the one you are interested in may not meet all of your needs), and the degree to which you feel he or she understands and aligns with your needs and desires. Taking such factors into consideration, develop a plan for how you might use resources from this book and from online sources, as well as resources you think of yourself, to find the best possible clinician to work with you on your current goals.

3. Measure something about your stuttering for 1 week. This is perhaps a brash idea but one that may be well suited to people who stutter and chose to read this book. Whether you seek the help of a professional, a friend, or another stutterer or you decide to go it alone, you may be helped by learning more about your stuttering—what affects it and how it affects you. You may bridle at this idea, feeling that every minute of every day your attention is drawn painfully, relentlessly, and in excruciating detail to all aspects of your stuttering. However, you may also find that pushing yourself into the role of observer can provide you with different and powerful insights that you can share with others or use yourself.

PARENTS OF CHILDREN WHO STUTTER

Where You Are Now

We can hope that your reading of sections or all of this book has given you a sense that you can make a positive contribution to the future of your child who now stutters, either by helping your child regain his or her status as a fluent speaker or by helping your child firmly establish his or her status as an effective communicator—stuttering not withstanding! However, we understand that coming to terms with those features of a child that may cause him or her pain is not a quick journey and perhaps never a complete one. Nonetheless, the rosy picture facing most children who begin to stutter can probably not be overstated. Information about the biologic underpinnings and potential social consequences of stuttering has burgeoned to an extent that even the small number of children who do not regain fluency face far, far better outcomes than adults who have continued to stutter. And many of them will be the first to say that their lot is not all that bad, either!

Regardless of whether you are currently working with a speech-language pathologist or seeking one, there is a great deal that your knowledge of stuttering can do to improve your interactions with your child as well as your own peace of mind. Consequently, we have some resources to recommend to you—even beyond those you were given in Chapter 1 and those listed up to this point in the chapter. Table 20.3 lists some resources related to more information about treatments, clinicians, and things you can do to advocate for your child and other children with stuttering.

Two Exercises to Take You Further

Below are two exercises that are intended to take your thinking further, possibly using materials you have identified within this book or by examining some of the materials from Table 20.3.

1. Look back through the chapters that you have considered most relevant to you and your child. As you do so, try to identify one thing that you might do in your daily interaction with your child that might help him or her deal with some aspect of stuttering. Try to implement it for 1 week and note what effect it has on your child, on the aspect of

Table 20.3. *Web-Based and Other Resources on Stuttering for Parents of Children Who Stutter*

Pamphlets and videos for parents
- **Pamphlet for Parents** from the Specialty Board on Fluency Disorders (http://www.fluencyspecialists.org/). This publication provides guidance about finding a speech-language pathologist for your child and getting the most out of therapy.
- Brochures such as **Talking with Your Child**, **Brochure for Teens**, and numerous others. Available as a pdfs or linked content on the Stuttering Foundation website (http://www.stutteringhelp.org/).
- Streaming video called "**Stuttering and Your Child: Help for Parents**" is available on the Stuttering Foundation website (http://www.stutteringhelp.org/).

Affording treatment
- **Special Education Law and You** under headings related to parents and therapy in the school on the Stuttering Foundation website.
- **Obtaining Reimbursement for Stuttering Treatment** under headings related to parents and insurance coverage on the Stuttering Foundation website

Materials to share with your child's teacher or speech-language pathologist
- **Tips for Teachers,** available as a pdf on the Stuttering Foundation of America website (http://www.stutteringhelp.org/).
- **Presentation on Stuttering**, available from the National Stuttering Association's website (http://www.westutter.org/) in the area for educators. This brochure gives suggestions for a presentation that could be given to your child's class by your child and his or her speech-language pathologist. A PowerPoint template for such a presentation is also available on the Stuttering Foundation website (http://www.stutteringhelp.org).
- **How Do I Handle Teasing?** is also available from the National Stuttering Association website (http://www.westutter.org/).

Support Groups for You and Your Child
- Two organizations associated with the **National Stuttering Association**
  - **NSAKids:** groups for children from 5 to 12 years old, their parents, and speech-language pathologists.
  - **TWST (Teens Who STutter):** groups for teenagers 13 to 19 years old.
- **Friends: The National Association of Young People Who Stutter** (http://www.friendswhostutter.org/) is an organization that sponsors a national convention and has a website that includes many personal statements by children who stutter.

your child's stuttering that you were interested in affecting, and, finally, on you.

2. If your child is not yet in therapy, you may have developed ideas about what treatment or treatments might be most helpful to your child and most congruent with your values and resources. Although some clinicians adopt and use a specific intervention described in this book, others will draw upon numerous approaches to devise an eclectic treatment approach. And some clinicians will, in fact, have little experience with stuttering and would be unlikely to represent the best choice for your child. Consequently, you will want to develop a plan for finding a clinician whose expertise, philosophy, and demeanor fit you and your child's needs. Resources from Chapter 1 and from Table 20.3 may help you develop a set of questions to ask and people to talk to as a means of finding the right clinician.

PROFESSORS WHO TEACH STUDENTS ABOUT STUTTERING
Where We Are Now

While some of you are reading this section of this final chapter because you always finish books you assign to your class, others may be here because you are in the same position as the first author of this chapter; namely, you may be relatively inexperienced as an instructor on the topic of stuttering and you are looking for help wherever it may be found. As editors, we hope that we have blended a mix of perspectives that should be of special help to those of you in the latter group. Specifically, we represent a combination of the relative inexperience offered by the first author and vast experience offered by the second author. Consequently, we hope that you have already been given some ideas that will help you present information about stuttering treatments in a way

Table 20.4. *Resources for Professors Teaching Courses in Stuttering*

- PowerPoints and quiz questions for *Treatment of Stuttering* are available from the faculty resource area of the thePoint, **Wolters Kluwer Lippincott Williams & Wilkins website** (http://www.lww.com/).
- Sample syllabi, PowerPoint presentations, blogs, podcasts, and therapy materials are all accessible from the link entitled Resources for Professors, Stuttering Course Materials on the **Stuttering Homepage** website (http://www.mnsu.edu/comdis/kuster/stutter.html).

that balances attention to technique, theory, and evidence within a critical perspective that views current inadequacies in treatments as the impetus for continued learning and work.

Regardless of your level of experience, you probably already have ideas about how you will organize your course and what its special features will need to be in order to address the experience, needs, and interests of your particular group of students. Should you follow a conventional class organization in which you focus on the nature, assessment, and treatment of stuttering, you will surely find it necessary to sample from each of the main sections of the text. However, we hope you will also take the opportunity to let students compare interventions intended for similar populations—a task facilitated by the shared organizational plan of each treatment chapter. If you are teaching a course focusing on treatment of stuttering, we would suggest that some of the resources highlighted in the Additional Readings section may increase the depth of information provided in the course, combined, of course, with the most recent publications on stuttering and its treatment.

Still, specifics are always helpful as one faces hours of instruction to plan, execute, and evaluate. Table 20.4 lists a variety of resources; some are provided in association with this book on the publisher's website, and others represent a mere sampling of the supports available on the World Wide Web and elsewhere. The generosity represented by the availability of syllabi, PowerPoint lectures, and videotaped materials should add to the energy that instructors often feel when they are preparing to teach a class for the first or twenty-first time—this time, it will be the best ever!

RECOMMENDATIONS FOR FURTHERING RESEARCH

In this final section of the book, we want to address a new audience—one that is likely to be well aware of much of the research evidence described in this volume—namely, researchers. Despite their familiarity with the research in stuttering, however, we hope that the context in which it is treated here may allow them to see what they know in a new light. Here, as we end our work on this project, we will briefly touch upon some of the conclusions we have reached about some good next steps for researchers. Although some are quite general, others are very specific

First, there is a considerable need for research evidence supporting treatments for each age group. We hope that this statement is not greeted by too many groans from readers, given that "more research is needed" amounts to an almost hackneyed, yet reasonable sentence for any research report. To justify the lack of groaning (or end it sooner), let's also be more specific. Research for preschool interventions would benefit from more consistent attention to the possibility that natural recovery, rather than effects of the treatment, is captured in studies designed to show treatment efficacy. This would entail more consistently using children who have not shown natural recovery for a period of time (e.g., 6 to 12 months) as participants and, ideally, incorporating random assignment and control groups of similar children. For school-age children, even basic demonstrations of treatment efficacy may help families and clinicians more easily secure school-based services or funding for private treatment through insurance. The challenge for research on adolescent and adult treatments is to determine which outcomes clients value most (e.g., reduced severity of stuttering; greater freedom to speak out, whether stuttering or not; and/ or better communication skills) and to develop valid long-term measures of these outcomes. It may also be particularly valuable for this group of clients to examine variables beyond techniques, especially those focusing on clinician characteristics, to find ways to increase the value of interventions (Zebrowski, 2007).

As a second recommendation, we hope researchers will respond to the rich opportunities for research related to the posttreatment changes in brain activity described in Chapters 17 (drug therapies for stuttering) and 19 (neuroimaging). These changes apparently enhance some speech-language processing capacities that underlie increased fluency, but what are they?

Some answers to this question are suggested in Chapters 17 and 19 and in other publications on posttreatment brain activity changes (De Nil et al., 2003; Neumann et al., 2003). It is clear that speech and language processing areas of the left hemisphere that have been underactive prior to treatment become more active after treatment. This shift has been described as resulting in "optimized sequencing and timing of articulatory, phonatory and respiratory movements gained through fluency-shaping therapy" (Neumann et al., 2003, p. 385). De Nil et al. (2003) have emphasized the increase in voluntariness of treated stutterers' "control over the execution and sequencing of their articulatory movements" (p. 375) and has noted the left hemisphere's specialization in "monitoring, sequencing and timing of sequential movements" (p. 374). The treatments studied by both groups were modified versions of the Precision Fluency Shaping Program (Webster, 1974), which requires clients to "reconstruct" their speech production through highly conscious monitoring of respiratory, phonatory, and articulatory movements, at first in slow motion and then at more normal rates in increasingly normal contexts (see Chapter 15 for a detailed description). Given the left hemisphere's specialization described earlier, it is likely that this intervention approach uses left hemisphere pathways to achieve this highly conscious fluency. What does this suggest about research needs?

One obvious need is to find the best, most efficient and effective therapy procedures to activate these left hemisphere structures. Are the best ones those used in the Precision Fluency Shaping approach? Are there other alternatives, such as those described in Chapter 14 on the Camperdown Program, that should be studied with neuroimaging? Retraining speech production using motor learning principles may have much to offer, both in terms of establishing new patterns of speech production as well as helping clients transfer the skills to daily life situations (Maas et al., 2008).

Treatment procedures used by stuttering modification approaches, including the use of highly conscious voluntary stuttering and proprioception (Van Riper, 1973), may also activate left hemisphere networks supporting accurate timing of sequential movements. It is not accidental that some of Van Riper's procedures may activate left hemisphere networks because they were based on his belief that "when a person stutters on a word, there is a temporal disruption of the simultaneous and successive programming of muscular movements required to produce one of the word's integrated sounds" (Van Riper, 1982, p. 415). His speculation about the nature of stuttering (and thus what his treatment attempts to overcome) is similar to the suggestions about what may change in treatment made by De Nil et al. (2003) and Neumann et al. (2003), quoted earlier.

In addition to studies of treatment procedures that make speech production more highly conscious and controlled, both groups have suggested the need for research into the comparative brain activity changes in those clients who continue to maintain fluency and those who do not. There may be several possibilities; different individuals may use different strategies to maintain fluency, and these may be reflected in different changes in brain structure and function. Some individuals may be able to develop new pathways (close to dysfunctional pathways) for neural loops that support fluency—pathways that link speech planning, execution, and feedback so that spontaneous automatized speech is possible. These may appear as new left hemisphere areas of activation in the immediate neighborhood of tracts used by normal speakers. Other individuals may maintain fluency only by long-term use of highly controlled fluency skills, such as slow rate and easy onset of voicing. The voluntary nature of this speech control may create more activity in the left hemisphere than seen prior to treatment, as well as activation in right hemisphere homologous areas, because the effort of such highly conscious control would involve many areas of the brain. These two scenarios might be in contrast to those individuals who relapse after treatment. In individuals who relapse, more right than left hemisphere activation—akin to patterns prior to treatment—may be typical. These would be individuals who can only maintain fluency by using highly voluntary speech but who are unable to meet this demand long term.

The chapters in this book describing treatments that may compensate for dysfunctions in the left hemisphere may not be limited to Chapters 14 (Camperdown) and 15 (Fluency Plus). Chapter 16 (SpeechEasy) describes a device that may circumvent auditory feedback deficits resulting from inactivity in left sensorimotor and auditory processing areas. Perhaps neural tissue nearby these damaged areas can be temporarily recruited while wearing this device and attending to the auditory signal. It is noteworthy that the device seems to have little carryover effect and requires the wearer to continue to attend to the signal, suggesting that new brain activity stimulated by the device does not change the habitual (perhaps right hemisphere) patterns used by the client.

Chapter 17 (pharmacologic treatment) suggests that one basic dysfunction in stuttering is inactivity in the striatum, part of the basal ganglia that serves as a way station in a loop between the speech motor cortex and subcortical structures, including other components of the basal ganglia involved in temporal regulation of speech. Brain imaging studies described in Chapter 17 indicate that both left cortical speech motor areas and subcortical areas such as the striatum are not as active in stutterers as in nonstutterers. Drugs that decrease the effect of dopamine, which is hypothesized to decrease striatal activity, appear to reduce stuttering. It does not appear that brain imaging studies have been done after the administration of these drugs to see which areas appear to be activated by the drug. It would be of interest to perform neuroimaging studies of both fluency-shaping therapies and pharmacotherapies to see if similar left hemisphere reactivations occur.

FINAL COMMENTS

We hope our brief remarks to researchers—present and future—provide a good beginning. In some ways, the paths ahead are clear. More research of the kind already undertaken to add to the support for existing interventions is needed. At the same time, new paths are opening. The tools available to researchers to examine the nature of stuttering have never been richer—from psychological tools for understanding the effects of stuttering on the lives of those who stutter to imaging techniques designed to examine the physiologic underpinnings of stuttering. Clinicians and researchers, using these tools, may lead us not just to a better understanding of the nature of stuttering, but also to increasingly effective methods for meeting the needs of those who already stutter and preventing persistent stuttering in future generations of children. The journey ahead has never been more promising.

APPENDIX 11.1

Assessment of the Audiovisual Session

Participants use this sheet to provide self-assessment and feedback for other participants regarding their quality of Smooth Speech and how socially appropriate they were during the speech.

Name _____ Date _____

Self-Assessment

	Self	Clinician	Agreement
Airflow continuity during the phrase Poor airflow / reasonable airflow / excellent airflow			
Phrasing and pausing (P+P) Poor P+P / reasonable P+P / excellent P+P			
Speech rate Slow speech rate / correct speech rate / fast speech rate			
Intonation Poor or boring / interesting / excellent intonation			
Presentation (eye contact, facial expression, posture) Poor / reasonable / excellent presentation			

Other Assessment

	Other	Clinician	Agreement
Airflow continuity during the phrase Poor airflow / reasonable airflow / excellent airflow			
Phrasing and pausing (P+P) Poor P+P / reasonable P+P / excellent P+P			
Speech rate Slow speech rate / correct speech rate / fast speech rate			

(CONTINUED)	Other	Clinician	Agreement
Intonation Poor or boring / interesting / excellent intonation			
Presentation (eye contact, facial expression, posture) Poor / reasonable / excellent presentation			

	Other	Clinician	Agreement
Airflow continuity during the phrase Poor airflow / reasonable airflow / excellent airflow			
Phrasing and pausing (P+P) Poor P+P / reasonable P+P / excellent P+P			
Speech rate Slow speech rate / correct speech rate / fast speech rate			
Intonation Poor or boring / interesting / excellent intonation			
Presentation (eye contact, facial expression, posture) Poor / reasonable / excellent presentation			

	Other	Clinician	Agreement
Airflow continuity during the phrase Poor airflow / reasonable airflow / excellent airflow			
Phrasing and pausing (P+P) Poor P+P / reasonable P+P / excellent P+P			
Speech rate Slow speech rate / correct speech rate / fast speech rate			
Intonation Poor or boring / interesting / excellent intonation			
Presentation (eye contact, facial expression, posture) Poor / reasonable / excellent presentation			

APPENDIX 14.1

Fluency Cycles Record Form

Fluency Cycles Record Form

Date	Cycle	Practice		Trial						Evaluation / Strategies
				Aim		Result				
		What ratings I give myself when I try to copy the pattern		*What ratings I am hoping to achieve in the next trial*		*What ratings I think I achieved in that trial*		*What ratings I think I achieved after listening to the recording of my trial. What is my strategy for the next trial? SR>2-P; SR<3-P/T; Every third cycle-P.*		
		SR	NAT	SR	NAT	SR	NAT	SR	NAT	
Clinic	1	1	7	1	4	2	3	2	2	More practice & consolidation
	2	1	7	1	5	1	5	1	5	Consolidate
	3	–	–	1	5	1	5	1	4	→ Home
Home day 1	4	1	7	1	5	1	4	1	4	Increase NAT
	5	–	–	1	4	1	4	2	3	Try to eliminate stuttering
	6	–	–	1	3	2	3	2	3	Stutter still there so more technique
	7	1	7	1	4	1	4	1	4	Consolidate
Home day 2	8	1	7	1	4	1	4	1	4	Less prolonged speech
	9	1	7	1	3	1	3	1	3	Less prolonged speech
	10	1	7	1	2	2	2	2	2	Too much stuttering → more prolonged speech
	11	1	7	1	3	1	3	1	3	Good consolidation
	12	–	–	1	3	1	3	1	3	

Neuroimaging Techniques

Regardless of functional neuroimaging technology, the final image of the working brain is the result of a statistical computation process. This procedure ("statistical parametric mapping") calculates whether the activity changes in a specific brain region are significant. The scanner produces an activity "map," represented as voxels, of the target area. A voxel (derived from *volumetric* and *pixel*) is a volume element that is represented by coordinate values on a regular grid in three-dimensional space. It is the three-dimensional equivalent of a pixel in a two-dimensional image.

To evaluate which brain regions are significantly more active during performance of a task compared with another task or with a relative rest state, special statistical procedures have to be carried out stepwise to accommodate for random effects and factors other than the task differences that may contribute to activation changes and to highlight the areas of activity linked specifically to the process under investigation (e.g., to look for the most significant difference to background brain activity). Regions of interest can be defined as specific brain regions that are expected to change their activity during a particular task.

Before the statistical analysis, the images have to be preprocessed. This procedure includes realignment, spatial normalization, and smoothing. Realignment corrects the images for head motions between scans. With spatial normalization, the brain images of the individual participants are adjusted for differences in brain shape and size. This process involves translation, rotation, and nonlinear warping of the brain surface to match a standard brain template. Such standard brain maps are the Talairach-Tournoux map and the templates from the Montreal Neurological Institute. Smoothing is a procedure to enhance the signal-to-noise ratio by relating voxel values to neighboring voxel values, using a Gaussian filter or a wavelet transformation.

After preprocessing, the proper statistical analysis is performed by assuming parametric statistical models at each voxel. The statistical method of general linear model is carried out to describe the respective variability in the data due to experimental and confounding effects and the residual variability. Hypotheses expressed in terms of the model parameters are assessed at each voxel with univariate statistics. Analyses may also examine correlations between a task variable and brain activity in a certain area over time, using linear convolution models. Because many statistical tests are being conducted, corrections for multiple comparisons have to be made.

The data are presented either as a table displaying coordinates of the significant differences in activities between tasks or as color-coded images. The latter are shown as MRI brain "slices" or three-dimensional reconstructions of the brain with the colors representing the location of voxels that have shown statistically significant differences between conditions. The color gradients are mapped according to statistical t or z values, resulting in an intuitively understandable visualization of the statistical strength of activation. Activation differences may also be represented as a "glass brain"—a representation of three outline views of the brain as if it were transparent, in which regions of activation are visible as areas of shading.

In the following sections, neuroimaging methods that have been applied in stuttering research are described.

POSITRON EMISSION TOMOGRAPHY

PET is a method to observe brain metabolism and changes in blood flow. Its principle is as follows. A radioactive solution containing atoms that emit positrons (positively charged electrons) is mixed with a chemical and infused as a tracer into the bloodstream. The tracer disintegrates in the body and emits positrons wherever the blood goes. The positrons interact with electrons to create photons emitted as electromagnetic radiation. The locations of those positron-emitting atoms are found by detectors that pick up the photons (Bear, Connors, & Paradiso, 2007).

The positron-emitting radioisotopes are produced in cyclotrons by bombarding atoms of stable chemical elements with protons. The resulting isotopes (for example, oxygen-15, carbon-11, nitrogen-13, or fluorine-18) have short half-lives. They shed their excess positive charge (more positive charge in the nuclei of the isotopes than can be balanced by the negative charge of their orbiting electrons) in the form of discrete positron emission (Huesing, Jaencke, & Tag, 2006). These radionuclides are incorporated into compounds normally used by the body, such as glucose (or glucose analogs), water, or ammonia, or into molecules that bind to receptors or other sites of drug action, depending on the research question. Such labeled compounds are called radiotracers. PET technology can be used to trace the biologic pathway of any compound in humans, provided that it can be radiolabeled with a PET isotope. Thus, hundreds of radiotracers are in use, either clinically or in research.

After the injection of the radiotracer into a vein, a waiting period follows while the active molecule becomes concentrated in tissues of interest. In functional neuroimaging, when the radiation has reached its maximum in the brain, images of regional cerebral blood flow are taken in a PET scanner. The PET signal is the result of the collision of the positrons that broke off from their unstable isotopes with electrons. The collision produces two gamma rays or photons moving in opposite directions. The photons are captured by the PET scanner, which identifies the source of these gamma rays along the line connecting the two sensors that had detected the beams. Increased neural activities in a brain region lead to increases in metabolism and blood flow and can be visualized as a denser distribution of gamma rays. The volume of metabolic activity, which can be measured by PET scans, amounts to 4 to 6 mm^3, which is enough to identify activated cortical and subcortical areas and to show variations within cortical areas.

PET can locate active regions in the brain involved, for instance, in speaking and listening.

The activations are visible by comparing images taken before and during a particular task. In functional neuroimaging, PET is used to study brain activations during cognitive tasks, as well as the nature and symptoms of depression, Parkinson's disease, and other diseases affecting the brain. The impact of drugs on brain activity can also be evaluated. In addition, PET can be used to study the distribution of receptors, as well as their interaction with certain drugs and neurotransmitters (there are more than 300 different kinds of receptors in the human brain that interact with approximately 100 identifiable neurotransmitters).

After data collection and preprocessing, statistical data analysis and three-dimensional reconstructions are performed. PET results can be seen as changes in the regional cerebral blood flow between different experimental conditions. Because PET has low spatial resolution, modern PET scanners integrate CT scanners, and both PET and CT are performed in one session, so that PET findings can be correlated more precisely with anatomic structures. The PET method also presents some additional disadvantages; specifically, it has limited temporal resolution. Moreover, it is invasive and exposes the examined subject to radioactive tracers, which limits its repeatability. Because only a few PET images per subject can be acquired, it is necessary to conduct group studies.

SINGLE PHOTON EMISSION COMPUTED TOMOGRAPHY

SPECT is similar to PET in its use of radioactive tracers and detection of gamma rays. However, SPECT detects a different type of photon, and the tracer used in SPECT emits gamma radiation that is measured directly. In contrast, recall that the PET tracer emits positrons that annihilate electrons up to a few millimeters away, causing two gamma photons to be emitted in opposite directions. A PET scanner detects these emissions almost in real time, which provides more radiation event localization information and thus, with a resolution of approximately 0.5 mm, produces higher resolution images than SPECT, which produces images with a resolution of approximately 1 cm.

As with PET, SPECT is based on conventional nuclear medicine imaging and tomographic reconstruction methods (Committee on the Mathematics and Physics of Emerging Dynamic Biomedical Imaging & National Research Council, 1996). Like PET, SPECT requires an injection of radiotracers to examine their spatial concentration in the brain. The intensity with which radiotracers are absorbed by different organs and tissue types depends on their biodistribution properties. The imaging device is a scintillation camera system that provides a two-dimensional projection image of the three-dimensional radioactivity distribution or radiopharmaceutical uptake in the brain. Because images are taken during the rotation of the gamma camera at different views around the patient, a three-dimensional model from multiple projections can be constructed. Images are acquired at certain points during the rotation, typically every 3 to 6 degrees.

As with PET, the range of SPECT application includes not only functional imaging but any gamma ray–based imaging where three-dimensional representations are necessary, such as the imaging of thyroid, bone, heart disease, tumors, infections, or brain injuries. In functional brain imaging, SPECT is used, for instance, to support the diagnosis of dementia.

SPECT is less expensive than PET because it does not require an accelerator nearby to produce tracers (due to the long half-life of SPECT tracers compared with PET tracers). Disadvantages of SPECT are distortions of the CT-similar reconstructed images due to poor spatial resolution, statistical noise fluctuations, and low contrast. Gamma ray photons may undergo photoelectric interactions that cause absorption of photons before exiting the patient. Other photons undergo Compton scattering, an effect that changes the direction and energy of the original photons. In stuttering research, SPECT has been used several times for the identification of the sites of lesions that are associated with acquired stuttering (Heuer et al. 1996; Turgut, Utku, & Balci, 2002).

FUNCTIONAL MAGNETIC RESONANCE IMAGING

fMRI reflects local changes in cerebral blood oxygenation evoked by sensory, motor, or cognitive tasks. It has revolutionized our understanding of the functioning brain because hundreds of high-resolution images can be obtained from a single subject, permitting a detailed analysis of brain activity. The principle of fMRI is as follows. MRI is based on the detection of electromagnetic signals (radiofrequency [RF] waves) that emanate from spinning hydrogen protons when they are excited by an RF pulse applied in the presence of an externally generated static magnetic field. The RF pulse excites the spinning protons and causes the spines to become synchronized (phase-locked), which is the precondition for the production of a strong signal. Magnetic inhomogeneities within the tissue cause minute shifts in the RFs of neighboring hydrogen protons within each voxel, causing them to fall out of synchronization (dephasing), which leads to a reduction of the RF signal. Differences in the rate of dephasing (called T2*) indirectly reflect neuronal activity (DeYoe et al., 1994).

The so-called blood oxygenation level dependent (BOLD) mechanism explains how changes in neuronal activity affect the magnetic resonance signal. Each sensory, motor, or cognitive task produces a localized increase in neuronal activity. This activity causes a local vasodilatation followed by a rapid increase in blood flow either by production of metabolites or by a direct effect on local blood vessels. This change in blood flow causes strong oxygen delivery, and an excess of oxygenated hemoglobin is delivered to the activated region, thereby reducing the concentration of deoxy-hemoglobin. Deoxy-hemoglobin is paramagnetic, whereas oxy-hemoglobin is not, and the change in the amount of deoxy-hemoglobin causes a dephasing of spinning hydrogen proteins and a resulting change of the RF signal, which appears as bright regions in the final fMRI images. Images are obtained in an magnetic resonance scanner designed for rapid gradient field switching. Scanners with higher magnetic field power produce images of higher resolution. Currently, 1.5-, 3-, and 9.4-tesla scanners (the latter for research aims only) are available. A subject is positioned supine inside the magnetic resonance scanner with his head inside a head coil and then engages in a series of tasks, which are presented either by a visual or by an acoustic system. A temporal series of usually several hundred images is obtained for each slice of the brain. The statistically significant voxels are color-coded and overlaid on anatomic images.

The most widespread fMRI technique is the BOLD-fMRI. It can provide images in a temporal resolution of approximately 1 second and a spatial resolution of 1 to 2 mm, which is much higher than that of PET and SPECT images. Approximately 30 images of brain slices are taken approximately every 2 seconds. Because images taken during different cognitive states are compared, these states should differ, if possible, in only one aspect. Several periods of rest alternate with several periods of activation. BOLD-fMRI is of special interest for studies dealing with language, vision, movement, hearing, and memory. One of the biggest problems with this technique is its sensitivity to movement, making speech production difficult to examine. Furthermore, brain regions located adjacent to large draining veins are sometimes more activated than the sites of neuronal activation. BOLD-fMRI measures regional differences in oxygenated blood. Another fMRI technique is the perfusion fMRI, which measures the regional blood flow (Huesing, Jaencke, & Tag, 2006).

Because fMRI is noninvasive, has no significant risks, is available in many clinics, and can be used in presurgical planning when the mapping of language, motor, and memory functions is necessary, it is used in a wide range of studies and clinical applications and has become the most important driving force of cognitive neurosciences. fMRI can make precise images of transient cognitive events and small structures, does not involve injection of radioactive materials, is suitable for investigations in healthy children due to its low risk, and allows statistical statements when comparing different mental and cognitive states within an individual in a single session.

fMRI is not rapid enough to observe the transient coordinations and oscillations of neuronal activities occurring across certain cortical areas during the performance of cognitive tasks. The temporal resolution needed for that is within the order of milliseconds. Because this resolution is only accessible by electromagnetic source imaging using surface recordings of multichannel EEG or MEG that allow true real-time measurements, such techniques are increasingly combined with fMRI to produce a relatively precise estimation of sensory, motor, and cognitive processes (Momjian et al., 2003).

DIFFUSION TENSOR IMAGING

DTI measures the directionality and magnitude of water diffusion in brain tissue. This technique can be applied to the assessment of white matter maturation, tract-specific localization of white matter lesions anf localization of tumors in relation to the white matter tracts, and localization of the main white matter tracts (tractography) for purposes such as neurosurgical planning.

DTI exploits the finding that the random diffusion-driven displacement of molecules in tissues, in particular of water molecules, may be anisotropic or "directionally dependent." The observation of this displacement provides clues to the structure and geometric organization of tissues. What does this mean? Molecular diffusion, which refers to the random translational motion of molecules, also called Brownian motion, is a truly three-dimensional process. However, because of the peculiar physical arrangement of the medium or the presence of obstacles that limit molecular movement in some directions, mobility of molecules in tissues may not be the same in all directions. This effect, called diffusion anisotropy, can be detected by DTI. If diffusion gradients are applied in at least three directions, a tensor for each voxel can be calculated that describes the three-dimensional shape of molecule diffusion. Only molecular displacements that occur along the direction of the gradient are visible. Diffusion anisotropy in white matter can be explained as a result of a specific organization of the fibers in bundles of more or less myelinated axonal fibers running in parallel. Exact mechanisms are still unknown, but it is clear that diffusion in the direction of the fibers is faster than in the perpendicular direction. This helps to map the spatial orientation of the white matter tracts in the brain given the assumption that the direction of fastest diffusion indicates the overall orientation of the fibers. Hence, DTI enables fiber tracking in the white matter of the brain by exploiting diffusion anisotropy effects (Le Bihan et al., 2001). It gives access both to superficial and deep organs with high resolution, providing details on tissue microstructure beyond the usual imaging resolution. In addition, it does not interfere with the diffusion process itself and, therefore, is noninvasive.

MAGNETOENCEPHALOGRAPHY

In areas of neural activity, electricity is generated and produces weak magnetic fields. MEG measures the magnetic fields generated by small electrical currents in neurons. Thus, MEG provides direct information about the dynamics of evoked and spontaneous neural activity and the location of their sources in the brain (Hämäläinen, 2007). MEG and EEG are closely related; EEG measures the electric potentials associated with neuronal currents, whereas MEG detects the corresponding magnetic fields.

Primary sources of the magnetic fields in the brain are excitatory postsynaptic potentials produced by the apical dendrites of pyramidal cells that extend vertically to the surface of the cerebral cortex. These excitatory potentials cause electric currents (dipoles). The dipoles are generated in a perpendicular direction to the cortex and produce magnetic fields. MEG selectively records activity oriented parallel to the surface of the brain (activity of pyramidal cells in the superficial parts of the sulci), whereas EEG records electrical activity oriented perpendicular to the surface of the brain (activity of pyramidal cells in cortical gyri and in the depth of the sulci). Thus, MEG is suitable for examination areas such as the auditory cortex located deep in the sylvian fissure.

Because magnetic fields produced by the neural activities are extremely weak, a highly sensitive magnetic flux densitometer is necessary to measure them, called a superconducting quantum interference device (SQUID). The SQUID requires cryogenic temperatures for operation. In modern MEG devices, an array of more than 300 SQUIDs is contained in a helmet-shaped liquid helium–containing vessel, allowing simultaneous measurements at many points over the head (Hämäläinen, 2007).

Advantages of MEG are many. It is noninvasive and nonhazardous. Signals can be recorded over the whole cortex, yet it does not require the placement of many electrodes on the scalp, as with EEG. The data can be collected in the natural seated position. Unlike PET and fMRI, which index brain activity only indirectly by way of blood flow and thus have a low temporal resolution, MEG has an extremely high temporal resolution (milliseconds), which allows a real-time recording of the brain activity. It also provides a good spatial resolution, from several millimeters to a couple of centimeters. However, its spatial resolution is not as good as that of fMRI. Finally, the measurement environment is completely silent, which especially facilitates auditory studies.

Major limitations of MEG are as follows: the localization of sources of electrical activity within the brain from magnetic measurement outside the head is complicated, and it is difficult to provide reliable information about subcortical sources of brain activity. Because MEG does not provide structural information, MEG data often have to be combined with magnetic resonance data into a composite image of function overlaid on anatomy to obtain activation maps. MEG is used for clinical purposes (e.g., to localize epileptiform spiking activity in epilepsy patients) and research purposes (e.g., to study language perception).

VOXEL-BASED MORPHOMETRY

VBM is one of the techniques developed to detect anatomic group differences in the stereotactic distribution of tissue types in the brain (Huesing, Jaencke, & Tag, 2006), where "stereotactic" means in relation to a special coordinate system used in the study and treatment of brain structures. It is used to investigate focal differences in brain anatomy using statistical parametric mapping. VBM analyzes gray matter, but for the analysis, white matter and cerebrospinal fluid volumes have to be segmented too. Although it is predominantly a tool to examine gray matter, it is also sometimes used for analyzing white matter. However, the white matter results are biased, and VBM is not the method of choice here, instead DTI is. Analyses are carried out after linear alignment of individual MRI scans to an image template in a standard brain map (Talairach space). The goal of the comparative analyses is to find group tissue differences at each stereotaxic voxel by computing a statistical parametric map in which each voxel is assessed by statistically quantifying the differences between groups at that particular stereotaxic position. Calculated values are compared with a reference distribution, which gives a probability value indicating whether such differences could occur by chance.

VBM has become an established tool in morphometry since 1995. VBM can be used not only for examining differences across subjects, but also for examining neuroanatomic differences between hemispheres in order to detect brain asymmetry. Originally, it was devised to detect cortical thinning in a way that was not confounded by volume changes, a problem characteristic of classical volumetric analyses of large brain structures. This result can be achieved by removing positional and volume differences through spatial normalization (Ashburner & Friston, 2001).

REFERENCES FOR ALL CHAPTERS

Achenbach, T. M. (1988). *Child Behavior Checklist for Ages 2–3*. Burlington, VT: University of Vermont.

Achenbach, T. M. (1991). *Manual for the Child Behavior Checklist/4-18 and 1991 Profile*. Burlington, VT: Department of Psychiatry, University of Vermont.

Ackermann, H., & Riecker, A. (2004). The contribution of the insula to motor aspects of speech production: A review and a hypothesis. *Brain and Language, 89*, 320–328.

Adams, M. R. (1977). A clinical strategy for differentiating the normally nonfluent child and the incipient stutterer. *Journal of Fluency Disorders, 2*, 141–148.

Adams, M. R. (1984). The differential assessment and direct treatment of stuttering. In J. Costello (Ed.), *Speech Disorders in Children* (pp. 261–290). San Diego, CA: College Hill.

Adams, M. R. (1984) The young stutterer: Diagnosis, treatment and assessment of progress. In W. Perkins (Ed.), *Stuttering Disorders: Current Therapy of Communication Disorders* (pp. 41–56). New York: Thieme.

Adams, M. R. (1990). The demands and capacities model I: Theoretical elaborations. *Journal of Fluency Disorders, 15*, 135–141.

Adams, M. R. (1991). The assessment and treatment of the school-age stutterer. *Seminars in Speech and Language, 12*, 279–290.

Adams, M. R. (1993). The home environment of children who stutter. *Seminars in Speech and Language, 14*, 185–191.

Adams, M. R., & Ramig, P. R. (1980). Vocal characteristics of normal speakers and stutterers during choral reading. *Journal of Speech and Hearing Research, 23*, 257–269.

Ahadi, S. A., & Rothbart, M. K. (1994). Temperament, development, and the Big Five. In G. A. Kohnstamm, C. F. Halverson, et al (Eds.), *The Developing Structure of Temperament and Personality from Infancy to Adulthood* (pp. 189–207). Hillsdale, NJ: Erlbaum.

Allen, G. D., & Hawkins, S. (1980). Phonological rhythm: Definition and development. In G. H. Yen-Komshian, J. F. Kavanagh, & C. A. Ferguson (Eds.), *Child Phonology* (Vol. 1, pp. 227–256). New York: Academic Press.

Alm, P. A. (2004). Stuttering and the basal ganglia circuits: a critical review of possible relations. *Journal of Communication Disorders, 37*, 325–369.

Alm, P. A. (2005). On the causal mechanisms of stuttering. Doctoral thesis. Department of Clinical Neuroscience, Lund University, Lund, Sweden.

Alm, P., & Risberg, J. (2007). Stuttering in adults: The acoustic startle response, temperamental traits and biological factors. *Journal of Communication Disorders, 40*, 1–41.

Amaro E., Jr., Williams, S. C., Shergill, S. S., Fu, C. H., MacSweeney, M., Picchioni, M. M., Brammer, M. J., & McGuire, P. K. (2002). Acoustic noise and functional magnetic resonance imaging: current strategies and future prospects. *Journal of Magnetic Resonance Imaging, 16*, 497–510.

Ambrose, N. G., Cox, N., & Yairi, E. (1993). Genetic aspects of early childhood stuttering. *Journal of Speech and Hearing Research, 36*, 701–706.

Ambrose, N. G., Cox, N. J., & Yairi, E. (1997). The genetic basis of persistence and recovery in stuttering. *Journal of Speech, Language and Hearing Research, 40*, 567–580.

Ambrose, N. G., & Yairi, E., (1999). Normative disfluency data for early childhood stuttering. *Journal of Speech, Language, and Hearing Research, 42*, 895–909.

American Psychiatric Association. (1994). *Diagnostic and Statistical Manual of Mental Disorders*. Washington, DC: American Psychiatric Association Publication.

American Psychiatric Association. (2000). *Diagnostic and Statistical Manual of Mental Disorders: DSM-IV-TR*. (4th ed.). Washington, DC: American Psychiatric Association.

American Psychiatric Association. (2000). Practice guidelines for the treatment of patients with major depressive disorder (revision). *American Journal of Psychiatry, 157*, 1–45.

American Speech-Language-Hearing Association. (1995). Guidelines for practice in stuttering treatment. *ASHA, 37* (Suppl 14), 26–35.

American Speech-Language-Hearing Association. (2001). *Scope of Practice in Speech Language Pathology*. Rockville, MD: American Speech-Language-Hearing Association.

American Speech-Language-Hearing Association. (2003). Code of ethics. http://www.professional.asha.org/resources/deskrefs.

Amster, B. (1984). The development of speech rate in normal preschool children. Unpublished doctoral dissertation, Temple University, Philadelphia, PA.

Anderson, J., & Conture, E. G. (2000). Language abilities of children who stutter: A preliminary study. *Journal of Fluency Disorders, 25*, 283–304.

Anderson, J., & Conture, E. G. (2004). Sentence-structure priming in young children who do and do not stutter. *Journal of Speech, Language, and Hearing Research, 47*, 552–571.

Anderson, J., Pellowski, M., & Conture, E. (2005). Childhood stuttering and dissociations across linguistic domains. *Journal of Fluency Disorders, 30*, 219–253.

Anderson, J., Pellowski, M., Conture, E., & Kelly, E. (2003). Temperamental characteristics of young children who stutter. *Journal of Speech, Language and Hearing Research, 46*, 1221–1223.

Andrews, G., & Craig, A. (1988). Prediction of outcome after treatment for stuttering. *The British Journal of Psychiatry, 153*, 236–240.

Andrews, G., Craig, A., Feyer, A., Hoddinott, S., Howie, P., & Neilson, M. (1983). Stuttering: a review of research findings and theories circa 1982. *Journal of Speech and Hearing Disorders, 48*, 226–246.

Andrews, G., & Cutler, J. (1974). Stuttering therapy: The relation between changes in symptom level and attitudes. *Journal of Speech and Hearing Disorders, 39*, 312–319.

Andrews, G., & Dosza, M. (1977). Haloperidol and the treatment of stuttering. *Journal of Fluency Disorders, 2*, 217–224.

Andrews, G., Guitar, B., & Howie, P. (1980). Meta-analysis of the effects of stuttering treatment. *Journal of Speech and Hearing Disorders, 45*, 287–307.

Andrews, G., Howie, P. M., Dozsa, M., & Guitar, B. (1982). Stuttering: Speech pattern characteristics under fluency-inducing conditions. *Journal of Speech and Hearing Research, 25*, 208–216.

Andrews, G., & Ingham, R. J. (1972). Stuttering: An evaluation of follow-up procedures for syllable-timed speech/token system therapy. *Journal of Communication Disorders, 5*, 307–319.

Andrews, G., Morris-Yates, A., Howie, P., & Martin, N. (1991). Genetic factors in stuttering confirmed. *Archives of General Psychiatry, 48*, 1034–1035.

Andrews, G., & Tanner, S. (1982). Stuttering: The results of 5 days treatment with an airflow technique. *Journal of Speech and Hearing Disorders, 47*, 427–429.

Appelt, A. (1945). *Stammering and Its Permanent Cure: A Treatise on Individual Psychological Lines*. London: Methuen.

Armson, J., Foote, S., Witt, C., Kalinowski, J., & Stuart, A. (1997). Effect of frequency altered feedback and audience size on stuttering. *European Journal of Disorders of Communication, 32*, 359–366.

Armson, J., Kiefte, M., Mason, J., & De Croos, D. (2006). The effects of SpeechEasy on stuttering frequency in laboratory conditions. *Journal of Fluency Disorders, 31*, 137–152.

Armson, J., & Stuart, A. (1998). Effect of extended exposure to frequency-altered feedback on stuttering during reading and monologue. *Journal of Speech, Language, and Hearing Research, 41*, 479–490.

Arndt, J., & Healey, E. C. (2001). Concomitant disorders in school-age children who stutter. *Language, Speech, and Hearing Services in Schools, 32*, 68–78.

Arnold, H. S., Conture, E. G., & Ohde, R. N. (2005). Phonological neighborhood density in the picture naming of young children who stutter: Preliminary study. *Journal of Fluency Disorders, 30*, 125–148.

Aron, M. L. (1967). The relationships between measurements of stuttering behavior. *Journal of the South African Speech and Hearing Association, 14*, 15–34.

Ashburner, J., & Friston, K. J. (2001). Why voxel-based morphometry should be used. *NeuroImage, 14*, 1238–1243.

Atack, J. R., Pike, A., Marshall, G., Stanley, J., Lincoln, R., Cook, S. M., Lewis, R. T., Blackaby, W. P., Goodacre, S. C., McKernan, R. M., Dawson, G. R., Wafford, K. A., & Reynolds, D. S. (2006). The in vivo properties of pagoclone in rat are most likely mediated by 5'-hydroxy pagoclone. *Neuropharmacology, 50*, 677–689.

Atlas, R., & Pepler, D. (1997). *Observations of Bullying in the Classroom*. Toronto: LaMarsh Centre for Research on Violence and Conflict Resolution, York University.

Attanasio, J. (2003). Some observations and reflections. In M. Onslow, A. Packman, & E. Harrison (Eds.), *The LP of Early Stuttering Intervention: A Clinician's Guide* (pp. 207–214). Austin, TX: Pro-Ed.

Au-Yeung, J., & Howell, P. (1998). Lexical and syntactic context and stuttering. *Clinical Linguistics and Phonetics, 12*, 67–78.

Azrin, N., & Nunn, R. (1974). A rapid method of eliminating stuttering by a regulated breathing approach. *Behavior Research and Therapy, 12*, 279–286.

Azrin, N., Nunn, R., & Frantz, S. (1979). Comparison of regulated-breathing versus abbreviated desensitization on reported stuttering episodes. *Journal of Speech and Hearing Disorders, 44*, 331–339.

Badgaiyan, R. D., Schacter, D. L., & Alpert, N. M. (2002) Retrieval of relational information: a role for the left inferior prefrontal cortex. *NeuroImage, 17*, 393–400.

Baer, D. M. (1988). If you know why you're changing a behavior, you'll know when you've changed it enough. *Behavioral Assessment, 10*, 219–223.

Baer, D. M. (1990). The critical issue in treatment efficacy is knowing why treatment was applied: A student's response to Roger Ingham. In L.B. Olswang, C.K. Thompson, S. F. Warren, & N. J. Minghetti

(Eds.), *Treatment Efficacy Research in Communication Disorders* (pp. 31–39). Rockville, MD: American Speech-Language-Hearing Foundation.

Bakker, K., Brutten, G. J., Janssen, P., & van der Meulen, S. (1991). An eyemarking study of anticipation and dysfluency among elementary school stutterers. *Journal of Fluency Disorders, 16,* 25–33.

Bakker, K., & Riley, G. (1997). *Computerized Scoring of Stuttering Severity.* Austin, TX: Pro-Ed.

Bär, K. J., Häger, F., & Sauer, H. (2004). Olanzapine- and clozapine-induced stuttering. A case series. *Pharmacopsychiatry, 37,* 131–134.

Barlow, D. H., & Hersen, M. (1984). *Single-Case Experimental Designs: Strategies for Studying Behavior Change* (2nd ed.). New York: Pergamon.

Barnes, T. R. (1989). A rating scale for drug-induced akathisia. *British Journal of Psychiatry, 154,* 672–676.

Barrett, P. M., Dadds, M. R., & Rapee, R. M. (1996). Family treatment of childhood anxiety: A controlled trial. *Journal of Consulting and Clinical Psychology, 64,* 333–342.

Bates, E., Appelbaum, M., Salcedo, J., Saygin, A. P., & Pizzamiglio, L. (2003). Quantifying dissociations in neuropsychological research. *Journal of Clinical and Experimental Neuropsychology, 25,* 1128–1153.

Beal, D. S., Gracco, V. L., Lafaille, S. J., & De Nil, L. F. (2007). Voxel-based morphometry of auditory and speech-related cortex in stutterers. *NeuroReport, 18,* 1257–1260.

Bear, M. B., Connors, B. W., & Paradiso, M. A. (2007). *Neuroscience. Exploring the Brain* (3rd ed.). Philadelphia: Lippincott.

Beck, A. (1976). *Cognitive Therapy and Emotional Disorders.* New York: New American Library.

Beck, J. S. (1995). *Cognitive Therapy: Basics and Beyond.* New York: The Gilford Press.

Beeson, P.M. & Robey, R.R. (2006). Evaluating single-subject treatment research: Lessons learned from the aphasia literature. *Neuropsychology* Review, 16, 161–169.

Beidel, D. C., Turner, S. M., & Morris, T. L. (2000). *SPAI-C. Social Phobia & Anxiety Inventory for Children.* New York: Multi-Health Systems Inc.

Beitchman, J. H., Wilson, B., Johnson, C. J., Atkinson, L., Young, A., Adlar, E., et al. (2001). Fourteen-year follow-up of speech/language impaired and control children: Psychiatric outcome. *Journal of American Academy of Child and Adolescent Psychiatry, 40,* 75–82.

Bennett, E. M. (2006). *Working with People Who Stutter: A Lifespan Approach.* Englewood Cliffs, NJ: Merrill-Prentice Hall.

Bennett, M. K., & Harrison, E. (2005). Using SMS technology to collect early childhood stuttering data prior to treatment: Pilot study. In C. Heine & L. Brown (Eds.), *Proceedings of the 2005 Speech Pathology Australia National Conference, Practicality and Impact: Making a Difference in the Real World* (pp. 97–103). Melbourne, Australia: Speech Pathology Australia.

Berman, R., & Slobin, D. (1994). *Relating Events in Narrative: A Crosslinguistic Developmental Study.* Hillsdale, NJ: Lawrence Erlbaum Associates.

Bernstein Ratner, N. (1995). Language complexity and stuttering in children. *Topics in Language Disorders, 15,* 42–57.

Bernstein Ratner, N. (1997). Stuttering: A psycholinguistic perspective. In R. Curlee & G. Siegel (Eds.), *Nature and Treatment of Stuttering: New Directions* (2nd ed.) (pp. 99–127). Needham, MA: Allyn & Bacon.

Bernstein Ratner, N. (1997). Leaving Las Vegas: Clinical odds and individual outcomes. *American Journal of Speech Language Pathology, 6,* 29–33.

Bernstein Ratner, N., & Sih, C. (1987). The effects of gradual increases in sentence length and complexity on children's disfluency. *Journal of Speech and Hearing Research, 52,* 278–287.

Bhatnagar, S. C., & Andy, O. J. (1989). Alleviation of acquired stuttering with human centremedian thalamic stimulation. *Journal of Neurology, Neurosurgery, and Psychiatry, 52,* 1182–1184.

Biermann-Ruben, K., Salmelin, R., & Schnitzler, A. (2005). Right rolandic activation during speech perception in stutterers: A MEG study. *NeuroImage, 25,* 793–801.

Bishop, J. H., Williams, H. G., & Cooper, W. A. (1991). Age and task complexity variables in motor performance of children with articulation-disordered, stuttering, and normal speech. *Journal of Fluency Disorders, 16,* 219–228.

Black, J. W. (1955). The persistence of the effects of delayed side-tone. *Journal of Speech and Hearing Disorders, 20,* 65–68.

Block, S., Onslow, M., Roberts, R., & White, S. (2004). Control of stuttering with EMG feedback. *Advances in Speech-Language Pathology, 6,* 100–106.

Blomgren, M., McCormick, C., & Gneiting, S. (2002). P300 ERPs in stutterers and nonstutterers: Stimulus and treatment effects. *The ASHA Leader, 7* (Abstr), 106.

Blomgren, M., Nagarajan, S. S., Lee, J. N., Li, T., & Alvord, L. (2003). Preliminary results of a functional MRI study of brain activation patterns in stuttering and nonstuttering speakers during a lexical access task. *Journal of Fluency Disorders, 28,* 337–356.

Blood, G. W. (1995). A behavioral-cognitive therapy program for adults who stutter: Computers and counseling. *Journal of Communication Disorders, 28,* 165–180.

Blood, G. W., & Blood, I. M. (2004). Bullying in adolescents who stutter: Communicative competence and self-esteem. *Contemporary Issues in Communication Science and Disorders, 31,* 69–79.

Blood, G. W., Blood, I. M., Bennett, S., Tellis, G., & Gabel, R. (2001). Communication apprehension and self-perceived communication competence in adolescents who stutter. *Journal of Fluency Disorders, 26,* 161–178.

Blood, G. W., Ridenour, V. J., Qualls, C. D., & Hammer, C. S. (2003) Co-occurring disorders in children who stutter. *Journal of Communication Disorders, 36,* 427–448.

Blood, G. W., & Seider, R. (1981). The concomitant problems of young stutters. *Journal of Speech and Hearing Disorders, 24,* 31–33.

Blood, I. M., & Blood, G. W. (1984). Relationship between stuttering severity and brainstem-evoked response testing. *Perceptual and Motor Skills, 59,* 935–938.

Bloodstein, O. (1950). Hypothetical conditions under which stuttering is reduced or absent. *Journal of Speech and Hearing Disorders, 15,* 142–153.

Bloodstein, O. (1970). Stuttering and normal nonfluency—A continuity hypothesis. *British Journal of Disorders of Communication, 5,* 30–39.

Bloodstein, O. (1975). *A Handbook on Stuttering.* Chicago: National Easter Seal Society for Crippled Children and Adults.

Bloodstein, O. & Grossman, M. (1981). Early stutterings: Some aspects of their form and distribution. *Journal of Speech and Hearing Research, 24,* 298–302.

Bloodstein, O. (1987). *A Handbook on Stuttering* (4th ed.). Chicago: National Easter Seal Society for Crippled Children and Adults.

Bloodstein, O. (1993). *Stuttering: The Search for a Cause and Cure.* Needham Heights, MA: Allyn & Bacon.

Bloodstein, O. (1995) *A Handbook on Stuttering* (5th ed.). San Diego, CA: Singular Publishing Group.

Bloodstein, O. & Berstein Ratner, N. (2007). *A Handbook on Stuttering* (6th ed.). Clifton Park, NY: Thomson Delmar.

Boberg, E. (1976). Intensive group therapy program for stutterers. *Human Communication, 1,* 29–42.

Boberg, E., Howie, P., & Woods, L. (1979). Maintenance of fluency: A review. *Journal of Fluency Disorders, 4,* 93–116.

Boberg, E., & Kully, D. (1985). *Comprehensive Stuttering Treatment Program.* San Diego, CA: College-Hill Press.

Boberg, E., & Kully, D. (1994). Long-term results of an intensive treatment program for adults and adolescents who stutter. *Journal of Speech and Hearing Research, 37,* 1050–1059.

Boberg, E., Yeudall, L. T., Schopflocher, D., & Bo-Lassen, P. (1983). The effect of an intensive behavioral program on the distribution of EEG alpha power in stutterers during the processing of verbal and visuospatial information. *Journal of Fluency Disorders, 8,* 254–263.

Boey, R. (2008). *Stuttering: Phenomenological-epidemiological and behavioral therapy considerations.* Doctoral dissertation. University of Antwerp, Belgium.

Boey, R., Wuyts, F., van de Heyning, P. H., De Bodt, M., & Heylen, L. (2007). Characteristics of stuttering-like disfluencies in Dutch-speaking children. *Journal of Fluency Disorders, 32,* 310–329.

Bonelli, P., Dixon, M., Bernstein Ratner, N., & Onslow, M. (2000). Child and parent speech and language following the Lidcombe Program of Early Stuttering Intervention. *Clinical Linguistics and Phonetics, 14,* 427–446.

Bosshardt, H.-G. (2006). Cognitive processing load as a determinant of stuttering: Summary of a research programme. *Clinical Linguistics and Phonetics, 20,* 371–385.

Bothe, A. K. (2002). Speech modification approaches to stuttering treatment in schools. *Seminars in Speech and Language, 23,* 181–186.

Bothe, A. K. (2003). Evidence-based treatment of stuttering: V. The art of clinical practice and the future of clinical research. *Journal of Fluency Disorders, 28,* 247–258.

Bothe, A. K. (2004a). Evidence-based treatment of stuttering: An introduction. In A. K. Bothe (Ed.), *Evidence-Based Treatment of Stuttering: Empirical Bases and Clinical Applications* (pp. 3–13). Mahwah, NJ: Lawrence Erlbaum.

Bothe, A. K. (2004b). Evidence-based, outcomes-focused decisions about stuttering treatment: Clinical recommendations in context. In A. K. Bothe (Ed.), *Evidence-Based Treatment of Stuttering: Empirical Bases and Clinical Applications* (pp. 261–270). Mahwah, NJ: Lawrence Erlbaum.

Bothe, A. K. (in press). Evidence-based practice: Basic steps and application to stuttering. In M. Onslow (Ed.), *Evidence Based Clinical Management of Stuttering.* Austin, TX: Pro-Ed.

Bothe, A. K., Davidow, J. H., Bramlett, R. E., Franic, D. M., & Ingham, R. J. (2006). Stuttering treatment research 1970–2005: II. Systematic review incorporating trial quality assessment of pharmacological approaches. *American Journal of Speech Language Pathology, 15,* 342–352.

Bothe, A. K., Davidow, J. H., Bramlett, R. E, & Ingham, R. J. (2006). Stuttering treatment research 1970–2005: I. Systematic review incorporating trial quality assessment of behavioral, cognitive, and related approaches. *American Journal of Speech Language Pathology, 15,* 321–341.

Botterill, W., Biggart, A., & Cook, F. (2006). An evaluation of a National Teaching Programme. *Proceedings of the Fifth World Congress on Fluency Disorders.* Dublin, Ireland.

Bradberry, A. (1997). The role of support groups and stuttering therapy. *Seminars in Speech and Language, 18*, 391–399.

Brady, J. P. (1991). The pharmacology of stuttering: A critical review. *American Journal of Psychiatry, 148*, 1309–1316.

Brady, J. P., Mcallister, T. W., & Price, T. R. (1990). Verapamil in stuttering. *Biological Psychiatry, 27*, 680–681.

Bramlett, R. E., Bothe, A. K., & Franic, D. F. (2006). Using preference based measures to assess quality of life in stuttering. *Journal of Speech, Language, and Hearing Research, 49*, 381–394.

Braun, A. R., Varga, M., Stager, S., Schulz, G., Selbie, S., Maisog, J. M., Carson, R. E., & Ludlow, C. L. (1997). Altered patterns of cerebral activity during speech and language production in developmental stuttering. An H215O positron emission tomography study. *Brain, 120*, 761–784.

Brisk, D. J., Healey, E. C., & Hux, K. A. (1997). Clinician's training and confidence associated with treating school-age children who stutter: A national survey. *Language, Speech, and Hearing Services in Schools, 28*, 164–176.

Brown, C. J., Zimmermann, G. N., Linville, R. N., & Hegmann, J. P. (1990). Variations in self-paced behaviors in stutterers and nonstutterers. *Journal of Speech and Hearing Research, 33*, 317–323.

Brown, S. F. (1938). Stuttering with relation to word accent and word position. *Journal of Abnormal Social Psychology, 33*, 112–120.

Brown, S. F. (1945). The loci of stuttering in the speech sequence. *Journal of Speech Disorders, 10*, 181–192.

Brown, S., Ingham, R. J., Ingham, J. C., Laird, A. R., & Fox, P. T. (2005). Stuttered and fluent speech production: an ALE meta-analysis of functional neuroimaging studies. *Human Brain Mapping, 25*, 105–117.

Brutten, G. J., & Dunham, S. (1989). The Communication Attitude Test. A normative study of grade school children. *Journal of Fluency Disorders, 14*, 371–377.

Brutten, G. J., & Janssen, P. (1979). An eye-marking investigation of anticipated and observed stuttering. *Journal of Speech and Hearing Research, 22*, 22–28.

Brutten, G. J., & Shoemaker, D. J. (1967). *The Modification of Stuttering*. Englewood Cliffs, NJ: Prentice-Hall.

Brutten, G. J., & Shoemaker, D. J. (1974). *Speech Situation Checklist*. Carbondale, IL: Speech Clinic, Southern Illinois University.

Brutten, G. J., & Vanryckeghem, M. (2006). *The Behavior Assessment Battery for School-Aged Children Who Stutter*. San Diego, CA: Plural Publishers.

Buchel, C., & Sommer, M. (2004). What causes stuttering? *PloS Biology, 2*, 159–163.

Buhr, A., & Zebrowski, P. (2007). Linguistic factors in stuttering. Manuscript to be submitted for publication.

Bunge, S. A., Ochsner, K. N., Desmond, J. E., Glover, G. H., & Gabrieli, J. D. (2001). Prefrontal regions involved in keeping information in and out of mind. *Brain, 124*, 2074–2086.

Burghaus, L., Hilker, R., Thiel, A., Galldiks, N., Lehnhardt, F. G., Zaro-Weber, O., Sturm, V., & Heiss, D. W. (2006). Deep brain stimulation of the subthalamic nucleus reversibly deteriorates stuttering in advanced Parkinson's disease. *Journal of Neural Transmission, 113*, 625–631.

Byrd, C., Conture, E., & Ohde, R. (2007). Phonological priming in young children who stutter: Holistic versus incremental processing. *American Journal of Speech-Language Pathology, 16*, 43–53.

Byrd, C., Wolk, L., & Davis, B. (2007). Phonological considerations in developmental stuttering. In E. Conture & R. Curlee (Eds.), *Stuttering and Related Fluency Disorders* (pp. 163–182). New York: Thieme Medical.

Caccamo, J. M. (1973). Accountability: A matter of ethics. *ASHA, 15*, 411–412.

Cantwell, D., & Baker, L. (1985). Psychiatric and learning disorders in children with speech and language disorders: A descriptive analysis. *Advances in Learning and Behavioral Disabilities, 2*, 29–47.

Carey, B., O'Brian, S., Onslow, M., Block, S., & Jones, M. (in press). A randomised controlled non-inferiority trial of a telehealth treatment for chronic stuttering: The Camperdown Program. *International Journal of Language and Communication Disorders*.

Carlberg, C. G., & Walberg, H. J. (1984). Techniques of research synthesis. *The Journal of Special Education, 18*, 11–26.

Carney, B. (2006, December 22). Parenting as therapy for children's mental disorders. *The New York Times*, pp. A1, A24.

Caruso, A. J., Max, L., McClowry, T. M. (1999). Perspectives on stuttering as a motor speech disorder. In A. J. Caruso & E. A. Strand (Eds.), *Clinical Management of Motor Speech Disorders in Children* (pp. 319–344). New York: Thieme.

Chalmers, I., Hedges, L. V., & Cooper, H. (2002). A brief history of research synthesis. *Evaluation and the Health Professions, 25*, 12–37.

Chambless, D. L., & Hollon, S. D. (1998). Defining empirically supported therapies. *Journal of Consulting and Clinical Psychology, 66*, 12–37.

Chang, S. E., Erickson, K. I., Ambrose, N. G., Hasegawa-Johnson, M. A., & Ludlow, C. L. (2008). Brain anatomy differences in childhood stuttering. *Neuroimage, 39*, 1333–1344.

Chase, R. A., Sutton, S., & Raphin, I. (1961). Sensory feedback influences on motor performance. *Journal of Auditory Research, 1,* 212–223.

Cheek, J., Onslow, M., & Cream, A. (2004). Beyond the divide: Comparing and contrasting aspects of qualitative and quantitative research approaches. *Advances in Speech Language Pathology, 6,* 147–152.

Chmela, K., & Reardon, N. (2001). *The School-Age Child Who Stutters: Working Effectively with Attitudes and Emotions.* Memphis, TN: Stuttering Foundation of America.

Christoffels, I. K., Formisano, E., & Schiller, N. O. (2007). Neural correlates of verbal feedback processing: An fMRI study employing overt speech. *Human Brain Mapping, 28,* 868–879.

Cimorell-Strong, J. M., Gilbert, H. R., & Frick, J. V. (1983). Dichotic speech perception: A comparison between stuttering and nonstuttering children. *Journal of Fluency Disorders, 8,* 77–91.

Classen, J., Liepert, J., Wise, S. P., Hallett, M., & Cohen, L. G. (1998). Rapid plasticity of human cortical movement representation induced by practice. *Journal of Neurophysiology, 79,* 1117–1123.

Cocomazzo, N. (submitted for publication). An evaluation of a student-delivered Camperdown Program for adults who stutter. Manuscript submitted for publication.

Cohen, J. (1988). *Statistical Power Analysis for the Behavioral Sciences.* Mahwah, NJ: Lawrence Erlbaum Associates.

Cohen, J. (1992). A power primer. *Psychological Bulletin, 112,* 155–159.

Cole, L. (Ed.) (1986). *The ASHA Manual on the Prevention of Speech and Language Disorders.* Rockville, MD: American Speech, Language and Hearing Association.

Cole, P., Martin, S., & Dennis, T. (2004). Emotion regulation as a scientific construct: Methodological challenges and directions for child development research. *Child Development, 75,* 317–333.

Coleman, C., Yaruss, J. S., & Hammer, D. (2007). Clinical research involving preschoolers who stutter: Real-world applications of evidence based practice. *Language, Speech, and Hearing Services in Schools, 38,* 286–289.

Coloroso, B. (2003). *The Bully, the Bullied, and the Bystander.* New York: Harper Collins Publishers, Inc.

Comings, D. E., Wu, S., Chiu, C., Ring, R. H., Gade, R., Ahn, C., MacMurray, J. P., Dietz, G., & Muhleman, D. (1996). Polygenic inheritance of Tourette syndrome, stuttering, attention deficit hyperactivity, conduct, and oppositional defiant disorder: The additive and subtractive effect of the three dopaminergic genes—DRD2, D beta H, and DAT1. *American Journal of Medical Genetics, 67,* 264–288.

Committee on the Mathematics and Physics of Emerging Dynamic Biomedical Imaging, and National Research Council. (1996). *Mathematics and Physics of Emerging Biomedical Imaging.* Washington, DC: National Academy Press.

Conture, E. G. (1982). *Stuttering.* Englewood Cliffs, NJ: Prentice Hall.

Conture, E. G. (1990). *Stuttering: Its Nature, Diagnosis, and Treatment* (2nd ed.). Boston: Allyn & Bacon.

Conture, E. G. (1991). Young stutterers' speech production: A critical review. In H. F. M. Peters, W. Hulstijn, & C. W. Starkweather (Eds.), *Speech Motor Control and Stuttering: Proceedings of the 2nd International Conference on Speech Motor Control and Stuttering* (pp. 365–384). New York: Elsevier.

Conture, E. G. (1996). Treatment efficacy: Stuttering. *Journal of Speech and Hearing Research, 39,* S18-S26.

Conture, E. G. (1997). Evaluating childhood stuttering. In R. Curlee and G. Siegel (Eds.), *Nature and Treatment of Stuttering: New Directions* (2nd ed., pp. 239–256). Boston: Allyn & Bacon.

Conture, E. G. (2001). *Stuttering: Its Nature, Diagnosis and Treatment.* Boston: Allyn & Bacon.

Conture, E. G., & Caruso, A. (1987). Assessment and diagnosis of childhood disfluency. In L. Rustin, D. Rowley, & H. Purser (Eds.), *Progress in the Treatment of Fluency Disorders* (pp. 57–82). London: Taylor & Francis.

Conture, E. G., & Guitar, B. E. (1993). Evaluating efficacy of treatment of stuttering: School-age children. *Journal of Fluency Disorders, 18,* 253–287.

Conture, E. G., & Kelly, E. M. (1991). Young stutterers' nonspeech behaviors during stuttering. *Journal of Speech and Hearing Research, 34,* 1041–1056.

Conture, E. G., Louko, L., & Edwards, M. L. (1993). Simultaneously treating stuttering and disordered phonology in children: Experimental treatment, preliminary findings. *American Journal of Speech-Language Pathology, 2,* 72–81.

Conture, E. G., & Melnick, K. S. (1999). Parent-child group approach to stuttering in preschool children. In M. Onslow & A. Packman (Eds.), *The Handbook of Early Stuttering Intervention* (pp. 17–52). London: The Singular Publishing Group Inc.

Conture, E. G., Rothenberg, M., & Molitor, R. D. (1986). Electroglottographic observations of young stutterers' fluency. *Journal of Speech and Hearing Research, 29,* 384–393.

Conture, E. G., Walden, T., Arnold, H., Graham, C., Karrass, J., & Hartfield, K. (2006). Communication-emotional model of stuttering. In N. Bernstein Ratner & J. Tetnowski (Eds.), *Current Issues in Stuttering Research and Practice* (pp. 17–46). Mahwah, NJ: Lawrence Erlbaum Associates, Publishers.

Conture, E. G., & Yaruss, J. S. (1993). *A Handbook for Childhood Stuttering: A Second Opinion.* Tucson, AZ: Bahill Intelligent Computer Systems.

Conture, E. G., & Yaruss, J. S. (2007). Treatment efficacy summary: Stuttering. A publication of the American Speech-Language-Hearing Association. Available at: http://www.asha.org/NR/rdonlyres/85BCEC0C-FBF5-43C7-880D-EF2D3219F807/0/TESStuttering.pdf.

Conture, E. G., & Zebrowski, P. (1992). Can childhood speech disfluencies be mutable to the influences of speech-language pathologists, but immutable to the influences of parents? *Journal of Fluency Disorders, 17*, 121–130.

Cook, D. J., Guyatt, G. H., Laupacis, A., Sackett, D. L., & Goldberg, R. J. (1995). Clinical recommendations using levels of evidence for antithrombotic agents. *Chest, 108* (Suppl), 227S-230S.

Cook, F., & Botterill, W. (1999). A profile of risk for generalist therapists. In *Proceedings of the Fifth Oxford Dysfluency Conference* (pp. 154–159). Leicester, United Kingdom: Kevin L. Baker.

Cook, F., & Botterill, W. (2005). Family based approach to therapy with primary school children: 'throwing the ball back.' In R. Lees & C. Stark (Eds.), *The Treatment of Stuttering in the Young School-Aged Child* (pp. 81–108). London: Whurr.

Cook, F., & Rustin, L. (1997). Commentary on the Lidcombe Programme of early stuttering intervention. *European Journal of Disorders of Communication, 32*, 250–258.

Cook, M. J., & Smith, L. M. (2006). *Outcomes for Adult Males Using the SpeechEasy Fluency Device for One Year*. Presented to the American Speech-Language-Hearing Association, Miami, FL.

Cooper, E. B. (1976). *Personalized Fluency Control Therapy*. Boston: Teaching Resources.

Cooper, E. B. (1993). Chronic perseverative stuttering syndrome: A harmful or helpful construct? *American Journal of Speech-Language Pathology, 2*, 11–15.

Cooper, E. B., & Cooper, C. S. (1985). Clinician attitudes toward stuttering: A decade of change (1973–1983). *Journal of Fluency Disorders, 10*, 19–33.

Cooper, E. B., & Cooper, C. S. (1985). *Cooper Personalized Fluency Control Therapy-Revised*. Allen, TX: DLM.

Cooper, E. B., & Cooper, C. S. (1996). Clinician attitudes towards stuttering: Two decades of change. *Journal of Fluency Disorders, 21*, 119–136.

Cooper, E. B., & Cooper, C. S. (1998). Multicultural considerations in the assessment and treatment of stuttering. In D. Battle (Ed.), *Communication Disorders in Multicultural Populations* (2nd ed.; pp. 247–274). Boston: Butterworth-Heinemann.

Cooper, H. M. (1982). Scientific principles for conducting integrative research reviews. *Review of Educational Research, 52*, 291–302.

Cooper, H., & Hedges, L. V. (1994). *The Handbook of Research Synthesis*. New York: Russell Sage.

Cooper, S. (2000). *Sticks and Stones*. New York: Times Books.

Cordes, A. K. (1998). Current status of the stuttering treatment literature. In A. K. Cordes & R. J. Ingham (Eds.), *Treatment Efficacy for Stuttering: A Search for Empirical Bases* (pp. 117–144). San Diego, CA: Singular.

Cordes, A. K. (2000). Individual and consensus judgments of disfluency types in the speech of persons who stutter. *Journal of Speech, Language, and Hearing Research, 43*, 951–964.

Cordes, A. K., & Ingham, R. J. (1994). The reliability of observational data: II. Issues in the identification and measurements of stuttering events. *Journal of Speech and Hearing Research, 37*, 279–294.

Cordes, A. K., & Ingham, R. J. (1998). *Treatment Efficacy for Stuttering: A Search for Empirical Bases*. San Diego, CA: Singular Publishing Group, Inc.

Costa, D. (1992). Antidepressants and the treatment of stuttering. *American Journal of Psychiatry, 149*, 1281.

Costello, J. M. (1975). Time-out procedures for the modification of stuttering: Three case studies. *Journal of Speech and Hearing Disorders, 40*, 216–231.

Costello, J. M. (1983). Current behavioral treatments for children. In D. Prins & R. J. Ingham (Eds.), *Treatment of Stuttering in Early Childhood: Methods and Issues* (pp. 69–112). San Diego, CA: College-Hill.

Costello, J. M., & Ingham, R. J. (1984). Assessment strategies for stuttering. In R. F. Curlee & W. H. Perkins (Eds.), *Nature and Treatment of Stuttering: New Directions*. San Diego, CA: College-Hill Press.

Coulter, C., Anderson, J., & Conture, E. (2009). Childhood stuttering and dissociations across linguistic domains: A replication and extension. Submitted for publication.

Cox, N., Cook, E., Ambrose, N., Yairi, E., Rydmarker, S., Lundstrom, C., et al. (2000). The Illinois-Sweden-Israel Genetics of Stuttering Project. Paper presented at the Third World Congress on Fluency Disorders, Nyborg, Denmark.

Craig, A. (1990). An investigation into the relationship between anxiety and stuttering. *Journal of Speech and Hearing Disorders, 55*, 290–294.

Craig, A. (1998a). *Treating Stuttering in Older Children, Adolescents and Adults: A Guide for Clinicians, Parents and Those Who Stutter*. Gosford, Australia: Feedback Publications Press.

Craig, A. (1998b). Relapse following treatment for stuttering: A critical review and correlative data. *Journal of Fluency Disorders, 23*, 1–30.

Craig, A. (2000). The developmental nature and effective treatment of stuttering in children and adolescents. *Journal of Developmental and Physical Disabilities, 12*, 173–186.

Craig, A. (2003). Clinical psychology and neurological disorders: Psychological therapies for stuttering. *Clinical Psychologist, 7*, 93–103.

Craig, A., & Calver, P. (1991). Following up on treated stutterers. Studies of perceptions of fluency and job status. *Journal of Speech and Hearing Research, 34*, 279–284.

Craig, A., & Cleary, P. (1982). Reduction of stuttering by young male stutterers using EMG feedback. *Biofeedback and Self-Regulation, 7*, 241–255.

Craig, A., Feyer, A. M., & Andrews, G. (1987). An overview of a behavioral treatment for stuttering. *Australian Psychologist, 22*, 53–62.

Craig, A., Franklin, J., & Andrews, G. (1984). A scale to measure locus of control of behavior. *British Journal of Medical Psychology, 57*, 173–180.

Craig, A., & Hancock, K. (1996). Anxiety in children and young adolescents who stutter. *Australian Journal of Human Communication Disorders, 24*, 29–38.

Craig, A., Hancock, K., Chang, E., McCready, C., Shepley, A., McCaul, A., Costello, D., Harding, S., Kehren, R., Masel, C., & Reilly, K. (1996). A controlled clinical trial for stuttering in persons aged 9 to 14 years. *Journal of Speech and Hearing Research, 39*, 808–826.

Craig, A., Hancock, K., & Cobbin, D. (2002). Managing adolescents who relapse following treatment for stuttering. *Journal of Speech Language and Hearing: Asia Pacific, 7*, 79–91.

Craig, A., Hancock, K., Tran, Y., & Craig, M. (2003). Anxiety levels in people who stutter: A randomised population study. *Journal of Speech, Language, and Hearing Research, 46*, 1197–1206.

Craig, A., Hancock, K., Tran, Y., Craig, M., & Peters, K. (2002). Epidemiology of stuttering in the community across the entire lifespan. *Journal of Speech, Language and Hearing Research, 45*, 1097–1105.

Craig, A., & Tran, Y. (2006).Chronic and social anxiety in people who stutter. *Advances in Psychiatric Treatment, 12*, 63–68.

Craig, W. M., & Pepler, D. J. (1995). Peer processes in bullying and victimization: An observational study. *Exceptionality Education in Canada, 5*, 81–95.

Craven, D. C., & Ryan, B. P. (1984). The use of a portable delayed auditory feedback unit in stuttering therapy. *Journal of Fluency Disorders, 9*, 237–243.

Cream, A., Onslow, M., Packman, A., & Llewellyn, G. (2003). Protection from harm: The experience after prolonged-speech treatment for stuttering. *International Journal of Language and Communication Disorders, 38*, 379–395.

Cream, A., Packman, A., & Llewellyn, G. (2004). The playground rocker: A metaphor for communication after treatment for adults who stutter. *Advances in Speech Language Pathology, 6*, 182–187.

Crichton-Smith, I. (2002). Changing conversational dynamics: A case study in parent-child interaction therapy. In *Proceedings of The Sixth Oxford Dysfluency Conference* (pp. 129–136). Leicester, United Kingdom: Kevin L. Baker.

Crilly, M. (2001). Evidence based bloodletting. *British Medical Journal, 322*, 854.

Crowe, T. A., & Cooper, E. B. (1977). Parental attitudes toward and knowledge of stuttering. *Journal of Communication Disorders, 10*, 343–357.

Crowe, T. A., & Walton, J. H. (1981). Teacher attitudes toward stuttering. *Journal of Fluency Disorders, 6*, 163–174.

Crystal, D. (1987). Towards a "bucket" theory of language disability: Taking account of interaction between linguistic levels. *Clinical Linguistics and Phonetics, 1*, 7–22.

Cuadrado, E. M., & Weber-Fox, C. M. (2003). Atypical syntactic processing in individuals who stutter: Evidence from event-related brain potentials and behavioral measures. *Journal of Speech, Language, and Hearing Research, 46*, 960–976.

Culatta, R., & Goldberg, S. (1995). *Stuttering Therapy: An Integrated Approach to Theory and Practice.* Boston: Allyn & Bacon.

Cullinan, W. L., & Prather, E. M. (1968). Reliability of "live" ratings of the speech of stutterers. *Perceptual and Motor Skills, 27*, 403–409.

Cullinan, W. L., Prather, E. M., & Williams, D. E. (1963). Comparison of procedures for scaling severity of stuttering. *Journal of Speech and Hearing Research, 6*, 187–194.

Curlee, R. F. (1981). Observer agreement on disfluency and stuttering. *Journal of Speech and Hearing Research, 24*, 595–600.

Curlee, R. F. (1993). Evaluating treatment efficacy for adults: Assessment of stuttering disability. *Journal of Fluency Disorders, 18*, 319–331.

Curlee, R. F. (1993). Identification and management of beginning stuttering. In R. F. Curlee (Ed.), *Stuttering and Related Disorders of Fluency* (pp. 1–22). New York: Thieme Medical Publishers, Inc.

Curlee, R. F. (2007). Identification and case selection guidelines for early childhood stuttering. In E.G. Conture & R. F. Curlee (Eds.), *Stuttering and Related Disorders of Fluency* (3rd ed., pp. 3–22). New York: Thieme Medical Publishers.

Curlee, R. F., & Perkins, W. H. (1969). Conversational rate control therapy for stutterers. *Journal of Speech and Hearing Disorders, 34*, 245–250.

Curlee, R. F., & Perkins, W. H. (1973). Effectiveness of a DAF conditioning program for adolescent and adult stutterers. *Behaviour Research and Therapy, 11*, 395–401.

Curran, M., & Hood, S. (1977). The effect of instructional bias on listener ratings of specific disfluency types in children. *Journal of Fluency Disorders, 2*, 99–107.

Curry, F. K. W., & Gregory, H. H. (1969). The performance of stutterers on dichotic listening tasks thought to reflect cerebral dominance. *Journal of Speech and Hearing Research, 12*, 73–82.

Cykowski, M. D, Kochunov, P. V., Ingham, R. J., Ingham, J. C., Mangin, J. F., Rivière, D., Lcaster, J. L., & Fox, P. T. (2007). Perisylvian sulcal morphology and cerebral asymmetry patterns in adults who stutter. *Cerebral Cortex, 18*, 571–583.

Damasio, A. (1994). *Descartes' Error: Emotion, Reason and the Human Brain*. New York: Avon Books.

Dapretto, M., & Bookheimer, S. Y. (1999). Form and content: Dissociating syntax and semantics in sentence comprehension. *Neuron, 24*, 292–293.

Darley, F. L., & Spriestersbach, D. C. (1978). *Diagnostic Methods in Speech Pathology* (2nd ed.). New York: Harper & Row.

Davidow, J. H., Bothe, A. K., & Bramlett R. E. (2006). The Stuttering Treatment Research Evaluation and Assessment Tool (STREAT): Evaluating treatment research as part of evidence-based practice. *American Journal of Speech-Language Pathology, 15*, 126–141.

Davis, S., Howell, P., & Cook, F. (2002). Sociodynamic relationships between children who stutter and their non-stuttering classmates. *Journal of Child Psychology and Psychiatry and Allied Disciplines, 69*, 141–158.

de Craen, A. J. M., van Vliet, H. A. A. M., & Helmerhorst, F. M. (2005). An analysis of systematic reviews indicated low incorporation of results from clinical trial quality assessment. *Journal of Clinical Epidemiology, 58*, 311–313.

de Kindkelder, M., & Boelens, H. (1998). Habitat-reversal treatment for children's stuttering: Assessment in three settings. *Journal of Behavioral Therapy in Experimental Psychiatry, 29*, 261–265.

Dell, C. W. (1993). Treating school-age stutterers. In R. F. Curlee (Ed.), *Stuttering and Related Disorders of Fluency* (pp. 45–67). New York: Thieme Medical Publishers.

Dell, C. W. (2000). *Treating the School-Age Stutterer: A Guide for Clinicians* (2nd ed.). Memphis, TN: Stuttering Foundation.

De Nil, L. F. (1999a). Uncovering the neural basis of stuttering: Recent contributions from functional neuroimaging. In E. Manders, D. Lembrechts, & P. Bastijns (Eds.), *Stotteren. Recente Inzichten* [Stuttering. Recent Insights] (pp. 75–91). Leuven/Amersfoort, The Netherlands: ACCO.

De Nil, L. F. (1999b). Stuttering: A neurophysiological perspective. In N. Bernstein Ratner & C. Healey (Eds.), *Stuttering Research and Practice: Bridging the Gap* (pp. 85–102). Mahwah, NJ: Erlbaum.

De Nil, L. F., Beal, D. S., Lafaille, S. J., Kroll, R. M., Crawley, A. P., & Gracco, V. L. (2008). The effects of simulated stuttering and prolonged speech on the neural activation patterns of stuttering and nonstuttering adults. *Brain and Language, 107*, 114–123.

De Nil, L. F., & Bosshardt, H. G. (2001). Studying stuttering from a neurological and cognitive information processing perspective. In H. G. Bosshardt, J. S. Yaruss, & H. F. M. Peters (Eds.), *Fluency Disorders: Theory, Research, Treatment and Self-Help* (pp. 53–58). Nijmegen, The Netherlands: Nijmegen University Press.

De Nil, L. F., & Brutten, G. J. (1991). Speech-associated attitudes of stuttering and nonstuttering children. *Journal of Speech and Hearing Research, 34*, 60–65.

De Nil, L. F, & Kroll, R. M. (1995). The relationship between locus of control and long-term treatment outcome in adults who stutter. *Journal of Fluency Disorders, 20*, 345–364.

De Nil, L. F., & Kroll R. M. (2001). Searching for the neural basis of stuttering treatment outcome: Recent neuroimaging studies. *Clinical Linguistics and Phonetics, 15*, 163–168.

De Nil, L. F., & Kroll, R. M. (2001). Understanding the neural basis of treatment using positron emission tomography. In H. G. Bosshardt, J. S. Yaruss, & H. F. M. Peters (Eds.), *Fluency Disorders: Theory, Research, Treatment and Self-Help* (pp. 43–46). Nijmegen, The Netherlands: Nijmegen University Press.

De Nil, L. F., Kroll, R. M., & Houle, S. (2001). Functional neuroimaging of cerebellar activation during single-word reading and verb generation in stuttering and nonstuttering adults. *Neuroscience Letters, 302*, 77–80.

De Nil, L. F., Kroll, R. M., Kapur, S., & Houle, S. (2000). A positron emission tomography study of silent and oral single word reading in stuttering and nonstuttering adults. *Journal of Speech, Language, and Hearing Research, 43*, 1038–1053.

De Nil, L. F., Kroll, R. M., Lafaille, S. J., & Houle, S. (2003). A positron emission tomography study of short- and long-term treatment effects on functional brain activation in adults who stutter. *Journal of Fluency Disorders, 28*, 357–380.

Desmond, J. E., & Fiez, J. A. (1998). Neuroimaging studies of the cerebellum: Language, learning, and memory. *Trends in Cognitive Science, 9*, 355–365.

Dewar, A, Dewar, A. W., Austin, W. T. S., & Brash, H. M. (1979). The long-term use of an automatically triggered auditory feedback masking device in the treatment of stammering. *British Journal of Disorders of Communication, 14*, 219–229.

DeYoe, E. A., Bandettini, P., Neitz, J., Miller, D., & Winans, P. (1994). Functional magnetic resonance imaging (FMRI) of the human brain. *Journal of Neuroscience Methods, 54*, 171–187.

DiLollo, A., Neimeyer, R. A., & Manning, W. H. (2002). A personal construct psychology view of relapse: Indications for a narrative therapy component to stuttering treatment. *Journal of Fluency Disorders, 27,* 19–40.

Dolcos, F., & McCarthy, G. (2006). Brain systems mediating cognitive interference by emotional distraction. *The Journal of Neuroscience, 26,* 2072–2079.

Dollaghan, C. (2004, April 13). Evidence-based practice myths and realities. *The ASHA Leader,* pp. 12.

Dollaghan, C. A. (2007). *The Handbook of Evidence-Based Practice in Communication Disorders.* Baltimore: Paul H. Brookes Publishing Co.

Dorsaint-Pierre, R., Penhune, V. B., Watkins, K. E., Neelin, P., Lerch, J. P., Bouffard, M., & Zatorre, R. J. (2006). Asymmetries of the planum temporale and Heschl's gyrus: Relationship to language lateralization. *Brain, 129,* 1164–1176.

Drayna, D. T. (1997). Genetic linkage studies of stuttering: Ready for prime time? *Journal of Fluency Disorders, 22,* 237–241.

Drayna, D. T. (2004). Results of a genome-wide linkage scan for stuttering. *American Journal of Medical Genetics, 124A,* 133–135.

Dunn, L. M. (1965). *The Peabody Picture Vocabulary Test.* Circle Pines, MN: American Guidance Science.

Dunn, L., & Dunn, L. (1981). *The Peabody Picture Vocabulary Test- Revised (PPVT-R)* (2nd ed.). Circle Pines, MN: American Guidance Service.

Dunn, L., & Dunn, L. (1997). *The Peabody Picture Vocabulary Test-III (PPVT-III)* (3rd ed.). Circle Pines, MN: American Guidance Service.

Dunn, L., & Dunn, L. (2006). *The Peabody Picture Vocabulary Test-4 (PPVT-4)* (4th ed.). Circle Pines, MN: American Guidance Service.

Dunn, L. M, Dunn, L. M., Whetton, C. C., & Burley, J. (1997). *British Picture Vocabulary Scale* (2nd ed.). Windsor, United Kingdom: NFER-Nelson.

Dunteman, G. (1989). *Principal Components Analysis.* Newbury Park, CA: Sage Publications Inc.

Egan, G. (2002). *The Skilled Helper: A Problem Management Approach to Helping* (7th ed.). Pacific Grove, CA: Brooks/Cole.

Einarsdóttir, J. (2009). The identification and measurement of stuttering in preschool children. Doctoral dissertation, University of Iceland, Reykjavik.

Eisenberg, N., & Fabes, R. (1992). Emotion, regulation, and the development of social competence. In M. S. Clark (Ed.), *Review of Personality and Social Psychology. Volume 14: Emotion and Social Behavior* (pp. 119–150). Newbury Park, CA: Sage.

Embrechts, M., Ebben, H., Franke, P., & van de Poel, C. (1998). Temperament: A comparison between children who stutter and children who do not stutter. In E. C. Healey & H. F. M. Peters (Eds.), *Stuttering: Proceedings of the Second World Congress on Fluency Disorders* (Vol. 2). Nijmegen, The Netherlands: University Press Nijmegen.

Eve, C., Onslow, M., Andrews, C., & Adams, R. (1995). Clinical measurement of early stuttering severity: The reliability of a 10-point scale. *Australian Journal of Human Communication Disorders, 23,* 26–39.

Evesham, M., & Fransella, F. (1985). Stuttering relapse: The effects of a combined speech and psychological reconstruction programme. *British Journal of Disorders of Communication, 20,* 237–248.

Faber, A., & Mazlish, E. (1980). *How to Talk So Kids Will Listen and Listen So Kids Will Talk.* New York: Avon Books.

Fairbanks, G. (1960). *Voice and Articulation Drillbook.* New York: Harper & Row.

Feldman, K. A. (1971). Using the work of others: Some observations on reviewing and integrating. *Sociology of Education, 44,* 86–102.

Felsenfeld, S. (1996). Progress and needs in the genetics of stuttering. *Journal of Fluency Disorders, 21,* 77–103.

Felsenfeld, S. (1997). Epidemiology and genetics of stuttering. In R. Curlee & G. M. Siegel (Eds.), *Nature and Treatment of Stuttering: New Directions* (2nd ed., pp. 3–22). Boston: Allyn and Bacon.

Ferreira, F., & Swets, B. (2002). How incremental is language production? Evidence from the production of utterances requiring the computation of arithmetic sums. *Journal of Memory and Language, 46,* 57–84.

Fiedler, P., & Standop, R. (1994). *Stottern: Ätiologie—Diagnose—Behandlung* [Stuttering: Etiology, Diagnosis, Treatment]. Weinheim, Germany: Urban & Schwarzenberg.

Finn, P. (1997). Adults recovered from stuttering without formal treatment: Perceptual assessment of speech normalcy. *Journal of Speech, Language, and Hearing Research, 40,* 821–831.

Finn, P. (2004). Establishing the validity of stuttering treatment effectiveness: The fallibility of clinical experience. *Perspectives on Fluency and Fluency Disorders* [Newsletter of Special Interest Division 4, American Speech-Language Hearing Association], October, 9–12.

Finn, P., Bothe, A. K., & Bramlett, R. E. (2005). Science and pseudoscience in communication disorders: Criteria and applications. *American Journal of Speech-Language Pathology, 14,* 172–186.

Finn, P., & Ingham, R. J. (1994). Stutterer's self-ratings of how natural speech sounds and feels. *Journal of Speech and Hearing Research, 37,* 326–340.

Finn, P., Ingham, R., Ambrose, N., & Yairi, E. (1997). Children recovered from stuttering without formal treatment: Perceptual assessment of speech normalcy. *Journal of Speech, Language, and Hearing Research, 40,* 867–876.

Flanagan, B., Goldiamond, I., & Azrin, N. (1958). Operant stuttering: The control of behaviour through response-contingent consequences. *Journal of the Experimental Analysis of Behavior, 1,* 173–178.

Flasher, L. V., & Fogle, P. T. (2004). *Counseling Skills for Speech-Language Pathologists and Audiologists.* Clifton Park, NY: Thomson/Delmar Publishing.

Forsnot, S. M. (1992). *Fluency Development for Young Stutterers: Differential Diagnosis and Treatment.* Buffalo, NY: EDUCOM Associates.

Fosnot, S. M., & Woodford, L. L. (1992). *The Fluency Development System for Young Children.* Buffalo, NY: United Educational Services.

Foundas, A. L., Bollich, A. M., Corey, D. M., Hurley, M., & Heilman, K. M. (2001). Anomalous anatomy of speech-language areas in adults with persistent developmental stuttering. *Neurology, 57,* 207–215.

Foundas, A. L., Bollich, A. M., Feldman, J., Corey, D. M., Hurley, M., Lemen, L. C., & Heilman, K. M. (2004). Aberrant auditory processing and atypical planum temporale in developmental stuttering. *Neurology, 63,* 1640–1646.

Foundas, A. L., Corey, D. M., Angeles, V., Bollich, A. M., Crabtree-Hartman, E., & Heilman, K. (2003). Atypical cerebral laterality in adults with persistent developmental stuttering. *Neurology, 61,* 1378–1385.

Fox, P. T., Ingham, R. J., Ingham, J. C., Hirsch, T. B., Downs, J. H., Martin, C., Jerabek, P., Glass, T., & Lancaster, J. L. (1996). A PET study of the neural systems of stuttering. *Nature, 382,* 158–162.

Fox, P. T., Ingham, R. J., Ingham, J. C., Zamarripa, F., Xiong, J.-H., & Lancaster, J. L. (2000). Brain correlates of stuttering and syllable production. A PET performance-correlation analysis. *Brain, 123,* 1985–2004.

Franic, D. M., & Bothe, A. K. (2007). Psychometric evaluation of condition-specific instruments used to assess health-related quality of life, attitudes, and related constructs in stuttering. Unpublished manuscript.

Franken, M.-C., Kielstra-Van der Schalk, C. J., & Boelens, H. (2005). Experimental treatment of early stuttering: A preliminary study. *Journal of Fluency Disorders, 30,* 189–199.

Frattali, C. (1998). Measuring modality-specific behaviors, functional abilities, and quality of life. In C. Frattali (Ed.), *Outcome Measurement in Speech-Language Pathology* (pp. 55–88). New York: Thieme Medical Publishers.

Freeman, F. J., & Ushijima, T. (1975). Laryngeal activity accompanying the moment of stuttering: A preliminary report of EMG investigations. *Journal of Fluency Disorders, 1,* 36–45.

Freeman, F. J., & Ushijima, T. (1978). Laryngeal muscle activity during stuttering. *Journal of Speech Hearing Research, 21,* 538–562.

Freund, H. (1966). *Psychopathology and the Problems of Stuttering.* Springfield, IL: Charles C. Thomas.

Friedman, A. (1992). *Let the Words Flow with Dr. Fluency.* Retrieved May 28, 2007, from http://www.dfluency.com.

Frisch, S., Kotz, S. A., von Cramon, D. Y., & Friederici, A. D. (2003). Why the P600 is not just a P300: The role of the basal ganglia. *Clinical Neurophysiology, 114,* 336–340.

Gaines, N. D., Runyan, C. M., & Meyers, S. C. (1991). A comparison of young stutterers' fluent versus stuttered utterances on measures of length and complexity. *Journal of Speech and Hearing Research, 34,* 37–42.

Gaura, V., Bachoud-Levi, A. C., Ribeiro, M. J., Nguyen, J. P., Frouin, V., Baudic, S., Brugières, P., Mangin, J. F., Boissé, M. F., Palfi, S., Cesaro, P., Samson, Y., Hantraye, P., Peschanski, M., & Remy, P. (2004). Striatal neural grafting improves cortical metabolism in Huntington's disease patients. *Brain, 127,* 65–72.

Gerfen, C. R. (2000). Molecular effects of dopamine on striatal-projection pathways. *Trends in Neuroscience, 10* (Suppl), 64–70.

Gerfen, C. R., Engber, T. M., Mahan, L. C., Susel, Z., Chase, T. N., Monsma, F. J. Jr., & Sibley, D. R. (1990). D1 and D2 dopamine receptor-regulated gene expression of striatonigral and striatopallidal neurons. *Science, 250,* 1429–1432.

Gertner, B. L., Rice, M. L., & Hadley, P. A. (1994). Influence of communicative competence on peer preferences in a preschool classroom. *Journal of Speech and Hearing Research, 37,* 913–923.

Giraud, A. L., Neumann, K., Bachoud-Levi, A.-C., von Gudenberg, A., Euler, H. A., Lanfermann, H., & Preibisch, C. (2008). Severity of dysfluency correlates with basal ganglia activity in persistent developmental stuttering. *Brain and Language, 104,* 190–199.

Goberman, A. M., & Blomgren, M. (2003). Parkinsonian speech disfluencies: Effects of L-dopa-related fluctuations. *Journal of Fluency Disorders, 28,* 55–70.

Goebel, M. D. (1984). A computer-aided fluency treatment program for adolescents and adults. Paper presented at the American Speech-Language Association Convention, San Francisco, CA.

Goldberg, G. (1985). Supplementary motor area structure and function. *The Behavioral and Brain Sciences, 8,* 567–616.

Goldberg, G. (1991). Microgenetic theory and the dual premotor systems hypothesis: Implications for rehabilitation of the brain-damaged subject. In

R. E. Hanlon (Ed.), *Cognitive Microgenesis: A Neuropsychological Perspective*. New York: Springer.

Goldiamond, I. (1965). Stuttering and fluency as manipulatable operant response classes. In L. Krasner & L. P. Ullman (Eds.), *Research in Behavior Modification*. New York: Holt, Rinehart & Winston.

Goldman, R. (1996). The use of Mellaril as an adjunct to the treatment of stuttering. In *Proceedings of the IV World Congress of Psychiatry*. Amsterdam: Excerpta Medica.

Goldman, R., & Fristoe, M. (2000). *Goldman-Fristoe Test of Articulation-2 (GFTA-2)*. Circle Pines, MN: American Guidance Service, Inc.

Goldman-Eiser, F. (1954). On the variability of the speed of talking and on its relation to the length of utterances in conversation. *British Journal of Psychology, 45*, 94–107.

Goldman-Eisler, F. (1956). The determinants of the rate of speech output and their mutual relations. *Journal of Psychosomatic Research, 1*, 137–143.

Goldsmith, H., Buss, A., Plomin, R., Rothbart, M., Thomas, A., Chess, S., Hinde, R., & McCall, R. (1987). Roundtable: What is temperament? Four approaches. *Child Development, 58*, 505–529.

Goodman, C. M. (1987). The Delphi technique: A critique. *Journal of Advanced Nursing, 12*, 729–734.

Gordon, C., Cotelingam, G., Stager, S., Ludlow, C., Hamburger, S., & Rapoport, J. (1995). A double-blind comparison of clomipramine and desipramine in the treatment of developmental stuttering. *Journal of Clinical Psychiatry, 56*, 238–242.

Gordon, P. A., & Luper, H. L. (1992). The early identification of beginning stuttering I: Protocols. *American Journal of Speech-Language Pathology, 1*, 43–53.

Gottwald, S. R., & Hall, N. E. (2003). Stuttering treatment in schools: Developing family and teacher partnerships. *Seminars in Speech and Language, 24*, 41–46.

Gottwald, S. R., & Starkweather, C. W. (1995). Fluency intervention for preschoolers and their families in the public schools. *Language, Speech and Hearing Services in Schools, 11*, 117–126.

Gottwald, S. R., & Starkweather, C. W. (1999). Stuttering prevention and early intervention: A multi-process approach. In M. Onslow & A. Packman (Eds.), *The Handbook of Early Stuttering Intervention* (pp. 53–82). San Diego, CA: Singular Publishing Company.

Grafman, J. (2000). Conceptualizing functional neuroplasticity. *Journal of Communication Disorders, 33*, 345–355.

Graham, C. G., & Conture, E. G. (2005). Occurrence of concomitant problems in families of children who stutter. Poster presented at the Annual American Speech-Language Hearing Association Conference, San Diego, CA.

Graham, C. G., & Hartfield, K. N. (2006). Relation of SES, language, and parent education CWS and CWNS. Poster presented at the Annual American Speech-Language Hearing Association Conference, Miami, FL.

Gregory, H. H. (1979). The controversies: Analysis and current status. In H. H. Gregory (Ed.), *Controversies about Stuttering Therapy*. Baltimore: University Park Press.

Gregory, H. H. (1999). Developmental intervention: Differential strategies. In M. Onslow & A. Packman (Eds.), *The Handbook of Early Stuttering Intervention* (pp. 83–102). San Diego, CA: Singular Press.

Gregory, H. H. (2003). *Stuttering Therapy: Rationale and Procedures*. Boston: Allyn & Bacon.

Gregory, H. H., & Hill, D. (1980). Stuttering therapy for children. *Seminars in Speech Language and Hearing, 1*, 351–364.

Gregory, H. H., & Hill, D. (1992). Differential evaluation-differential therapy for stuttering children. In R. F. Curlee (Ed.), *Stuttering and Related Disorders of Fluency* (pp. 23–44). New York: Thieme Medical Publishers, Inc.

Gregory, H. H., & Hill, D. (1999). Differential evaluation-differential therapy for stuttering children. In R. F. Curlee (Ed.), *Stuttering and Related Disorders of Fluency* (2nd ed., pp. 22–42). New York: Thieme Medical Publishers, Inc.

Groopman, J. (2007). *How Doctors Think*. Boston: Houghton Mifflin.

Guitar, B. (1976). Pretreatment factors associated with the outcome of stuttering therapy. *Journal of Speech and Hearing Research, 19*, 590–600.

Guitar, B. (1998). *Stuttering: An Integrated Approach to Its Nature and Treatment* (2nd ed.). Baltimore: William & Wilkins.

Guitar, B. (2003). Acoustic startle responses and temperament in individuals who stutter. *Journal of Speech, Language and Hearing Research, 46*, 233–241.

Guitar, B. (2003). The Lidcombe program in historical context. In M. Onslow, A. Packman, & E. Harrison (Eds.), *The Lidcombe Program of Early Stuttering Intervention* (pp. 27–39). Austin, TX: PRO-ED.

Guitar, B. (2005). *Stuttering: An Integrated Approach to Its Nature and Treatment* (3rd ed.). Baltimore: Williams & Wilkins.

Guitar, B. (2006). *Stuttering: An Integrated Approach to Its Nature and Treatment* (3rd ed.). Baltimore: Lippincott, Williams & Wilkins.

Guitar, B., & Bass, C. (1978). Stuttering therapy: The relation between attitude change and long-term outcome. *Journal of Speech and Hearing Disorders, 43*, 392–400.

Guitar, B., & Marchinkoski, L. (2001). Influence of mothers' slower speech on their children's speech rate. *Journal of Speech, Language, and Hearing Research, 44,* 853–861.

Guitar, B., Schaefer, H. K., Donahue-Kilburg, G., & Bond, L. (1992). Parent verbal interactions and speech rate: A case study in stuttering. *Journal of Speech and Hearing Research, 35,* 742–754.

Guralnick, M. J., Connor, R. T., Hammond, M. A., Gottman, J. M., & Kinnish, K. (1996). The peer relations of preschool children with communication disorders. *Child Development, 67,* 471–489.

Gurmankin, A. D., Baron, J. M., Hershey, J. C., & Ubel, P. A. (2002). The role of physicians' recommendations in medical treatment decisions. *Medical Decision Making, 22,* 262–271.

Guyatt, G., & Rennie, D. (Eds.) (2002). *Users' Guides to the Medical Literature: Essentials of Evidence-Based Practice.* Chicago: AMA Press.

Hall, J. W., & Jerger, J. (1978). Central auditory function in stutterers. *Journal of Speech and Hearing Research, 21,* 324–337.

Hall, N. E. (1996). Language and fluency in child language disorders: Changes over time. *Journal of Fluency Disorders, 21,* 1–32.

Hall, N. E. (2004). Lexical development and retrieval in treating children who stutter. *Language, Speech and Hearing Services in Schools, 35,* 57–69.

Hall, N. E., & Burgess, S. D. (2000). Exploring developmental changes in fluency as related to language acquisition: A case study. *Journal of Fluency Disorders, 25,* 119–141.

Hall, N. E., Wagovich, S., & Bernstein Ratner, N. (2007). Language considerations in childhood stuttering. In E. Conture & R. Curlee (Eds.), *Stuttering and Related Disorders of Fluency* (3rd ed., pp. 153–167). New York: Thieme Medical Publishers.

Hall, N. E., Yamashita, T. S., & Aram, D. M. (1993). Relationship between language and fluency in children with developmental language disorders. *Journal of Speech and Hearing Research, 36,* 568–579.

Hämäläinen M. (2007). Martinos Center for Biomedical Imaging. Retrieved December 23, 2008, from http://www.nmr.mgh.harvard.edu/martinos/research/technologiesMEG.php.

Hammett, L. A. (1994). An intensive therapy program in the public schools. Unpublished master's thesis, James Madison University, Harrisonburg, VA.

Hancock, K., & Craig, A. (2002). The effectiveness of re-treatment for adolescents who stutter. *Journal of Speech, Language, Hearing, Asia-Pacific, 7,* 138–156.

Hancock, K., Craig, A., Campbell, K., Costello, D., Gilmore, G., McCaul, A., & McCready, C. (1998). Two to six year controlled trial stuttering outcomes for children and adolescents. *Journal of Speech and Hearing Research, 41,* 1242–1252.

Hannley, M., & Dorman, M. (1982). Some observations on auditory function and stuttering. *Journal of Fluency Disorders, 7,* 93–108.

Hargrave, S., Kalinowski, J., Stuart, A., Armson, J., & Jones, K. (1994). Effect of frequency-altered feedback on stuttering frequency at normal and fast speech rates. *Journal of Speech and Hearing Research, 37,* 1313–319.

Harris, V., Onslow, M., Packman, A., Harrison, E., & Menzies, R. (2002). An experimental investigation of the impact of the Lidcombe Program on early stuttering. *Journal of Fluency Disorders, 27,* 203–214.

Harrison, E., Kingston, M., & Shenker, R. (2007). Management of stuttering preschoolers: Case studies in evidence based treatment. In M. Onslow & S. O'Brian (Eds.), *Evidence Based Treatment of Stuttering.* Manuscript in preparation.

Harrison, E. Onslow, M. Andrews, C. Packman, A., & Webber, M. (1998). Control of stuttering with prolonged speech: Development of a one-day instatement program. In A. Cordes & R. Ingham (Eds.), *Treatment Efficacy in Stuttering.* San Diego, CA: Singular Publishing Group.

Harrison, E., Onslow, M., & Menzies, R. (2004). Dismantling the Lidcombe Program of early stuttering intervention: Verbal contingencies for stuttering and clinical measurement. *International Journal of Language and Communication Disorders, 39,* 257–267.

Harrison, E., Onslow, M., & Rousseau (2007). The Lidcombe Program 2007: Clinical tales and clinical trials. In E. G. Conture & R. F. Curlee (Eds.), *Stuttering and Related Disorders of Fluency* (3rd ed., pp. 55–75). New York: Thieme.

Harrison, E., Wilson, L., & Onslow, M. (1999). Distance intervention for early stuttering with the Lidcombe Programme. *Advances in Speech-Language Pathology, 1,* 31–36.

Hartfield, K., & Conture, E. (2006). Effects of perceptual and conceptual similarity in lexical priming of young children who stutter: Preliminary findings. *Journal of Fluency Disorders, 31,* 303–324.

Harvey, J., Culatta, R., Halikas, J., Sorenson, J., Luxenberg, M., & Pearson, V. (1992). The effects of carbamazepine on stuttering. *Journal of Nervous and Mental Disease, 180,* 451–457.

Hashimoto, Y., & Sakai, K. L. (2003). Brain activations during conscious self-monitoring of speech production with delayed auditory feedback: An fMRI study. *Human Brain Mapping, 20,* 22–28.

Haupt, D. W., & Newcomer J. W. (2001). Hyperglycemia and antipsychotic medications. *Journal of Clinical Psychiatry, 62* (Suppl 27), 15–26.

Hayes, S. C., Barlow, D. H., & Nelson-Gray, R. O. (1999). *The Scientist Practitioner: Research and*

Accountability in the Age of Managed Care (2nd ed.). Boston: Allyn and Bacon.

Hayes, W., & Pindzola, R. (2004). *Diagnosis and Evaluation in Speech Pathology* (6th ed., pp. 191–216). Boston: Allyn & Bacon.

Hayhow, R., Cray, A. M., & Enderby, P. (2002). Stammering and therapy views of people who stammer. *Journal of Fluency Disorder, 27*, 1–16.

Hayhow, R., Kingston, M., & Ledzion, R. (1998). The use of clinical measures in the Lidcombe Programme for children who stutter. *International Journal of Language and Communication Disorders, 33*, 364–369.

Hayhow, R., Kingston, M., & Ledzion, R. (2003). The United Kingdom. In M. Onslow, A. Packman, & E. Harrison (Eds.), *The Lidcombe Program of Early Stuttering Intervention: A Clinician's Guide* (pp. 147–159). Austin, TX: Pro-Ed.

Haynes, R. B., Sackett, D. L., Gray, J. M., Cook, D. J., & Guyatt, G. H. (1996). Transferring evidence from research into practice: I. The role of clinical care research evidence in clinical decisions. *ACP Journal Club, 125*, A14-A16.

Haynes, R. B., Sackett, D. L., Guyatt, G. H., & Tugwell, P. (2006). *Clinical Epidemiology: How to Do Clinical Practice Research* (3rd ed.). Philadelphia: Lippincott Williams & Wilkins.

Healey, E. C., & Reid, R. (2003). ADHD and stuttering: A tutorial. *Journal of Fluency Disorders, 28*, 79–82.

Healey, E. C., & Scott, L. A. (1995). Strategies for treating elementary school-age children who stutter: An integrative approach. *Language, Speech, and Hearing Services in Schools, 26*, 151–161.

Hearne, A. (2006). Developing treatments for adolescents who stutter. Unpublished doctoral dissertation, University of Sydney, Sydney, Australia.

Heilman, K. M., Voeller, K., & Alexander, A. W. (1996). Developmental dyslexia: A motor-articulatory feedback hypothesis. *Annals of Neurology, 39*, 407–412.

Heiss, W. D, Kessler, J., Thiel, A., Ghaemi, M., & Karbe, H. (1999). Differential capacity of left and right hemispheric areas for compensation of post-stroke aphasia. *Annals of Neurology, 45*, 430–438.

Helliesen, G. (2006). *Speech Therapy for the Severe Adolescent and Adult Stutterer.* Newport News, VA: Apollo Press.

Herath, P., Klingberg, T., Young, J., Amunts, K., & Roland, P. (2001). Neural correlates of dual task interference can be dissociated from those of divided attention: An fMRI study. *Cerebral Cortex, 11*, 796–805.

Herder, C., Howard, C., Nye, C., & Vanryckeghem, M. (2006). Effectiveness of behavioral stuttering treatment: A systematic review and meta-analysis.

Contemporary Issues in Communication Science and Disorders, 33, 61–73.

Herring, J. P. (1986). *Fluency Criterion Program: A Stuttering Management System for Children and Adults.* Tucson, AZ: Communication Skill Builders, Inc.

Hersen, M. (2002). *Clinical Behavior Therapy: Adults and Children.* New York: John Wiley & Sons, Inc.

Heuer, R. J., Sataloff, R. T., Mandels, S., & Travers, N. (1996). Neurogenic stuttering: Further corroboration of site of lesion. *Ear, Nose and Throat Journal, 75*, 161–168.

Hewat, S., Harris, V., & Harrison, E. (2003). Special case studies. In M. Onslow, A. Packman, & E. Harrison (Eds.), *The Lidcombe Program of Early Stuttering Intervention: A Clinician's Guide* (pp. 119–136). Austin, TX: Pro-Ed.

Hewat, S., Onslow, M., Packman, A., & O'Brian, S. (2006). A Phase II clinical trial of self-imposed time-out treatment for stuttering in children and adults. *Disability and Rehabilitation, 28*, 33–42.

Hill, C. E., & O'Brien, K. M. (2000). *Helping Skills: Facilitating Exploration, Insight, and Action.* Washington, DC: American Psychological Association.

Hillis, J. W., & McHugh, J. (1998). Theoretical and pragmatic considerations for extraclinical generalization. In: A. K. Cordes and R. J. Ingham (Eds.), *Treatment Efficacy for Stuttering: A Search for Empirical Bases* (pp. 243–292). San Diego, CA: Singular.

Hodson, B. (2004). *The Hodson Assessment of Phonological Patterns–Third Edition (HAPP-3).* Austin, TX: PRO-ED, Inc.

Homzie M. J., Lindsay J. S., Simpson J., & Hasenstab S. (1988). Concomitant speech, language, and learning problems in adult stutterers and in members of their families. *Journal of Fluency Disorders, 13*, 261–277.

Howell, P. (2004). Assessment of some contemporary theories of stuttering that apply to spontaneous speech. *Contemporary Issues of Communication Science Disorders, 39*, 122–139.

Howell, P., & Au-Yeung, J. (1995). Syntactic determinants of stuttering in the spontaneous speech of normally fluent and stuttering children. *Journal of Fluency Disorders, 20*, 317–330.

Howell, P., & Au-Yeung, J. (2002). The EXPLAN theory of fluency control and the diagnosis of stuttering. In E. Fava (Ed.), *Pathology and Therapy of Speech Disorders* (pp. 75–94). Amsterdam, The Netherlands: John Benjamins.

Howell, P., Au-Yeung, J., & Sackin, S. (1999). Exchange of stuttering from function words to content words with age. *Journal of Speech, Language and Hearing Research, 42*, 345–354.

Howell, P., El-Yaniv, N., & Powell, D. (1987). Factors affecting fluency in stutterers when speaking under altered auditory feedback. In H. M. Peters &

W. Hulstijn (Eds.), *Speech Motor Dynamics in Stuttering* (pp. 361–369). New York: Springer Press.

Howie, P. M., Tanner, S., & Andrews, G. (1981). Short- and long-term outcome in an intensive treatment program for adult stutterers. *Journal of Speech and Hearing Disorders, 46,* 104–109.

Hresko, W., Reid, D., & Hamill, D. (1991). *Test of Early Language Development-2.* Austin, TX: Pro-Ed.

Hresko, W., Reid, D., & Hamill, D. (1999). *Test of Early Language Development-3.* Austin, TX: Pro-Ed.

Huang, S. C., Yu, D. C., Barrio, J. R., Grafton, S., Melega, W. P., Hoffman, J. M., Satyamurthy, N., Mazziotta, J. C., & Phelps, M. E. (1991). Kinetics and modeling of L-6[18F] fluoro-dopa in human positron emission tomographic studies. *Journal of Cerebral Blood Flow Metabolisms, 11,* 898–913.

Hubbard, C.P., & Prins, D. (1994). Word familiarity, syllabic stress pattern, and stuttering. *Journal of Speech and Hearing Research, 37,* 564–571.

Huesing, B., Jaencke, L., & Tag, B. (2006). *Impact Assessment of Neuroimaging. Final Report.* Zurich, Switzerland: vdf Hochschulverlag.

Hugh-Jones, S., & Smith, P. K. (1999). Self-reports of short- and long-term effects of bullying on children who stammer. *British Journal of Educational Psychology, 69,* 141–158.

Hulstijn, W., Peters, H., & van Lieshout, P. (1997). *Speech Production: Motor Control, Brain Research and Fluency Disorders.* Amsterdam: Elsevier Press.

Immordino-Yang, M. H., & Damasio, A. (2007). We feel therefore we learn: The relevance of affective and social neuroscience to education. *Mind, Brain and Education, 1,* 3–10.

Indefrey, P., & Levelt, W. J. M. (2000). The neural correlates of language production. In M. Gazzaniga (Ed.), *The New Cognitive Neuroscience* (2nd ed., pp. 845–865). Chicago, IL: MIT Press.

Indefrey, P., & Levelt, W. J. M. (2004). The spatial and temporal signatures of word production components. *Cognition, 92,* 101–144.

Indevus Pharmaceuticals. (2006). EXPRESS: Examining Pagoclone for Persistent Developmental Stuttering Study. Clinical trials.gov Identifier: NCT00216255. Announced May 24, 2006.

Ingham, J. C. (1999). Behavioral treatment of young children who stutter: An extended length of utterance method. In R. F. Curlee (Ed.), *Stuttering and Related Disorders of Fluency* (2nd ed., pp. 80–109). New York: Thieme Medical Publishers.

Ingham, J. C. (2003). Evidence-based treatment of stuttering: I. Definition and application. *Journal of Fluency Disorders, 28,* 197–207.

Ingham, J. C., & Riley, G. (1998). Guidelines for documentation of treatment efficacy for young children who stutter. *Journal of Speech Language and Hearing Research, 41,* 753–770.

Ingham, R. J. (1982). The effects of self-evaluation training on maintenance and generalization during stuttering treatment. *Journal of Speech and Hearing Disorders, 47,* 271–280.

Ingham, R. J. (1984). Generalization and maintenance of treatment. In R. F Curlee, & W. H. Perkins (Eds.), *Nature and Treatment of Stuttering: New Directions.* San Diego, CA: College-Hill Press.

Ingham, R. J. (1984). *Stuttering and Behavior Therapy: Current Status and Experimental Foundations.* San Diego, CA: College-Hill Press.

Ingham, R. J. (1987). *Residential Prolonged Speech Stuttering Therapy Manual.* Santa Barbara, CA: Department of Speech and Hearing Sciences, University of California.

Ingham, R. J. (1990). Research on stuttering treatment for adults and adolescents: A perspective on how to overcome a malaise. In J. A. Cooper (Ed.), *Research Needs in Stuttering: Roadblocks and Future Directions* (pp. 91–95). Rockville, MD: American Speech-Language-Hearing Association.

Ingham, R. J. (1999). Performance-contingent management of stuttering in adolescents and adults. In R. F. Curlee (Ed.), *Stuttering and Related Disorders of Fluency* (2nd ed., pp. 200–211). New York: Thieme Medical Publishers.

Ingham, R. J. (2001). Brain imaging studies of developmental stuttering. *Journal of Communication Disorders, 34,* 493–516.

Ingham, R. J. (Ed.) (2003). Brain imaging and stuttering [Special Issue]. *Journal of Fluency Disorders, 28* (4).

Ingham, R. J., & Andrews, G. (1973). Behavior therapy and stuttering therapy: A review. *Journal of Speech and Hearing Disorders, 38,* 406–441.

Ingham, R. J., & Andrews, G. (1973). Details of a token economy stuttering therapy programme for adults. *Australian Journal of Human Communication Disorders, 1,* 13–20.

Ingham, R. J., Bakker, K., Moglia, R., & Kilgo, M. (2001). *The Stuttering Measurement System Training Program.* Santa Barbara, CA.

Ingham, R. J., & Cordes, A. (1992). Interclinic differences in stuttering event counts. *Journal of Fluency Disorders, 17,* 171–176.

Ingham, R. J., & Cordes, A. (1997). Self-measurement and evaluating stuttering treatment efficacy. In R. F. Curlee & G. M. Siegel (Eds.), *Nature and Treatment of Stuttering: New Directions* (2nd ed., pp. 413–437). Boston: Allyn & Bacon.

Ingham, R. J., & Cordes, A. K. (1998). Treatment decisions for young children who stutter: Further concerns and complexities. *American Journal of Speech-Language Pathology, 7,* 10–19.

Ingham, R. J., & Cordes, A. K. (1999). On watching a discipline shoot itself in the foot: Some observations on current trends in stuttering treatment. In N. B. Ratner & E. C. Healey (Eds.), *Stuttering Research and Practice: Bridging the Gap* (pp. 211–230). Mahwah, NJ: Lawrence Erlbaum.

Ingham, R. J., Cordes, A., & Finn, P. (1993). Time-interval measurement of stuttering: Systematic replication of Ingham, Cordes & Gow (1993). *Journal of Speech and Hearing Research, 36,* 1168–1176.

Ingham, R. J., & Costello, J. M. (1984). Stuttering treatment outcome evaluation. In J. M. Costello (Ed.), *Speech Disorders in Children: Recent Advances* (pp. 313–346). San Diego, CA: College-Hill.

Ingham, R. J., & Costello, J. M. (1985). Stuttering treatment outcome evaluation. In J. M. Costello (Ed.), *Speech Disorders in Adults: Recent Advances* (pp. 189–223). San Diego, CA: College-Hill.

Ingham, R. J., Fox, P. T., Ingham, J. C., Collins, J., & Pridgen, S. (2000). TMS in developmental stuttering and Tourette syndrome. In M. S. George & R. H. Belmaker (Eds.), *Transcranial Magnetic Stimulation in Neuropsychiatry* (pp. 223–236). Washington, DC: American Psychiatric Press.

Ingham, R. J., Fox, P. T., Ingham, J. C., Xiong, J., Zamarripa, F., Hardies, L. J., & Lancaster, J. L. (2004). Brain correlates of stuttering and syllable production: Gender comparison and replication. *Journal of Speech, Language, and Hearing Research, 47,* 321–341.

Ingham, R. J., Fox, P. T., Ingham, J. C., Zamarripa, F. (2000). Is overt stuttered speech a prerequisite for the neural activations associated with chronic developmental stuttering? *Brain and Language, 75,* 163–194.

Ingham, R. J., Gow, M., & Costello, J. M. (1985). Stuttering and speech naturalness: Some additional data. *Journal of Speech and Hearing Disorders, 50,* 217–219.

Ingham, R. J., Ingham, J. C., Onslow, M., & Finn, P. (1989). Stutterers' self-ratings of speech naturalness: Assessing effects and reliability. *Journal of Speech and Hearing Research, 32,* 419–431.

Ingham, R. J., Kilgo, M., Ingham, J. C., Moglia, R., Belknap, H., & Sanchez, T. (2001). Evaluation of a stuttering treatment based on reduction of short phonation. *Journal of Speech, Language, and Hearing Research, 44,* 1229–1244.

Ingham, R. J., Martin, R. R., Haroldson, S. K., Onslow, M., & Leney, M. (1985). Modification of listener-judged naturalness in the speech of stutterers. *Journal of Speech and Hearing Research, 28,* 495–504.

Ingham, R. J., Moglia, R., Frank, P., Ingham, J., & Cordes, A. (1997). Experimental investigations of the effects of frequency-altered auditory feedback on the speech of adults who stutter. *Journal of Speech, Language, and Hearing Research, 40,* 361–372.

Ingham, R. J., & Onslow, M. (1985). Measurement and modification of speech naturalness during stuttering therapy. *Journal of Speech and Hearing Disorders, 50,* 261–281.

Ingham, R. J., & Onslow, M. (1987). Generalization and maintenance of treatment benefits for children who stutter. *Seminars in Speech and Language, 8,* 303–326.

Jackson, G. B. (1980). Methods for integrative reviews. *Review of Educational Research, 50,* 438–460.

James, J. E. (1981). Behavioral self-control of stuttering using time-out from speaking. *Journal of Applied Behavior Analysis, 14,* 25–37.

James, J. E. (2007). Claims of a "new" stuttering treatment using time-out from speaking are exaggerated: A brief review of the literature and commentary on Hewat et al. (2006). *Disability and Rehabilitation, 29,* 1057–1060.

James, J., Ricciardelli, L., Hunter, C., & Rogers, P. (1989) Relative efficacy of intensive and spaced behavioral treatment of stuttering. *Behavior Modification, 13,* 376–395.

Jäncke, L., Hanggi, J., & Steinmetz, H. (2004). Morphological brain differences between adult stutterers and non-stutterers. *BioMed Central Neurology, 4,* 23.

Jäncke, L., Shah, N. J., Posse, S., Grosse-Ryuken, M., & Muller-Gartner, H. W. (1998). Intensity coding of auditory stimuli: An fMRI study. *Neuropsychologia, 36,* 875–883.

Johannsen, H. S. (2000). Design of the longitudinal study and influence of symptomatology; heredity; sex ratio and lateral dominance on the further development of stuttering. In *Proceedings of the Third World Congress of Fluency Disorders: Theory, Research, Treatment and Self Help* (pp. 183–186). Nijmegen, The Netherlands: University Press Nijmegen.

Johnson, K., Conture, E., Karrass, J., & Walden, T. (2009). Influence of variations in stuttering frequency on talker group classification. *Journal of Communication Disorders, 42,* 195–210.

Johnson, W. (1942). A study of the onset and development of stuttering. *Journal of Speech and Hearing Disorders, 7,* 251–257.

Johnson, W. (1961). *Stuttering and What You Can Do about It.* Danville, IL: Interstate Printers and Publishers, Inc.

Johnson, W., & Associates. (1959). *The Onset of Stuttering.* Minneapolis, MN: University of Minneapolis Press.

Johnson, W., & Rosen, L. (1937). Studies in the psychology of stuttering: VII. Effects of certain changes in speech pattern upon the frequency of stuttering. *Journal of Speech Disorders, 2,* 105–109.

Jones, B., & Nagin, D. (2006). Advances in group-based trajectory modeling and a SAS procedure for estimating them. Unpublished manuscript.

Jones, B., Nagin, D., & Roeder, K. (2001). A SAS procedure based on mixture models for estimating developmental trajectories. *Sociological Methods and Research, 29,* 374–393.

Jones, M., Blakeley, M., & Ormond, T. (2003). New Zealand. In M. Onslow, A. Packman, & E. Harrison (Eds.), *The Lidcombe Program of Early Stuttering Intervention: A Clinician's Guide* (pp. 173–182). Austin, TX: Pro-Ed.

Jones, M., Gebski, V., Onslow, M., & Packman, A. (2001). Design of randomized controlled trials: Principles and methods applied to a treatment for early stuttering. *Journal of Fluency Disorders, 26,* 247–267.

Jones, M., Hearne, A., Onslow, M., Ormond, T., Williams, S., Schwarz, I., & O'Brian, S. (2007). Extended follow up of a randomised controlled trial of the LP of Early Stuttering Intervention. Manuscript submitted for publication.

Jones, M., Onslow, M., Harrison, E., & Packman, A. (2000). Treating stuttering in children: Predicting outcome in the Lidcombe Program. *Journal of Speech, Language, and Hearing Research, 43,* 1440–1450.

Jones, M., Onslow, M., Packman, A., Williams, S., Ormond, T., Schwarz, I., & Gebski, V. (2005). Randomised controlled trial of the Lidcombe Program of early stuttering intervention. *British Medical Journal, 331,* 7518.

Jones, M., Onslow, M., Packman, A., Williams, S., Ormond, T., Schwarz, T., & Gebski, V. (2005). A randomised controlled trial of the Lidcombe Program for early stuttering intervention. *British Medical Journal, 331,* 659–661.

Jones, P. H., & Ryan, B. P. (2001). Experimental analysis of the relationship between speaking rate and stuttering during mother-child conversation. *Journal of Developmental and Physical Disabilities, 13,* 279–305.

Jones, R. K. (1966). Observations on stammering after localized cerebral injury. *Journal of Neurology, Neurosurgery, and Psychiatry, 29,* 192–195.

Jones, R. K. (1967). Dypraxic ambiphasia. A neurophysiologic theory of stammering. *Transactions of the American Neurological Association, 92,* 197–201.

Kagan, J. (1994). *Galen's Prophecy: Temperament in Human Nature.* New York: Basic Books.

Kahneman, D. P., Slovic, P., & Tversky, A. (Eds.) (1982). *Judgment Under Uncertainty: Heuristics and Biases.* Cambridge, United Kingdom: Cambridge University Press.

Kahneman, D. P., & Tversky, A. (1996). On the reality of cognitive illusions: A reply to Gigerenzer's critique. *Psychological Review, 103,* 582–591.

Kalinowski, J., Armson, J., Roland-Mieszkowski, M., & Stuart, A. (1993). Effects of alterations in auditory feedback and speech rate on stuttering frequency. *Language and Speech, 36,* 1–16.

Kalinowski, J., Stuart, A., Rastatter, M., Miller, R., Zimmerman, S., & Shine, R. (1998). Examination of altered auditory feedback: Therapeutic implications. In E. C. Healey & H. F. M. Peters (Eds.), *Proceedings from the Second World Congress on Fluency Disorders* (pp. 54–57). Nijmegen, The Netherlands: University Press Nijmegen.

Kalinowski, J., Stuart, A., Sark, S., & Armson, J. (1996). Stuttering amelioration at various auditory feedback delays and speech rates. *European Journal of Disorders of Communication, 31,* 259–269.

Kamhi, A.G. (2006). Treatment decisions for children with speech-sound disorders. *Language, Speech, and Hearing Services in Schools, 37,* 271–279.

Karrass, J., Walden, T., Conture, E., Arnold, H., Graham, C., & Hartfield, K. (2005). Relation of emotional reactivity and regulation to childhood stuttering across multiple measures of emotional reactivity and regulation in children. Manuscript in preparation.

Karrass, J., Walden, T., Conture, E., Graham, C., Arnold, H., Hartfield, K., & Schwenk, K. (2006). Relation of emotional reactivity and regulation to childhood stuttering. *Journal of Communication Disorders, 39,* 402–423.

Kassubek, J., Juengling, F. D., Kioschies, T., Henkel, K., Karitzky, J., Kramer, B., Ecker, D., Andrich, J., Saft, C., Kraus, P., Aschoff, A. J., Ludolph, A. C., & Landwehrmeyer, G. B. (2004). Topography of cerebral atrophy in early Huntington's disease: A voxel based morphometric MRI study. *Journal of Neurology, Neurosurgery, and Psychiatry, 75,* 213–220.

Kaufman, G. (1985). *Shame: The Power of Caring.* Rochester, VT: Schenkman.

Kaufman, G., Raphael, L., & Espeland, P. (1999). *Stick Up for Yourself.* Minneapolis, MN: Free Spirit Publishing, Inc.

Kazdin, A. E. (1982). *Single Case Research Designs: Methods for Clinical and Applied Settings.* New York: Oxford University Press.

Kelly, E. M. (1993). Speech rates and turn-taking behaviors of children who stutter and their parents. *Seminars in Speech and Language, 14,* 203–214.

Kelly, E. M. (1994). Speech rates and turn-taking behaviors of children who stutter and their fathers. *Journal of Speech and Hearing Research, 37,* 1284–1294.

Kelly, E. M., & Conture, E. G. (1992). Speaking rates, response time latencies, and interrupting behaviors of young stutterers, nonstutterers, and their mothers. *Journal of Speech and Hearing Research, 35,* 1256–1267.

Kelly, E. M., Martin, J. S, Baker, K. I., Rivera, N. J., Bishop, J. E., Kriziske, C. B., Stettler, D. S., &

Stealy, J. M. (1997). Academic and clinical preparation and practices of school speech-language pathologists with people who stutter. *Language, Speech and Hearing Services in the Schools, 28,* 195–212.

Kelman, E., & Nicholas, A. (2008). *Practical Intervention for Early Childhood Stammering: Palin PCI.* Milton Keynes, United Kingdom: Speechmark Publishing Limited.

Kelman, E., & Schneider, C. (1994) Parent-child interaction: An alternative approach to the management of children's language difficulties. *Child Language Teaching and Therapy, 10,* 81–96.

Kent, L. R. (1963). The use of tranquilizers in the treatment of stuttering. *Journal of Speech and Hearing Disorders, 28,* 288–294.

Kent, L. R., & Williams, D. E. (1959). Use of meprobamate as an adjunct to stuttering therapy. *Journal of Speech and Hearing Disorders, 24,* 64–69.

Khan, L., & Lewis, N. (2002). *Khan-Lewis Phonological Analysis-Second Edition (KLPA-2).* Bloomington, MN: Pearson Assessments

Kim, S. W. (1996). Opioid antagonists in the treatment of impulse-control disorders. *Journal of Clinical Psychiatry, 59,* 159–164.

Kingston, M., Huber, A., Onslow, M., Jones, M., & Packman, A. (2003). Predicting treatment time with the Lidcombe Program: Replication and meta-analysis. *International Journal of Language and Communication Disorders, 38,* 165–177.

Klassen, T. R., & Kroll, R. M. (2005). Opinions on stuttering and its treatment: A follow-up survey and cross-cultural comparison. *Journal of Speech-Language Pathology and Audiology, 29,* 73–82.

Klee, T., Schaffer, M., May, S., Membrino, I., & Mougey, K. (1989). A comparison of the age-MLU relation in normal and specifically language impaired preschool children. *Journal of Speech and Hearing Disorders, 54,* 226–233.

Kline, M. I., & Starkweather, C. W. (1979). Receptive and expressive language performance in young stutterers. *ASHA, 21* (Abstr), 797.

Kloth, S. A. M., Janssen, P., Kraaimaat, F., & Brutten, G. J. (1998). Child and mother variables in the development of stuttering among high-risk children: A longitudinal study. *Journal of Fluency Disorders, 23,* 217–230.

Kloth, S. A. M., Kraaimaat, F. W., Janssen, P., & Brutten, G. J. (1999). Persistence and remission of incipient stuttering among high-risk children. *Journal of Fluency Disorders, 24,* 253–265.

Koushik, S., Shenker, R. C., Onslow, M., & Adaman, B. (2007). Follow-up of school-age children after Lidcombe Program treatment. Poster presented at the meeting of the American Speech and Hearing Association, Boston, MA.

Kowal, A., O'Connell, D. C., & Sabin, E. G. (1975). Development of temporal patterning and vocal hesitations in spontaneous narratives. *Journal of Psycholinguistic Research, 4,* 195–207.

Kraaimaat, F. W., Vanryckeghem, M., & Van Dam-Baggen, R. (2002). Stuttering and social anxiety. *Journal of Fluency Disorders, 27,* 319–330.

Krall, T. (2001). The International Stuttering Association—Objectives, activities, outlook: Our dreams for self-help and therapy. In H.-G. Bosshardt, J. S. Yaruss, & H. F. M. Peters (Eds.), *Fluency Disorders: Theory, Research, Treatment, and Self-Help—Proceedings of the Third World Congress on Fluency Disorders* (pp. 30–40). Nijmegen, The Netherlands: Nijmegen University Press.

Kroll, R. (1991). *Manual of Fluency Maintenance: A Guide for Ongoing Practice.* Toronto: Clarke Institute of Psychiatry.

Kroll, R.., & Beitchman, J. H. (2005). Stuttering. In B. J. Sadock & V. A. Sadock (Eds.), *Comprehensive Textbook of Psychiatry* (pp. 3154–3159). Philadelphia: Lippincott Williams & Wilkins.

Kroll, R. M., Cook, F., De Nil, L., & Ratner, N. B. (2006). Preparing clinicians to treat stuttering effectively: An interactive panel discussion. Paper presented at the 5th World Congress on Fluency Disorders, Dublin, Ireland.

Kroll, R. M., & De Nil, L. F. (1995). Locus of control and client performance variables as predictors of stuttering treatment outcome. In C. W. Starkweather & H. M. F. Peters (Eds.), *Proceedings of the First World Congress on Stuttering: Volume 1* (pp. 375–379). Munich, Germany: International Fluency Association.

Kroll, R. M., & De Nil, L. F. (1998). Positron emission tomography studies of stuttering: Their relationship to our theoretical and clinical understanding of the disorder. *Journal of Speech Language Pathology and Audiology, 22,* 261–270.

Kroll, R. M., & De Nil, L. F. (2000). Research using PET scans identifies neural bases of stuttering and its treatment. *Stuttering Foundation of America Newsletter, Summer Edition,* 1–3.

Kroll, R.M., De Nil, L. F., & Houle, S. (1999). Toward a scientific understanding of stuttering & treatment: PET-scan studies. Paper presented at the Annual Convention of the American Speech-Language-Hearing Association, San Francisco, CA.

Kroll, R. M., De Nil, L. F., Kapur, S., & Houle, S. (1997). A positron emission tomography investigation of post-treatment brain activation in stutterers. In H. F. M. Peters, W. Hulstijn, & P. H. H. M. Van Lieshout (Eds.), *Speech Production: Motor Control, Brain Research and Fluency Disorders* (pp. 307–320). Amsterdam: Elsevier.

Kroll, R. M., Gaulin, B., & Tammsalu, A. (1981). Fluency maintenance: Follow-up data on a model for post-treatment. Paper presented at the Annual Convention of the American Speech-Language-Hearing Association, Los Angeles, CA.

Kroll, R. M., & Klassen, T.R. (in press). Perspectives on the academic and clinical education in stuttering. *Canadian Journal of Speech-Language Pathology and Audiology, 31,* 92–100.

Kroll, R. M., & O'Keefe, B. M. (1990). Opinions on stuttering therapy: A survey of CASLPA members. *Journal of Speech-Language Pathology and Audiology, 14,* 59–63.

Kroll, R. M., & Scott-Sulsky, L. (2006). *Fluency Plus Program: A Comprehensive Treatment Program for School Aged Children Who Stutter.* Toronto: Speech Foundation of Ontario.

Kully, D., & Boberg, E. (1988). An investigation of inter-clinic agreement in the identification of fluent and stuttered syllables. *Journal of Fluency Disorders, 13,* 309–318.

Kully, D., & Boberg, E. (1991). Therapy for school-age children. In E. Perkins (Ed.), *Seminars in Speech and Language: Stuttering: Challenges of Therapy.* New York: Thieme Medical Publishers.

Kully, D., & Langevin, M. (1999). Intensive treatment for stuttering adolescents. In R. F. Curlee (Ed.), *Stuttering and Related Disorders of Fluency* (2nd ed., pp. 139–159). New York: Thieme Medical Publishers.

Kully, D., & Langevin, M. (2005). Evidence-based practice in fluency disorders. *The ASHA Leader, 10,* 10–11, 23.

Kunz, R., & Oxman, A. D. (1998). The unpredictability paradox: Review of empirical comparisons of randomised and non-randomised clinical trials. *British Medical Journal, 317,* 1185–1190.

Ladouceur, R., Boudreau, L., & Theberge, S. (1981). Awareness training and regulated-breathing method in modification of stuttering. *Perceptual and Motor Skills, 53,* 187–194.

Ladouceur, R., Caron, C., & Caron, G. (1989). Stuttering severity and treatment outcome. *Journal of Behavior Therapy and Experimental Psychiatry, 20,* 49–56.

Ladouceur, R., & Martineau, G. (1982). Evaluation of regulated-breathing method with and without parental assistance in the treatment of child stutterers. *Journal of Behavior Therapy and Experimental Psychiatry, 13,* 301–306.

Laiho, A., & Klippi, A. (2007). Long- and short-term results of children's and adolescents' therapy courses for stuttering. *International Journal of Language and Communication Disorders, 42,* 367–382.

Langevin, M. (1997). Peer teasing project. In E. Healey & H. F. M. Peters (Eds.), *Second World Congress on Fluency Disorders: Proceedings* (pp. 169–171). Nijmegen, The Netherlands: Nijmegen University Press.

Langevin, M. (2000). *Teasing and Bullying: Unacceptable Behaviour. The TAB Program.* Edmonton, Alberta, Canada: Institute for Stuttering Treatment and Research.

Langevin, M., Bortnick, K., Hammer, T., & Wiebe, E. (1998). Teasing/bullying experienced by children who stutter: Toward development of a questionnaire. *Contemporary Issues in Communication Science and Disorders, 25,* 12–24.

Langlois, A., & Long, S. H. (1988). A model for teaching parents to facilitate fluent speech. *Language, Speech and Hearing Services in Schools, 32,* 68–78.

Lass, N. J., Ruscello, D. M., Schmitt, J. F., Pannbacker, M. D., Orlando, M. B., Dean, K. A., Ruziska, J. C., & Bradshaw, K. H. (1992). Teachers' perceptions of stutterers. *Language, Speech, and Hearing Services in Schools, 23,* 78–81.

Lattermann, C., Euler, H. A., & Neumann, K. A. (2007). Randomized control trial to investigate the impact of the LP on early stuttering in German-speaking preschoolers. Manuscript submitted for publication.

Lattermann, C., Euler, H. A., & Neumann, K. A. (2008). A randomized control trial to investigate the impact of the Lidcombe Program on early stuttering in German-speaking preschoolers. *Journal of Fluency Disorders, 33,* 52–65.

Latterman, C., Shenker, R. C., & Thorardottir, E. (2005). Progression of language complexity during treatment with the LP for early stuttering intervention. *American Journal of Speech-Language Pathology, 14,* 242–253.

Le Bihan, D., Mangin, J. F., Poupon, C., Clark, C. A., Pappata, S., Molko, N., & Chabriat, H. (2001). Diffusion tensor imaging: concepts and applications. *Magnetic Resonance Imaging, 13,* 534–546.

Lee, B. S. (1951). Artificial stutter. *Journal of Speech and Hearing Disorders, 16,* 53–55.

Lee, L. (1974). *Developmental Sentence Analysis: A Grammatical Assessment Procedure for Speech and Language Clinicians.* Evanston, IL: Northwestern University Press.

Lehéricy, S., Benali, H., Van de Moortele, P. F., Pélégrini-Issac, M., Waechter, T., Ugurbil, K., & Doyon, J. (2005). Distinct basal ganglia territories are engaged in early and advanced motor sequence learning. *Proceedings of the National Academy of Sciences of the United States of America, 102,* 12566–12571.

Leibovitz, S., & Kroll, R. M. (1980). Intensive stuttering therapy: Retrospective data and current maintenance considerations. Paper presented at the Annual Convention of the American Speech-Language-Hearing Association, Detroit, MI.

Leichnetz, G. R. (2001). Connections of the medial posterior parietal cortex (area 7m) in the monkey. *The Anatomical Record, 263,* 215–236.

Leith, W. R. (1984). *Handbook of Stuttering Therapy for the School Clinician.* San Diego, CA: College Hill

Levelt, W. J. M. (1989). *Speaking: From Intention to Articulation.* Cambridge, MA: MIT Press.

Levelt, W. J. M., Roelofs, A., & Meyer, A. S. (1999). A theory of lexical access in speech production. *Behavioral and Brain Sciences, 22,* 1–49.

Levelt, W. J. M., & Wheeldon, L. (1994). Do speakers have access to mental syllabary? *Cognition, 50,* 239–269.

Lewis, C., Onslow, M., Packman, A., Jones, M., & Simpson, J. M. (in press). A phase II trial of telehealth delivery of the LP of early stuttering intervention. *American Journal of Speech-Language Pathology.*

Lewis, D., & Sherman, D. (1951). Measuring the severity of stuttering. *Journal of Speech and Hearing Disorders, 16,* 320–326.

Liebotwitz, M. R. (1993). Pharmacotherapy of social phobia. *Journal of Clinical Psychiatry, 54* (Suppl 3), 1–5.

Lincoln, M., & Onslow, M. (1997). Long-term outcome of an early intervention for stuttering. *American Journal of Speech-Language Pathology, 6,* 51–58.

Lincoln, M., Onslow, M., Lewis, C., & Wilson, L. (1996). A clinical trial of an operant treatment for school-age children who stutter. *American Journal of Speech-Language Pathology, 5,* 73–85.

Lincoln, M., Onslow, M., & Reed, V. (1997). Social validity in the treatment outcomes of an early intervention for stuttering: The Lidcombe Program. *American Journal of Speech-Language Pathology, 6,* 77–84.

Lincoln, M., & Packman, A. (2003). Measuring stuttering. In M. Onslow, A. Packman, & E. Harrison (Eds.), *The Lidcombe Program of early Stuttering Intervention: A Clinician's Guide.* Austin, TX: Pro-Ed.

Linde, K., Scholz, M., Ramirez, G., Clausius, N., Melchart, D., & Jonas, W. B. (1999). Impact of study quality on outcome in placebo-controlled trials of homeopathy. *Journal of Clinical Epidemiology, 52,* 631–636.

Littell, J. H. (2005). Lessons from a systematic review of effects of multisystemic therapy. *Children and Youth Services Review, 27,* 445–463.

Logan, K. J., & Conture, E. G. (1995). Length, grammatical complexity, and rate differences in stuttered and fluent conversational utterances of children who stutter. *Journal of Fluency Disorders, 20,* 35–61.

Logan, K. J., & Conture, E. G. (1997). Selected temporal, grammatical, and phonological characteristics of conversational utterances produced by children who stutter. *Journal of Speech, Language, and Hearing Research, 40,* 107–120.

Logan, K. J., & LaSalle, L. R. (1999). Grammatical characteristics of children's conversational utterances that contain disfluency clusters. *Journal of Speech, Language and Hearing Research, 42,* 80–91.

Logan, K. J., & Yaruss, J. S. (1999). Helping parents address attitudinal and emotional factors with young children who stutter. *Contemporary Issues in Communication Science and Disorders, 26,* 69–81.

Louko, L. J., Edwards, M. L., & Conture, E. G. (1990). Phonological characteristics of young stutterers and their normally fluent peers: Preliminary observations. *Journal of Fluency Disorders, 15,* 191–210.

Ludlow, C., & Dooman, A. (1992). Genetic aspects of idiopathic speech and language disorders. *Otolaryngology Clinicians in North America, 25,* 979–994.

Luper, H. I., & Mulder, R. I. (1964). *Stuttering Therapy for Children.* Englewood Cliffs, NJ: Prentice-Hall.

Luterman, D. (2001). *Counseling Persons with Communicative Disorders and Their Families* (5th ed.). Austin, TX: Pro-Ed.

Lynd, R. S. (1939). *Knowledge for What? The Place of Social Science in American Culture.* Princeton, NJ: Princeton University Press.

Maansson, H. (2007). Complexity and diversity in early childhood stuttering. In J. Au-Yeung & M. Healey (Eds.), *Research, Treatment and Self-Help in Fluency Disorders: New Horizons. Proceedings of the Fifth World Congress on Fluency Disorders.* Nyborg, Denmark.

Maas, E., Robin, D., Austermann Hula, S., Freedman, S., Wulf, G., Ballard, K., & Schmidt, R. (2008). Principles of motor learning in treatment of motor speech disorders. *American Journal of Speech-Language Pathology, 17,* 277–298.

MacLean, P. D. (1993). Perspectives on cingulate cortex in the limbic system. In B. Vogt & M. Gabriel (Eds.), *Neurobiology of Cingulate Cortex and the Limbic Thalamus* (pp. 1–15). Boston: Birkhauser.

Macleod, J., Kalinowski, J., Stuart, A., & Armson, J. (1995). Effect of single and combined altered auditory feedback on stuttering frequency at two speech rates. *Journal of Communication Disorders, 28,* 217–228.

Maguire G. A. (2002). Prolactin elevation with antipsychotic medications: Mechanisms of action and clinical consequences. *Journal of Clinical Psychiatry, 63* (Suppl 4), 56–62.

Maguire, G. A., Riley, G. D., Franklin, D. L., & Gottschalk, L. A. (2000). Risperidone for the treatment of stuttering. *Journal of Clinical Psychopharmacology, 20,* 479–482.

Maguire, G. A., Riley, G. D., Franklin, D. L., Maguire, M., & Brojeni, P. (2000). The dopamine hypothesis of stuttering and its treatment implications. *International Journal of Neurophychopharmacology, 3* (Suppl 1), S12.

Maguire, G. A., Riley, G. D., Franklin, D. L., Maguire, M., & Brojeni, P. (2004). Olanzapine in the treatment of developmental stuttering: A double-blind, placebo-controlled trial. *Annals of Clinical Psychiatry, 16,* 63–67.

Maguire, G. A., Riley, G. D., & Yu B. P. (2002). A neurological basis of stuttering? *The Lancet Neurology, 1,* 407.

Maguire, G. A., Yu, B. P., Franklin, D. L., & Riley, G. D. (2004). Alleviating stuttering with pharmacological interventions. *Expert Opinion Pharmacotherapy, 7,* 1565–1571.

Mahr, G. C., & Torosian, T. (1999). Anxiety and social phobia. *Journal of Fluency Disorders, 24,* 119–126.

Mallard, A. R., Gardner, L. S., & Downey, C. S. (1988). Clinical training in stuttering for school clinicians. *Journal of Fluency Disorders, 13,* 253–259.

Manning, W. H. (1991). Sports analogies in the treatment of stuttering: Taking the field with your client. *Public School Caucus, 10,* 10–11.

Manning, W. H. (1999). Progress under the surface and over time. In N. Bernstein Ratner & E. C. Healey (Eds.), *Stuttering Research and Practice: Bridging the Gap* (pp. 123–130). Mahwah, NJ: Lawrence Erlbaum Associates, Inc.

Manning, W. H. (2001). *Clinical Decision Making in Fluency Disorders* (2nd ed.). San Diego, CA: Singular/Thompson Learning.

Marinkovic, K., Dhond, R. P., Dale, A. M., Glessner, M., Carr, V., & Halgren, E. (2003). Spatiotemporal dynamics of modality-specific and supramodal word processing. *Neuron, 38,* 487–497.

Martin, R. R., & Berndt, L. A. (1970). The effects of time-out on stuttering in a 12-year-old boy. *Exceptional Children, 36,* 303–304.

Martin, R. R., & Haroldson, S. K. (1971). Time-out as a punishment for stuttering during conversation. *Journal of Communication Disorders, 4,* 15–19.

Martin, R. R., & Haroldson, S. K. (1977). Effects of vicarious punishment on stuttering frequency. *Journal of Speech and Hearing Research, 20,* 21–26.

Martin, R., & Haroldson, S.K. (1992). Stuttering and speech naturalness: Audio and audiovisual judgments. Journal of Speech and Hearing Research, 35, 521–528.

Martin, R. R., Haroldson, S. K., & Triden, K. A. (1984). Stuttering and speech naturalness. *Journal of Speech and Hearing Disorders, 49,* 53–58.

Martin, R.R., & Ingham, R. J. (1973). Stuttering. In B. Lahey (Ed.), Modification of Speech and Language. Springfield, IL: Charles C. Thomas.

Martin, R. R., Kuhl, P., & Haroldson, S. K. (1972). An experimental treatment with two preschool stuttering children. *Journal of Speech and Hearing Research, 15,* 743–752.

Martin, R. R., & Siegel, G. M. (1966a). The effects of response contingent shock on stuttering. *Journal of Speech and Hearing Research, 9,* 340–352.

Martin, R. R., & Siegel, G. M. (1966b). The effects of simultaneously punishing stuttering and rewarding fluency. *Journal of Speech and Hearing Research, 9,* 466–475.

Martin, R. R., St Louis, K., Haroldson, S., & Hasbrouck, J. (1975). Punishment and negative reinforcement of stuttering using electric shock. *Journal of Speech and Hearing Research, 18,* 478–490.

Marx, C. E., Van Doren, M. J., Duncan, G. E., Liebermann, J. A., & Morrow, A. L. (2003). Olanzapine and clozapine increase the GABAergic neuroactive steroid allopregnanolone in rodents. *Neuropsychopharmacology, 28,* 1–13.

Matthews, S., Williams, R., & Pring, T. (1997). Parent-child interaction therapy and dysfluency: A single-case study. *European Journal of Disorders of Communication, 32,* 346–357.

Max, L. (2004). Stuttering and internal models for sensorimotor control: A theoretical perspective to generate testable hypotheses. In B. Maassen, R. Kent, H. Peters, P. van Lieshout, & W. Hulstijn (Eds.), *Speech Motor Control in Normal and Disordered Speech* (pp. 357–387). New York: Oxford University Press.

Max, L., & Caruso, A. J. (1998). Adaptation of stuttering frequency during repeated readings: Associated changes in acoustic parameters of perceptually fluent speech. *Journal of Speech, Language, and Hearing Research, 41,* 165–181.

Max, L., Caruso, A. J., & Gracco, V. L. (2003). Kinematic analyses of speech, orofacial nonspeech, and finger movements in stuttering and nonstuttering adults. *Journal of Speech, Language, and Hearing Research, 46,* 215–232.

Max, L., Guenther, F. H., Gracco, V. L., Ghosh, S. S., & Wallace, M. E. (2004). Internal models and feedback-biased motor control as sources of dysfluency: A theoretical model of stuttering. *Contemporary Issues in Communication Science and Disorders, 31,* 105–122.

May, A., & Gaser, C. (2006). Magnetic resonance-based morphometry: A window into structural plasticity of the brain. *Current Opinion in Neurology, 19,* 407–411.

McCauley, R. J., & Fey, M. E. (2006). Chapter 1: Introduction. In R. J. McCauley & M. E. Fey (Eds.), *Treatment of Language Disorders in Children* (pp. 1–20). Baltimore: Paul H. Brookes Publishing Company.

McCauley, R. J., & Fey, M. E. (Eds.) (2006). *Treatment of Language Disorders in Children*. Baltimore: Brookes Publishing, Inc.

McColl, T., Onslow, M., Packman, A., & Menzies, R. G. (2001). A cognitive behavioral intervention for social anxiety in adults who stutter. *Proceedings of the 2001 Speech Pathology Australia National Conference*, 93–98.

McDearmon, J. R. (1968). Primary stuttering at the onset of stuttering: A reexamination of data. *Journal of Speech and Hearing Research, 11*, 631–637.

McNair, D. M., Lorr, M., & Droppleman, L. F. (1971). *Profile of Mood States Manual*. San Diego, CA: Educational and Industrial Testing Service.

McReynolds, L. V. (1990). Historical perspective of treatment efficacy research. In L. B. Olswang, C. K. Thompson, S. F. Warren, & N. J. Minghetti (Eds.), *Treatment Efficacy Research in Communication Disorders*. Rockville, MD: American Speech-Language-Hearing Foundation.

McReynolds, L. V., & Kearns, K. P. (1983). *Single-Subject Experimental Design in Communicative Disorders*. Baltimore: University Park Press.

Meade, M. O., & Richardson, W. S. (1997). Selecting and appraising studies for a systematic review. *Annals of Internal Medicine, 127*, 531–537.

Melnick, K. S., & Conture, E. G. (1999). Parent-child group approach to stuttering in preschool and school-age children. In M. Onslow & A. Packman (Eds.), *Early Stuttering: A Handbook of Intervention Strategies* (pp. 17–51). San Diego, CA: Singular Publishing.

Melnick, K. S., & Conture, E. G. (2000). Relationship of length and grammatical complexity to the systematic and nonsystematic speech errors and stuttering of children who stutter. *Journal of Fluency Disorders, 25*, 21–45.

Melnick, K. S., Conture, E. G., & Ohde, R. N. (2003). Phonological priming in picture naming of young children who stutter. *Journal of Speech, Language and Hearing Research, 46*, 1428–1443.

Menzies, R. G., Onslow, M., & Packman, A. (1999) Anxiety and stuttering: Exploring a complex relationship. *American Journal of Speech-Language Pathology, 8*, 3–10.

Menzies, R., O'Brian, S., Onslow, M., Packman, A., St Clare, T., & Block, S. (2008). An experimental clinical trial of a cognitive behavior therapy package for chronic stuttering. *Journal of Speech, Language, and Hearing Research, 51*, 1451–1464.

Messenger, M., Onslow, M., Packman, A, & Menzies, R. (2004). Social anxiety in stuttering: Measuring negative social expectancies. *Journal of Fluency Disorders, 29*, 201–212.

Mesulam, M. M., & Mufson, E. J. (1982). Insula of the old world monkey. I. Architectonics in the insulo-orbito-temporal component of the paralimbic brain. *Journal of Comparative Neurology, 212*, 1–22.

Meyer, M., Friederici, A. D., & von Cramon, D. Y. (2000). Neurocognition of auditory sentence comprehension: Event related fMRI reveals sensitivity to syntactic violations and task demands. *Cognitive Brain Research, 9*, 19–33.

Meyers, S., & Woodfood, L. (1992). *The Fluency Development System for Young Children*. Buffalo, NY: United Educational Services.

Meyers, S. C., & Freeman, F. J. (1985). Are mothers of stutterers different? An investigation of social-communicative interaction. *Journal of Fluency Disorders, 10*, 193–209.

Meyers, S. C., & Freeman, F. J. (1985). Interruptions as a variable in stuttering and disfluency. *Journal of Speech and Hearing Research, 28*, 428–435.

Meyers, S. C., & Freeman, F. J. (1985). Mother and child speech rates as a variable in stuttering and disfluency. *Journal of Speech and Hearing Research, 28*, 436–444.

Mikheev, M., Mohr, C., Afanasiev, S., Landis, T., & Thut, G. (2002). Motor control and cerebral hemispheric specialization in highly qualified judo wrestlers. *Neuropsychologia, 40*, 1209–1219.

Miles, S., & Bernstein Ratner, N. B. (2001). Parental language input to children at stuttering onset. *Journal of Speech, Language and Hearing Research, 44*, 1116–1130.

Millard, S. K. (2002). Therapy outcome: Parents' perspectives. In *Proceedings of The Sixth Oxford Dysfluency Conference* (pp. 89–98). Leicester, United Kingdom: Kevin L. Baker.

Millard, S. K., Edwards, S., & Cook, F. M. (2009). Parent-child interaction therapy: Adding to the evidence. *International Journal of Speech and Language Pathology, 11*, 1–15.

Millard, S. K., Nicholas, A., & Cook, F. (2008). Is parent-child interaction therapy effective in reducing stuttering? *Journal of Speech, Language and Hearing Research, 51*, 636–650.

Miller, B., & Guitar, B. (2009). Relationship of length and grammatical complexity to the systematic and nonsystematic speech errors and stuttering of children who stutter -term outcome of the LP of early stuttering intervention. *American Journal of Speech-Language Pathology, 18*, 42–49.

Miller, J. F. (1981). *Assessing Language Production in Children: Experimental Procedures*. Austin, TX: Pro-Ed.

Mink, J. W. (2003). The basal ganglia and involuntary movements: Impaired inhibition of competing motor patterns. *Archives of Neurology, 60*, 1365–1368.

Moher, D., Schulz, K. F., & Altman, D. G. (2001). The CONSORT statement: Revised recommendations for improving the quality of reports of parallel-group randomised trials. *The Lancet, 357,* 1191–1194.

Molt, L. (2005). A brief historical review of assistive devices for treating stuttering. Presented at the 8th International Stuttering Awareness Day Online Conference (ISAD8). Available at: www.mnsu.edu/comdis/isad8/isadcon8.html.

Molt, L. (2006a). SpeechEasy AAF device long-term clinical trial: Attitudinal/perceptual measures. Poster presented to the American Speech-Language-Hearing Association, Miami, FL.

Molt, L. (2006b). SpeechEasy AAF device long-term clinical trial: Speech fluency and naturalness measures. Poster presented to the American Speech-Language-Hearing Association, Miami, FL.

Molt, L. (2006c). SpeechEasy AAF device long-term clinical trial: Usage patterns and satisfaction ratings. Poster presented to the American Speech-Language-Hearing Association, Miami, FL.

Molt, L. (2007a). Auditory processing measures as predictors for altered auditory feedback success. Poster presented to the American Speech-Language-Hearing Association, Boston, MA.

Molt, L. (2007b). Indicators for long-term successful usage of altered auditory feedback devices. Poster presented to the American Speech-Language-Hearing Association, Boston, MA.

Momjian, S., Seghier, M., Seeck, M., & Michel, C. M. (2003). Mapping of the neuronal networks of human cortical brain functions. *Advances and Technical Standards in Neurosurgery, 28,* 91–142.

Moncrieff, J. (1998). Research synthesis: Systematic reviews and meta-analysis. *International Review of Psychiatry, 10,* 304–311.

Montgomery, C. (2006). The treatment of stuttering: From the hub to the spoke. In N. Bernstein Ratner & J. Tetnowski (Eds.), *Current Issues in Stuttering Research and Practice* (pp. 159–204). Mahwah, NJ: Lawrence Erlbaum.

Montgomery, D. C. (1997). *Introduction to Statistical Quality Control* (3rd ed.). New York: John Wiley & Sons Inc.

Moore, W. H. Jr. (1984). Hemispheric alpha asymmetries during an electromyographic biofeedback procedure for stuttering: A single-subject experimental design. *Journal of Fluency Disorders, 9,* 143–162.

Moore, W. H. Jr. (1986). Hemispheric alpha asymmetries of stutterers and nonstutterers for the recall and recognition of words and connected reading passages: Some relationships to severity of stuttering. *Journal of Fluency Disorders, 11,* 71–89.

Moore, W. H. Jr., & Haynes, W. O. (1980). Alpha hemispheric asymmetry and stuttering: Some support for a segmentation dysfunction hypothesis. *Journal of Speech and Hearing Research, 23,* 229–247.

Morgan, S., & Simons, A. (1991). Diathesis-stress theories in the context of life stress research: Implications for the depressive disorders. *Psychological Bulletin, 110,* 406–425.

Moscicki, E. K. (1993). Fundamental methodological considerations in controlled clinical trials. *Journal of Fluency Disorders, 18,* 183–196.

Mosley, L., & Mead, D. (2001). Considerations in using the Delphi approach: Design, questions and answers. *Nurse Researcher, 8,* 24–37.

Movsessian, P. (2005). Neuropharmacology of theophylline induced stuttering: The role of dopamine, adenosine and GABA. *Medical Hypotheses, 64,* 290–297.

Mowrer, D. (1972). Accountability and speech therapy. *ASHA, 14,* 111–115.

Murphy, B. C., & Dillon, C. (2003). *Interviewing in Action: Relationships, Process and Change.* Belmont, CA: Brooks/Cole.

Murphy, B., Quesal, R. W., & Gulker, H. (2007). Covert stuttering. *Perspectives in Fluency and Fluency Disorders, 17,* 4–9

Murphy, W. P., (1989). *The School-Age Child Who Stutters: Dealing Effectively with Shame and Guilt* [Videotape No. 86]. Memphis, TN: Stuttering Foundation of America.

Murphy, W. P. (1999). A preliminary look at shame, guilt, and stuttering. In N. Bernstein-Ratner & C. Healey (Eds.), *Stuttering Research and Practice: Bridging the Gap* (pp. 131–143). Mahwah, NJ: Lawrence Erlbaum Associates.

Murphy, W. P., & Quesal, R. W. (2002). Strategies for addressing bullying with the school-age child who stutters. *Seminars in Speech and Language, 23,* 205–211.

Murphy, W. P., Reardon, N. A., & Yaruss, J. S. (2004). A classroom presentation about stuttering [Brochure]. New York: National Stuttering Association.

Murphy, W. P., Yaruss, J. S., & Quesal, R. W. (2007a). Enhancing treatment for school-age children who stutter. I: Reducing negative reactions through desensitization and cognitive restructuring. *Journal of Fluency Disorders, 32,* 121–138.

Murphy, W. P., Yaruss, J. S., & Quesal, R. W. (2007b). Enhancing treatment for school-age children who stutter. II: Reducing bullying through role-playing and self-disclosure. *Journal of Fluency Disorders, 32,* 139–162.

Mysak, E. D. (1960). Servo theory and stuttering. *Journal of Speech and Hearing Disorders, 25,* 188–195.

Naylor, R. V. (1953). A comparative study of methods of estimating the severity of stuttering. *Journal of Speech and Hearing Disorders, 18,* 30–37.

Neilson, M. (1999). Cognitive-behavioral treatment of adults who stutter: The process and the art. In R. F. Curlee (Ed.), *Stuttering and Related Disorders of Fluency* (2nd ed., pp. 181–199). New York: Thieme Medical Publishers.

Neilson, M., & Andrews, G. (1993). Intensive fluency training of chronic stutterers. In R. F. Curlee (Ed.), *Stuttering and Related Disorders of Fluency* (pp. 139–165). New York: Thieme Medical Publishers.

Neumann, K., Euler, H. A., Wolff, V., Gudenberg, A., Giraud, A.-L., Lanfermann, H., Gall, V., & Preibisch, C. (2003). The nature and treatment of stuttering as revealed by fMRI: A within- and between-group comparison. *Journal of Fluency Disorders, 28,* 381–410.

Neumann, K., Preibisch, C., Euler, H. A., Wolff von Gudenberg, A., Lanfermann, H., Gall, V., & Giraud, A.-L. (2005). Cortical plasticity associated with stuttering therapy. *Journal of Fluency Disorders, 30,* 23–39.

Newman, L. L., & Smit, A. B. (1989). Some effects of variations in response time latency on speech rate, interruptions, and fluency in children's speech. *Journal of Speech and Hearing Research, 32,* 635–644.

Nicholas, A., Millard, S. K., & Cook, F. (2003). Parent-child interaction therapy: Child and parent variables pre and post therapy. In *Proceedings of the Fourth World Congress of Fluency Disorders, Montreal* (p. 108). Nijmegen, The Netherlands: University Press Nijmegen.

Nippold, M. (1990). Concomitant speech and language disorders in stuttering children: A critique of the literature. *Journal of Speech and Hearing Disorders, 55,* 51–60.

Nippold, M. (2002). Stuttering and phonology: Is there an interaction? *American Journal of Speech-Language Pathology, 11,* 99–110.

Nippold, M., & Rudzinski, M. (1995). Parents' speech and children's stuttering: A critique of the literature. *Journal of Speech-Language-Hearing Research, 38,* 978–989.

Nittrouer, S., & Chaney, C. (1984). Operant techniques used in stuttering therapy: A review. *Journal of Fluency Disorders, 9,* 169–190.

Nudelman, H. B., Herbrich, K. E., Hoyt, B. D., & Rosenfield, D. B. (1992). A model of the phonatory response times of stutterers and fluent speakers to frequency-modulated tones. *Journal of the Acoustical Society of America, 92,* 1882–1888.

Nudelman, H. B., Hoyt H. B., Herbrich K. E., & Rosenfield D. B. (1989). A neuroscience model of stuttering. *Journal of Fluency Disorders, 14,* 399–427.

Nudo, R. J. (2003). Adaptive plasticity in motor cortex: implications for rehabilitation after brain injury. *Journal of Rehabilitative Medicine, 41* (Suppl), 7–10.

O'Brian, S., Cream, A., Onslow, M., & Packman, A. (2001). A replicable, nonprogrammed, instrument-free method for the control of stuttering with prolonged-speech. *Asia Pacific Journal of Speech, Language, and Hearing, 6,* 91–96.

O'Brian, S., Onslow, M., Cream, A., & Packman, A. (2003). Camperdown Program: Outcomes of a new prolonged-speech treatment model. *Journal of Speech, Language, and Hearing Research, 46,* 933–946.

O'Brian, S., Packman, A., & Onslow, M. (2004). Self-rating of stuttering severity as a clinical tool. *American Journal of Speech-Language Pathology, 13,* 219–226.

O'Brian, S., Packman, A., & Onslow, M. (2008). Telehealth delivery of the Camperdown program for adults who stutter: A phase I trial. *Journal of Speech, Language, and Hearing Research, 51,* 184–195.

O'Brian, S., Packman, A., Onslow, M., Cream, A., O'Brian, N., & Bastock, K. (2003). Is listener comfort a viable construct in stuttering research? *Journal of Speech, Language, and Hearing Research, 46,* 503–509.

O'Brian, S., Packman, A., Onslow, M., & O'Brian, N. (2004). Measurement of stuttering in adults: Comparison of stuttering-rate and severity-scaling methods. *Journal of Speech, Language, and Hearing Research, 47,* 1081–1087.

O'Donnell, J. J., Armson, J., & Kiefte, M. (2008). The effectiveness of SpeechEasy during situations of daily living. Journal of Fluency Disorders, 33, 99–119.

Ojemann, G. A., & Ward, A. A. Jr. (1971). Speech representation in ventrolateral thalamus. *Brain, 94,* 669–680.

Onslow, M. (2003). From laboratory to living room: The origins and development of the Lidcombe Program. In M. Onslow, A. Packman, & E. Harrison (Eds.), *The Lidcombe Program of Early Stuttering Intervention: A Clinician's Guide* (pp. 21–25). Austin, TX: Pro-Ed.

Onslow, M. (2003). Overview of the Lidcombe Program. In M. Onslow, A. Packman, & E. Harrison (Eds.), *The Lidcombe Program of Early Stuttering Intervention: A Clinician's Guide* (pp. 3–20). Austin, TX: Pro-Ed.

Onslow, M. (2004). Treatment of stuttering in preschool children. *Behaviour Change, 21,* 201–214.

Onslow, M., Andrews, C., & Costa, L. (1990). Parental severity scaling of early stuttered speech: Four case studies. *Australian Journal of Human Communication Disorders, 18,* 47–61.

Onslow, M., Andrews, C., & Lincoln, M. (1994). A control/experimental trial of an operant treatment for early stuttering. *Journal of Speech and Hearing Research, 37,* 1244–1259.

Onslow, M., Costa, L., Andrews, C., Harrison, E., & Packman, A. (1996). Speech outcomes of a prolonged-speech treatment for stuttering. *Journal of Speech and Hearing Research, 39*, 734–749.

Onslow, M., Costa, L., & Rue, S. (1990). Direct early intervention with stuttering: Some preliminary data. *Journal of Speech and Hearing Disorders, 55*, 405–416.

Onslow, M., Harrison, E., Jones, E., & Packman, A. (2002). Beyond-clinic speech measures during the LP of early stuttering intervention. *Acquiring Knowledge in Speech, Language and Hearing, 4*, 82–85.

Onslow, M., Jones, M., O'Brian, S., & Menzies. (2007). Biostatistics for clinicians: Defining, identifying, and evaluating clinical trials of stuttering treatments. Manuscript submitted for publication.

Onslow, M., & O'Brian, S. (1998). Reliability of clinician's judgments about prolonged speech targets. *Journal of Speech, Language and Hearing Research, 41*, 969–975.

Onslow, M., O'Brian, S., Packman, A., & Rousseau, I. (2004). Long-term follow up of speech outcomes for a prolonged-speech treatment for stuttering: The effects of paradox on stuttering treatment research. In A. K. Bothe (Ed.), *Evidence-Based Treatment of Stuttering: Empirical Bases and Clinical Applications* (pp. 231–244). Mahwah, NJ: Lawrence Erlbaum.

Onslow, M., & Packman, A. (1999). The Lidcombe program of early stuttering intervention. In N. Bernstein Ratner & E. C. Healey (Eds.), *Stuttering Treatment and Research: Bridging the Gap* (pp. 193–210). Mahwah, NJ: Erlbaum Press.

Onslow, M., Packman, A., & Harrison, E. (2003). *The Lidcombe Program of Early Stuttering Intervention: A Clinician's Guide*. Austin, TX: Pro-Ed.

Onslow, M., Packman, A., & Payne, P. (2007). Clinical identification of early stuttering: Methods, issues, and future directions. *Asia Pacific Journal of Speech Pathology and Audiology, 10*, 15–31.

Onslow, M., Ratner, N. B., & Packman, A. (2001). Changes in linguistic variables during operant, laboratory control of stuttering in children. *Clinical Linguistics and Phonetics, 15*, 651–662.

Onslow, M., Stocker, S., Packman, A., & McLeod, S. (2002). Speech timing in children after the Lidcombe Program of early stuttering intervention. *Clinical Linguistics and Phonetics, 16*, 21–33.

Ornstein, A. F., & Manning, W. H. (1985). Self-efficacy scaling by adult stutterers. *Journal of Communication Disorders, 18*, 313–320.

Orton, S. T. (1927). Studies in stuttering. *Archives of Neurological Psychiatry, 18*, 671–672.

Orton, S. T., & Travis, L. E. (1929). Studies in stuttering: IV. Studies of action currents in stutterers. *Archives of Neurology and Psychiatry, 21*, 61–68.

Oyler, M. E. (1996a). Temperament: Stuttering and the behaviorally inhibited child. Seminar conducted at the meeting of the American Speech-Language-Hearing Association Annual Convention.

Oyler, M. E. (1996b). Vulnerability in stuttering children. *Dissertation Abstracts International*, UMI No. 9602431.

Oyler, M. E., & Ramig, P. R. (1995). Vulnerability in stuttering children. Paper presented at the Annual Meeting of the American Speech, Language and Hearing Association, Orlando, FL.

Packman, A. (2003). Issues. In M. Onslow, A. Packman, & E. Harrison (Eds.), *The Lidcombe Program of Early Stuttering Intervention: A Clinician's Guide* (pp. 199–206). Austin, TX: Pro-Ed.

Packman, A., & Attanasio, J. (2005). *Theoretical Issues in Stuttering*. Hove, United Kingdom: Psychology Press.

Packman, A., Code, C., & Onslow, M. (in press). On the cause of stuttering: Integrating theory with behavioral and brain research. *Journal of Neurolinguistics*.

Packman, A., Hansen, E. J., & Herland, M. (2007). Parents' experiences of the LP: The Norway-Australia connection. In J. Au-Yeung & M. M. Leahy (Eds.), *Research, Treatment, and Self-Help in Fluency Disorders: New Directions* (pp. 418–422). Dublin: International Fluency Association.

Packman, A., & Onslow, M. (1995). Reliability of listeners' stuttering counts: The effects of instructions to count agreed stuttering. *Australian Journal of Human Communication Disorders, 23*, 35–47.

Packman, A., Onslow, M., & Attanasio, J. (2003). The timing of early intervention in the Lidcombe Program. In M. Onslow, A. Packman, & E. Harrison (Eds.), *The Lidcombe Program of Early Stuttering Intervention: A Clinician's Guide* (pp. 41–55). Austin, TX: Pro-Ed.

Packman, A., Onslow, M., & Menzies, R. G. (2000). Novel speech patterns and the control of stuttering. *Disability and Rehabilitation, 22*, 65–79.

Packman, A., Onslow, M., Richard, F., & van Doorn, J. (1996). Linguistic stress and variability: A model of stuttering. *Clinical Linguistics and Phonetics, 10*, 235–263.

Packman, A., Onslow, M., & van Doorn, J. (1994). Prolonged-speech and modification of stuttering: Perceptual, acoustic and electroglottographic data. *Journal of Speech and Hearing Research, 37*, 724–734.

Packman, A., Rousseau, I., Onslow, M., Dredge, R., Harrison, E., & Wilson, L. (2003). Australia. In M. Onslow, A. Packman, & E. Harrison (Eds.), *The Lidcombe Program of Early Stuttering Intervention: A Clinician's Guide* (pp. 139–146). Austin, TX: Pro-Ed.

Packman, A., van Doorn, J., & Onslow, M. (1992). Stuttering treatments: What is happening to the acoustic signal? In J. Pittam (Ed.), *Proceedings of the Fourth Australian International Conference on Speech Science and Technology* (pp. 402–407). Brisbane, Australia.

Paden, E. P., Yairi, E., & Ambrose, N. G. (1999). Early childhood stuttering II: Initial status of phonological abilities. *Journal of Speech, Language, and Hearing Research, 42,* 1113–1124.

Paus, T. (2001). Primate anterior cingulate cortex: where motor control, drive and cognition interface. *Nature Reviews Neuroscience, 2,* 417–424.

Pellowski, M., & Conture, E. G. (2002). Characteristics of speech disfluency and stuttering behaviors in 3- and 4-year-old children. *Journal of Speech-Language and Hearing Research, 45,* 20–34.

Pellowski, M., & Conture, E. (2005). Lexical priming in picture naming of young children who do and do not stutter. *Journal of Speech, Language, and Hearing Research, 48,* 278–294.

Pellowski, M., Conture, E., Anderson, J., & Ohde, R. (2001). Articulatory and phonological assessment of children who stutter. In H.-G. Bosshardt, J. Scott Yaruss, & H. F. M. Peters (Eds.), *Fluency Disorders: Theory, Research Treatment and Self-Help: Proceedings of the Third World Congress of Fluency Disorders* (pp. 248–252). Nijmegen, The Netherlands: Nijmegen University Press.

Penfield, W., & Welch, K. (1951). The supplementary motor area of the cerebral cortex. *Archives of Neurology and Psychiatry, 66,* 289–317.

Perkins, W. H. (1979). From psychoanalysis to discoordination. In H. H. Gregory (Ed.), *Controversies about Stuttering Therapy* (pp. 97–127). Baltimore: University Park Press.

Perkins, W. H. (1990). What is stuttering? *Journal of Speech and Hearing Disorders, 55,* 379–382.

Perkins, W. H. (1992). *Stuttering Prevented.* San Diego, CA: Singular Publishing Group.

Peters, H., Hulstijn, W., & Van Lieshout, P. (2000). Recent developments in speech motor research it on stuttering. *Folia Phoniatrica et Logopaedica, 52,* 103–119.

Peters, H. F. M., & Starkweather, C. W. (1990). The interaction between speech motor coordination and language processes in the development of stuttering: Hypotheses and suggestions for research. *Journal of Fluency Disorders, 15,* 115–125.

Peters, T. J., & Guitar, B. G. (1991). *Stuttering: An Integrated Approach to Its Nature and Treatment.* Baltimore, MD: Williams & Wilkins.

Peterson, G., & Gordon, P. (1982). The effects of syntactic complexity on the occurrence of disfluencies in five-year-old children. Paper presented at the Annual Meeting of the American Speech, Language, and Hearing Association.

Petrides, M., & Pandya, D. N. (2002). Comparative cytoarchitectonic analysis of the human and the macaque ventrolateral prefrontal cortex and corticocortical connection patterns in the monkey. *European Journal of Neuroscience, 16,* 291–310.

Phillips, B., Ball, C., Sackett, D., Badenoch, D., Straus, S., Haynes, B., & Dawes, M. (1998/2006). Oxford Centre for Evidence Based Medicine Levels of Evidence and Grades of Recommendation [described as "produced by" Phillips et al. "since November 1998"; last retrieved March 3, 2006, from http://www.cebm.net/levels_of_evidence.asp].

Pindzola, R. H. (1986). A description of some selected stuttering instruments. *Journal of Childhood Communication Disorders, 9,* 183–200.

Pindzola, R. H. (1987). *Stuttering Intervention Program: Age 3 to Grade 3.* Austin, TX: Pro-Ed.

Pindzola, R. H. (1999). The stuttering intervention program. In M. Onslow & A. Packman (Eds.), *The Handbook of Early Stuttering Intervention* (pp. 119–138). San Diego, CA: Singular Press.

Pindzola, R. H., Jenkins, M., & Lokken, K. (1989). Speaking rates of young children. *Language, Speech, and Hearing Services in Schools, 20,* 133–138.

Pindzola, R. H., & White, D. (1986). A protocol for differentiating the incipient stutterer. *Language, Speech, and Hearing Services in School, 17,* 2–15.

Pollard, R., Ellis, J. B., Finan, D., & Ramig, P. R. (2009). A six-month, phase I clinical trial of the effects of the SpeechEasy on objective and perceived aspects of stuttering in naturalistic environments. *Journal of Speech, Language and Hearing Research, 52,* 516–533.

Pollard, R., Ramig, P. R., Ellis, J. B., & Finan, D. (2007). Case study of SpeechEasy use combined with traditional stuttering treatment. Technical session presented at the 2007 American Speech-Language-Hearing Association Convention, Boston, MA.

Pool, K. D., Devous, M. D., Freeman, F. J., Watson B. C., & Finitzo, T. (1991). Regional cerebral blood flow in developmental stutterers. *Archives of Neurology, 48,* 509–512.

Postma, A., & Kolk, H. (1993). The covert repair hypothesis: Prearticulatory repair processes in normal and stuttered disfluencies. *Journal of Speech and Hearing Research, 36,* 472–487.

Power, M. (2002). Research based stuttering therapy. *Perspectives on Fluency and Fluency Disorders* [Newsletter of Special Interest Division 4, American Speech-Language Hearing Association], *12* (1).

Preibisch, C., Neumann, K., Raab, P., Euler, H. A., Wolff von Gudenberg, A., Lanfermann, H., & Giraud, A.-L. (2003). Evidence for compensation for stuttering by the right frontal operculum. *NeuroImage, 20,* 1356–1364.

Preibisch, C., Raab, P., Neumann, K., Euler, H. A., Wolff von Gudenberg, A., Gall, V., Lanfermann, H., & Zanella, F. (2003). Event-related fMRI for the suppression of speech-associated artifacts in stuttering. *NeuroImage, 19*, 1076–1084.

Price, C. J. (2000). The anatomy of language: Contributions from functional neuroimaging. *Journal of Anatomy, 197*, 335–359.

Pring, T. (2005). *Research Methods in Communication Disorders*. London: Whurr Publishers Ltd.

Prins, D., & Hubbard, C. P. (1988). Response contingent stimuli and stuttering: Issues and implications. *Journal of Speech and Hearing Research, 31*, 696–709.

Prins, D., & Miller, M. (1973). Personality, improvement, and regression in stuttering therapy. *Journal of Speech and Hearing Research, 16*, 685–690.

Prins, D., Mandelkorn, T., & Cerf, F. (1980). Principal and differential effects of haloperidol and placebo treatments upon speech disfluencies in stutters. *Journal of Speech and Hearing Research, 23*, 614–629.

Pugh, K. R., Mencl, W. E., Jenner, A. R., Katz, L., Frost, S. J., Lee, J. R., Shaywitz, S. E., & Shaywitz, B. A. (2001). Neurobiological studies of reading and reading disability. *Journal of Communication Disorders, 34*, 479–492.

Purcell, R., & Runyan, C.M. (1980). Normative study of speech rates of children. *Journal of the Speech and Hearing Association of Virginia, 21*, 6–14.

Quesal, R. W., Yaruss, J. S., & Molt, L. (2004). Many types of data: Stuttering treatment outcomes beyond fluency. In A. Packmann, A. Meltzer, and H. F. M. Peters (Eds.), *Theory, Research, and Therapy in Fluency Disorders: Proceedings of the Fourth World Congress on Fluency Disorders* (pp. 218–224). Nijmegen, The Netherlands: Nijmegen University Press.

Quinn, P. T. (1972). Stuttering: Cerebral dominance and the dichotic word test. *The Medical Journal of Australia, 2*, 639–643.

Quinn, P. T., & Peachey, E. C. (1973). Haloperidol in the treatment of stutterers. *British Journal of Psychiatry, 123*, 247–248.

Rajput, A. H., Fenton, M., Birdi, S., & Macaulay, R. (1997). Is levodopa toxic to human substantia nigra? *Movement Disorders, 12*, 634–638.

Ramig, P. R. (1984). Rate changes in the speech of stutterers after therapy. *Journal of Fluency Disorders, 9*, 285–294.

Ramig, P. R. (1993). The impact of self-help groups on persons who stutter: A call for research. *Journal of Fluency Disorders, 18*, 351–361.

Ramig, P. R., & Bennett, E. M. (1995). Working with 7–12 year old children who stutter: Ideas for intervention in the public schools. *Language, Speech and Hearing Services in Schools, 26*, 138–150.

Ramig, P. R., & Bennett, E. M. (1997). Clinical management of children: Direct management strategies. In R. F. Curlee & G. M. Siegel (Eds.), *Nature and Treatment of Stuttering: New Directions* (2nd ed., pp. 292–312). Needham Heights, MA: Allyn & Bacon.

Ramig, P. R., & Dodge, D. M. (2005). *The Child and Adolescent Stuttering Treatment and Activity Resource Guide*. Clifton Park, NY: Thompson Delmar Learning.

Rantala, S. L., & Petri-Larmi, M. (1976). Haloperidol (serenase) in the treatment of stuttering. *Folia Phoniatrica, 28*, 354–361.

Rapee, R. M., & Wignall, A., Psych, M., Hudson, J. L., & Schniering, C. A. (2000). *Treating Anxious Children and Adolescents: An Evidence-Based Approach*. Oakland, CA: New Harbinger Publications, Inc.

Ratner, N. B. (1992). Measurable outcomes of instructions to modify normal parent-child verbal interactions: Implications for indirect stuttering therapy. *Journal of Speech and Hearing Research, 35*, 14–20.

Reardon, N., & Reeves, L. (2002). Stuttering therapy in partnership with support groups: The best of both worlds. *Seminars in Speech and Language, 23*, 213–218.

Reardon-Reeves, N. A., & Yaruss, J. S. (2004). *The Source for Stuttering: Ages 7–18*. East Moline, IL: LinguiSystems.

Reed, C. G., & Godden, A. L. (1977). An experimental treatment using verbal punishment with two preschool stutterers. *Journal of Fluency Disorders, 2*, 225–233.

Reeves, P. L. (2006). The role of self-help/mutual aid in addressing the needs of individuals who stutter. In N. Bernstein Ratner & J. Tetnowski (Eds.), *Current Issues in Stuttering Research and Practice* (pp. 255–278). Mahwah, NJ: Lawrence Erlbaum.

Renfrew, C. E. (1997). *Action Picture Test*. Oxon, United Kingdom: Winslow Press Ltd.

Rettew, D. C., Stanger, C., McKee, L., Doyle, A., & Hudziak, J. J. (2006). Interactions between child and parent temperament and child behavior problems. *Comprehensive Psychiatry, 47*, 412–420.

Reynolds, C. R., & Richmond, B. O. (2000). *Revised Children's Manifest Anxiety Scale (RCMAS)*. Los Angeles, CA: Western Psychological Services.

Reynolds, C. R., Richmond, B. O., & Lowe, P. A. (2003). *AMAS. The Adult Manifest Anxiety Scale*. Los Angeles, CA: Western Psychological Services.

Richels, C. G., & Conture, E. G. (2007). An indirect treatment approach for early intervention for childhood stuttering. In E. Conture and R. Curlee (Eds.), *Stuttering and Related Disorders of Fluency* (3rd ed., pp. 77–99). New York: Thieme Publishers.

Riley, G. D. (1972). A stuttering severity instrument for children and adults. *Journal of Speech and Hearing Disorders, 37*, 314–320.

Riley, G. D. (1981). *The Stuttering Prediction Instrument.* Trigard, OR: C.C. Publications.

Riley, G. D. (1994). *Stuttering Severity Instrument for Children and Adults* (3rd ed.). Austin, TX: Pro-Ed.

Riley, G. D., & Ingham, J. (2000). Acoustic duration changes associated with two types of treatment for children who stutter. *Journal of Speech, Language and Hearing Research, 43*, 965–978.

Riley, G. D., Maguire, G., & Wu, J. C. (2001). Brain imaging to examine a dopamine hypothesis in stuttering. In B. Maassen, W. Hulstijn, R. D. Kent, H. F. M. Peters, & P. H. H. M. van Lieshout (Eds.), *Speech Motor Control in Normal and Disordered Speech* (pp. 156–158). Nijmegen, The Netherlands: Vantilt.

Riley, G. D., & Riley, J. (1980). Motoric and linguistic variables among children who stutter: A factor analysis. *Journal of Speech and Hearing Disorders, 45*, 504–513.

Riley, G. D., & Riley, J. (1984). A component model for treating stuttering in children. In M. Peins (Ed.), *Contemporary Approaches in Stuttering Therapy* (pp. 123–172). Boston: Little, Brown.

Riley, G. D., & Riley, J. (1991). Treatment implications of oral motor discoordination. In H. F. M. Peters, W. Hulstijn, & C. W. Starkweather (Eds.), *Speech Motor Control and Stuttering* (pp. 471–476). Amsterdam: Elsevier Science Publishers.

Riley, J., Riley, G., & Maguire, G. (2004). Subjective screening of stuttering severity, locus of control and avoidance: Research edition. *Journal of Fluency Disorders, 29*, 51–62.

Robb, M. P., Lybolt, J. T., & Price, H. A. (1985). Acoustic measures of stutterers' speech following an intensive therapy program. *Journal of Fluency Disorders, 10*, 269–279.

Robey, R. R. (2004). Reporting point and interval estimates of effect-size for planned contrasts: Fixed within effect analyses of variance. *Journal of Fluency Disorders, 29*, 307–341.

Robey, R. R. (2005). An introduction to clinical trials. *ASHA Leader, May 24*, 6–7, 22.

Robey, R. R., & Schultz, M. C. (1998). A model for conducting clinical-outcome research: An adaptation for use in aphasiology. *Aphasiology, 12*, 787–810.

Rommel, D. (2000). The influence of psycholinguistic variables on stuttering in childhood. In *Proceedings of the Third World Congress on Fluency Disorders in Nyborg, Denmark* (pp. 195–202). Nijmegen, The Netherlands: University Press Nijmegen.

Rommel, D., Hage, P., Kalehne, P., & Johannsen, H. (2000). Development, maintenance and recovery of childhood stuttering: Prospective longitudinal data 3 years after first contact. In K. L. Baker, L. Rustin, & F. Cook (Eds.), *Proceedings of the Fifth Oxford Conference, 7th-10th July, 1999* (pp. 168–182). Berkshire, United Kingdom: Kevin L. Baker.

Rosen, H. J., Petersen, S. E., Linenweber, M. R., Snyder, A. Z., White, D. A., Chapman, L., Dromerick, A. W., Fiez, J. A., & Corbetta, M. D. (2000). Neural correlates of recovery from aphasia after damage to left inferior frontal cortex. *Neurology, 55*, 1883–1894.

Rossini, P. M., & Dal Forno, G. (2004). Integrated technology for evaluation of brain function and neural plasticity. *Physical Medicine and Rehabilitation Clinics of North America, 15*, 263–306.

Rothbart, M., Ahadi, S., Hershey, K., & Fischer, P. (2001). Investigations of temperament at 3–7 years: The Children's Behavior Questionnaire. *Child Development, 72*, 1394–1408.

Rothbart, M., & Bates, J. (1998). Temperament. In W. Damon (Series Ed.) & N. Eisenberg (Volume Ed.), *Handbook of Child Psychology: Volume 3. Social, Emotional and Personality Development* (pp. 105–176). Newbury Park, CA: Sage.

Rousey, C. L., Goetzinger, C. P., & Dirks, D. (1959). Sound localization ability of normal, stuttering, neurotic, and hemiplegic subjects. *Archives of General Psychiatry, 1*, 640–645.

Rousseau, I., Packman, A., Onslow, M., Harrison, E., & Jones, M. (2007). An investigation of language and phonological development and the responsiveness of preschool age children to the Lidcombe Program. *Journal of Communication Disorders, 40*, 382–397.

Rovee-Collier, C., Hayne, H., & Colombo, M. (2001). *The Development of Implicit and Explicit Memory.* Philadelphia: John Benjamin Publishing Co.

Runyan, C. M., Bell, J. N., & Prosek, R. A. (1990). Speech naturalness ratings of treated stutterers. *Journal of Speech and Hearing Disorders, 55*, 434–438.

Runyan, C. M., & Bennett, C. W. (1982). Results of a survey of public school speech language pathologists in Virginia. *Journal of the Speech and Hearing Association of Virginia, 23*, 91–95.

Runyan, C. M., & Runyan, S. E. (1986). A Fluency Rules therapy program for young children in the public schools. *Language, Speech, and Hearing Services in Schools, 17*, 276–284.

Runyan, C. M., & Runyan, S. E. (1991). A fluency rules therapy program for young children in the public schools. In E. C. Healey (Ed.), *Readings on Research in Stuttering* (pp. 190–194). New York: Longman Publishing Group.

Runyan, C. M., & Runyan, S. E. (1993). A Fluency Rules therapy program for school-age stutterers: An update on the Fluency Rules program. In R. Curlee (Ed.), *Stuttering and Related Disorders of Fluency* (pp. 101–114). New York: Thieme Medical Publishers, Inc.

Runyan, C. M., & Runyan, S. E. (1999). Therapy for school-age stutterers: An update on the Fluency Rules program. In Richard F. Curlee (Ed.), *Stuttering and Related Disorders of Fluency* (2nd ed., pp. 110–123). New York: Thieme Medical Publishers.

Runyan, C. M., & Runyan, S. E. (2007). Therapy for school-aged stutterers: An update on the fluency rules program. In E. G. Conture & R. F. Curlee (Eds.), *Stuttering and Related Disorders of Fluency* (pp. 100–114). New York: Thieme Medical Publishers.

Runyan, C. M., Runyan, S. E., & Hibbard, S. (2006). The Speech Easy device: A three year study. Poster presented to the American Speech-Language-Hearing Association, Miami, FL.

Rustin, L. (1987) The treatment of childhood disfluency through active parental involvement. In L. Rustin, H. Purser, & D. Rowley (Eds.) *Progress in the Treatment of Fluency Disorders* (pp. 166–180). London: Taylor and Francis.

Rustin, L., Botterill, W., & Kelman, E. (1996). *Assessment and Therapy for Young Dysfluent Children: Family Interaction*. London: Whurr Publishers Ltd.

Rustin, L., & Cook, F. (1995). Parental involvement in the treatment of stuttering. *Language, Speech and Hearing Disorders in Schools, 26*, 127–137.

Ryan, B. (1971). Operant procedures applied to stuttering therapy for children. *Journal of Speech and Hearing Disorders, 36*, 264–280.

Ryan, B. (1974). *Programmed Therapy for Stuttering in Children and Adults*. Springfield, IL: Charles C. Thomas.

Ryan, B. (1979). Stuttering therapy in a framework of operant conditioning and programmed learning. In H. H. Gregory (Ed.), *Controversies about Stuttering Therapy*. Baltimore: University Park Press.

Ryan, B. (2000). Speaking rate, conversational speech acts, and linguistic complexity of 20 preschool stuttering and nonstuttering children and their mothers *Clinical Linguistics and Phonetics, 14*, 25–51.

Ryan, B. P. (2000). *Programmed Therapy for Stuttering in Children and Adults* (2nd ed.). Springfield, IL: C.C. Thomas.

Ryan, B. P. (2001). A longitudinal study of articulation, language, rate and fluency of 22 preschool children who stutter. *Journal of Fluency Disorders, 26*, 107–127.

Ryan, B. P., & Ryan, B. (1983). Programmed stuttering therapy for children: Comparison of four establishment programs. *Journal of Fluency Disorders, 8*, 291–321.

Ryan, B. P., & Ryan, B. (1995). Programmed stuttering treatment for children: Comparison of two establishment programs through transfer, maintenance, and follow-up. *Journal of Speech and Hearing Research, 38*, 61–75.

Ryan, B. P., & Van Kirk, B. (1971). *Programmed Conditioning for Fluency: Program Book*. Monterey, CA: Behavioral Sciences Institute.

Sackett, D. L., Straus, S. E., Richardson, W. S., Rosenberg, W., & Haynes, R. B. (2000). *Evidence Based Medicine: How to Practice and Teach EBM* (2nd ed.). New York: Elsevier Churchill Livingstone.

Sadock, B. J., & Sadock, V. A. (2000). *Kaplan and Sadock's Comprehensive Textbook of Psychiatry* (7th ed.). Baltimore: Lippincott Williams & Wilkins.

Saint-Laurent, L., & Ladouceur, R. (1987). Massed versus distributed application of the regulated-breathing method for stutterers and its long-term effect. *Behavior Therapy, 18*, 38–50.

Salmelin, R., Schnitzler, A., Schmitz, F., & Freund, H. J. (2000) Single word reading in developmental stutterers and fluent speakers. *Brain, 123*, 1184–1202.

Salmelin, R., Schnitzler, A., Schmitz, F., Jäncke, L., Witte, O. W., & Freund, H.-J. (1998). Functional organization of the auditory cortex is different in stutterers and fluent speakers. *NeuroReport, 9*, 2225–2229.

Saltuklaroglu, T., Dayalu, V., & Kalinowski, J. (2002). Reduction of stuttering: The dual inhibition hypothesis. *Medical Hypotheses, 58*, 67–71.

Sander, E. K. (1961). Reliability of the Iowa speech disfluency test. *Journal of Speech and Hearing Disorders, Monograph Supplement, 7*, 21–30.

Schaal, S., Sternad, D., Osu, R., & Kawato, M. (2004). Rhythmic arm movement is not discrete. *Nature Neuroscience, 7*, 1136–1143.

Schiavetti, N., & Metz, D. E. (2002). *Evaluating Research in Communicative Disorders* (4th ed.). Boston: Allyn and Bacon.

Schulpher, M., Gafni, A., & Watt, I. (2002). Shared decision making in a collectively funded health care system: Possible conflicts and some potential solutions. *Social Science and Medicine, 54*, 1369–1377.

Schulz, K. F., Chalmers, I., Haynes, R. J., & Altman, D. G. (1995). Empirical evidence of bias: Dimensions of methodological quality associated with estimates of treatment effects in controlled trials. *Journal of the American Medical Association, 273*, 408–412.

Schwartz, H. D. (1999). *A Primer for Stuttering Therapy*. Boston: Allyn & Bacon.

Schwartz, H. D., & Conture, E. G. (1988). Subgrouping young stutterers: Preliminary behavioral observations. *Journal of Speech and Hearing Disorders, 31*, 62–71.

Schwenk, K. A., Conture, E. G., & Walden, T. A. (2007). Reaction to background stimulation of preschool children who do and do not stutter. *Journal of Communication Disorders, 40*, 129–141.

Seider, R. A., Gladstien, K. L., & Kidd, K. K. (1983). Recovery and persistence of stuttering among relatives of stutterers. *Journal of Speech and Hearing Disorders, 48*, 402–409.

Seltzer, H., & Culatta, R. (1979). A modeling approach to stuttering therapy for young children. *Journal of Childhood Communication Disorders, 3*, 103–110.

Semel, E., Wiig, E. H., & Secord, W. A. (2003). *Clinical Evaluation of Language Fundamentals–4 (CELF-4)*. San Antonio, TX: Harcourt Assessment, Inc.

Semel, E., Wiig, E. H., & Secord, W. A. (2004). *Clinical Evaluation of Language Fundamentals–Preschool 2 (CELF-P2)*. San Antonio, TX: Harcourt Assessment, Inc.

Shames, G. H., & Florance, C. L. (1980). *Stutter-Free Speech: A Goal for Therapy*. Columbus, OH: Charles E. Merrill.

Shames, G. H., & Sherrick, C. E. Jr. (1963). A discussion of nonfluency and stuttering as operant behaviour. *Journal of Speech and Hearing Disorders, 28*, 3–18.

Shapiro, D. (1999). *Stuttering Intervention: A Collaborative Journey to Fluency Freedom*. Austin, TX: Pro-Ed.

Sheehan, J. G. (1958). Conflict theory and avoidance-reduction therapy. In J. Eisenson (Ed.), *Stuttering: A Second Symposium* (pp. 97–198). New York: Harper & Row, Publishers.

Sheehan, J. G. (1970). *Stuttering: Research and Therapy*. New York: Harper & Row.

Shenker, R. C., & Finn, P. (1985). An evaluation of the effects of supplemental "fluency" training during maintenance. *Journal of Fluency Disorders, 10*, 257–267.

Shenker, R. C., Koushik, S., Mostlova, A., Taggart, L., & Lawlor, D. (2005). Evaluation of treatment efficacy with The Lidcombe Program for early stuttering: Results of long term follow up. Paper presented at the 5th Oxford Dysfluency Conference, Oxford, United Kingdom.

Shenker, R. C., & Wilding, J. (2003). Canada. In M. Onslow, A. Packman, & E. Harrison (Eds.), *The Lidcombe Program of Early Stuttering Intervention: A Clinician's Guide*. Austin, TX: Pro-Ed.

Sherman, D. (1952). Clinical and experimental use of the Iowa scale of severity of stuttering. *Journal of Speech and Hearing Disorders, 17*, 316–320.

Sherman, D. (1955). Reliability and utility of individual ratings of severity of audible characteristics of stuttering. *Journal of Speech and Hearing Disorders, 20*, 11–16.

Shine, R. E. (1980). Direct management of the beginning stutterer. *Seminars in Speech, Language and Hearing, 1*, 339–350.

Shine, R. E. (1981). *Systematic Fluency Training for Young Children*. Tigarad, OR: C.C. Publications.

Shine, R. E. (1988). *Systematic Fluency Training for Young Children* (3rd ed.). Austin, TX: Pro-Ed.

Shugart, Y. Y., Mundorff, J., Kilshaw, J., Doheny, K., Doan, B., Wanyee, J., Green, E. D., & Drayna, D. (2004). Results of a genome-wide linkage scan for stuttering. *American Journal of Medical Genetics, 124A*, 133–135.

Shumak, I. C. (1955). A speech situation rating sheet for stutterers. In W. Johnson (Ed.), *Stuttering in Children and Adults: Thirty Years of Research at the University of Iowa* (pp. 341–347). Minneapolis, MN: University of Minnesota Press.

Siegel, G. M. (1976). The high cost of accountability. *ASHA, 17*, 796–797.

Silverman, F. H. (1974). Disfluency behavior of elementary-school stutterers and nonstutterers. *Language, Speech, and Hearing Services in Schools, 5*, 32–37.

Silverman, S. W., & Ratner, N. B. (1997). Syntactic complexity, fluency, and accuracy of sentence imitation in adolescents. *Journal of Speech-Language and Hearing Research, 40*, 95–106.

Simon, J., Pilling, S., Burbeck, R., & Goldberg, D. (2006). Treatment options in moderate and severe depression: Decision analysis supporting a clinical guideline. *The British Journal of Psychiatry, 189*, 494–501.

Simpson, G. M., & Angus, J. W. (1970). A rating scale for extrapyramidal side effects. *Acta Psychiatrica Scandinavica Supplement, 212*, 11–19.

Smith, A., & Kelly, E. (1997). Stuttering: A dynamic, multifactorial model. In R. Curlee & G. M. Siegel (Eds.), *Nature and Treatment of Stuttering: New Directions* (2nd ed., pp. 204–216). Boston: Allyn & Bacon.

Smith, B., & Kroll, R. (1979). A precision fluency shaping feedback system. Paper presented at the 32nd Annual Conference on Engineering in Medicine and Biology, Denver, CO.

Smith, J. M., Kucharski, L. T., Eblen, C., Knutsen, E., & Linn, C. (1979). An assessment of tardive dyskinesia in schizophrenic outpatients. *Psychopharmacology, 64*, 99–104.

Smith, P. K., & Sharp, S. (1994). *School Bullying: Insights and Perspectives*. New York: Routledge.

Smits-Bandstra, S., De Nil, L., & Rochon, E. (2006). The transition to increased automaticity during finger sequence learning in adult males who stutter. *Journal of Fluency Disorders, 31*, 22–42.

Smits-Bandstra, S., De Nil, L., & Saint-Cyr, J. A. (2006). Speech and nonspeech sequence skill learning in adults who stutter. *Journal of Fluency Disorders, 31,* 116–136.

Sommer, M., Koch, M. A., Paulus, W., Weiller, C., & Buchel, C. (2002). Disconnection of speech-relevant brain areas in persistent developmental stuttering. *Lancet, 360,* 380–383.

Sommers, R. K., & Caruso, A. J. (1995). In-service training in speech-language pathology: Are we meeting the needs for fluency training? *American Journal of Speech-Language Pathology, 4,* 22–28.

Song, L. P., Peng, D. L., Jin, Z., Yao, L., Ning, N., Guo, X. J., & Zhang, T. (2007). Gray matter abnormalities in developmental stuttering determined with voxel-based morphometry. *Zhonghua Yi Xue Za Zhi, 87,* 2884–2888.

SpeechEasy Consumer Information Packet. (2006). Available from Janus Development Group, Inc. 112 Staton Road Greenville, NC 27834. Phone: 866–551–9042. Email: customerserv@janusdevelopment.com.

SpeechEasy Policy and Procedure Manual. (2006). Available from the Janus Development Group, Inc. 112 Staton Road Greenville, NC 27834. Phone: 866–551–9042. Email: customerserv@janusdevelopment.com.

SpeechEasy Training Manual. (2006). Available from Janus Development, Inc. 112 Staton Road Greenville, NC 27834. Phone: 866–551–9042. Email: customerserv@janusdevelopment.com.

Spielberger, C. D., Gorsuch, R. L., & Lushene, R. E. (1970). *Manual for the State-Trait Anxiety Inventory (Self-Evaluation Questionnaire).* Palo Alto, CA: Consulting Psychologists Press.

Spielberger, C. D., Gorsuch, R. L., Luschene, R. E., Vagg, P. R., & Jacobs, G. A. (1983). *STAI Manual for the State-Trait Anxiety Inventory.* New York: Consulting Psychologists Press.

Stager, S. V., Calis, K., Grothe, D., Bloch, M., Turcasso, N., Ludlow, C., & Braun, A. (1997). A double-blind trial of pimozide and paroxetine for stuttering. In W. Hulstijn, H. Peters, & P. H. H. M. Van Lieshout (Eds.), *Speech Production: Motor Control, Brain Research and Fluency Disorders* (pp. 371–381). Amsterdam: Excerpta Medica.

Stager, S. V., & Ludlow, C. L. (1993). Speech production changes under fluency-evoking conditions in nonstuttering speakers. *Journal of Speech and Hearing Research, 36,* 245–253.

Stager, S. V., Ludlow, C., Gordon, C., Cotelingam, M., & Rapoport, J. (1995). Fluency changes in persons who stutter following a double blind trial of clomipramine and desipramine. *Journal of Speech and Hearing Research, 38,* 516–525.

Starke, A. (1994). The Van Riper program as intensive interval therapy. In C. W. Starkweather & H. F. M. Peters (Eds.), *Proceedings of the First World Congress on Fluency Disorders* (pp. 425–428). Nijmegen, The Netherlands: University of Nijmegen,

Starkweather, C. W. (1987). *Fluency and Stuttering.* Englewood Cliffs, NJ: Prentice-Hall.

Starkweather, C. W. (2002). The epigenesis of stuttering. *Journal of Fluency Disorders, 27,* 269–287.

Starkweather, C. W., & Givens-Ackerman, J. (1997). *Stuttering.* Austin, TX: Pro-Ed.

Starkweather, C. W., & Gottwald, S. R. (1990). The demands and capacities model II: Clinical applications. *Journal of Fluency Disorders, 15,* 143–157.

Starkweather, C. W., & Gottwald, S. R. (1993). A pilot study of relations among specific measures obtained at intake and discharge in a program of preventions and early intervention for stuttering. *American Journal of Speech-Language Pathology, 2,* 51–58.

Starkweather, C. W., Gottwald, S. R., & Halfond, M. H. (1990). *Stuttering Prevention: A Clinical Method.* Englewood Cliffs, NJ: Prentice-Hall.

Stein, M. B., Baird, A., & Walker, J. R. (1996). Social phobia in adults with stuttering. *American Journal of Psychiatry, 153,* 278–280.

Stephenson-Opsal, D., & Bernstein-Ratner, N. (1988). Maternal speech rate modification and childhood stuttering. *Journal of Fluency Disorders, 13,* 49–56.

Stier, E. (1911). *Untersuchungen über die Linkshändigkeit und die Funktionellen Differenzen der Hirnhälften* [*Investigations about Left-Handedness and the Functional Differences of the Brain Halves*]. Jena, Germany: Fischer.

St. Louis, K. O., & Durrenberger, C. H. (1992). Clinician preferences for managing various communication disorders. Paper presented at the American Speech-Language-Hearing Association Convention, San Antonio, TX.

St. Louis, K. O., & Durrenberger, C. H. (1993). What communication disorders do experienced clinicians prefer to manage? *ASHA, 35,* 23–31.

St. Louis, K. O., & Lass, N. J. (1980). A survey of university training in stuttering. *Journal of the National Student Speech-Language-Hearing Association, 10,* 88–97.

St. Louis, K. O., & Lass, N. J. (1981). A survey of communicative disorders students' attitudes toward stuttering. *Journal of Fluency Disorders, 6,* 49–79.

St. Louis, K. O., & Westbrook, J. B. (1987). The effectiveness of treatment for stuttering. In L. Rustin, H. Purser, & D. Rowley (Eds.), *Progress in the Treatment of Fluency Disorders* (pp. 235–257). London: Whurr.

Stocker, B. (1977). *The Stocker-Probe Technique.* Tulsa, OK: Modern Education Program.

Straus, S. E., Richardson, W. S., Glasziou, P., & Haynes, R. B. (2005). *Evidence Based Medicine: How to*

Practice and Teach EBM (3rd ed.). New York: Elsevier Churchill Livingstone.

Stuart, A., & Kalinowski, J. (1996). Fluent speech, fast articulatory rate, and delayed auditory feedback: Creating a crisis for a scientific revolution? *Perceptual and Motor Skills, 82*, 211–218.

Stuart, A., Kalinowski, J., Armson, J., Stenstrom, R., & Jones, K. (1996). Fluency effect of frequency alterations of plus/minus one-half and one-quarter octave shifts in auditory feedback of people who stutter. *Journal of Speech and Hearing Research, 39*, 396–401.

Stuart, A., Kalinowski, J., & Rastatter, M. (1997). Effect of monaural and binaural altered auditory feedback on stuttering frequency. *Journal of the Acoustical Society of America, 101*, 3806–3809.

Stuart, A., Kalinowski, J., Rastatter, M., & Lynch, K. (2002). Effect of delayed auditory feedback on normal speakers at two speech rates. *Journal of the Acoustical Society of America, 111*, 2237–2240.

Stuart, A., Kalinowski, J., Rastatter, M., Saltuklaroglu, T., & Dayalu, V. (2004). Investigations of the impact of altered auditory feedback in-the-ear devices on the speech of people who stutter: Initial fitting and 4-month follow-up. *International Journal of Language and Communication Disorders, 39*, 93–113.

Stuart, A., Kalinowski, J., Saltuklaroglu, T., & Guntupalli, V. K. (2006). Investigations of the impact of altered auditory feedback in-the-ear devices on the speech of people who stutter: One-year follow-up. *Disability and Rehabilitation, 28*, 1–9.

Stuart, A., Xia, S., Jiang, Y., Jiang, T., Kalinowski, J., & Rastatter, M. P. (2003). Self-contained in-the ear device to deliver altered auditory feedback: Applications for stuttering. *Annals of Biomedical Engineering, 31*, 233–237.

Sugimoto, T., Sugimoto, M., Uchida, I., Mashimo, T., & Okada, S. (2001). Inhibitory effects of theophylline on recombinant GABA (A) receptors. *Neuroreport, 12*, 489–493.

Suresh, R., Ambrose, N., Roe, C., Pluzhnikov, A., Wittke-Thompson, J. K., Ng, M. C., Wu, X., Cook, E. H., Lundstrom, C., Garsten, M., Ezrati, R., Yairi, E., & Cox, N. J. (2006). New complexities in the genetics of stuttering: Significant sex-specific linkage signals. *American Journal of Human Genetics, 78*, 554–563.

Swift, W., Swift, E., & Arellano, M. (1975). Haloperidol as a treatment for adult stuttering. *Comprehensive Psychiatry, 16*, 61–67.

Taylor, I. K. (1966). What words are stuttered? *Psychological Bulletin, 65*, 233–242.

Teesson, K., Packman, A., & Onslow, M. (2003). The Lidcombe behavioral data language of stuttering. *Journal of Speech, Language, and Hearing Research, 46*, 1009–1015.

Thomas, C., & Howell, P. (2001). Assessing efficacy of stuttering treatments. *Journal of Fluency Disorders, 26*, 311–333.

Thompson, R. A. (1994). Emotion regulation: A theme in search of definition. *Monographs of the Society for Research in Child Development, 59* (2–3, Serial No. 240), 25–52.

Thompson-Schill, S. L., D'Esposito, M., & Kan, I. P. (1999). Effects of repetition and competition on activity in left prefrontal cortex during word generation. *Neuron, 23*, 513–522.

Torrance, G. W. (1987). Utility approach to measuring health-related quality of life. *Journal of Chronic Disease, 40*, 593–600.

Toscher, M. M., & Rupp, R. R. (1978). A study of the central auditory processes in stutterers using the Synthetic Sentence Identification (SSI) Test battery. *Journal of Speech and Hearing Research, 21*, 779–792.

Travis, L. E. (1931). *Speech Pathology*. New York: Appleton-Century.

Travis, L. E. (1957). The unspeakable feelings of people with special reference to stuttering. In L. E. Travis (Ed.), *Handbook of Speech Pathology* (pp. 916–946). New York: Appleton-Century-Crofts, Inc.

Travis, L. E., & Knott, J. R. (1936). Brain potentials from normal speakers and stutterers. *Journal of Psychology, 2*, 137–150.

Travis, L. E., & Knott, J. R. (1937). Bilaterally recorded brain potentials from normal speakers and stutterers. *Journal of Speech Disorders, 2*, 239–241.

Trinder, L. (2000). A critical appraisal of evidence-based practice. In L. Trinder & S. Reynolds (Eds.), *Evidence-Based Practice: A Critical Appraisal* (pp. 212–241). Oxford, United Kingdom: Blackwell Science.

Tulving, E. (1983). *Elements of Episodic Memory*. New York: Oxford University Press.

Turgut, N., Utku, U., & Balci, K. (2002). A case of acquired stuttering resulting from left parietal infarction. *Acta Neurologica Scandinavica, 105*, 408–410.

Turner, S. M., Beidel, D. C., & Dancu, C. V. (1996). *SPAI. Social Phobia and Anxiety Inventory*. New York: Multi-Health Systems.

Tversky, A., & Kahneman, D. (1974). Judgment under uncertainty: Heuristics and biases. *Science, 185*, 1124–1131.

Tyler, A. A. (2006). Commentary on "Treatment decisions for children with speech-sound disorders": Revisiting the past in EBP. *Language, Speech, and Hearing Services in Schools, 37*, 280–283.

Ulrich, L., Pepe, E., Kroll, R., & De Nil, L. (1992). Client performance variables affecting stuttering treatment. Paper presented at the American Speech-Language-Hearing Association, San Antonio, TX.

United States Congress. (1997). *Individuals with Disabilities Education Act Amendments of 1997*. Washington, DC: Government Printing Office.

United States Department of Education. (2001). *Twenty-Third Annual Report to Congress on the Implementation of the Individuals with Disabilities Education Act*. Washington, DC: United States Department of Education.

United States Department of Education. (2002). *Twenty-Fourth Annual Report to Congress on the Implementation of the Individuals with Disabilities Education Act*. Washington, DC: United States Department of Education.

United States Food and Drug Administration. (2004). Safety data on Zyprexa (olanzapine): Hyperglycemia and diabetes [Dear Doctor letter]. Retrieved from the U.S. Food and Drug Administration MedWatch Website, January 8, 2007, http://www.fda.gov/medwatch/SAFETY/2004/zyprexa.htm.

Van Borsel, J., Reunes, G., & Van den Bergh, N. (2003). Delayed auditory feedback in the treatment of stuttering: clients as consumers. *International Journal of Language and Communication Disorders, 38*, 119–129.

Van Riper, C. (1958). Experiments in stuttering therapy. In J. Eisenson (Ed.), *Stuttering: A Symposium*. New York: Harper & Row.

Van Riper, C. (1971). *The Nature of Stuttering*. Englewood Cliffs, NJ: Prentice-Hall.

Van Riper, C. (1973). *The Treatment of Stuttering*. Englewood Cliffs, NJ: Prentice-Hall.

Van Riper, C. (1977). The public school specialist in stuttering. *Journal of the American Speech and Hearing Association, 19*, 467–469.

Van Riper, C. (1982). *The Nature of Stuttering* (2nd ed.). Englewood Cliffs, NJ: Prentice-Hall.

Vanryckeghem, M., & Brutten, G. J. (1996). The relationship between communication attitude and fluency failure of stuttering and nonstuttering children. *Journal of Fluency Disorders, 21*, 109–118.

Vanryckeghem, M., & Brutten, G. J. (1997). The speech-associated attitude of children who do and do not stutter and the differential effect of age. *American Journal of Speech-Language Pathology, 6*, 67–73.

Vanryckeghem, M., & Brutten, G. (2006). *Behavior Assessment Battery*. San Diego, CA: Plural Publishing, Inc.

Vanryckeghem, M., Brutten, G. J., & Hernandez, L. (2005). A comparative investigation of the speech-associated attitude of preschool and kindergarten children who do and do not stutter. *Journal of Fluency Disorders, 30*, 307–318.

Vanryckeghem, M., Hylebos, C., Brutten, G. J., & Peleman, M. (2001). The relationship between communication attitude and emotion of children who stutter. *Journal of Fluency Disorders, 26*, 1–15.

Ventry, I. M., & Schiavetti, N. (1980). *Evaluating Research in Speech Pathology and Audiology*. Reading, MA: Addison-Wesley.

von Neumann, J., & Morgenstern, O. (1947). *Theories of Games and Economic Behavior*. Princeton, NJ: Princeton University Press.

Vuust, P., Roepstorff, A., Wallentin, M., Mouridsen, K., & Ostergaard, L. (2006). It don't mean a thing... Keeping the rhythm during polyrhythmic tension, activates language areas (BA47). *NeuroImage, 31*, 832–841.

Wahlhaus, M. M., Girson, J., & Levy, C. (2003). South Africa. In M. Onslow, A. Packman, & E. Harrison (Eds.), *The Lidcombe Program of Early Stuttering Intervention: A Clinician's Guide* (pp. 183–190). Austin, TX: Pro-Ed.

Walker, J. F., Archibald, L. M. D., Cherniak, S. R., & Fish, V. G. (1992). Articulation rate in 3- and 5-year-old children. *Journal of Speech and Hearing Research, 35*, 4–13.

Wall, M. J., & Myers, F. L. (1995). *Clinical Management of Childhood Stuttering* (2nd ed.). Austin, TX: Pro-Ed..

Wall, M. J., Starkweather, C. W., & Cairns, H. S. (1981). Syntactic influences on stuttering in young child stutterers. *Journal of Fluency Disorders, 6*, 283–298.

Ward, N. S, Brown, M. M., Thompson, A. J., & Frackowiak, R. S. (2003). Neural correlates of outcome after stroke: A cross-sectional fMRI study. *Brain, 126*, 1430–1434.

Watkins, K. E., Smith, S. M., Davis, S., & Howell, P. (2008). Structural and functional abnormalities of the motor system in developmental stuttering. *Brain, 131*, 50–59.

Watkins, R. V., & Yairi, E. (1997). Language production abilities of children whose stuttering persisted or recovered. *Journal of Speech, Language and Hearing Research, 40*, 385–399.

Watkins, R. V., Yairi, E., & Ambrose, N. (1999). Early childhood stuttering III: Initial status of expressive language abilities. *Journal of Speech, Language and Hearing Research, 42*, 1125–1135.

Watson, J. B. (1988). A comparison of stutterers' and nonstutterers' affective, cognitive, and behavioral self-reports. *Journal of Speech and hearing Research, 31*, 377–385.

Watts, F. (1973). Mechanisms of fluency control in stutterers. *British Journal of Disorders of Communication, 8*, 131–138.

Webber, M., & Onslow, M. (2003). Maintenance of treatment effects. In M. Onslow, A. Packman, & E. Harrison (Eds.), *The Lidcombe Program of Early*

Stuttering Intervention: A Clinician's Guide. Austin, TX: Pro-Ed.

Weber, C., & Smith, A. (1990). Autonomic correlates of stuttering and speech assessed in a range of experimental tasks. *Journal of Speech and Hearing Research, 33,* 690–706.

Weber-Fox, C., & Hampton, A. (2008). Stuttering and natural speech processing of semantic and syntactic constraints on verbs. *Journal of Speech, Language, and Hearing Research, 51,* 1058–1071.

Weber-Fox, C., Spencer, R. M. C., Spruill III, J. E., & Smith, A. (2004). Phonologic processing in adults who stutter: Electrophysiological and behavioral evidence. *Journal of Speech, Language, and Hearing Research, 47,* 1244–1258.

Webster, R. L. (1974). *The Precision Fluency Shaping Program: Speech Reconstruction for Stutterers.* Roanoke, VA: Communications Development Corporation.

Webster, R. L. (1979). Empirical considerations regarding stuttering therapy. In H. H. Gregory (Ed.), *Controversies about Stuttering Therapy.* Baltimore: University Park Press.

Webster, R. L. (1980). Evolution of a target based behavioral therapy for stuttering. *Journal of Fluency Disorders, 5,* 303–320.

Webster, R. L., & Lubker, B. B. (1968). Interrelationships among fluency producing variables in stuttered speech. *Journal of Speech and hearing Research, 11,* 754–766.

Webster, R. L., Morgan, B. T., & Cannon, M. W. (1987). Voice onset abruptness in stutterers before and after therapy. In H. F. M. Peters & W. Hulstijn (Eds.), *Speech Motor Dynamics in Stuttering* (pp. 295–305). Wein, Germany: Springer-Verlag.

Webster, W. G. (1993). Hurried hands and tangled tongues. In E. Boberg (Ed.), *Neuropsychology of Stuttering* (pp. 73–127). Edmonton, Alberta, Canada: The University of Alberta Press.

Weiss, A. L., & Zebrowski, P. M. (1992). Disfluencies in the conversations of young children: Some answers about questions. *Journal of Speech and Hearing Research, 35,* 1230–1238.

Wells, P. G., & Malcolm, M. T. (1971). Controlled trial of the treatment of 36 stutterers. *British Journal of Psychiatry, 119,* 603–604.

Wexler, K. B., & Mysack, E. D. (1982). Disfluency characteristics of 2-, 4-, and 6-year old males. *Journal of Fluency Disorders, 7,* 37–46.

Wildgruber, D., Ackermann, H., & Grodd, W. (2001). Differential contributions of motor cortex, basal ganglia, and cerebellum to speech motor control: Effects of syllable repetition rate evaluated by fMRI. *NeuroImage, 13,* 101–109.

Wilkenfeld, J. R., & Curlee, R. F. (1997). The relative effects of questions and comments on children's

stuttering. *American Journal of Speech-Language Pathology, 6,* 79–89.

William, K. T. (1997). *Expressive Vocabulary Test (EVT).* Circle Pines, MN: American Guidance Services, Inc.

William, K. T. (2006). *Expressive Vocabulary Test-2 (EVT- 2).* Circle Pines, MN: American Guidance Services, Inc.

Williams, D. E. (1957). A point of view about 'stuttering.' *Journal of Speech and Hearing Disorders, 22,* 390–397.

Williams, D. E. (1971). Stuttering therapy for children. In L. E. Travis (Ed.), *Handbook of Speech Pathology and Audiology* (pp. 1073–1093). New York: Appleton-Century-Crofts.

Williams, D. E. (1983). Talking with children who stutter. In *Counseling Stutterers* (Publication No. 18). Memphis, TN: Speech Foundation of America.

Williams, D. F., & Dugan, P. M. (2002). Administering stuttering modification therapy in school settings. *Seminars in Speech and Language, 23,* 187–194.

Wilson, L., Onslow, M., & Lincoln, M. (2004). Telehealth adaptation of the Lidcombe Program of early stuttering intervention: Five case studies. *American Journal of Speech-Language Pathology, 13,* 81–93.

Wingate, M. E. (1964). A standard definition of stuttering. *Journal of Speech and Hearing Disorders, 29,* 484–489.

Wingate, M. E. (1964). Recovery from stuttering. *Journal of Speech and Hearing Disorders, 29,* 312–321.

Wingate, M. E. (1970). Effect on stuttering of changes in audition. *Journal of Speech and Hearing Research, 13,* 861–873.

Wingate, M. E. (1971). The fear of stuttering. *Journal of the American Speech-Language-Hearing Association, 13,* 3–5.

Wingate, M. E. (1976). *Stuttering: Theory and Treatment.* New York: Irvington Publishers.

Wingate, M. E. (1988). *The Structure of Stuttering. A Psycholinguistic Analysis.* New York: Springer.

Winslow, H., & Guitar, B. (1994). The effects of structured turn-taking on disfluencies: A case study. *Language, Speech and Hearing Services in Schools, 25,* 251–257.

Wohlert, A. B., & Smith, A. (2002). Developmental change in variability of lip muscle activity during speech. *Journal of Speech Language and Hearing Research, 45,* 1077–1087.

Wood, F., & Stump, D. (1980). Patterns of regional cerebral blood flow during attempted reading aloud by stutters both on and off haloperidol medication: Evidence for inadequate left frontal activation during stuttering. *Brain and Language, 9,* 141–144.

Wood, M. J. S., & Ryan, B. (2000). Experimental analysis of speaking and stuttering rate in a child who stutters. *Journal of Developmental and Physical Disabilities, 12,* 267–289.

Woods, S., Shearsby, J., Onslow, M., & Burnham, D. (2002). The psychological impact of the Lidcombe Program of early stuttering intervention: Eight case studies. *International Journal of Language and Communication Disorders, 37,* 31–40.

Woolf, G. (1967). The assessment of stuttering as struggle, avoidance and expectancy. *The British Journal of Disorders of Communication, 2,* 158–171.

World Health Organization. (2001). *International Classification of Functioning, Disability and Health.* Geneva, Switzerland: World Health Organization

World Health Organization. (2002). *Towards a Common Language for Functioning, Disability, and Health: The International Classification of Functioning, Disability, and Health (ICF).* Geneva, Switzerland: World Health Organization.

Wright, L., & Ayre, A. (2000). *The Wright & Ayre Stuttering Self-Rating Profile (WASSP).* Bicester, United Kingdom: Winslow Press.

Wu, J. C., Maguire, G., Riley, G., Fallon, J., LaCasse, L., Chin, S., Klein, E., Tang, C., Cadwell, S., & Lottenberg, S. (1995). A positron emission tomography [18F]deoxyglucose study of developmental stuttering. *NeuroReport, 6,* 501–505.

Wu, J. C., Maguire, G., Riley, G., Lee, A., Keator, D., Tang, C., Fallon, J., & Najafi, A. (1997). Increased dopamine activity associated with stuttering. *NeuroReport, 8,* 767–770.

Yairi, E. (1981). Disfluencies of normally speaking two-year old children. *Journal of Speech and Hearing Research, 24,* 490–495.

Yairi, E. (1983). The onset of stuttering in two and three year old children: A preliminary report. *Journal of Speech and Hearing Disorders, 48,* 171–177.

Yairi, E. (1997a). Disfluency characteristics of childhood stuttering. In R. Curlee & G. Siegel (Eds.), *Nature and Treatment of Stuttering: New Directions* (2nd ed., pp. 3–23). Boston: Allyn & Bacon.

Yairi, E. (1997b) Home environments of stuttering children. In R. Curlee & G. Siegel (Eds.), *Nature and Treatment of Stuttering: New Directions* (2nd ed., pp. 49–78). Boston: Allyn & Bacon.

Yairi, E. (2007). Subtyping stuttering I: A review. *Journal of Fluency Disorders, 32,* 165–196.

Yairi, E., & Ambrose, N. (1992). A longitudinal study of stuttering in children: A preliminary report. *Journal of Speech and Hearing Research, 35,* 755–760.

Yairi, E., & Ambrose, N. (1992). Onset of stuttering in preschool children: Selected factors. *Journal of Speech and Hearing Research, 35,* 782–788.

Yairi, E., & Ambrose, N. (1999). Early childhood stuttering I: Persistency and recovery rates. *Journal of Speech, Language and Hearing Research, 42,* 1097–1112.

Yairi, E., & Ambrose, N. (2002). Evidence for genetic etiology in stuttering. *Perspectives, 12,* 10–15.

Yairi, E., & Ambrose, N. (2005). *Early Childhood Stuttering: For Clinicians by Clinicians.* Austin, TX: Pro-Ed.

Yairi, E., Ambrose, N., & Cox, N. (1996). Genetics of stuttering: A critical review. *Journal of Speech and Hearing Research, 39,* 771–784.

Yairi, E., Ambrose, N. G., Paden, E. P., & Throneburg, R. N. (1996). Predictive factors of persistence and recovery: Pathways of childhood stuttering. *Journal of Communication Disorders, 29,* 51–77.

Yairi, E., Watkins, R., Ambrose, N., & Paden, E. (2001). What is stuttering? *Journal of Speech Language and Hearing Research, 44,* 585–592.

Yaruss, J. S. (1997). Clinical implications of situational variability in preschool children who stutter. *Journal of Fluency Disorders, 22,* 187–203.

Yaruss, J. S. (1997). Clinical measurement of stuttering behaviors. *Contemporary Issues in Communication Science and Disorders, 24,* 33–44.

Yaruss, J. S. (1997). Utterance timing and childhood stuttering. *Journal of Fluency Disorders, 22,* 263–286.

Yaruss, J. S. (1998). Describing the consequences of disorders: Stuttering and the International Classification of Impairments, Disabilities, and Handicaps. *Journal of Speech, Language, and Hearing Research, 41,* 249–257.

Yaruss, J. S. (1998). Real-time analysis of speech fluency: Procedures and reliability training. *American Journal of Speech-Language Pathology, 7,* 25–37.

Yaruss, J. S. (1999). Utterance length, syntactic complexity, and childhood stuttering. *Journal of Speech, Language, and Hearing Research, 42,* 329–344.

Yaruss, J. S. (2007). Application of the ICF in fluency disorders. *Seminars in Speech and Language, 28,* 312–322.

Yaruss, J. S., Coleman, C., & Hammer, D. (2006). Treating preschool children who stutter: Description and preliminary evaluation of a family-focused treatment approach. *Language, Speech and Hearing Services in Schools, 37,* 118–136.

Yaruss, J. S., Coleman, C. E., & Quesal, R. W. (2007a). Overall Assessment of the Speaker's Experience of Stuttering—School-Age. Unpublished assessment instrument.

Yaruss, J. S., Coleman, C. E., & Quesal, R. W. (2007b). Overall Assessment of the Speaker's Experience of Stuttering—Teenage. Unpublished assessment instrument.

Yaruss, J. S., & Conture, E. G. (1995). Mother and child speaking rates and utterance lengths in adjacent fluent utterances: Preliminary observations. *Journal of Fluency Disorders, 20,* 257–278.

Yaruss, J. S., LaSalle, L. R., & Conture, E. G. (1998). Evaluating stuttering in young children: Diagnostic data. *American Journal of Speech-Language Pathology,* 7, 62–76.

Yaruss, J. S., Murphy, W. P., Quesal, R. W., & Reardon, N. A. (2004). *Bullying and Teasing: Helping Children Who Stutter.* New York: National Stuttering Association.

Yaruss, J. S., & Quesal, R. W. (2002). Academic and clinical education in fluency disorders: An update. *Journal of Fluency Disorders,* 27, 43–63.

Yaruss, J. S., & Quesal, R. W. (2002). Research-based stuttering therapy revisited. *Perspectives on Fluency and Fluency Disorders* [Newsletter of Special Interest Division 4, American Speech-Language Hearing Association], 12, 22–24.

Yaruss, J. S., & Quesal, R. W. (2004). Stuttering and the International Classification of Functioning, Disability, and Health (ICF): An update. *Journal of Communication Disorders,* 37, 35–52.

Yaruss, J. S., & Quesal, R. W. (2006). Overall Assessment of the Speaker's Experience of Stuttering (OASES): Documenting multiple outcomes in stuttering treatment. *Journal of Fluency Disorders,* 31, 90–115.

Yaruss, J. S., Quesal, R. W., & Reeves, L. (2007). Self-help and mutual aid groups as an adjunct to stuttering therapy. In E. G. Conture & R. F. Curlee (Eds.), *Stuttering and Related Disorders of Fluency* (3rd ed.). New York: Thieme Medical Publishers.

Yaruss, J. S., Quesal, R. W., Reeves, L., Molt, L., Kluetz, B., Caruso, A. J., Lewis, F., & McClure, J. A. (2002). Speech treatment and support group experiences of people who participate in the National Stuttering Association. *Journal of Fluency Disorders,* 27, 115–135.

Yaruss, J. S., & Reardon, N. A. (2003). Fostering generalization and maintenance in school settings. *Seminars in Speech and Language,* 24, 33–40.

Young, M. A. (1961). Predicting ratings of severity of stuttering. *Journal of Speech and Hearing Disorders, Monograph Supplement,* 7, 31–54.

Young, M. A. (1969). Observer agreement: Cumulative effects of repeated ratings of the same samples and of knowledge of group results. *Journal of Speech and Hearing Research,* 12, 144–155.

Zackheim, C. T., & Conture, E. G. (2003). Childhood stuttering and speech disfluencies in relation to children's mean length of utterance: A preliminary study. *Journal of Fluency Disorders,* 28, 115–142.

Zackheim, C. T., Conture, E. G., Ohde, R. N., Graham, C. G., & Gregory, L. J. (2003). Holistic (word level) vs. incremental (sound level) processing in young children who stutter: Pre- vs. post-treatment. Annual American Speech-Language Hearing Association Conference, Chicago, IL

Zebrowski, P. (1994). Stuttering. In J. Tomblin, H. Morris, & D. Spriestersbach (Eds.), *Diagnosis in Speech-Language Pathology* (pp. 215–245). San Diego, CA: Singular Publishing Group, Inc.

Zebrowski, P. M. (2007). Beyond technique: What makes therapy work. Presentation at the Annual Meeting of the Council of Academic Programs in Communication Sciences and Disorders, Palm Springs, CA.

Zebrowski, P. M. (2007). Treatment factors that influence therapy outcomes of children who stutter. In R. Curlee & E. G. Conture (Eds.), *Stuttering and Related Disorders of Fluency* (3rd ed., pp. 23–38). New York: Thieme.

Zebrowski, P. M., Weiss, A. L., Savelkoul, E. M., & Hammer, C. S. (1996). The effect of maternal rate reduction on the stuttering, speech rates and linguistic productions of children who stutter: Evidence from individual dyads. *Clinical Linguistics and Phonetics,* 10, 189–206.

Zebrowski, P. M., & Kelly, E. M. (2002). *Therapy for Stuttering.* San Diego, CA: Singular Publishing Group.

Zenner, A. A., Ritterman, S. I., Bowen, S., & Gronhord, K. D. (1978). Measurement and comparison of anxiety levels of parents of stuttering, articulatory defective and non-stuttering children. *Journal of Fluency Disorders,* 3, 273–283.

Zimmerman, I. L., Steiner, V., & Pond, I. E. (1997). *Preschool Language Scale–3.* San Antonio, TX: Harcourt Assessment, Inc.

Zimmerman, S., Kalinowski, J., Stuart, A., & Rastatter, M. (1997). Effect of altered auditory feedback on people who stutter during scripted telephone conversations. *Journal of Speech, Language, and Hearing Research,* 40, 1130–1134.

Note: Page numbers referencing definitions are bolded.